GASTROINTESTINAL ONCOLOGY

Gastrointestinal Oncology

Evidence and Analysis

Edited by

Peter McCulloch
University of Oxford
Oxford, UK

Martin S. Karpeh
Stony Brook University Medical Center
Stony Brook, New York, USA

David J. Kerr
University of Oxford
Oxford, UK

Jaffer Ajani
University of Texas M.D. Anderson Cancer Center
Houston, Texas, USA

informa
healthcare

New York London

Informa Healthcare USA, Inc.
52 Vanderbilt Avenue
New York, NY 10017

Printed and bound by CPI Group (UK) Ltd, Croydon, CR0 4YY

Transferred to Digital Print 2012

International Standard Book Number-10: 1-4200-8638-3 (Paperback)
International Standard Book Number-13: 978-1-4200-8638-6 (Paperback)

Visit the Informa Web site at
www.informa.com

and the Informa Healthcare Web site at
www.informahealthcare.com

Preface

If you are reading this preface you are unusual. Most readers do not read prefaces. If you are reading it purposefully, you probably want to know why you should buy or read this book, what it contains, or why it has been put together in the way it has. So we will try to answer those questions.

This book is designed as a medium-sized reference providing up-to-date, evidence-based information on the management of the major problems in gastrointestinal oncology, both surgical and medical. It gives in-depth coverage of important current issues and controversies and clarifies the nature and quality of the evidence. It does not provide information on exotic rarities or superspecialist debates. It is designed for a busy clinician who needs practical support in dealing with the problems of oncological practice. It has a deliberately international authorship so that readers can appreciate both the commonalities in the approach to cancer treatment throughout the world as well as some of the interesting debates and differences.

It is to be hoped that it is no longer necessary to justify taking an evidence-based approach. In the decade since the evidence-based movement became internationally popular, there has been an enormous improvement in the general quality of the reporting of clinical research, largely stimulated by the pressure from clinical epidemiologists, who have pointed out the flaws and pitfalls of traditional reporting and study methods. We all now recognize that it is vital to evaluate the quality of the evidence on which our clinical practice and beliefs are based and to retain a healthy degree of doubt where the lack of good objective evidence calls for it. We asked our contributors to answer specific questions current in their field and to grade the supporting evidence for their answers according to an internationally accepted classification. We hope this will allow the reader to gain a much clearer perception of the scope of current knowledge than may be gained from reading the declarative statements in traditional textbooks, many of which would fail to stand up the scrutiny of an evidence-based examination. A pure summary of the evidence, without any significant expert commentary would, however, be unhelpful, as well as extremely dull. One of the things we are now quite clear about is the extent to which our knowledge of the efficacy of treatment is imperfect and incomplete. A simple account of the evidence would therefore leave many holes, gaps, and questions, unplugged and unanswered. Both the senior trainee and the practicing clinician need guidance in situations where the evidence is not sufficiently strong to provide an immediate answer, and help in interpreting the finer points of controversies and debate where the evidence is conflicting. We have therefore asked experts in each field to provide an account that mixes their own experience and broad understanding of the subject with a rigorous analysis of the available clinical trials.

We hope this book will appeal to a wide audience. We think it should be useful to senior trainees in gastrointestinal surgery, surgical oncology, clinical oncology, and gastroenterology. We have principally aimed it at practicing clinicians, who need an authoritative update on topics within their practice, but lack the time or resources to conduct an exhaustive review of the evidence themselves. We hope that patients and their relatives with a desire to understand the detailed arguments and evidence behind proposed treatments will also gain from reading the relevant chapters.

The controversies and hot topics discussed in the book include the surgical approaches to multiple liver metastases and hepatoma, to esophageal, gastric, and rectal cancers, as well as the oncological evidence on adjuvant and neoadjuvant therapy for these tumors and for the pancreas. We also have excellent advice on the management of malignant and premalignant disease in Barrett's esophagus and a comprehensive monograph on the management of carcinoid tumors of the GI tract. We have been fortunate in that this elite group of contributors have agreed to help us with this volume. While we emphasize the importance of the objective evidence, many readers will be particularly interested to also read the opinions of internationally recognized authorities such as Glyn Jamieson, Yuman Fong, Masatoshi Makuuchi and Hubert Stein on the surgical side, and Michel Ducreux, Joel Tepper, Eric Van Cutsem and Carol Portlock among oncologists. We express our sincere thanks to all our chapter authors for their hard work and for cooperating with us in working in an unfamiliar format.

We hope you do find this book useful and are very happy to receive feedback on how it can be improved.

Peter McCulloch
Martin S. Karpeh
David J. Kerr
JafferAjani

Acknowledgments

The editors would like to thank Geoffrey Greenwood, who initiated this project, as well as Sherri Niziolek, Andrea Seils, and Joseph Stubenrauch for their hard work in helping us to put it together. We are particularly indebted to our personal assistants Ms. Sue Boyt and Ms. Patricia Pugliani. Thanks are also due to our institutions, the Universities of Oxford and New York, and to our families and loved ones for their forbearance over a long gestation period. Finally, thanks to Informa Healthcare for commissioning this book and bringing it to a successful conclusion.

Contents

Contributors

Cletus A. Arciero Fox Chase Cancer Center, Philadelphia, Pennsylvania, U.S.A.

Stephen Attwood Department of Upper GI Surgery, North Tyneside General Hospital, North Shields, U.K.

Dimitra G. Barabouti James H. Quillen VA Medical Center, Mountain Home, Tennessee, U.S.A.

Hugh Barr Cranfield Health, Gloucestershire Hospitals NHS Foundation Trust, Gloucester, U.K.

Johanna Bendell Division of Oncology and Transplantation, Duke University Medical Center, Durham, North Carolina, U.S.A.

Valérie Boige Gastrointestinal Tract Oncology Service, Gustave Roussy Institute, Villejuif, France

Abigail S. Caudle Department of Surgery/Division of Surgical Oncology, University of North Carolina School of Medicine, Chapel Hill, North Carolina, U.S.A.

Pierre Chan Department of Medicine, Queen Mary Hospital, University of Hong Kong, Hong Kong, China

Tom Crosby Velindre Cancer Centre, Cardiff, U.K.

Steven A. Curley Department of Surgical Oncology, The University of Texas MD Anderson Cancer Center, Houston, Texas, U.S.A.

Ronald DeMatteo Department of Surgery, Memorial Sloan-Kettering Cancer Center, New York, New York, U.S.A.

Michel Ducreux Gastrointestinal Tract Oncology Service, Gustave Roussy Institute and Medical Oncology Service, Paul Brousse Hospital, Villejuif, France

Yuman Fong Department of Surgery, Memorial Sloan-Kettering Cancer Center and Weill Cornell Medical College, New York, New York, U.S.A.

Andrew Hartley Cancer Centre, University Hospital Birmingham, Birmingham, U.K.

R. Hardwick Addenbrooke's Hospital, Cambridge, U.K.

Karin Haustermans Digestive Oncology Unit, University Hospital Gasthuisberg, Leuven, Belgium

J. D. Hayden Department of Surgery, University of Adelaide and Royal Adelaide Hospital, Adelaide, South Australia, Australia

John P. Hoffman Fox Chase Cancer Center, Philadelphia, Pennsylvania, U.S.A.

James R. Howe Department of Surgery, University of Iowa College of Medicine, Iowa City, Iowa, U.S.A.

G. G. Jamieson Department of Surgery, University of Adelaide and Royal Adelaide Hospital, Adelaide, South Australia, Australia

Janusz A. Z. Jankowski Department of Cancer and Molecular Medicine, Medical School and University Hospitals Trust, Leicester, U.K.

William Jarnagin Division of Surgical Oncology, Department of Surgery, University of California, Los Angeles, Los Angeles, California, U.S.A.

Catherine R. Jephcott Department of Oncology, Churchill Hospital, Oxford, U.K.

Hong Jin Kim Department of Surgery/Division of Surgical Oncology, University of North Carolina School of Medicine, Chapel Hill, North Carolina, U.S.A.

Louise E. Jones Department of Surgery, University Hospital Aintree, Liverpool, U.K.

Nancy E. Kemeny Gastrointestinal Oncology Service, Solid Tumor Division, Department of Medicine, Memorial Sloan-Kettering Cancer Center, New York, New York, U.S.A.

David J. Kerr Department of Clinical Pharmacology, Radcliffe Infirmary, University of Oxford, Oxford, U.K.

Alison G. Killelea State University of New York, Downstate Medical Center, Brooklyn, New York, U.S.A.

Andrew H. Ko Comprehensive Cancer Center, University of California, San Francisco, San Francisco, California, U.S.A.

Norihiro Kokudo Hepatobiliary Pancreatic Surgery Division, Department of Surgery, University of Tokyo, Tokyo, Japan

Ching Lung Lai Department of Medicine, Queen Mary Hospital, University of Hong Kong, Hong Kong, China

Stéphanie Laurent Digestive Oncology Unit, University Hospital Gasthuisberg, Leuven, Belgium

John S. Macdonald Gastrointestinal Oncology Service, Saint Vincent's Comprehensive Cancer Center, New York, New York, U.S.A.

Masatoshi Makuuchi Hepatobiliary Pancreatic Surgery Division, Department of Surgery, University of Tokyo, Tokyo, Japan

David Malka Gastrointestinal Tract Oncology Service, Gustave Roussy Institute, Villejuif, France

Peter McCulloch Nuffield Department of Surgery, University of Oxford, Oxford, U.K.

Nikhil Misra Addenbrooke's Hospital, Cambridge, U.K.

Somnath Mukherjee Velindre Cancer Centre, Cardiff, U.K.

Kerri A. Nowell Department of Surgery, University of Iowa College of Medicine, Iowa City, Iowa, U.S.A.

Colette R. J. Pameijer Division of Surgical Oncology and Colon and Rectal Surgery, State University of New York at Stony Brook, Stony Brook, New York, U.S.A.

Dorothy C. Pan Department of Medicine, Memorial Sloan-Kettering Cancer Center, New York, New York, U.S.A.

Kyriakos Papadopoulos South Texas Accelerated Research Therapeutics, South Texas Oncology and Hematology, San Antonio, Texas, U.S.A.

David Peake Cancer Centre, University Hospital Birmingham, Birmingham, U.K.

Carol S. Portlock Department of Medicine, Memorial Sloan-Kettering Cancer Center, New York, New York, U.S.A.

Graeme J. Poston Department of Surgery, University Hospital Aintree, Liverpool, U.K.

David E. Rivadeneira Division of Surgical Oncology and Colon and Rectal Surgery, State University of New York at Stony Brook, Stony Brook, New York, U.S.A.

J. R. Siewert Departments of Surgery, Paracelsus Private Medical University, Salzburg, Austria and Klinikum rechts der Isar, Technical University, Munich, Germany

Paramjeet Singh Department of Surgery, Memorial Sloan-Kettering Cancer Center, New York, New York, U.S.A.

H. J. Stein Departments of Surgery, Paracelsus Private Medical University, Salzburg, Austria and Klinikum rechts der Isar, Technical University, Munich, Germany

Margaret A. Tempero Comprehensive Cancer Center, University of California, San Francisco, San Francisco, California, U.S.A.

Joel E. Tepper Department of Radiation Oncology, University of North Carolina School of Medicine, NC Clinical Cancer Center, Chapel Hill, North Carolina, U.S.A.

Charles R. Thomas Department of Radiation Medicine, Oregon Health and Sciences University, Portland, Oregon, U.S.A.

James S. Tomlinson Division of Surgical Oncology, Department of Surgery, University of California, Los Angeles, Los Angeles, California, U.S.A.

Archie N. Tse Gastrointestinal Oncology Service, Solid Tumor Division, Department of Medicine, Memorial Sloan-Kettering Cancer Center, New York, New York, U.S.A.

Eric Van Cutsem Digestive Oncology Unit, University Hospital Gasthuisberg, Leuven, Belgium

B. H. A. von Rahden Departments of Surgery, Paracelsus Private Medical University, Salzburg, Austria and Klinikum rechts der Isar, Technical University, Munich, Germany

Lawrence D. Wagman Liver Tumor Program, Division of Surgery, City of Hope National Medical Center, Duarte, California, U.S.A.

Kevin T. Watkins Department of Surgery, State University of New York at Stony Brook, Stony Brook, New York, U.S.A.

Christopher Willett Department of Radiation Oncology, Duke University Medical Center, Durham, North Carolina, U.S.A.

W. Douglas Wong Department of Surgery, Memorial Sloan-Kettering Cancer Center and Cornell University Medical College, New York, New York, U.S.A.

Y. Nancy You Department of Surgery, Mayo Clinic, Rochester, Minnesota, U.S.A.

P. L. Youd Department of Gastroenterology, St. Mark's Hospital, Harrow, U.K.

Man Fung Yuen Department of Medicine, Queen Mary Hospital, University of Hong Kong, Hong Kong, China

1 Surgical and Ablative Treatment of Barrett's Esophagus and Its Complications

Hugh Barr
Cranfield Health, Gloucestershire Hospitals NHS Foundation Trust, Gloucester, U.K.

Stephen Attwood
Department of Upper GI Surgery, North Tyneside General Hospital, North Shields, U.K.

INTRODUCTION

The columnar-lined (Barrett's) esophagus, named after Norman "Pasty" Barrett has become one of the most fascinating conditions in gastrointestinal oncology. It has a very distinctive endoscopic appearance and is an intriguing pathological change. It would be of academic interest only were it not for its potential to degenerate to esophageal adenocarcinoma. There is currently a worrying rise in the annual incidence of this cancer (1,2), which is matched by little change in the effects of treatment on the mortality. The median survival was 0.75 years (1973–1977) and has improved to 0.9 years (1993–1999) (3). Various risk factors for degeneration to cancer have been identified, and it is a particular and increasing problem for white men in England and Scotland (4). Currently, 0.5% to 1% of adults with Barrett's metaplasia will progress to cancer. The annual conversion to adenocarcinoma for patients with long segments (>3 cm of Barrett's metaplasia) is 1% in the United Kingdom (5). Despite family clusters, there seem no obvious inheritable genetic factors. If this trend continues, there is little prospect of altering the impact modern medicine will have on this disease, despite the introduction of neoadjuvant therapy with chemoradiation and improved surgical outcomes. It is postulated that the incidence and mortality will remain closely matched (Fig. 1).

Surveillance programs for patients detected with Barrett's are widely used, but at present, carry little conviction even among proponents since they are not justified on cost effectiveness grounds. Nevertheless, some individuals with early cancers are identified sooner and offered curative surgery (6,7). Thus, surveillance really represents a "current coping strategy" to pragmatically offer patients and their physicians some hope of preventing lethal symptomatic cancer (8,9).

Symptomatic adenocarcinoma is a lethal disease: fifty percent of patients have extensive locoregional or metastatic disease at presentation. It has been found that of those selected and considered fit for resection, 73% have invasive tumors (>pT2), 60% have lymph node metastases, and 18% have other metastases (10). In unselected series, the overall operative mortality remains high at 11% (11).

The clinical risk factors for the identification of the "bad Barrett's metaplasia," which will progress to dysplasia and adenocarcinoma, are undergoing intense investigation, as are the molecular risk factors. These have yet to be proven in a randomized, controlled study to be beneficial to stratify the risks within an individual patient or indeed the population (12–23).

However, the identification of the Barrett's premalignant phenotype may allow strategies of early intervention to prevent cancer rather than awaiting the detection of cancer. This is most appropriate at the identification of dysplasia, which is currently the best indicator of malignant degeneration.

PATHOLOGICAL CONSIDERATIONS

The normal esophagus is lined by squamous epithelium, but it is readily damaged by the chronic injury of duodeno-gastroesophageal reflux disease. Repair is affected in this abnormal environment by columnar intestinal and gastric cells, an example of phenotypic plasticity. The mucosa has adapted to hostile environmental conditions by a metaplastic response. Three distinct

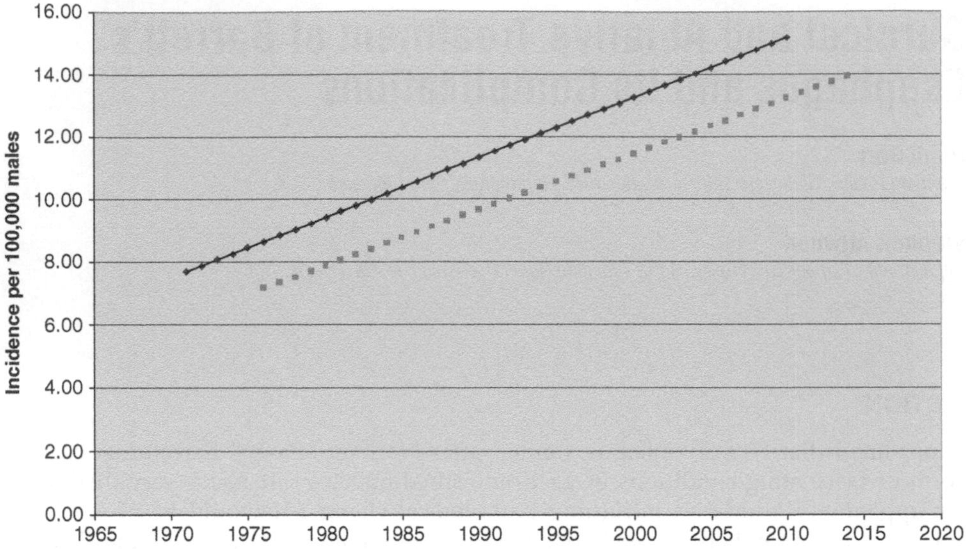

FIGURE 1 The current situation regarding the incidence and mortality of esophageal adenocarcinoma in white U.K. men.

types of columnar metaplasia are recognized. The commonest and clinically most important is intestinal metaplasia, and it is most likely to undergo malignant transformation to adenocarcinoma. The malignant potential of cardiac and fundic metaplasia is uncertain (24). The malignant degeneration within a segment of Barrett's esophagus occurs in a probabilistic rather than in an inevitably deterministic manner. Yet Barrett's does appear to be a necessary intermediary step, allowing interventional opportunities to stabilize the epithelium or destroy it. There is often a relatively long time sequence prior to the development of cancer. This may allow early intervention with endoscopic ablation, chemo, or surgical prophylaxis.

Pathological diagnosis is dependent on the endoscopist clearly identifying the site of biopsy in the gastric cardia, a hiatus hernia, or in the esophagus. The endoscopic problem is that the anatomy and position of the gastroesophageal junction is difficult to define. There is a lack of a universally accepted and reproducible set of criteria to endoscopically identify the cardia of the stomach from the distal esophagus. During endoscopy, it is important to identify certain important landmarks in order to allow some delineation of abnormal columnar-lined esophagus. The squamo-columnar junction is usually visible as the pale squamous epithelium merges into redder columnar mucosa. The gastroesophageal junction is imaginary, but, at present, is defined endoscopically as the level of the most proximal gastric fold. Some patients with an hiatus hernia have defective and weak lower-esophageal sphincters, and, therefore, there is no clear-cut flare as one enters the stomach with the endoscope. The proximal margin of the gastric folds must be determined when the distal esophagus is minimally inflated. Overinflation will flatten and obscure all the gastric folds. If the squamo-columnar and gastro-esophageal junction coincides, the entire esophagus is lined with squamous mucosa. When the squamo-columnar junction is proximal to the gastroesophageal junction, there is a columnar-lined segment or Barrett's esophagus. Pathology can give a clear indication of esophageal origin when an esophageal gland or, more usually (in a biopsy sample), a duct from these glands is seen. The depth of biopsy required makes these findings unusual. The requirement of the presence of intestinal metaplasia in a biopsy to diagnose Barrett's esophagus is difficult, as it can be found in the macroscopically normal squamocolumnar junction in up to 18% of patients undergoing endoscopy. The debate has deepened as the cytokeratin immunoreactivity (CK7/CK20 pattern) may be able to differentiate the intestinal metaplasia associated with Barrett's esophagus from that associated with *Helicobacter pylori* gastritis (24,25).

Dysplasia, "the unequivocal neoplastic alteration of the gastrointestinal epithelium which has the potential to progress to invasive malignancy that remains confined within the basement membrane of the gland within which it arose" (28) remains the best predictor for the development of invasive malignancy. The classification of neoplastic change in the gastrointestinal mucosa has five categories: negative for dysplasia, indefinite for dysplasia, low-grade dysplasia, high-grade dysplasia, and invasive carcinoma (26–29). Inter- and intraobserver studies have demonstrated that pathologists can demonstrate acceptable levels of agreement for the two major comparative groups of high-grade dysplasia combined with carcinoma, against negative for dysplasia combined with indefinite and low-grade dysplasia (kappa values of 0.8). However, the division into the four groups of negative for dysplasia, combined indefinite for dysplasia and low-grade dysplasia, high-grade dysplasia, and carcinoma has revealed that there are poorer levels of agreement (intraobserver kappa values of 0.64 and interobserver kappa values of 0.43) (30). The vital separation of high-grade dysplasia from intramucosal cancer depends on the penetration of neoplastic cells through the basement membrane. This classification is also difficult with interobserver agreement between all pathologists and specific gastrointestinal pathologists for high-grade dysplasia and intramucosal carcinoma having a kappa value of 0.42 and 0.56, respectively, even from resection specimens. These data have serious consequences for patients undergoing endoscopic surveillance, when the number of biopsies are often collected in a hurried fashion, small, and difficult to orientate correctly (31,32).

RATIONALE AND CRITERIA FOR CONSIDERATION OF ABLATION TREATMENT

At what stage should consideration be given to the ablation of the Barrett's epithelium? This is a subject of much debate, but, generally, intervention is considered following the diagnosis of dysplasia. The pathological difficulties make radical therapy at the time of diagnosis of dysplasia difficult. Initially, the diagnosis of high-grade dysplasia should be confirmed by further biopsies and a second, preferably expert, pathologist. The natural history of dysplasia remains uncertain, with contradictory and confusing data. There are arguments for rigorous-protocol endoscopic surveillance of patients with high-grade dysplasia with jumbo biopsy and intervention at the diagnosis of cancer (33). Recently, a very large study has demonstrated a cumulative cancer incidence over five years of only 9%, with only 12 of 75 (16%) of patients developing cancer during 13.9 years of surveillance. This U.S. group adopted a very aggressive approach to the diagnosis of synchronous cancer with three-monthly endoscopic biopsy in the first year before the patient was categorized as having pure high-grade dysplasia (34). Others have found dysplasia is a marker for occult invasive cancer and argue that a diagnosis of high-grade dysplasia should still be the end point of surveillance and the patient offered definitive radical therapy. This is usually surgical excision if the patient is considered fit to undergo the procedure. This view is justified, not only as a prophylactic measure but also because approximately 30% of these patients will have a coexistent cancer, which is only identified after surgical excision (35).

THEORETICAL AND PRACTICAL CONSIDERATIONS FOR ENDOSCOPIC MUCOSAL ABLATION

There are important considerations in the choice of endoscopic mucosal ablation. The most important being the depth of destruction that can be obtained to destroy both Barrett's mucosa and neoplastic tissue and, at the same time, allow safe healing. The mean thickness of nondysplastic Barrett's mucosa is about 0.6 mm. This figure has been derived by measurement in various ways. Histopathology measured Barrett's mucosa to be 0.5 mm (range 0.39–0.59 mm) compared with a normal squamous epithelium of 0.49 (range 0.42–0.58 mm) (36). It was assumed that fixation produces a 10% shrinkage with a further 10% reduction which was caused by processing—producing a shrinkage of 20%. Thus, the mean thickness of Barrett's mucosa is approximately 0.6 mm. Optical coherence tomography (OCT) of excised unfixed specimens has recorded a depth of between 0.45 mm and 0.5 mm (37). Dysplasia and mucosal cancer are thicker and in OCT appear optically denser. This represents approximately 15% of the thickness of the distal esophageal wall, which is approximately 4 mm, as measured by endoscopic ultrasound (38). It is important to understand that the technique of ablation must not produce full-thickness necrosis and risk perforation, particularly in the distended esophagus.

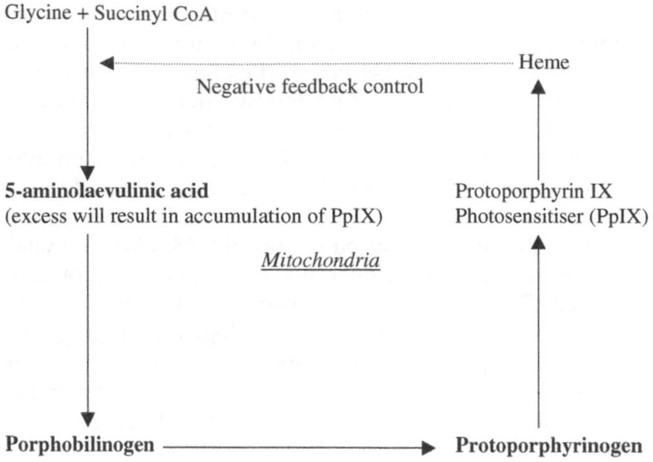

FIGURE 2 Diagram to illustrate the pathway of endogenous photosensitization with 5-aminolaevulinic acid to generate the photosensitizer protoporphyrin IX.

The conditions for safe healing are of crucial importance. In a canine model of gastroesophageal reflux, columnar-lined esophagus could be induced and was thought to be associated with regrowth from the proximal columnar-lined portion of the deep esophageal glands (39). After full reflux control, an acute injury to the esophageal mucosa was still associated with some regeneration by columnar cells, as well as squamous islands from the distal squamous part of the esophageal gland ducts. It was postulated that stems cells, possibly in the esophageal gland duct have multipotential for cell differentiation and could produce columnar or squamous cells depending on environmental conditions. Squamous re-epithelialization could be encouraged by full reflux control. Recent detailed, human morphological studies have confirmed that squamous regeneration is universally associated with esophageal ducts (40).

However, studies of a rodent model (does not have esophageal glands) of Barrett's-like esophagus have suggested that the ductal epithelium may not be so crucial (41). The multipotential stem cells may not be exclusively located in the duct epithelium but reside in the basal layer of the squamous and the regenerative columnar villi epithelium. The depth of the mucosal injury appears to be crucial to the type of regeneration. It has been suggested, but not established, that for squamous cells to predominate, as well as environmental control of reflux being essential, some part of the distal squamous-lined–esophageal-gland duct must survive. As this duct is the most distal portion, and thus the part most likely to destroyed by ablation techniques, the empirical evidence does not support this hypothesis. Certainly, multipotential stem cells must survive to regenerate the epithelium, but, at present, the site and source of these cells are unknown, and they may reside deeper in the esophageal duct. It is very important that reflux control is adequate. Patients with long segments of Barrett's esophagus ablated, who have persistent acid and bile reflux, are more prone to recurrence at 1-year follow-up (42).

METHODS OF ENDOSCOPIC ABLATION: PHOTODYNAMIC THERAPY

Exogenous Photosensitization

Exogenous photodynamic therapy with an administered photosensitizer will destroy sufficient depth to eradicate early T1 and some T2 cancers (43). Up to 30% of patients may develop esophageal strictures, and cutaneous photosensitivity is a problem. This form of therapy is ideal if there is nodularity and possible early occult cancer is present. The depth of necrosis may be approximately 6 mm (44,45), which clearly implies full-thickness damage to the esophagus. Perforation does not occur because the damage spares the tissue architecture, with collagen remaining intact and the bursting strength of the intestine maintained (46). There is, however, an increased risk of stricture formation. The patient receives light irradiation for 48 hours after the administration of 2 mg/kg of Photofrin (porfimer sodium) by slow intravenous injection (47).

The clinical protocol for tetra(m-hydroxyphenyl)chlorine (mTHPC) proposes a drug dose of 0.15 mg/kg administered intravenously four days before irradiation (48).

Endogenous Photosensitization

Endogenous photodynamic therapy (PDT) with orally administered 5-aminolaevulinic acid (ALA) is ideal if there is no visible lesion. The mechanism for the generation of the endogenous photosensitizer is shown in Figure 2. There is a much-reduced risk of stricture or cutaneous photosensitivity. The depth of tissue necrosis is limited to 2 mm. The patient receives 30 mg/kg to 75 mg/kg ALA dissolved in orange juice or lemonade, and the maximum dosage used is 75 mg/kg (49–52). The prodrug is administered three to six hours prior to endoscopic light irradiation. The dose may be fractionated into two aliquots of 30 mg/kg each ingested four hours and three hours prior to PDT.

Endoscopic Technique of Photodynamic Therapy

Endoscopy is usually performed with topical anesthesia and intravenous sedation of between 1 and 10 mg of midazolam. In our practice, we have found that analgesia is occasionally administered (pethidine 50–100 mg intravenously). Patients photosensitized using 5-ALA often require a prolonged endoscopy (20–40 minutes) and notice local discomfort and irritation during light irradiation. Throughout treatment, oxygen is delivered via a nasal sponge at a rate of 4 to 5 L/min. Repeat sedation may be necessary. The treatment times are considerably shorter for Photofrin (8–10 minutes) and tetra(*m*-hydroxyphenyl)chlorine (mTHPC) (2 minutes) photosensitization than for ALA, and there appears no problem of discomfort. It is very important to pay close attention to light dosimetry and use an appropriate light-centering device (53). The aim is to deliver an even light dose to a defined circumferential area of the esophagus; treating long areas and repeated sequential areas are irradiated in 5 to 7 cm lengths. Usually windowed balloons are the easiest to use. These inflatable, transparent polyurethrane balloons can be passed over a guide wire, or through the biopsy channel of the endoscope. A small video endoscope is passed down beside the device to ensure positional stability throughout treatment. Light is usually delivered by a laser fiber, which is inserted and the correct wavelength of light chosen PpIX-630 nm, Photofrin-630 nm, and mTHPC-652 nm. Nonlaser light devices are also highly effective.

Thermal, Photothermal (Laser), Cryotherapy, and Mechanical Ablation

Thermal and photothermal methods often require repeated application and endoscopic therapy. They are usually cheaper, more readily available and may be as effective as PDT. In areas of large field change, PDT offers some advantages as a large surface area can be treated. The potassium titanyl phosphate (KTP) laser has tissue penetration characteristics that should allow safe thermal treatment of mucosal disease. Irradiation with the KTP laser with a power of 15 to 20 W for a 1-second pulse produces mucosal temperatures of greater than 65°C with a temperature of 21°C on the outer surface of the esophagus. It was extremely difficult to generate high temperatures on the external surface of the esophagus, using this laser. The diode laser (25 W for 5 seconds) could produce surface temperatures of 90°C but with external temperature of 38°C. The Nd:YAG laser tended to produce worrying temperatures through to the external surface at energy levels that were sufficient to produce thermal destruction on the mucosa (54). It has proved to be highly effective for the treatment of dysplasia and early cancer (55). The Nd: YAG laser has been used very effectively, but the risk of perforation and full-thickness damage is greater.

There are two other widely used method of thermal ablation. The most commonly used is argon beam plasma coagulation (APC). This transfers electrical energy to the tissue by means of an ionized, electrically conducting plasma of argon gas, delivered at between 1 L/min and 2 L/min. The APC has certain theoretical safety advantages. The current causing very high temperatures on the surface produce a zone of devitalization, surrounded by zones of coagulation, desiccation, and tissue shrinkage. As soon as the area on the surface loses electrical conductivity as a result of this desiccation, the plasma beam has to change direction in order to remain electrically conductive. Therefore, the depth effect is limited, and full-thickness necrosis and perforation are unlikely to occur. Five perforations have been reported, two resolved with conservative medical therapy, and three had operations following which two patients died. Strictures are reported in 0% to 9% of patients, and fever may also occur (56–59). Another important method is multipolar electrocoagulation (MPEC). This device depends on the heat of a current passing between electrodes in contact with the tissue. An endoscopic probe is used to produce a surface white coagulum over the entire circumferential area of Barrett's esophagus. Strictures requiring dilatation have occurred in less than 1% of patients. Residual areas of Barrett's occur in 8% (0–28%), and the other complications of pain and fever are transient and mild (60,61).

Endoscopic Mucosal Resection

Endoscopic mucosal resection is an excellent method for the eradication of focal lesions in the esophagus and does allow accurate pathological assessment and staging. The ideal lesions are (*i*) less than 20 mm in diameter; (*ii*) well- or moderately differentiated carcinomas (grading G1/G2); (*iii*) areas of focal high-grade dysplasia; (*iv*) endoscopic macroscopic appearance types I (polypoid), IIa (flat raised), IIb (flat at mucosal level), and IIc (slightly depressed). Larger areas that are ulcerated (type III); poorly differentiated; or infiltrating the mucosa can be treated but there is an increased risk of recurrence (62,63). In addition, the management of multifocal areas of high-grade dysplasia may be technically difficult, requiring multiple interventions, although with experience very substantial areas can be removed (64). There are essentially two standard methods—the "lift-and-cut" and the "suck-and-cut" technique (Figs. 3–5).

A standard forward-viewing endoscope is fitted with a transparent guttered cap. The cap, holding open snare within the gutter, is used to aspirate the tissue to form a polyp. It is usual to form a pseudopolyp by submucosal injection. This has the benefit of allowing the area to be assessed for invasion and reduces the chance of inadvertent perforation. If the area fails to lift then there is a definite possibility of submucosal invasion. The area of tissue is then removed with the snare. An alternative method is to use a variceal banding initially to ligate the base and form the pseudopolyp. Resections of esophageal lesions can be with a double channel endoscopy. A grasping forceps is used to pull the lesion into the loop of the snare, following elevation with a submucosal injection. Recently, a ceramic tip resection device, predominantly developed for use in the treatment of early gastric cancer, has been used in the esophagus.

Chromoendoscopy may be useful to identify early cancer and dysplasia. The dyes that may be used are methylene blue, which has proved useful in the identification of dysplasia and cancer, which stain less than the surrounding intestinal metaplasia. Lugol's solution can be used to identify residual columnar epithelium with squamous mucosa. Toludine blue will stain columnar mucosa and indigo carmine can be used as a nonabsorbed stain to enhance magnification endoscopic discrimination of suspect lesions.

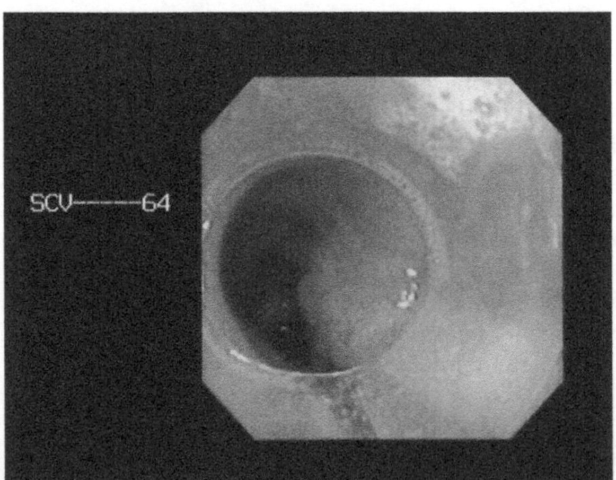

FIGURE 3 A nodule of intramucosal carcinoma in a segment of Barrett's esophagus viewed at endoscopy through the transparent endoscopic mucosal resection cap prior to resection.

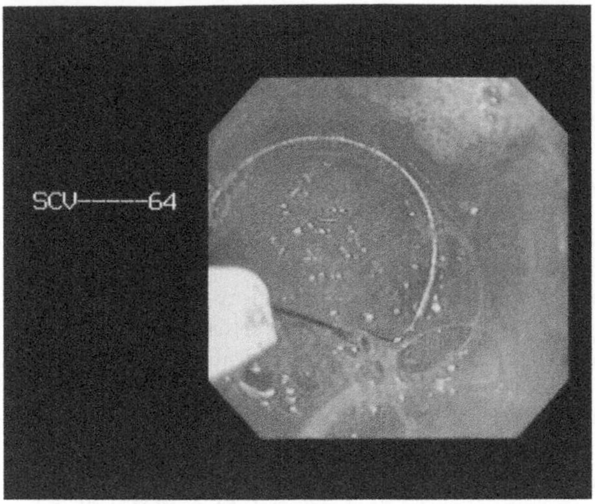

FIGURE 4 The same lesion as in Figure 3. This endoscopic picture is taken after submucosal injection as the lesion is being aspirated into the cap prior to snare resection.

In a series of 295 patients, 31% of patients with lesions less than 2 cm, had them removed with a single resection. Overall 80% had intramucosal carcinoma, 16% were invasive into the submucosa and the remaining 4% had dysplasia. Lymphatic invasion was present in 3.5% usually associated with submucosal invasion (65).

The major concern is that metachronous tumors can occur in up to 14% of patients. Patients must therefore continue with endoscopic surveillance (62,63). It is important for all these patients to receive acid-suppressing therapy with proton pump inhibitors (PPIs).

The question remains as to how much of the neoplastic or preneoplastic segment can be removed by this technique. Piecemeal circumferential resections have been performed removing half the circumference at a time. The resections were performed one month apart, and complete eradication was possible in 83% of 21 patients. There was immediate endoscopically controllable bleeding in four patients, no perforations and no stricture formation (66).

Thus, the technique appears to be remarkably safe. The most worrying complications are bleeding and perforation. The overall complication rate for both the major complications of bleeding and stricture formation and other milder complications is 12.5%. To avoid the perforation, great care should be taken to ensure that the lesion lifts with submuosal injection and forms a pseudoployp following suction ligation. Large lesions can be treated with multistep piecemeal resection.

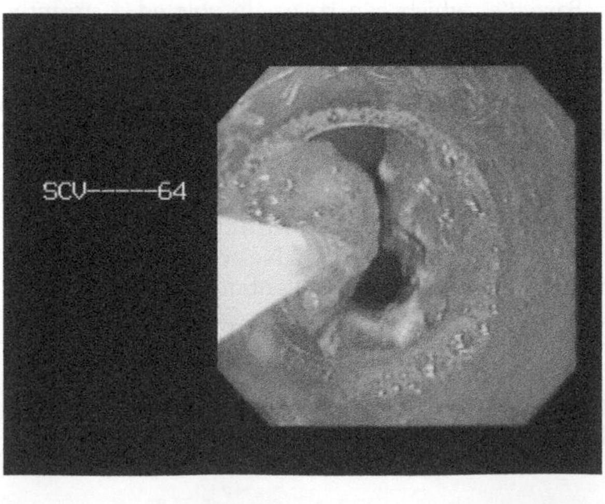

FIGURE 5 The same lesion as in Figures 3 and 4, immediately after resection. There are residual areas seen at the margins of the resection that will require further endoscopic mucosal resection.

INITIAL CLINICAL TRIALS

There has been a randomized partially blinded trial for prevention of cancer in Barrett's esophagus, which examined 208 patients with confirmed high-grade dysplasia. It is very instructive to note that over 485 patients (with a diagnosis of high-grade dysplasia) had to be screened to enter 208 patients with confirmed high-grade dysplasia. The patients were randomized (2:1) such that 138 had PDT and omeprazole (O) and 70 received omeprazole only. At the end of the minimum of 24-month follow-up, ablation of all areas of high-grade dysplasia was noted in 76.8% of patients in the PDT + O group ($n = 138$) versus 38.6% in the O group ($n = 70$) ($P < 0.0001$). After a mean follow-up of 24.2 months, 13.0% of patients in the PDT + O group had disease progression to cancer as compared to 28% in the O group after a mean follow-up of 18.6 months ($P = 0.006$). Strictures occurred in 37.1% of patients following PDT (67). This preliminary data establishes that PDT is now a highly effective treatment for the eradication of high-grade dysplasia in Barrett's esophagus.

A comparison of APC against Photofrin PDT. PDT showed that dysplasia was eradicated in 10 of 13 (77%) patients treated with PDT and 11 of 16 patients (69%) after APC. Photosensitivity was seen in two (15%) of PDT patients whereas three (19%) of patients treated with APC had dysphagia, pain, and fever (68). A further randomized trial compared ALA PDT following continuous light and fractionated irradiation and APC thermal coagulation for the ablation of patients with low-grade dysplasia [8] and no dysplasia [32] in Barrett's esophagus. The results showed that the mean endoscopic reduction of Barrett's esophagus at six weeks was 51% for ALA with continuous irradiation, 86% following fractionated irradiation, and 93% following APC treatment. Another randomized comparison demonstrated the complete ablation of Barrett's epithelium followed APC treatment occurred in 97% of patients compared with only 24% of patients treated with ALA PDT (69). A comparison of endoscopic devices, APC and multipolar thermocoagulation, has shown that the latter resulted in fewer treatment session with significantly more patients achieving histological ablation. The study examined 52 patients, with between 2 cm and 7 cm of Barrett's esophagus without cancer or high-grade dysplasia and followed up with six monthly endoscopies for up to four years (70).

The Quality of Evidence: 1B Recommendation Grade B. The randomized clinical trial with PDT is the major evidence for the effectiveness of mucosal ablation, yet further follow-up is necessary. The comparison of PDT with APC coagulation also indicates that this may be as effective as PDT.

THEORETICAL ANALYSIS

The management of Barrett's esophagus remains a controversial area. Most patients will die from Barrett's rather than from an esophageal adenocarcinoma. However, in a patient with Barrett's esophagus, it is now possible to remove abnormal areas and resurface the entire lower esophagus using a variety of endoscopic techniques. The question remains, who should be treated? Many studies have looked at treating metaplasic Barrett's, which can be easily ablated. Currently, ablation is not widely used nor recommended for patients with metaplasia only. Most usually, treatment is restricted to patients who are detected to have high-grade dysplasia, at risk of malignant degeneration, or patients with an early Barrett's adenocarcinoma. Other strategies are being explored for the large numbers of patients with Barrett's metaplasia. Treatment of dysplasia demands an "obsession with regression" whereas "prevention of progression" is the correct approach for metaplasia. Most patients in this latter group can have excellent symptom control on PPI therapy. It is highly appropriate that this is being formally addressed, at the epicenter of the epidemic, by Cancer Research U.K. and National Cancer Research Network in the United Kingdom. They are supporting a large randomized trial on chemoprevention using aspirin and esomeprazole—Aspirin and Esomeprazole Chemoprevention Trial (AspECT). The trial has commenced, and, due to its size, will inform many of our future management strategies (71).

It is appropriate, while awaiting long-term data, to conduct a "Gedanken" thought experiment. The purpose is to estimate the effect of endoscopic eradication of high-grade dysplasia xtrapolating from current data. This would involve detection and destruction of dysplasia followed by continued surveillance.

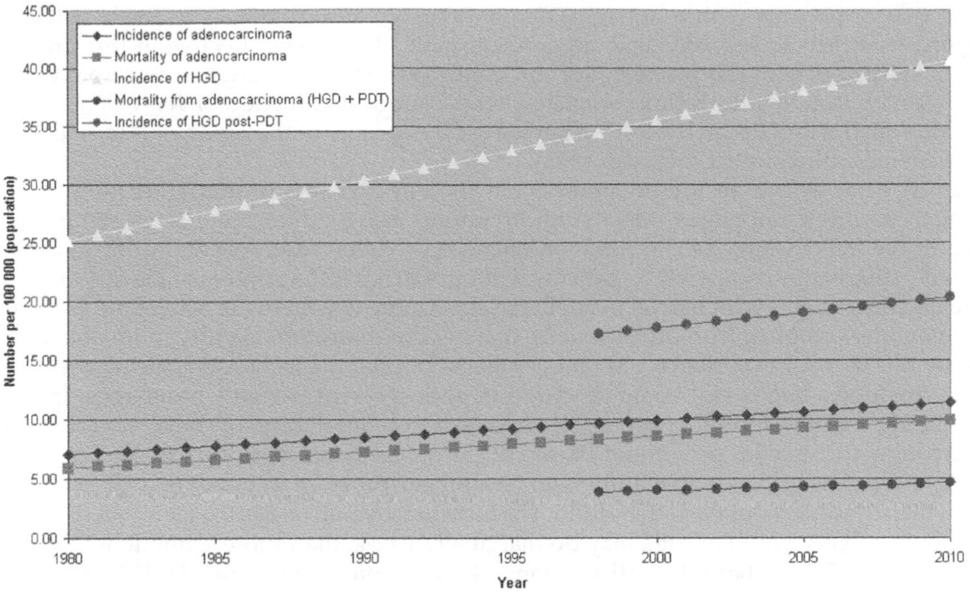

FIGURE 6 A "theoretical experiment" detection, destruction of dysplasia. The continuous lines indicate the incidence of high-grade dysplasia, esophageal adenocarcinoma, and the mortality from esophageal adenocarcinoma. The circles (blue and crimson) represent the data available from 1998, when trials of ablation started, and indicate that high-grade dysplasia could be eradicated and thus the incidence, and the mortality and incidence of esophageal adenocarcinoma considerably reduced. *Abbreviations*: HGD, high-grade dysplasia; PDT, photodynamic therapy.

The assumptions are:

1. Patients progression to adenocarcinoma is through detected Barrett's esophagus and high-grade dysplasia (72).
2. The incidence of esophageal cancer continues to rise, and the mortality continues to parallel the incidence.
3. Figure 6 presents the theoretical analysis and suggests that the mortality and possibly the incidence of esophageal adenocarcinoma could be considerably reduced.

This minimally invasive solution to the eradication of high-grade dysplasia in Barrett's esophagus has been subject to a detailed cost-effective analysis (73). It was compared with (*i*) no preventive strategy, (*ii*) elective surgical esophagectomy, (*iii*) endoscopic ablation, and (*iv*) surveillance endoscopy. The strategy of endoscopic ablation provided the longest quality-adjusted life expectancy. Endoscopic surveillance was cheaper but associated with shorter survival, and the authors conclude that optimal utilization of healthcare resources was achieved by endoscopic ablation (73).

Effect of Surgery on the Natural History of Barrett's Esophagus

The place of surgery in controlling the natural history of Barrett's esophagus relates to three areas. These are the symptoms, the benign and malignant complications. The majority of patients with Barrett's remain symptomatic for life with partial relief by taking acid suppression medication.

Effect on Surgery on the Natural History of Symptoms

The rationale for antireflux surgery in the management of patients with Barrett's esophagus comes from the understanding that the degree of reflux in these patients is at the severe end of the reflux spectrum (74). This has been best documented by pH and bile reflux monitoring (75). The degree of exposure of the esophagus to acid in the average patient with Barrett's is more than twice that of patients with esophagitis and an even greater difference to those without tissue injury. It is clear to see why acid suppression with PPIs is less effective in this group, compared to refluxers with less tissue injury and it creates a group of patients for whom there is more to gain by stopping the reflux completely with a surgical procedure. Even when symptoms are controlled with PPIs, there is still a pathological exposure of the esophagus to acid and to bile in patients with Barrett's esophagus (76).

There is some debate in the literature about the effectiveness of antireflux surgery in patients with Barrett's esophagus. Most surgical authors believe that there is no significant difference in the effectiveness of the common operation (Nissen fundoplication) for patients with Barrett's esophagus compared to patients without Barrett's. As surgeons, the authors do recognize that the patients with Barrett's esophagus have more edema in the wall of the esophagus, and more peri-esophagitis with adhesions, making the dissection slightly more demanding. Despite this it is our experience and that of others (77) that the technical achievement of a completed fundoplication is still straightforward in patients with Barrett's esophagus. In the laparoscopic approach to antireflux surgery, there is no difference in rates of conversion to open surgery among patients with or without Barrett's. The subsequent disruption of the repair or recurrence of reflux is said by some authors to be a bigger problem in patients with Barrett's esophagus than those without Barrett's (78,79). The literature overall favors the view that patients after antireflux surgery with Barrett's may do marginally worse than those without. Recurrent symptoms occur in 25% of Barrett's patients (range 45–155) compared to 10% (5–15%) in those without Barrett's. There is a wide range of opinion on this: Parrilla et al. (80) state that there is no difference between those refluxers with or without Barrett's metaplasia in terms of symptomatic and 24-hour pHmetry follow-up (8% failure with Barrett's vs. 10% without Barrett's). Others have documented anatomical disruption of the wrap, to be twice as common in Barrett's (12%) compared to those with uncomplicated gastroesophageal reflux disease (5%) (79).

Effect of Surgery on the Natural History of Benign Complications

The literature on the effect of antireflux surgery on complications in Barrett's esophagus is limited to peptic stricture. The other complications of bleeding and perforation are too rare for any useful cohort studies or prospective trials. Table 1 describes three studies which have looked at nonrandomized (81,82) and randomized (83) cohorts of patients with Barrett's esophagus who were treated by either continuation of acid suppression or by antireflux surgery. In the nonrandomized studies, it is important to look at the case selection. In both, the indication for surgery included a requirement for symptoms to persist despite acid suppression medication. Thus, the patient group who were offered surgery were initially those patients who were worse than those left on medical therapy. After successful antireflux surgery, patients in both groups were asymptomatic initially, and in each study, follow-up over three to five years showed a significant recurrence of symptoms of reflux and in symptomatic peptic stricture. The literature shows a clear benefit in both symptomatic outcome and prevention of stricture after antireflux surgery for patients with Barrett's esophagus (evidence level 1b and 2b, recommendation Grade B).

Effect of Surgery on the Natural History of Malignant Degeneration

From the standpoint of tumor biology, it has been believed for some time that patients with reflux injury in their esophageal epithelium are at an increased risk of developing adenocarcinoma through the metaplastic process of Barrett's esophagus. A logical hypothesis is that if the reflux

TABLE 1 Comparison of Medical Vs. Surgical Treatment of Reflux Disease and Barrett's Esophagus

Author	Number in study	Length F'up yrs	Recurrent stricture		Symptoms reflux	
			Med rx	Surg rx	Med rx	Surg rx
McEntee 1991	44	2	26%	12%	56%	32%
Attwood 1988	45	4	34%	10%	42%	16%
Ortiz 1996	59	4	30%	6%	44%	21%

is responsible for the injury then the complete abolition of reflux would allow healing and restoration of normal epithelial biology. Antireflux surgery has the potential to stop all reflux regardless of its quality, in contrast to acid suppression.

The natural history of cancer development in Barrett's esophagus is assumed to be a progression through intestinal metaplasia to low-grade dysplasia, high-grade dysplasia, and then ultimately cancer. This process is well-described and well-summarized by Woodman et al. (84). Although this is a neat categorization, the observation of this process in reality is very rare, as most patients with adenocarcinoma are diagnosed without previous documentation of the stepwise changes. Conversely, most patients with intestinal metaplasia or low-grade dysplasia do not progress to high-grade dysplasia or invasive cancer. Conversion of Barrett's to cancer varies from <0.5% per annum in the United States to 1% per annum in the United Kingdom. This makes the introduction of a therapeutic intervention such as surgery difficult to assess and with currently available data there is insufficient evidence to support a strategy of surgical correction of reflux to prevent cancer in Barrett's esophagus.

The timing of a cancer prevention intervention is important. In the generation of cancer, Barrett's metaplasia undergoes numerous mutations, changing its genetic structure to create heterozygosity, microsatellite instability, aneuploidy, and tetraploidy, all of which can be identified in many patients who have Barrett's epithelium but no identifiable cancer (85,86). These changes eventually create a histologically detectable lesion—either high-grade dysplasia or invasive adenocarcinoma through a process of clonal expansion whereby individual nuclear changes become replicated and self-perpetuating. The whole process may take many years, and if reflux injury is driving the process, it may be necessary to stop the reflux early in the process and then follow the outcome many years later. Currently, the literature on cancer development after antireflux surgery includes only short periods of follow-up for most patients, and the average ages of patients undergoing surgery is 50 to 60 years, and follow-up studies rarely average more than five years.

Regression of Metaplasia After Antireflux Surgery

Regression of the metaplastic process has been documented after antireflux surgery. Abbas et al. (87) quote 18% (9 of 49) to be completely regressing with a further 6% (3 of 49) partially regressing. Desai et al. (79) quote a similar figure for regression of 14%. Oelschlager (88) describes a 55% regression in patients who start out with short segment Barrett's (30 of 54) compared to none (0 of 36) who had long segments >3 cm. Gurski et al. (89) describe an even higher rate of regression—58% for short segment (19 of 33) and 20% for long segment Barrett's (9 of 44). One of the great difficulties in assessing the outcome of the length of Barrett's after antireflux surgery is the change in anatomy after repair of a hiatus hernia. It is difficult to know if the regression seen in a short segment of Barrett's metaplasia (less than 2 cm) is actual regression or simply anatomical rearrangement of the cardia by the surgical intervention.

Regression of Low-Grade Dysplasia After Antireflux Surgery

There are some important studies in the literature that deal specifically with surgical control of reflux in relation to the progression or resolution of low-grade dysplasia. In patients with low-grade dysplasia, Ackroyd (90) conducted a randomized controlled trial to compare antireflux surgery with medical therapy (proton pump inhibition) to look at the rate of regression of the dysplastic process. In this study, there was a statistically significant resolution of dysplasia after surgery and greater than that seen with medical therapy. This supports two previous nonrandomized studies (81,82) which had also shown better resolution of low-grade dysplasia after antireflux surgery.

Effect of Antireflux Surgery on Progression to High-Grade Dysplasia

Few reports comparing medical and surgical therapy for Barrett's esophagus have focused on the outcome of high-grade dysplasia. Parrilla (91) reports the outcome of a randomized trial of Barrett's treatment looking at 5-year follow-up after surgery or medical therapy with a PPI and showed that 2 of 43 (5%) progressed to high-grade dysplasia after PPI versus 2 of 58 (3%) after surgery—a difference that is not significant. The problem with considering antireflux surgery in the presence of high-grade dysplasia is that there may already be a focus of invasive cancer, and currently, the only therapeutic strategies accepted are observation, ablation, or resection as discussed early in this chapter.

The quality of evidence that surgery affects the natural history of complicated Barrett's esophagus remains very variable, and one cannot with confidence say that progression is halted or the phenotypic changes reversed or indeed stabilized. We are dependent on a substantial amount of observational and poorly controlled data. The evidence level is 2C to 3B, and recommendation Grade C.

The Effects of Antireflux Surgery Combined with Ablation Therapies

Antireflux surgery has been used as an adjunct to ablation therapies described above for low- and high-grade dysplasia (90,92,93). It seems clear that after ablation therapy the likelihood of recurrent metaplasia is less if the reflux is controlled by antireflux surgery rather than acid suppression medication, but there has been no data on any benefit in terms of cancer progression or resolution of high-grade dysplasia that relates to the method of reflux control.

THE PREVENTION OF CANCER DEVELOPING IN BARRETT'S ESOPHAGUS BY ANTIREFLUX SURGERY

The literature on cancer development after antireflux surgery for Barrett's esophagus clearly shows that cancers do occur. Without controlled studies, it is difficult to know if patients after surgery are at lower risk than those left on medication. Surgical authors discuss the reasons for malignant progression under two headings. Those cancers that were predetermined before the antireflux surgery tend to occur within the first few years after the antireflux operation, and those that occur late develop in patients whose reflux has continued after their operation. This is a consistent theme of rationalization whether the surgical authors advocate antireflux surgery or not. DeMeester and Oberg (74,94) both advocate antireflux surgery as a means of preventing cancers and quote low rates of cancer (mostly occurring in the first five years). Csendes (95) on the other hand argues that in his patient cohort the recurrence of reflux after simple fundoplication is too common and so he advocates a complex procedure that includes an antrectomy, a roux-en-Y biliary diversion and a fundoplication. This combination has the advantage of effectively removing bile from the stomach, and therefore the esophagus, while also reducing the acid production and preventing any material in the stomach from refluxing into the esophagus. From the work of Stein et al. (75) and Sarela et al. (76), it is clear that patients with Barrett's esophagus treated with PPIs have persistent severe degrees of both bile and acid exposure and the possibility that a combined bile diversion procedure with antireflux surgery has some theoretical value.

In the series of Csendes (95), he has shown six adenocarcinomas developing in 161 surgically treated patients with Barrett's esophagus (occurring at 4–6, 9, 17, and 18 years). Recurrent reflux was documented in those patients with late development of cancer after antireflux surgery. Numerous other authors have noted occasional cancer development in Barrett's after antireflux surgery and most comment on recurrent reflux (77,87).

An important epidemiological study of gastric and esophageal cancer after antireflux surgery was conducted in Sweden by Ye et al. (96) who examined 10,000 patients who had undergone antireflux surgery and a further 67,000 patients with gastroesophageal reflux disease who did not undergo surgery. Their study did not specifically address the issue of Barrett's esophagus. They found that cancer of the esophagus and cardia was elevated in both study groups (standardized incidence ratio of 6.3 for esophageal and 2.4 for gastric carcinoma in patients with gastroesophageal reflux, and 14.1 and 5.3, respectively, after surgery for reflux) compared to the rest of the population. This confirmed their previous report of a strong association between reflux symptoms and the development of carcinoma of the esophagus. The stronger association of cancer with the surgically treated population is more likely to relate to the severity of reflux, requiring surgical intervention rather than as a consequence of the intervention. In terms of cancer protection, the lack of benefit of antireflux surgery in this population does not answer the question in relation to Barrett's esophagus, but it does serve to caution proponents of surgery as a cancer protection until more direct data is available.

Corey et al. (97) in their literature review on data published up to 2001 found a cumulative 4678 patient years of follow up after antireflux surgery for Barrett's and documented a cancer rate of 3.8 per 1000 patient years compared to 5.3 per 1000 patient years after medical therapy. Although, this is a 30% reduction in the rate of cancer development after antireflux surgery, in their study, which was a meta-analysis, this difference did not reach statistical significance.

The combination of ablation with surgery has yet to be fully evaluated, as has the prophylactic and protective effect of surgery. The natural history of Barrett's esophagus remains variable, and prophylactic interventions are yet to be proven. Grade 3B. Recommendation C/D.

CONCLUSION

The role of antireflux surgery in Barrett's esophagus is of proven value to patients with significant symptoms and in the prevention of complications of stricture. Antireflux surgery is better than medical therapy at inducing resolution of metaplastic epithelium but this has yet to be proven of clinical value to the patient. Its role in cancer prevention is theoretically attractive, but studies so far have been disappointing in terms of cancer outcome. There is some value in using antireflux surgery as an adjunct to ablation, although even this should be in the context of controlled clinical trials. It is not advisable to recommend antireflux surgery for patients with Barrett's esophagus on the basis of potential protection against cancer development.

From a scientific standpoint, it would be of great interest if an early antireflux operation could be performed in the context of a randomized, controlled trial in patients in their 40s and followed for 25 years to the peak age of incidence of Barrett's adenocarcinoma. This would allow protection of the epithelium in the lower esophagus at the right time in the metaplasia-dysplasia cancer sequence and would at the same time offer the greatest number of years of improved quality-of-life. However, it is unlikely, with a cancer conversion rate of <1% per annum, that such a trial could be completed with sufficient numbers to provide a conclusive result.

REFERENCES

1. Wei JT, Shaheen NJ. The changing epidemiology of esophageal adenocarcinoma. Sem Gastrointest Dis 2003; 14:112–127.
2. el-Serag HB. The epidemic of esophageal adenocarcinoma. Gastroenterol Endosc Clin N Am 2002; 31:421–440.
3. Mason AC, Eloubeidi MA, el-Serag HB. Temporal trends in survival of patients with esophageal adenocarcinoma 1973–1997. Gastroenterology 2001; 122:A30.
4. Jankowski J, Harrison RF, Perry I, Balkwill F, Tselepis C. Seminar: Barrett's metaplasia. Lancet 2000; 356:2079–2085.
5. Jankowski J, Provenzale D, Moayyedi P. Oesophageal adenocarcinoma arising from Barrett's metaplasia has regional variations in the West. Gastroenterology 2002; 122:588–590.
6. Dulai GS. Surveying the case for surveillance. Gastroenterology 2002; 122:820–825.
7. Corley DA, Levin TR, Weiss NS, Buffer PA. Surveillance and survival in Barrett's adenocarcinoma: A population-based study. Gastroenterology 2002; 122:633–640.
8. Spechler SJ, Barr H. Review article: Screening and surveillance for Barrett's oesophagus: What is a cost-effective framework. Aliment Pharmacol Ther 2004; 19(suppl 1):49–53.
9. Barr H, Playford RJ. Endoscopic surveillance of patients with Barrett's oesophagus. Gut 2002; 51:313–315.
10. Farrow DC, Vaughan TL. Determinants of survival following the diagnosis of esophageal adenocarcinoma (United States). Cancer Causes Control 1996; 7:322–327.
11. Bachmann MO, Alderson D, Edwards D, et al. Cohort study in South and West England of the influence of specialization on the management and outcome of patients with oesophageal and gastric cancers. BJS 2002; 89:914–922.
12. Cameron AJ, Lomboy CT. Barrett's esophagus: Age, prevalence and extent of columnar epithelium. Gastroenterology 1992; 103:1241–1245.
13. Menke-Pluymers MBE, Hop WCJ, Dees J, van Blankenstein M, Tilanus HW. Risk factors for the development of an adenocarcinoma in Barrett's oesophagus. Cancer 1993; 72:1155–1158.
14. Lagergren J, Bergstrom R, Lindren A, et al. Symptomatic gastroesophageal reflux as a risk factor for esophageal adenocarcinoma. N Engl J Med 1999; 340:825–831.
15. Skinner DB, Walther BC, Riddell RH, Schmidt H, Iascone C, DeMeester T. Barrett's esophagus. Ann Surg 1983; 198:554–566.
16. Lagergren J, Berstrom R, Nyren O. Association between body mass and adenocarcinoma of the esophagus. Ann Intern Med 1999; 130:883–890.

17. Romero Y, Cameron AJ, Locke GR, et al. Familial aggregation of gastroesophageal reflux in patients with Barrett's esophagus and esophageal adenocarcinoma. Gastroenterology 1997; 113:1449–1456.
18. Lagergren J, Bergstrom R, Adami HO, Nyren O. Association between medications that relax the lower esophageal sphincter and risk for esophageal adenocarcinoma. Ann Intern Med 2000; 133:165–175.
19. Morgan G, Vainio H. Barrett's oesophagus, oesophageal cancer and colon cancer: An explanation of the association and cancer chemopreventative potential of non-steroidal anti-inflammatory drugs. Eur J Cancer Prev 1998; 7:195–199.
20. Weston AP, Badr AS, Topalovski M, Cherian R, Dixon A, Hassanein RS. Propective evaluation of the prevalence of gastric *Helicobacter pylori* infection in patients with GERD, Barrett's esophagus, Barrett's dysplasia, and Barrett's adenocarcinoma. Am J Gastroenterology 2000; 95:387–394.
21. Gray MR, Donnelly RJ, Kingsnorth AN. The role of smoking and alcohol in metaplasia and cancer risk in Barrett's oesophagus. Gut 1993; 34:727–731.
22. Spechler SJ, Sperber H, Doos WG, Schimmel EM. The prevalence of Barrett's esophagus in patients with chronic peptic esophageal strictures. Dig Dis Sci 1983; 28:769–774.
23. Morales TG, Sampliner RE. Barrett's esophagus: An update on screening, surveillance and treatment. Arch Intern Med 1999; 159:1411–1416.
24. Barr H. The pathological implications of surveillance, treatment and surgery for Barrett's oesophagus. Curr Diagnostic Pathol 2003; 9:242–251.
25. Couvelard A, Cauvin J-M, Goldfain D, Rotenberg A, Robaszkiewicz M, Flejou J-F. Cytokeratin immunoreactivity of intestinal metaplasia at normal oesophagogastric junction indicates its aetiology. Gut 2001; 49:761–766.
26. Riddell RH, Goldman H, Ransohoff D. Dysplasia in inflammatory bowel disease. Standardised classification with provisional clinical application. Hum Pathol 1983; 14:931–966.
27. Reid BJ, Haggitt RC, Rubin CE, et al. Observer variation in the diagnosis of dysplasia in Barrett's esophagus. Hum Pathol 1988; 19:166–178.
28. Haggitt RC. Barrett's esophagus, dysplasia, and adenocarcinoma. Hum Pathol 1994; 25:982–993.
29. Schlemper RJ, Riddell RH, Kato Y, et al. The Vienna classification of gastrointestinal epithelial neoplasia. Gut 2000; 47:251–255.
30. Montgomery E, Bronner MP, Goldblum JR, et al. Reproducibility of the diagnosis of dysplasia in Barrett's oesophagus: A reaffirmation. Hum Pathol 2001; 32:368–378.
31. Ormsby AH, Petras RE, Henricks WH, et al. Observer variation in the diagnosis of superficial oesophageal adenocarcinoma. Gut 2002; 51:671–676.
32. Alderson D. Observer variation in the diagnosis of superficial oesophageal adenocarcinoma: Another spanner in the works. Gut 2002; 51:620–621.
33. Levine DS, Haggitt RC, Blount PL, Rabinovitch PS, Rusch VW, Reid BJ. An endoscopic biopsy protocol can differentiate high-grade dysplasia from early adenocarcinoma in Barrett's esophagus. Gastroenterology 1993; 105:40–50.
34. Schnell TG, Sontag SJ, Chejfec G, et al. Long term non-surgical management of Barrett's esophagus with high-grade dysplasia. Gastroenterology 2001; 120:1607–1619.
35. Zaninotto G, Parenti AR, Ruol A, Costantini M, Merigliano S, Ancona E. Oesophageal resection for high-grade dysplasia in Barrett's oesophagus. BJS 2000; 87:1102–1105.
36. Ackroyd R, Brown NJ, Stephenson TJ, Stoddard CJ, Reed MW. Ablation treatment for Barrett oesophagus: What depth of tissue destruction is needed. J Clin Pathol 1999; 52:509–512.
37. Bamford K, James J, Barr H, Tatam R. Electromagnetic simulation of laser-induced fluorescence in bronchial tissue and predicted optical scattering behaviour. Optical Imaging Tech Biomonitoring IV 1998; 3567:18–28.
38. Johnston MH. Cryotherapy and other newer techniques. Gastrointest Endosc Clin N Am 2003; 13:491–504.
39. Li H, Walsh TN, O'Dowd G, Gillen P, Byrne PJ, Hennessy TPJ. Mechanisms of columnar metaplasia and squamous regeneration in experimental Barrett's esophagus Surgery 1994; 115:176–181.
40. Coad RA, Warner PJ, Barr H, Shepherd NA, Woodman AC. On the genesis of Barrett's oesophagus: A three dimensional study of the relationship between oesophageal gland ducts, Barrett's oesophagus and associated squamous islands. Br J Cancer 2004; 91:P105.
41. Van den Boogert J, Van Hillegersberg R, De Bruin RWF, Van Velthuysen MLF, Tilanus HW. A rat model for Barrett's oesophagus and prospects for photodynamic therapy. Eur J Gastroenterol Hepatol 1997; 9:A53.
42. Basu KK, Pick B, Bale R, West KP, de Caestecker JS. Efficacy and one year follow-up of argon plasma coagulation therapy for ablation of Barrett's oesophagus: Factors determining persistence and recurrence of Barrett's epithelium. Gut 2002; 51:776–780.
43. Sibille A, Lambert R, Souquet J-C, Sabben G, Descos F. Long-term survival after photodynamic therapy for esophageal cancer. Gastroenterology 1995; 108:337–344.
44. Heier SK, Rothman KA, Heier LM, Rosenthal WS. Photodynamic therapy for obstructing esophageal cancer: Light dosimetry and a randomized comparison with Nd:YAG laser therapy. Gastroenterology 1995; 109:63–72.

45. Barr H, Krasner N, Boulos PB, Chatlani PT, Bown SG. Photodynamic therapy for colorectal cancer: A quantitative pilot study. Brit J Surg 1990; 77:93–96.
46. Barr H, Tralau CJ, Boulos PB, MacRobert AJ, Tilly R, Bown SG. The contrasting mechanisms of colonic damage between photodynamic therapy and thermal injury. Photochem Photobiol 1987; 46:795–800.
47. Lightdale CJ. Role of photodynamic therapy in the management of advanced esophageal cancer. Gastrointest Endosc Clin N Am 2000; 10:397–408.
48. Radu A, Wagnieres G, van den Berg H, Monnier P. Photodynamic therapy of early squamous cell cancers of the esophagus. Gastrointest Endosc Clin N Am 2000; 10:439–460.
49. Barr H. Barrett's esophagus: Treatment with 5-aminolevulinic acid photodynamic therapy. Gastrointest Endosc Clin N Am 2000; 10:421–438.
50. Barr H, Shepherd NA, Dix A, Roberts DJH, Tan WC, Krasner N. Eradication of high-grade dysplasia in columnar-lined (Barrett's) oesophagus using photodynamic therapy with endogenously generated protoporphyrin IX. Lancet 1996; 348:584–585.
51. Barr H. Gastrointestinal tumours: Let there be light. Lancet 1998; 352:1242–1244.
52. Tan WC, Fulljames C, Stone N, et al. Photodynamic therapy using 5-aminolaevulinic acid for oesophageal adenocarcinoma associated with Barrett's metaplasia. J Photochem Photobiol B: Biology 1999; 53:75–80.
53. Panjehpour M, Overholt BF, Haydek JM. Light sources and delivery devices for photodynamic therapy in the gastrointestinal tract. Gastrointest Endosc Clin N Am 2000; 10:513–532.
54. Dix AJ, Barr H. Photothermal ablation of metaplastic columnar-lined (Barrett's) oesophagus, experimental studies for safe endoscopic laser therapy. Prog Biomed Optics (SPIE Proceedings) 1996; 2922:275–280.
55. Gossner L, May A, Stolte M, Seitz G, Hahn EG, Ell C. KTP laser destruction of dysplasia and early cancer in columnar-lined Barrett's esophagus. Gastrointest Endosc 1999; 49:8–12.
56. Barham CP, Shepherd N, Barr H. Regression of Barrett's epithelium using argon gas coagulation and acid suppression. Gut 1996; 39:T114.
57. Franchimont D, Van Laethem J-L, Deviere J. Argon plasma coagulation in Barrett's oesophagus. Gastrointest Endosc Clin N Am 2003; 13:457–466.
58. Deviere J. Argon plasma coagulation therapy for ablation of Barrett's oesophagus. Gut 2002; 51:763–764.
59. Morris CD, Byrne JP, Armstrong GRA, Attwood SEA. Prevention of neoplasticprogression of Barrett's oesophagus by endoscopc argon beam plasma ablation. BJS 2001; 88:1357–1362.
60. Sampliner RE, Fennerty MB, Garewal HS. Reversal of Barrett's esophagus with acid suppression and multipolar electrocoagulation: Preliminary results. Gastrointest Endosc 1996; 44:532–535.
61. Sampliner RE. Multipolar electrocoagulation. Gastrointest Endosc Clin N Am 2003; 13:449–455.
62. Ell C, May A, Gossner L, et al. Endoscopic mucosal resection of early cancer and high-grade dysplasia in Barrett's oesophagus. Gastroenterology 2000; 118:670–671.
63. May A, Gossner L, Pech P, et al. Local endoscopic therapy for intraepithelial high-grade neoplasia and early adenocarcinoma in Barrett's oesophagus: Acute-phase and intermediate results of a new treatment approach. Eur J Gastro Hep 2002; 14:1085–1091.
64. Seewald S, Akaraviputh T, Seitz U, et al. Circumferential endoscopic mucosal resection and complete removal of Barrett's epithelium: A new approach to management of Barrett's esophagus containing high-grade intraepithelial neoplasia and intramucosal carcinoma. Gastrointest Endosc 2003; 57:854–859.
65. Vieth M, Ell C, Gossner L. Histological analysis of endoscopic resection specimens from 326 patients with Barrett's esophagus and early neoplasia. Endoscopy 2004; 36:776–781.
66. Giovannini M, Bories E, Pesenti C, et al. Circumferential endoscopic mucosal resection in Barrett's esophagus with high-grade intraepithelial neoplasia or mucosal cancer. Preliminary results in 21 patients. Endoscopy 2004; 36:282–287.
67. Overholt BF, Lightdale CJ, Wang K, et al. International multicenter partially blinded randomised study of the efficacy of photodynamic therapy (PDT) using porfimer sodium (POR) for the ablation of high-grade dysplasia (HGD) in Barrett's esophagus (BE): Results of 24 month follow-up. Gastroenterology 2003; 124(suppl 1)A20:151.
68. Ragunath K, Krasner N, Raman VS, Haqqani MT, Phillips CJ, Cheung I. Endoscopic ablation of dysplastic Barrett's oesophagus comparing argon plasma coagulation and photodynamic therapy: Short term results of a randomized prospective trial assessing efficacy and cost effectiveness. Scand J Gastroenterol 2005; 40:750–758.
69. Hage M, Sieresma PD, van Dekken H, et al. 5-Aminolevulinic acid photodynamic therapy versus argon plasma coagulation for ablation of Barrett's oesophagus: A randomised trial. Gut 2004; 53:785–790.
70. Kelty CJ, Ackroyd R, Brown NJ, Stephenson TJ, Stoddard CJ, Reed MWR. Endoscopic ablation of Barrett's oesophagus: A randomised controlled trial of photodynamic therapy vs argon plasma coagulation. Br J Surg 2004; 91:42 (abstract).
71. Jankowski JA, Attwood S, Barr H, Moayyedi P, Watson P. Intervention and surveillance strategies for Barrett's oesophagus. In: Cunningham D, Jankowski J, Miles A, eds. The Effective Management of Upper Gastrointestinal Malignancies. Loc: Pub, (2004):54–61.

72. Solaymani-Dodaran M, Logan RFA, West J, Card T, Coupland C. Risk of oesophageal cancer in Barrett's oesophagus and gastro-oesophageal reflux. Gut 2004; 53:1070–1074.
73. Shaheen NJ, Inadomi JM, Overholt BF, Sharma P. What is the best management strategy for high-grade dysplasia in Barrett's oesophagus? A cost effectiveness analysis. Gut 2004; 53:1736–1744.
74. DeMeester TR, Attwood SEA, Smyrk TC, Therkildsen DH, Hinder RA. Surgical therapy in Barrett's esophagus. Ann Surg 1990; 212:628–642.
75. Stein HJ, Kauer WKH, Feussner H, Siewert JR. Bile reflux in benign and malignant Barrett's esophagus: Effect of medical acid suppression and Nissen fundoplication. J Gastrointest Surg 1998; 2:333–341.
76. Sarela AI, Hick DG, Verbeke CS, Casey JF, Guillou PJ, Clark GW. Persistent acid and bile reflux in asymptomatic patients with Barrett esophagus receiving proton pump inhibitor therapy. Arch Surg 2004; 139:547–551.
77. O'Riordan JM, Byrne PJ, Ravi N, Keeling PW, Reynolds JV. Long term clinical and pathologic response of Barrett's esophagus after antireflux surgery. Am J Surg 2004; 188:27–33.
78. Csendes A, Burdiles P, Braghetto I, Korn O. Adenocarcinoma appearing very late after anti-reflux surgery for Barret's esophagus: Long term follow up, review of the literature and addition of six patients. J Gastrointest Surg 2004; 8:434–441.
79. Desai KM, Soer NJ, Frisella MM, Quasebarth MA, Dunnegan DL, Brunt LM. Efficacy of laparoscopic antireflux surgery in patients with Barrett's esophagus. Am J Surg 2003; 186:652–659.
80. Parrilla P, Martinez de Haro LF, Ortiz A, Munitiz V, Serrano A, Torres G. Barrett's esophagus without esophageal stricture does not increase the rate of failure of Nissen fundoplication. Ann Surg 2003; 237:48–93.
81. McEntee GP, Stuart RC, Byrne PJ, Nolan N, Hennessy TPJ. An evaluation of surgical and medical treatment of Barrett's oesophagus. Gullet 1991; 1:169–172.
82. Attwood SEA, Barlow AP, Norris TL, Watson A. Barrett's oesophagus: The effect of anti-reflux surgery on symptom control and the development of complications. Br J Surg 1992; 79:1021–1024.
83. Ortiz A, Martinez de Haro LF, Parrilla P, et al. Conservative treatment versus antireflux surgery in Barrett's esophagus: Long term results of a prospective study. Br J Surg 1996; 83:274–278.
84. Woodman AC, Jankowski JA, Shepherd NA. The metaplasia–dysplasia-carcinoma sequence of Barrett's esophagus. In: Tilanus HW, Attwood SEA, eds. Barrett's Esophagus. Amsterdam: Kluwer Academic, 2001:167–180.
85. Rabinovich PS, Reid BJ, Haggitt C, Norwood TH, Rubin CE. Progression to cancer in Barrett's esophagus is associated with genomic instability. Lab Invest 1988; 60:65–71.
86. Reid BJ, Haggitt RC, Rubin CE, Rabinovich PS. Barrett's esophagus. Correlation between flow cytometry and histology n detection of patients at risk for adenocarinoma. Gastroenterology 1987; 93:1–11.
87. Abbas AE, Deschamps C, Cassivi SD, et al. Barrett's esophagus: The role of fundoplication. Ann Thorac Surg 2004; 77:393–396.
88. Oelschlager BK, Barreca M, Chang L, Oleynikov D, Pellegrini CA. Clinical and pathologic response of Barrett's esophagus to laparoscopic antireflux surgery. Ann Surg 2003; 238:458–464.
89. Gurski RR, Peters JH, Hagen JA, et al. Barrett's esophagus can and does regress after antireflux surgery: A study prevalence and predictive features. J Am Coll Surg 2003; 196:706–713.
90. Ackroyd R, Tam W, Schoeman M, Devitt PG, Watson DI. Prospective randomised controlled trial of argon plasma coagulation vs endoscopic surveillance of patients with Barrett's esophagus after antireflux surgery. Gastrointest Endosc 2004; 59:1–7.
91. Parrilla P, Martinez de Haro LF, Ortiz A, et al. Long term results of a prospective randomised study comparing medical and surgical treatment of Barrett's esophagus. Ann Surg 2003; 237:291–298.
92. Noberto L, Polese L, Angriman I, Erroi F, Cecchetto A, D'Amico DF. High energy laser therapy of Barrett's esophagus: Preliminary results. World J Surg 2004; 28:350–354.
93. Attwood SEA, Lewis CJ, Caplin S, Hemming K, Armstrong GR. Argon beam plasma coagulation as therapy for high-grade dysplasia in Barrett's esophagus. J Clin Gastroeterol Hepatol 2003; 1:258–263.
94. Oberg S, Johansson J, Wenner J, et al. Endoscopic surveillance of columnar lined esophagus: Frequency of intestinal metaplasia detection and impact of antireflux surgery. Ann Surg 2001; 234:619–626.
95. Csendes A. Surgical treatment of Barrett's esophagus, 1980–2003. World J Surg 2004; 28:225–231.
96. Ye W, Chow WH, Lagergren J, Yin L, Nyren O. Risk of adenocarcinoma of the esophagus and gastric cardia in patients with gastroesophageal reflux disease and after antireflux surgery. Gastroenterology 2001; 121:1506–1508.
97. Corey KE, Schmitz SM, Shaheen NJ. Does a surgical antireflux procedure decrease the incidence of esophageal adenocarcinoma in Barrett's esophagus? Am J Gastroenterol 2003; 98:2390–2394.

2 The Role of Drugs and Nutrition in the Prevention of Esophageal Adenocarcinoma Associated with Barrett's Esophagus

P. L. Youd
Department of Gastroenterology, St. Mark's Hospital, Harrow, U.K.

Janusz A. Z. Jankowski
Department of Cancer and Molecular Medicine, Medical School and University Hospitals Trust, Leicester, U.K.

INTRODUCTION

Chemoprevention of esophageal adenocarcinoma in Barrett's esophagus (BE) is an expanding area of research. This chapter will briefly discuss the histopathologic background of BE and its association with esophageal cancer. It will explore up-to-date research, looking at the potential chemotherapeutic drug groups, namely proton pump inhibitors (PPIs) and cyclo-oxygenase (COX) inhibitors, particularly focusing on the molecular basis of their action and any current evidence to support their use. The less well understood role of nutrition in the pathogenesis of esophageal cancer is also discussed, based mainly on case-control studies. We conclude with a summary for physicians seeking to optimize preventative strategies even as avoiding both overprescribing and unnecessary anxiety for patients.

BARRETT'S ESOPHAGUS AND ESOPHAGEAL ADENOCARCINOMA

Barrett's esophagus occurs when the normal squamous epithelium of the lower esophagus is replaced by columnar epithelium. This occurs when injury to the squamous epithelium heals by a metaplastic process. Chronic gastroesophageal reflux disease (GERD) has been strongly implicated in this process due to the interplay between the refluxate (acid and bile) and the esophageal mucosa. The resulting columnar cells are defined as specialized intestinal metaplasia consisting of cells with gastric, small intestinal, and colonic features.

Despite being more resistant to acid damage than esophageal squamous cells, the metaplastic epithelium of BE is associated with a 30- to 125-fold increased risk of esophageal adenocarcinoma (1). The incidence of esophageal adenocarcinoma in patients with BE in the United States is approximately 0.5% per annum (2). However, in the United Kingdom, it is about twice that at 1% (3). Factors believed to influence its incidence are summarized in Table 1.

A distinction has been made between short- and long-segment BE, that is, <3 cm and >/=3 cm. The long-segment BE has been reported to be associated with increased severity of gastroesophageal reflux, a more advanced age, and increased cancer risk. However, current expert consensus states that there is no evidence that a risk gradient may be demarcated at a particular segment length (level 5 evidence) (4). Evidence suggests that there is a progression from Barrett's metaplasia through low- and high-dysplasia to adenocarcinoma (5). The mechanism by which this occurs appears to depend on both genetic and environmental factors. Exposure of tissue explants to acid pulses has been demonstrated to induce histological and molecular change in Barrett's epithelium, such as increased cell proliferation, activation of the Na/H-exchange pump, activation of protein kinase C, increased COX-2 expression and mitogen-activated protein kinase (MAPK) activation.

Similarly, several cell-signaling pathways have been implicated in carcinogenesis of tissues, including that of the esophagus (Table 2). Examples of such pathways are those involved in cell cycle/checkpoint control (p53 and p27), apoptosis/caspase control (FasL, tumor necrosis factor, c-myc), growth-factor phosphorylation (phosphatidylinositol-3-kinase, PI3k), mitogen activated protein kinase (MAPK) activation [in particular, MAPK kinase kinase (MEKK)/p38],

TABLE 1 Factors Influencing the Risk of Esophageal Adenocarcinoma

Reduced risk	Increased risk
Chronic GERD aspirin	Barrett's metaplasia
Selective COX-2 inhibitors	Bile acid disease
Proton pump inhibitors	Chronic inflammation
Vitamin C	Smoking
Fiber	Obesity
Beta-carotene	Alcohol
Folic acid	High fat diet/cholesterol
Vitamin E	Dietary protein
Vitamin B6	Certain micronutrient deficiencies
Helicobacter pylori infection Gastrin	Vitamin B12
Congenital developmental syndromes	

Abbreviations: COX, cyclo-oxygenase; GERD, gastroesophageal reflux disease.

cytokine signaling [nuclear factor (NF)-kappaB, COX/prostaglandins (PGs)], chromatin regulation and methylation, beta-catenin expression, wnt signaling and gastrin (6). It would therefore follow that the medical interference with these molecular pathways could inhibit malignant change.

The incidence of esophageal adenocarcinoma is increasing rapidly, and has done so particularly over the course of the past two decades (7). Recently, there has been much debate whether the paralleled decrease in gastric adenocarcinoma reflects improved classification of this cancer (8).

Prompted by this rising incidence, several developing areas of research have focused on the reduction of malignant change in BE. These areas include medical management, surgical and endoscopic intervention for GERD and BE, dietary modification, endoscopic surveillance, and an early interest in molecular surveillance, for example, p53 and p16 mutations (9). Chemoprevention is currently looking the most promising option (10,11). It has a high level of patient acceptability and cost effectiveness as well as a low associated morbidity and mortality.

CHEMOPREVENTION OF ESOPHAGEAL ADENOCARCINOMA

Proton Pump Inhibitors

The role of acid suppression in GERD is still a matter for debate. The association between long-term GERD and BE has been established. The association between BE and esophageal adenocarcinoma has also been established. Whether there is any definite role of acid reflux in the progression from Barrett's epithelium to malignancy remains unclear.

It has been hypothesized that a reduction in esophagea-acid exposure should reduce the incidence of Barrett's adenocarcinoma by reducing mucosal irritation. One study looked at the 24-hour esophageal and gastric pH of 110 patients with GERD and BE who had been

TABLE 2 Cell-Signaling Pathways Implicated in Esophageal Carcinogenesis

Cell cycle/checkpoint control, e.g., p53 and p27
Apoptosis/caspase control, e.g., FasL, TNF, c-myc
Growth factor phosphorylation, e.g., PI3k
MAPK activation, in particular, MEKK/p38
Cytokine signalling, e.g., NF kappa B, COX/prostaglandins
Chromatin regulation and methylation
Beta-catenin
Wnt signaling
Gastrin

Abbreviations: COX, cyclo-oxygenase; MAPK, mitogen-activated protein kinase; MEKK, MAPK kinase kinase; NF-kappa B, nuclear factor-kappa B; TNF, tumor necrosis factor.

rendered asymptomatic on PPI therapy (12). It was found that, despite the absence of symptoms, only 56% of patients with GERD and 38% with BE normalized their esophageal pH. If acid suppression does indeed impact the development of esophageal adenocarcinoma, the question of more aggressive acid suppression in such patients is raised as an issue. The plausibility of this statement is discussed here.

The Role of Acid Suppression in Barrett's Chemoprevention: Scientific Data

Several studies have suggested indirect evidence for the role of acid suppression in the prevention of adenocarcinoma in BE.

1. Despite patients with GERD becoming asymptomatic with conventional PPI doses, pH manometry studies show that there may still be pathological levels of acid reflux occurring (13).
2. Cell proliferation in ex vivo BE specimens is higher than in normal esophageal tissue at all pH levels. Pulse acid exposure increases cell proliferation in BE, whereas continuous acid exposure results in a reduced rate of proliferation compared with a neutral pH (14). The implication might be that continuous and profound acid suppression or exposure in BE rarely, if ever, occurs.
3. Cultured biopsy specimens of Barrett's epithelium have been shown to exhibit hyperproliferation and increased COX-2 expression, a proliferation mediator, when exposed to acid for an hour (14,15).
4. Brief exposure to acid has been shown to activate the MAPK pathways that have a role in increasing proliferation and survival, and in decreasing apoptosis in BE (16). Acid has been shown to activate the MAPK pathways in BE in vivo suggesting that carcinogenesis in BE may occur in part through the activation of these pathways.
5. A small, clinical study showed a significant reduction in the proliferation marker proliferating-cell nuclear antigen (PCNA) in biopsy specimens taken from patients for whom PPI therapy had normalized esophageal acid exposure over a 24-hour period. This reduction in proliferation and improved differentiation was not demonstrated in specimens where this normalization had not occurred. However, they also indicated that incomplete acid suppression could result in short episodes of acid reflux leading to epithelial changes. This in turn could select for poorly differentiated cells with increased proliferative potential (17).

The Role of Acid Suppression in Barrett's Chemoprevention: Clinical Data

These referenced studies appear to support the argument in favor of acid suppression in the prevention of Barrett's-associated adenocarcinoma. However, there remains an absence of convincing clinical evidence to support the role of routine antisecretory therapy in BE when balanced against the price and inconvenience of prescriptions. Indeed, based on the absence of clinical data, a recent expert consensus rejected the statement that normalization of esophageal acid exposure by acid suppression reduces the risk for development of esophageal adenocarcinoma (4).

One study of 68 patients followed over a period of two years showed that, while reflux symptoms were controlled on both standard-dose ranitidine and high-dose omeprazole, the latter showed a statistically significant regression in both the area and length of Barrett's epithelium (evidence level 1b) (18). Although the magnitude of regression was small, the almost complete and prolonged acid suppression achieved invites speculation regarding the benefit of aggressive PPI therapy in BE. In contrast, a second study demonstrated no significant reduction in the length of BE on high-dose PPI therapy and concluded that control of pH alone is insufficient for the reversal of Barrett's epithelium (evidence level 4) (19). Several other studies have shown inconsistent and therefore inconclusive effects of PPI therapy in Barrett's regression.

Interestingly, even the speed of introduction of a PPI after diagnosis of BE has been suggested to influence the risk of dysplastic change. One study published a 5.6 times increased risk of developing low-grade dysplasia if PPI therapy was withheld for two years following diagnosis compared with those who started treatment in the first year (evidence level 2b) (20). They found similar results for high-grade dysplasia and adenocarcinoma.

A large, prospective, randomized controlled trial has also looked at the comparative role of antireflux surgery with antisecretory medication in the prevention of esophageal cancer (21). Two hundred and forty-seven patients with GERD were randomized to medical and surgical treatment groups. They were followed up for a mean of 10.6 (medical patients) and 9.1 (surgical patients) years. At the end of this period, 160 survivors were identified. Various outcome measures and endpoints were assessed, including the incidence of adenocarcinoma. They found that patients with BE at baseline developed esophageal adenocarcinoma at an annual rate of 0.4%, compared with 0.07% in those without BE. There was no difference between the medical and surgical groups, although the respective sizes of the groups and the sexual bias may have influenced results. Despite the absence of controls, they concluded that surgical intervention could not be expected to reduce the risk of esophageal adenocarcinoma or reduce the need for antisecretory medication postoperatively.

Cyclo-Oxygenase Inhibitors

COX is the rate-limiting enzyme in the conversion of arachidonic acid to PGs. There are two isoenzymes of COX. COX-1 is constitutively expressed in most tissues. Its role appears to be in the production of PGs controlling normal physiologic function. Conversely, COX-2 is usually undetectable in normal tissue. It is expressed during inflammation, reproduction, and carcinogenesis in response to cell activation by hormones, proinflamatory cytokines, growth factors, and tumor promoters. It is implicated in epithelial adaptation in injured or inflamed mucosa (5). It is now known that prostaglandin E2 (PGE2) activates the transcription-factor peroxisome proliferator-activated receptor (PPAR) through phosphatidylinositol-3-kinase (PI3K) signaling (22). Also, wild type p53 has been shown to suppress COX-2 transcription, raising the possibility that p53 is one of the determinants of COX-2 expression (23).

Two types of COX inhibitor exist, namely selective and nonselective. The former are specific to the COX-2 enzyme and the latter, for example, aspirin, inhibit both COX-1 and COX-2.

The Role of Prostaglandins in Carcinogenesis

PGE2 exerts carcinogenic effects on the esophagus (24), its contribution being related to other factors that predispose to esophageal carcinoma. The implication is that nonsteroidal anti-inflammatory drugs (NSAIDs) may be useful in the prevention of esophageal carcinoma.

The molecular basis of COX-2 expression and its product PGE2 is a growing area of understanding (25). COX -2 is induced by the oncogenes ras and scr, interleukin-1, hypoxia, benzo[a]pyrene, ultraviolet light, epidermal growth factor, transforming growth factor beta and tumor necrosis factor alpha. It is suppressed by dexamethasone, antioxidants and tumor-suppressor gene p53 (Fig. 1). PGE2 stimulates the antiapoptotic protein bcl-2. It also induces interleukin-6 (IL-6) that enhances haptoglobin synthesis, and is associated with tumor

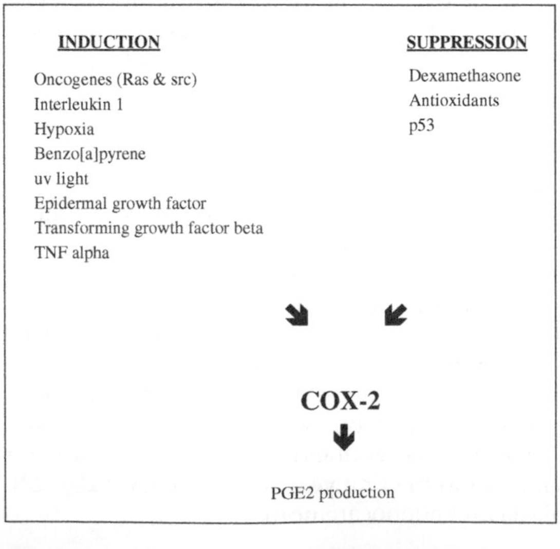

FIGURE 1 Induction and suppression of cyclo-oxygenase-2. *Abbreviations*: ras, reticular activating system; TNF, tumor necrosis factor.

metastases, IL-6 with cancer cell invasion and haptoglobin with implantation and angiogenesis. These processes, some of which are discussed in more detail later in this chapter, provide a basis for our understanding of both selective and nonselective COX-2 inhibitors in carcinogenesis.

Cyclo-Oxygenase-2 Inhibition in the Chemoprevention of Esophageal Cancer: Scientific Data

COX-2 overexpression has been reported in patients with both BE and esophageal adenocarcinoma. Several studies have demonstrated that COX-2 expression is increased serially along the BE-dysplasia-adenocarcinoma sequence. They consistently show absence of or negligible COX-2 in normal esophageal epithelium (26–30). While the Zimmerman study also demonstrated absence of COX-2 in Barrett's metaplasia cells, the other four studies reported expression of COX-2 in between 50% and 81% of Barrett's metaplasias. All five studies reported COX-2 expression in between 78% and 100% of esophageal adenocarcinomas. Interestingly, high COX-2 expression has also been shown as an independent prognostic variable in patient survival, suggesting that tumors with a high COX-2 content have a more aggressive course (30).

Most research into the role of COX-2 inhibition in carcinogenesis has concentrated on animal studies and human colonic cancers. The hypothesis for COX-2 inhibition as a preventative strategy for esophageal adenocarcinoma originated from supportive evidence for its role in colonic cancer (31,32). The implication is that the studies and mechanisms discussed in this chapter may be transferable in our understanding of esophageal carcinoma. Indeed, COX-2 inhibition has been shown to reduce the development of esophageal adenocarcinoma in animal models (33).

The role of COX-2 in carcinogenesis appears to be in resisting apoptosis, increasing cell proliferation, stimulating angiogenesis, modulating a cancer cell's invasive properties and increasing inflammation (Fig. 2). The molecular role of COX-2 inhibitors in these individual processes is discussed as follows:

Reduced Resistance to Apoptosis

Inhibition of programmed cell death can lead to the proliferation of abnormal cells. This results in clonal expansion of tumor cells. Most research to date has focused on human colonic cancer cells, and there are various mechanisms by which COX-2 has been implicated in this process. First, malignant cells expressing COX-2 have been shown to contain higher levels of the anti-apoptotic protein bcl-2 (34). NSAIDs have been seen to reverse the resistance to apoptosis by down regulation of bcl-2 (35). Second, COX inhibition has been shown to both actively induce apoptosis (36,37) and to reduce the expression of the transcriptional factor, nuclear factor kappa B (NF-kappa B), which prevents apoptosis (38).

Inhibition of Cell Proliferation

The Ras/Raf/MAPK pathway is a key growth-stimulating cascade which results in cellular proliferation. COX-2 is induced by activation of this pathway (39) and NSAIDs can inhibit this process. Selective COX-2 inhibitors can prevent epithelial cells progressing from the G0/G1 quiescent stage in the cycle to the S-phase of DNA replication, thereby reducing cell proliferation.

Inhibition of Angiogenesis

The growth of a tumor is dependent on its blood supply. A tumor's secretion of vascular growth factors is increased by its overexpression of COX-2 (40). Selective COX-2 inhibitors therefore inhibit angiogenesis (41). Selective COX-2 inhibitors also reduce angiogenesis via MAPK pathway inhibition (42).

Reduction in Invasion

COX-2 overexpression is shown to increase the invasive properties of cancer cells by increasing PG production (43), activating metalloproteinases 1 and 2 and by increasing the cell-surface receptor CD44 (44). It has also been seen to increase tumor dissemination in animals (43).

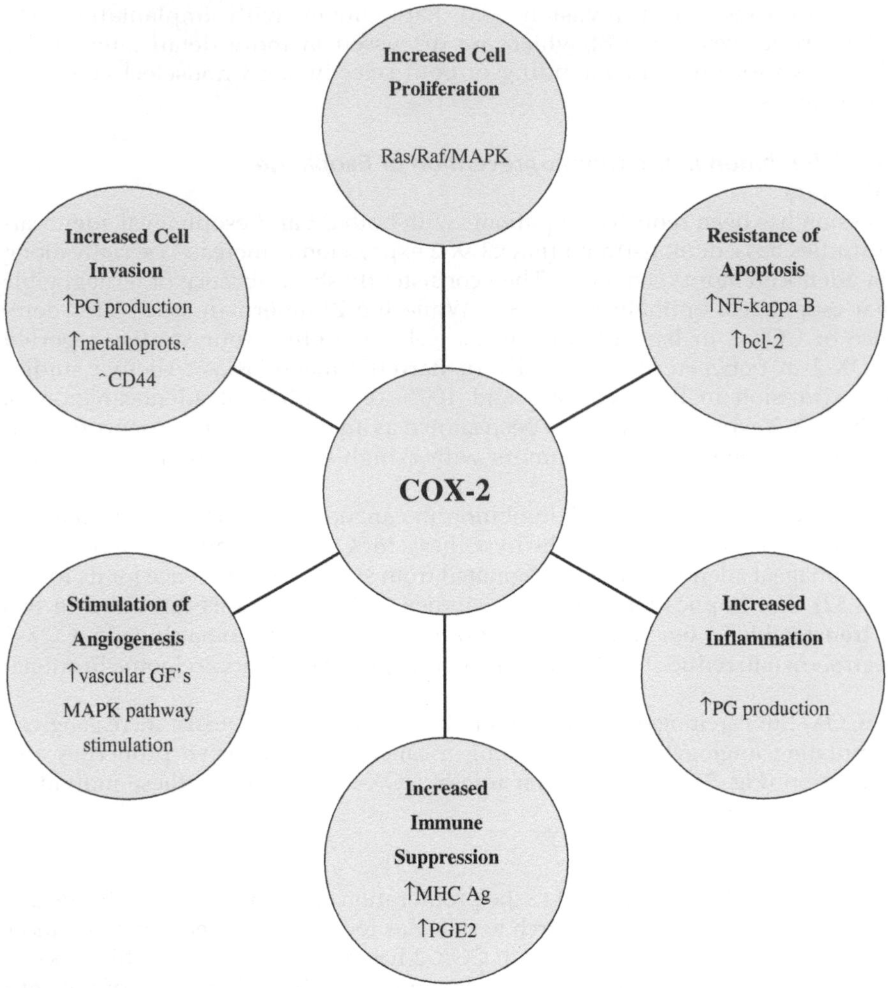

FIGURE 2 Role of cyclo-oxygenase-2 in carcinogenesis. *Abbreviations*: MAPK, mitogen-activated protein kinase; PG, prostaglandin; NF-kappa B, nuclear factor-kappa B; PGE2, prostaglandin E2; MHC Ag, major histocompatibility antigens.

Inhibition of Immunosuppression

Tumor cells release colony-stimulating factors that result in PGE2 production. PGE2 works at a cellular level allowing the tumor cells to escape normal immune surveillance. PG synthesis can by inhibited by NSAIDs, indirectly enhancing immune responses (45). They may also upregulate expression of major histocompatibility complex antigens (MHC Ag) (46).

Inhibition of Inflammation

The chronic inflammation of BE is a recognized risk factor for malignant change (47). It would therefore follow that reduction in cytokine-mediated induction of COX-2 and subsequent reduced synthesis of PGs would result in reduced carcinogenesis.

As an exeption, despite the evidence to support NSAID-associated chemoprevention as a COX-2-mediated phenomenon, several factors are likely to play a part in the process. Genetic predisposition is among these. Recently published data indicated that the role of NSAIDs is influenced by protein expression of the cyclin D1 gene in tumors (48). It was concluded that the risk for developing esophageal adenocarcinoma was reduced by aspirin and other NSAIDs only in patients with cyclin D+ tumors and not in cyclin D- tumors. Of note, this data was not specific to patients with previous BE.

Cyclo-Oxygenase-2 Inhibition in the Chemoprevention of Esophageal Cancer: Clinical Data

Many epidemiologic studies have shown a reduction in the development of malignant disease with the long-term use of NSAIDs, especially of gastrointestinal cancers (49). Statistically significant studies looking at the use of aspirin favor the drug as a chemopreventative agent in esophageal cancer. For example, Thun et al. demonstrated an approximately 40% lower risk of esophageal carcinoma in patients who used aspirin at least 16 times per month for at least a year (50). Occasional aspirin use has also been shown to reduce the risk of esophageal adenocarcinoma by 90%, according to data from the National Health and Nutrition Examination Survey and the National Epidemiological Follow-up Studies, which looked at over 14,000 patients (evidence level 2b) (51). This data was supported by a case-controlled study by Farrow et al., who reviewed 650 cases and 695 controls (52). They also reported a reduced incidence of esophageal squamous-cell carcinoma in aspirin users.

Two further case-controlled studies have looked at the role of NSAIDs in esophageal adenocarcinoma, but results differed. The first, a population-based study, found a protective effect of NSAIDs based on their 12,174 cases and 34,934 controls (53). These findings however were not supported by a single hospital-based study which found no significant reduction in cancer risk with NSAIDs (54).

The most conclusive data so far for the use of COX-2 inhibitors in the prevention of esophageal adenocarcinoma comes from a systematic review with meta-analysis of observational studies evaluating the association of aspirin/NSAID use and esophageal cancer (55). Nine studies (two cohort, seven case control) containing 1813 cancer cases were identified and independently reviewed. Pooled results support a protective association between aspirin and NSAIDs and esophageal cancer (of both histologic types). Results also provided evidence for a dose effect. They concluded that their findings would support the evaluation of these agents in clinical trials of high-risk patients (evidence level 2b).

One example of a high-risk group might include those patients with BE. The specific role of COX-2 inhibition in BE is discussed as follows.

Cyclo-Oxygenase-2 Inhibition and Chemoprevention of Malignant Change in Barrett's Esophagus

As the aforementioned in vivo studies have looked at the overall incidence of esophageal cancer, irrespective of the presence of Barrett's metaplasia, the role of COX-2 inhibitors in Barrett's metaplasia has also been studied in both in vitro and animal studies. In primary cultured endoscopic biopsy specimens of Barrett's tissue, selective COX-2 inhibitors were found to significantly decrease both COX-2 activity and proliferation of epithelial cells by 55% (56). Buttar's team also demonstrated a 55% reduced relative risk of developing esophageal adenocarcinoma and 79% reduction postesophagojejunostomy in rat models compared with controls. The prevalence of BE in the two groups was not significantly different (57).

A single completed in vivo study has demonstrated possible chemopreventative qualities of selective COX-2 inhibitors. Kaur et al. compared biopsy specimens of Barrett's epithelium with samples taken after 10 days of rofecoxib 25-mg daily. Rofecoxib resulted in a 77% reduction in COX-2 expression, 59% decrease in PGE2 content, and 62.5% reduction in proliferating-cell nuclear antigen expression (58).

These findings have initiated the start of two ongoing randomized clinical trials. One multicenter trial by Forastiere et al. (Baltimore, U.S.A.) is looking at the effect of selective COX-2 inhibitors in low- and high-grade dysplasia. The second is a European study being conducted by Attwood et al. comparing the effect of PPIs alone with the effect of a PPI plus a selective COX-2 inhibitor in the prevention of esophageal adenocarcinoma in Barrett's patients. Their outcomes are awaited.

Whether a selective or nonselective COX-2 inhibitor is preferable for chemoprevention in Barrett's patients is uncertain. Selective COX-2 inhibitors appear to have a lower side-effect profile than NSAIDs when used long term. In one study, the effects of a selective COX-2 inhibitor (rofecoxib) were compared with aspirin in BE patients on varying doses of the PPI esomeprazole (59). Biopsies of the BE segment and esophageal mucosa found that only the combination of PPI and aspirin resulted in a significant reduction in COX-2 and PGE2.

The Specific Role of Aspirin in Chemoprevention of Esophageal Cancer

It has been recognized for over a decade that aspirin, a nonselective COX inhibitor, reduces the risk of developing oesophageal cancer. Corley et al.'s meta-analysis referred to earlier concluded that there exists a protective association between aspirin and NSAIDs and oesophageal cancer of both histologic types, the effect of aspirin being greater (55). It also provided evidence for a dose effect, with greater protection being afforded by frequent compared with intermittent drug use. A similar conclusion for the chemopreventative role of aspirin was reached in recently published data of three case-controlled studies (60).

Whether this data can be accurately extrapolated to cover the role of aspirin in Barrett associated adenocarcinoma is of major importance in the management of BE. While aspirin is known to be associated with several complications, including gastrointestinal haemorrhage and strokes, a study looking at the cost-effectiveness and safety of aspirin in the prevention of Barrett's adenocarcinoma supported its use (61). It concluded that, regardless of whether the patient undergoes endoscopic surveillance, enteric-coated aspirin used in the management of BE is a cost-effective strategy for preventing malignant change.

The exact mechanism by which aspirin exerts its chemoprotective effect is uncertain. Various hypotheses exist and these are discussed in the following (Table 3). Some have already been outlined in relation to specific COX-2 inhibition.

Induction of Apoptosis

As previously stated, programmed cell death is essential for the prevention of clonal expansion of abnormal or malignant cells. The role of aspirin in this process was demonstrated by examining its effect on the growth and apoptosis of ten oesophageal cancer cell lines (62). Results showed that: (*i*) growth inhibition by aspirin was dose and time dependent and associated with the induction of apoptosis; (*ii*) bile acids could induce COX-2 expression in six out of eight cell lines tested, correlating to PGE2 production (a product of COX-2); (*iii*) aspirin could inhibit the enzymatic activity of COX-2 induced by bile acids; (*iv*) bcl-2 was downregulated by aspirin in the two cell lines tested. They thereby surmised that induction of apoptosis by aspirin may be one mechanism by which the drug interferes in esophageal carcinogenesis.

Inhibition of Prostaglandin E2

Both human and experimental esophageal tumors contain increased PGE2, probably resulting from activation of COX-2 in response to mitogens and growth factors. The increased level of PGE2 is thought to accelerate cell proliferation within the malignant tissue (63). The optimal dose of aspirin to suppress such an effect remains unclear.

The E-cadherin–Catenin Complex

Beta-catenin has an essential role in intercellular adhesion and signal transduction, functioning as a transcriptional activator downstream in the wnt signaling pathway. It has been implicated in the development of several cancers, including gastric (64), oesophageal squamous cell (65), and colorectal (66).

The E-cadherin-catenin complex is involved in adhesion of epithelial cells. Disruption of a part of this complex results in poor differentiation and increased invasiveness of cancers, as

TABLE 3 Hypothesized Chemotherapeutic Actions of Aspirin

Induction of apoptosis
bcl-2 down regulation
Inhibition of PGE2
Beta-catenin expression
E-cadherin expression
Transcription factor inhibition
NF-kappa B
AP-1
MAPK pathways

Abbreviations: MAPK, mitogen-activated protein kinase; NF, nuclear factor; PGE2, prostaglandin E2; AP-1, activating protein-1.

has been seen in gastric carcinoma (64). Tumors retaining normal membranous beta-catenin have a survival advantage, suggesting abnormal beta-catenin to be a poor prognostic marker. One study indicated that altered subcellular distribution of beta-catenin occurs frequently in dysplastic BE and possibly reflects the signaling function of this molecule (67).

Specific evidence for a relationship between aspirin and beta-catenin in esophageal adenocarcinoma has not been established. However, aspirin and indomethacin have been shown to downregulate beta-catenin/T-cell factor (Tcf) signaling in colorectal cancer cells via enhanced phosphorylation (66). The role of aspirin therefore remains a promising key target in esophageal anticancer therapy.

Nuclear Factor-Kappa B and AP-1 Inhibition

NF-kappa B and AP-1 are two important transcription factors governing the expression of many early response genes involved in inflammation and carcinogenesis. Environmental or occupational exposure to certain chromium particles can cause inflammation and malignancy. It has been suggested that these particles activate NF-kappa B and AP-1 expression and that aspirin substantially inhibits this process (68). The data suggests that the activation of AP-1 or NF-kappa B is through involvement of the MAPK or I kappa B kinase (IKK) pathways, respectively. This provides a further possible explanation for the molecular role of aspirin in the chemoprevention of esophageal cancer. Similar data in skin cancer supports the promising role of aspirin in chemoprevention by inhibition of ultraviolet light-induced AP-1 activity (69).

Mitogen-Activated Protein Kinase Pathways

The role of MAPK pathways have been discussed earlier in reference to acid exposure and are clearly not specific to aspirin. Both selective and nonselective NSAIDs inhibit angiogenesis through direct effects on epithelial cells. Angiogenesis is necessary for the growth and metastasis of solid tumors. The role of NSAIDs in this process involves inhibition of MAPK (ERK2) activity and interference with extracellular signal regulated kinase ERK nuclear translocation. It is independent of protein kinase C and has PG-dependent and PG-independent components (42).

Selective Cyclo-Oxygenase-2 Inhibitors as Neoadjuvant Therapy for Esophageal Cancer

In contrast to COX-1 inhibition, administration of a selective COX-2 inhibitor significantly suppresses cell growth and increases apoptosis in human esophageal cancer cell lines expressing COX-2 (70). In addition, survival benefit has been shown in patients with low COX-2 expression in esophageal adenocarcinoma after intentionally curative resection (30). These studies provide an experimental basis for clinical studies into the role of COX-2 inhibitors in the treatment of adenocarcinoma related to BE. They also provide supportive data for the initiation of therapeutic trials with selective COX-2 inhibitors as neoadjuvant therapy for esophageal adenocarcinoma. A small number of such trials are in process, although no large randomized control trials have yet published data with hard endpoints.

Helicobacter pylori and Esophageal Adenocarcinoma

It has been hypothesized that the increasing incidence of esophageal adenocarcinoma may in part reflect the decreasing prevalence of *H. pylori* in the developed world. A meta-analysis of 17 studies (published only in abstract) examined the prevalence of *H. pylori* and cagA+ strains of *H. pylori* in patients with BE or esophageal adenocarcinoma, along with controls (71). A study was made on 2162 patients and 3132 controls with a pooled *H. pylori* prevalence of 37.7% and 51.2%, respectively. The conclusion was that the prevalence of *H. pylori* and cagA+ *H. pylori* is negatively associated with BE and esophageal adenocarcinoma. The proposed mechanism is that *H. pylori* infection may lead to gastric body atrophy. This in turn would lead to reduced gastric acid secretion and its complications. Conversely, *H. pylori* infection would result in reduced acid secretion. It should be noted however that, despite this association, no protective effect has been proven between *H. pylori* infection and esophageal adenocarcinoma and the question of "friend or foe?" still remains.

Combination Drug Therapy

A PPI with a COX-2 inhibitor has been suggested as a promising combination in the prevention of adenocarcinoma secondary to BE. Preliminary results of a multicenter, randomized controlled trial however demonstrated no reduction in the cell proliferation index or development of dysplasia, despite a reduction in COX-2 expression (level 1b evidence) (72). Sixty-two patients with BE were followed up over a six-month period having been randomized to take either a PPI alone or in combination with rofecoxib. It was found that although initial introduction of rofecoxib reduced COX-2 expression, it did not significantly reduce cell proliferation. These results challenge the theory that COX-2 inhibition reduces malignant change, although the short follow-up period is acknowledged. Further work looking at combination drug therapy in esophageal chemoprevention is required.

NUTRITION AND ESOPHAGEAL ADENOCARCINOMA

The increasing incidence of esophageal adenocarcinoma over the course of the past 30 years has provoked scientific and epidemiologic interest. Most relevant, nutrition-based research to date consists of case-controlled studies. Nonetheless, certain dietary associations with the disease have emerged (Fig. 3). Obesity and a high fat diet have been seen to increase the risk of esophageal cancer, whereas several nutrients appear to reduce its incidence. These are discussed individually.

Obesity

Obesity is an established risk factor for both esophageal and gastric cardial adenocarcinoma, the association with the former being stronger. Obesity's etiological role in esophageal adenocarcinoma, in contrast to squamous cell carcinoma, was established in 1995 (73,74). An American study subsequently demonstrated a fourfold increased risk of esophageal adenocarcinoma in those in the highest quartile of body mass index (BMI) compared with the lowest quartile (75). Even more dramatic results published an eightfold increased risk for individuals in the highest quartile compared with the lowest BMI, along with a 16-fold increase between obese subjects (BMI > 30) and those with BMI <22 (level 1b evidence) (76).

A fairly bold statement is that "oesophageal adenocarcinoma is a largely preventable disease in women" (77). Nonetheless, having identified 74 affected women in the United Kingdom, Cheng et al. identified high BMI at the age of 20 years to be a significant risk factor for the condition. Having highlighted the incidence of esophageal adenocarcinoma in British women amongst the highest incidence in the country, they summarized that obesity and low fruit consumption had a population attributable risk of 90%.

The multifactorial nature of esophageal adenocarcinoma, probably involving both host and genetic factors, was highlighted in a recent review (78). It is logical to suppose that the strikingly

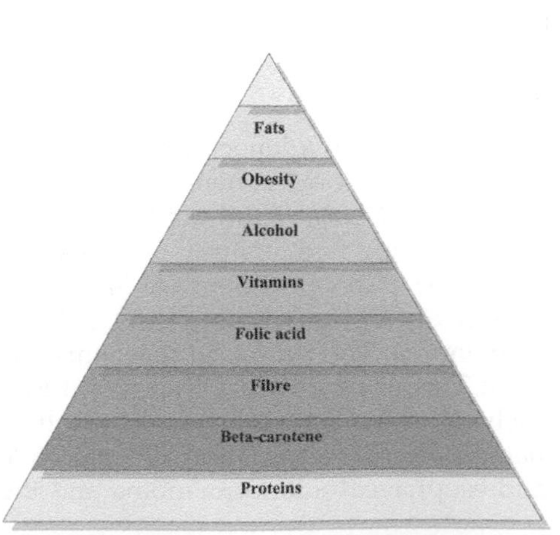

FIGURE 3 Dietary factors suggested to increase esophageal cancer risk.

increased risk of esophageal adenocarcinoma with both GERD and obesity may be attributed to the independent association of these two etiological factors with each other. This failed to be confirmed in one large case-controlled study from Sweden (79), thereby raising the possibility that hormonal effects may underlie the association of obesity and esophageal cancer.

High Fat Diet

Diets high in total fat, saturated fat, and cholesterol are associated with an increased risk of esophageal adenocarcinoma. The largest, population-based, case-control study was undertaken in the United States, and demonstrated that dietary fat was significantly associated with adenocarcinoma, although not squamous-cell carcinoma, of the esophagus (80).

Alcohol

The role of alcohol in esophageal carcinogenesis, specifically in the development of adenocarcinoma, remains somewhat controversial. It has been suggested that the main risk factors for the development of cancers of the oral cavity, pharynx, and esophagus in the developed world are tobacco and alcohol, together accounting for 75% of these cancers (81). The mechanism by which alcohol has this effect is not clear, although it is likely to be a direct effect on the endothelium (82).

A further study found a statistically significant increased risk of esophageal adenocarcinoma in smokers and a strong association of alcohol with squamous-cell carcinoma of the esophagus (83). However, neither beer nor liquor drinking was shown to be significantly associated with adenocarcinoma of the esophagus, and wine drinking was associated with a significant decrease in risk.

A meta-analysis of 14 studies conducted between 1966 and 2001 found the carcinogenic effects of alcohol and tobacco to be multiplicative on the relative-risk scale of cancers of the upper aerodigestive tract (84). Contrary to the conclusion of the aforementioned study, this meta-analysis also isolated alcohol as an independent risk factor for esophageal adenocarcinoma.

Micronutrient Deficiencies

Epidemiologic evidence indicates that diets high in fruits and vegetables are associated with a reduced risk of several carcinomas, including esophageal and gastric. It is believed that the vitamins and minerals in these foods may contribute to the reduced cancer risk.

A scientific review of 206 epidemiologic and 22 animal studies looked at the association of various cancers with fruit and vegetable consumption (85). Along with several other cancer sites, there appeared to be an evidence for the protective effect of these foods in esophageal cancer. The most protective effect seemed to be from raw vegetables, followed by allium vegetables, carrots, green vegetables, cruciferous vegetables, and tomatoes. The protective substances appeared to include dithiolthiones, isothiocyanates, indole-3-carbinol, allium compounds, isoflaveanes, protease inhibitors, saponins, phytosterols, inositol hexaphosphate, vitamin C, D-limonene, lutein, folic acid, beta carotene, lycopene, selenium , vitamin E, flavanoids, and dietary fiber.

One particular study observed that the dietary nutrients most beneficial in the prevention of esophageal adenocarcinoma are the antioxidants, principally vitamin C, beta-carotene, and vitamin E (86). In support of this finding is a scientific study that isolated lower levels of vitamin C in the plasma and mucosa of patients with BE compared with those with squamous mucosa (87). This would be consistent with the suggested role of oxidative stress in the pathogenesis and neoplastic progression of BE.

Interestingly, one of the case-controlled studies discussed earlier suggested a distinction between plant- and animal-derived nutrients (80). They concluded that nutrients associated with a lower risk of esophageal adenocarcinoma were predominantly derived from plant-based foods, whereas those derived from animal origin appeared to result in an increased risk. They also concluded that, of all the nutrients studied, dietary fiber had the greatest effect on risk reduction.

Whether micronutrient supplementation would influence cancer risk and mortality was investigated in a local community in China (88). The region studied has one of the highest esophageal and gastric cardia cancer rates in the world. Although the results were not definitive, the study of 29,584 adults did suggest that vitamin and mineral supplementation reduces esophageal cancer risk (level 1b evidence). The particular combination of beta carotene, vitamin E, and selenium was found to be most beneficial.

SUMMARY

Chemoprevention of esophageal adenocarcinoma by PPIs and NSAIDs remains a highly promising and rapidly developing field of medical research. Despite popular opinion and common practice amongst medical practitioners, expert consensus recently rejected the statement that normalization of esophageal acid exposure by acid suppression reduces the risk of developing esophageal adenocarcinoma from Barrett's epithelium (4).

The same expert opinion did, however, unanimously accept that epidemiologic studies show a significant risk reduction in esophageal adenocarcinoma for NSAID/aspirin users. Although the understanding of their clinical application is limited, many epidemiologic and experimental studies show promise for NSAIDs as anticancer drugs in the gastrointestinal tract. What remains uncertain is their exact mechanism of action, the appropriate doses and the risk–benefit ratio in long term.

Despite the promising role of COX-2 and selective COX-2 inhibitors, there is an urgent need for randomized controlled trials assessing their benefit in both low- and high-risk patients with BE. Although chemoprevention may be a viable alternative in patients at risk from surveillance endoscopy owing to comorbidity, prospective clinical trials are necessary before NSAIDs can be recommended in the prevention of Barrett's-related adenocarcinoma in the general population.

As stated in a recent review article, there is a great need for randomized controlled trials to assess the outcomes of chemopreventive therapy in patients with Barrett's metaplasia (89). Whether a combination of a COX-2 inhibitor and a PPI can work together to prevent malignant change in BE is being investigated in the 10-year Aspirin Esomeprazole Chemoprevention Trial (ASPECT) owing to finish in 2014 (www.digestivedisease.org). In the meantime, however, we conclude that there remains no data to convincingly support the role of drugs in the chemoprevention of esophageal adenocarcinoma secondary to BE.

The role of diet in the prevention of esophageal adenocarcinoma remains equally controversial. The existing data in this field has been drawn from the conclusions of case-controlled studies. Encouragingly, there remains promise for the protective effect of some foodstuffs, including certain micronutrients, fiber, antioxidants, and weight loss. As yet, however, there is certainly no convincing basis by which physicians can advise dietary manipulation or supplementation in the fight against this disease. Once again, randomized controlled trials are awaited.

REFERENCES

1. Stein HJ, Siewert JR. Barrett's esophagus: pathogenesis, epidemiology, functional abnormalities, malignant degeneration and surgical management. Dysphagia 1993; 8(3):276–288.
2. Shaheen NJ, Crosby MA, Bozymski EM, Sandler RS. Is there publication bias in the reporting of cancer risk in Barrett's oesophagus? Gastroenterology 2000; 199:333–338.
3. Jankowski JA, Provenzale D, Moayyedi P. Esophageal adenocarcinoma arising from Barrett's metaplasia has regional variations in the west. Gastroenterol 2002; 122(2):588–590.
4. Sharma P, McQuaid K, Dent J, et al. A critical review of the diagnosis and management of Barrett's esophagus: the AGA Chicago workshop. Gastroenterology 2004; 127:310–330.
5. Jankowski J, Harrison RF, Perry I, Balkwill F, Tselepis C. Seminar: Barrett's metaplasia. Lancet 2000; 356:2079–2085.
6. Harris JC, Clarke PA, Awan A, Jankowski J, Watson SA. An antiapoptotic role for gastrin and the gastrin/CCK-2 receptor in Barrett's esophagus. Cancer Res 2004; 64(6):1915–1919.
7. Blot WJ, Devesa SS, Kneller RW, Fraumeni JF. Rising incidence of adenocarcinoma of the oesophagus and gastric cardia. JAMA 1991; 265:1287–1289.
8. Corley DA, Kubo A. Influence of site classification on cancer incidence rates: an analysis of gastric cardia carcinomas. J Natl Cancer Inst 2004; 96(18):1383–1387.
9. Wijnhoven BP, Tilanus HW, Dinjens WN. Molecular biology of Barrett's adenocarcinoma. Ann Surg 2001; 233(3):332–337.

10. Corley DA, Kerlikowske K, Verma R, Buffler P. Protective association of aspirin/NSAIDs and oesophageal cancer: a systematic review and meta-analysis. Gastroenterology 2003; 124:47–56.
11. Thun MJ. NSAIDs and esophageal cancer: ready for trials but not yet broad clinical application. Gastroenterology 2003; 124:246–247.
12. Gerson LB, Boopari V, Ullah N, Triadafilopoulos G. Esophageal and gastric pH in patients with gastroesophageal reflux disease and Barrett's esophagus treated with proton pump inhibitors. Gastroenterology 2004; 126(suppl 2):A-57 [Abstract 452].
13. Ouatu-Lascar R, Triadafilopoulos G. Complete elimination of reflux symptoms does not guarantee normalisation of intra-oesophageal acid reflux in patients with Barrett's oesophagus. Am J Gastroenterol 1998; 93:711–716.
14. Fitzgerald RC, Omary MB, Triadafilopoulos G. Dynamic effects of acid on Barrett's esophagus. An ex vivo proliferation and differentiation model. J Clin Invest 1996; 98:2120–2128.
15. Shirvani VN, Ouatu-Lascar R, Kaur BS, Omary MB, Triadafilopoulos G. Cyclooxygenase-2 expression in Barrett's oesophagus and adenocarcinoma: ex vivo induction by bile salts and acid exposure. Gastroenterol 2000; 118:487–496.
16. Souza RF, Shewmake K, Terada LS, Spechler S. Acid exposure activates the mitogen activated protein kinase pathways in Barrett's oesophagus. Gastroenterology 2002; 122:299–307.
17. Ouata-Lascar R, Fitzgerald RC, Triadafilopoulos G. Differentiation and proliferation in Barrett's oesophagus and the effects of acid suppression. Gastroenterology 1999; 117:327–335.
18 Peters FT, Ganesh S, Kuipers EJ, et al. Endoscopic regression of Barrett's oesophagus during omeprazole treatment; a randomised double blind study. Gut 1999; 45(4):489–494.
19. Sharma P, Sampliner RE, Camargo E. Normalization of esophageal pH with high-dose proton pump inhibitor does not result in regression of Barrett's esophagus. Am J Gastroenterol 1997; 92(4): 582–585.
20. Hillman LC, Chiragakis L, Shadbolt B, Kaye GL, Clarke A. Proton-pump inhibitor therapy and the development of dysplasia in patients with Barrett's oesophagus. Cancer Epidemiol Biomarkers Prev 2004; 13(1):34–39.
21. Spechler SJ, Lee E, Ahnen D, et al. Long-term outcome of medical and surgical therapies for gastroesophageal reflux disease: follow-up of a randomised controlled trial. JAMA 2001; 285(18): 2331–2338.
22. Wang D, Wang H, Shi Q, et al. Prostaglandin E(2) promotes colorectal adenoma growth via transactivation of the nuclear peroxisome proliferator-activated receptor delta. Cancer Cell 2004; 6(3):285–295.
23. Subbaramaiah K, Altori N, Chung WJ, Mestre JR, Sampat A, Dannenberg AJ. Inhibition of cyclooxygenase-2 expression by p53. J Biol Chem 1999; 274:10911–10915.
24. Morgan G. Deleterious effects of prostaglandin E2 in oesophageal carcinogenesis. Med Hypotheses 1997; 48(2):177–181.
25. Fosslien E. Molecular pathology of cyclo-oxygenase-2 in neoplasia. Ann Clin Lab Sci 2000; 30(1):3–21.
26. Wilson KT, Fu S, Ramanujam KS, Meltzer SJ. Increased expression of inducible nitric oxide and cyclooxygenase-2 in Barrett's oesophagus and associated adenocarcinoma. Cancer Res 1998; 58:2929–2934.
27. Zimmerman KC, Sarbia M, Weber AA, Borchard F, Gabbert HE, Schror K. Cyclooxygenase-2 expression in human esophageal carcinoma. Cancer Res 1999; 59:198–204.
28. Shirvani VN, Ouatu-Lascar R, Kaur BS, Omary MB, Triadafilopoulos G. Cyclooxygenase-2 expression in Barrett's oesophagus and adenocarcinoma: ex vivo induction by bile salts and acid exposure. Gastroenterology 2000; 118:487–496.
29. Morris CD, Armstrong, GR, Bigley G, Green H, Attwood SEA. Cyclooxygenase-2 expression in the Barrett's metaplasia-dysplasia-adenocarcinoma sequence. Am J Gastroenterol 2001; 96:990–996.
30. Buskens CJ, Van Rees BP, Sivula A, et al. Prognostic significance of elevated cyclooxygenase-2 expression in patients with adenocarcinoma of the oesophagus. Gastroenterology 2002; 122:1800–1807.
31. Smalley WE, DuBois RN. Colorectal cancer and non-steroidal anti-inflammatory drugs. Adv Pharmacol 1997; 39:1–20.
32. Steinbach G, Lynch PM, Phillips RK, et al. The effect of celecoxib, a cyclo-oxygenase-2 inhibitor, in familial adenomatous polyposis. N Engl J Med 342:1946–1952.
33. Buttar NS, Wang KK, Leontovich O, et al. Chemoprevention of esophageal adenocarcinoma by COX-2 inhibitors in an animal model of Barrett's esophagus. Gastroenterology 2002; 112:1101–1112.
34. Sheng H, Shao J, Morrow JD, Beauchamp RD, DuBois RN. Modulation of apoptosis and Bcl-2 expression by prostaglandin E2 in human colon cancer cells. Cancer Res 1998; 58:362–366.
35. Liu XH, Yao S, Kirschenbaum A, Levine AC. NS398, a selective cyclooxygenase-2 inhibitor induces apoptosis and down-regulates bcl-2 expression in LCNaP cells. Cancer Res 1998; 58:4245–4249.
36. Zhang Z, DuBois RN. Par-4, a proapoptotic gene, is regulated by NSAIDs in human colonic carcinoma cells. Gastroenterology 2000; 18:1012–1017.
37. Chan TA, Morin PJ, Vogelstein B, Kinzler KW. Mechanisms underlying nonsteroidal anti-inflammatory drug-mediated apoptosis. Proc Natl Acad Sci USA 1998; 95:681–686.
38. Shao J, Fujiwara T, Kadowaki Y, et al. Overexpression of the wild-type p53 gene inhibits NF-kappa B activity and synergizes with aspirin to induce apoptosis in human colon cancer cells. Oncogene 2000; 19:726–736.

39. Subbaramaiah K, Chung WJ, Dannenberg AJ. Ceramide regulates the transcription of cyclo-oxygenase-2. Evidence for involvement of extracellular signal-regulated kinase/c-June N-terminal kinase and p38 mitogen-activeated protein kinase pathways. Curr Opin Cell Biol 1998; 273:32943–32949.
40. Tsujii M, Kawano S, Tsujii S, Sawaoka H, Hori M, DuBois RN. Cyclooxygenase regulates angiogenesis induced by colon cancer cells. Cell 1998; 93:705–716.
41. Masferrer JL, Leahy KM, Koki AT, Zweifel BS, Settle SL, Woerner BM. Antiangiogenic and antitumour activities of cyclooxygenase-2 inhibitors. Cancer Res 2000; 60:1306–1311.
42. Jones MK, Wang H, Peskar BM. Inhibition of angiogenesis by nonsteroidal anti-inflammatory drugs: insight into mechanisms and implications for cancer growth and ulcer healing. Nat Med 1999; 5(12): 1348–1349.
43. Tsujii M, Kawano S, DuBois RN. Cyclo-oxgenase-2 expression in human colon cancer cells increases metastatic potential. Proc Natl Acad Sci USA 1997; 92:3336–3340.
44. Dohadwala M, Luo J, Zhu L, Lin Y, Dougherty GJ, Sharma S. Non-small cell lung cancer cyclo-oxygenase-2 dependent invasion is mediated by CD44. J Biol Chem 2001; 276:20809–20812.
45. Schiff SJ, Rigas B. Nonsteroidal anti-inflammatory drugs and colorectal cancer: evolving concepts of their chemoprotective actions. Gastroenterol 1997; 113:1992–1998.
46. Rigas B, Tsioulias GJ, Allan C, Wali RK, Brasitus TA. The effect of bile acids and piroxicam on MHC antigen expression in rat colonocytes during colon cancer development. Immunology 1994; 83:319–323.
47. Weitzman SA, Gordon LI. Inflammation and cancer: role of phagocyte-generated oxidants in carcinogenesis. Blood 1990; 76:655–663.
48. Gammon MD, Terry MB, Arber N, et al. Nonsteroidal anti-inflammatroy drug use associated with reduced incidence of adenocarcinomas of the oesophagus and gastric cardia that overexpress cyclin D1: a population-based study. Cancer Epidemiol Biomarkers Prev 2004; 13(1):34–39.
49. Van Rees BP, Ristimaki A. COX-2 in carcinogenesis of the gastrointestinal tract. Scand J Gastroenterol 2001; 36:897–903.
50. Thun MJ, Namboodiri MM, Calle EE, Flanders WD, Heath CW, Jr. Aspirin use and risk of fatal cancer. Cancer Res 1993; 53:1322–1327.
51. Funkhouser EM, Sharp GB. Aspirin and reduced risk of oesophageal adenocarcinoma. Cancer 1995; 76:1116–1119.
52. Farrow DC, Vaughan TL, Hansten PD, Stanford JL, Risch HA, Gammon MD. Use of aspirin and other nonsteroidal anti-inflammatory drugs and risk of esophageal and gastric cancer. Cancer Epidemiol Biomarkers Prev 1998; 2:97–102.
53. Langman MJS, Cheng KK, Gilman EA, Lancashire RJ. Effect of anti-inflammatory drugs on overall risk of common cancer: a case control study in general practice research database. Br Med J 2000; 320:1642–1646.
54. Coogan PF, Rosenberg L, Palmer JR, Strom BL, Zauber AG. Nonsteroidal anti-inflamatory drugs and risk of digestive cancers at sites other than the large bowel. Cancer Epidemiol Biomarkers Prev 2000; 1:119–123.
55. Corley DA, Kerlikowske K, Verma R, Buffler P. Protective association of aspirin/NSAIDs and oesophageal cancer: a systematic review and meta-analysis. Gastroenterology 2003; 124:47–56.
56. Buttar NS, Wang KW, Anderson MA, et al. The effect of selective cyclooxygenase-2 inhibition in Barrett's epithelium: an in vitro study. J Natl Cancer Inst 2002; 94:422–429.
57. Buttar NS, Wang KK, Leontovich O, et al. Chemoprevention of oesophageal adenocarcinoma by COX-2 inhibition in an animal model of Barrett's oesophagus. Gastroenterology 2002; 122:1101–1112.
58. Kaur BS, Khamnehei N, Iravani M, Namburu SS, Lin O, Triadafilopoulos G. Rofecoxib inhibits cyclooxygenase-2 expression and activity and reduces cell proliferation in Barrett's oesophagus. Gastroenterology 2002; 123:60–67.
59. Triadafilopoulos G, Kaur B, Traxler B. The effects of esomeprazole combined with aspirin or rofecoxib on steady state prostaglandin E2 production in patients with Barrett's esophagus. Gastroenterology 2004; 126(suppl 2):A-617.
60. Bosetti C, Talamini R, Franceschi S, Negri E, Garavello W, La Vecchia C. Aspirin use and cancers of the upper aerodigestive tract. Br J Cancer 2003; 88(5):672–674.
61. Hur C, Nishioka NS, Gazelle GS. Cost-effectiveness of aspirin chemoprevention for Barrett's esophagus. J Natl Cancer Inst 2004; 96(4):316–325.
62. Li M, Lotan R, Levin B, Tahara E, Lippman SM, Xu XC. Aspirin induction of apoptosis in esophageal cancer: a potential for chemoprevention. Cancer Epidemiol Biomarkers Prev 2000; 9(6):545–549.
63. Sjodahl R. Nonsteroidal anti-inflammatory drugs and the gastrointestinal tract. Extent, mode and dose dependence of anticancer effects. Am J Med 2001; 110(1A):S66–S69.
64. Zhou YN, Xu CP, Han B, et al. Expression of E-cadherin and beta-catenin in gastric carcinoma and its correlation with the clinicopathological features and patient survival. World J Gastroenterol 2002; 8(6):987–993.
65. de Castro J, Gamallo C, Palacios J, et al. beta-catenin expression pattern in primary oesophageal squamous cell carcinoma. Relationship with clinicopathological features and clinical outcome. Virchows Arch 2000; 437(6):599–604.

66. Dihlmann S, Klein S, Doeberitz MK. Reduction of beta-catenin/T-cell transcription factor signalling by aspirin and indomethacin is caused by increased stabilization of phosphorylated beta-catenin. Mol Cancer Ther 2003; 2(6):509–516.
67. Seery JP, Syrigos KN, Karayiannakis AJ, Valizadeh A, Pignatelli M. Abonrmal expression of the E-cadherin-catenin complex in dysplastic Barrett's oesophagus. Acta Oncol 1999; 38(7):945–948.
68. Chen F, Ding M, Lu Y, et al. Participation of MAP kinase p38 and IkappaB kinase in chromium (VI)-induced NF-kappaB and AP-1 activation. J Environ Pathol Toxicol Oncol 2000; 19(3):231–238.
69. Ma WY, Huang C, Dong Z. Inhibition of ultraviolet C irradiation-induced AP-1 activity by aspirin is through inhibition of JNKs but not erks or P38 MAP kinase. Int J Oncol 1998; 12(3):565–568.
70. Souza R, Shewmake K, Beer DG, Cryer B, Spechler. Selective inhibition of cyclooxygenase-2 suppresses growth and induces apoptosis in human esophageal adenocarcinoma cells. Cancer Res 2000; 60:5767–5772.
71. Sharma VK, Crowell MD, Howden CW. Infection with H. pylori or CAGA+ H. pylori is protective against Barrett's oesophagus (BE): and esophageal adenocarcinoma (EAC): A meta-analysis. Gastroenterology 2004; 126(suppl 2): A-87 [Abstract 452].
72. Lanas AI, Ortega J, Sopena F. Long-term effects of COX-2 inhibitor on oesophageal epithelial proliferation of patients with Barrett's esophagus: Preliminary results of a randomized controlled trial. Gastroenterol 2004; 126(suppl 2):A-25.
73. Brown LM, Swanson CA, Gridley G. Adenocarcinoma of the oesophagus: role of obesity and diet. J Natl Cancer Inst 1995; 87:104–109.
74. International Agency for Research on Cancer. Overweight and lack of exercise linked to increased cancer risk. IARC Handbooks of Cancer Prevention. Vol. 6. Geneva: World Health Organisation, 2002.
75. Chow WH, Blot WJ, Vaughan TL, et al. Body mass index and risk of adenocarcinomas of the esophagus and gastric cardia. J Natl Cancer Inst 1998; 90:150–155.
76. Lagergren J, Bergstrom R, Nyren O. Association between body mass and adenocarcinoma of the esophagus and gastric cardia. Ann Intern Med 1999; 130(11):883–890.
77. Cheng KK, Sharp L, McKinney PA, et al. A case-control study of oesophageal adenocarcinoma in women: a preventable disease. Br J Cancer 2000; 83(1):127–132.
78. Mayne ST, Navarro SA. Diet, obesity and reflux in the etiology of adenocarcinomas of the esophagus and gastric cardia in humans. J Nutr 2002 Nov; 132(11 suppl):S3467–S3470. Review.
79. Lagergren J, Bergstrom R, Nyren O. No relation between body mass and gastro-oesophageal reflux symptoms in a Swedish population based study. Gut 2000; 47(1):26–29.
80. Mayne ST, Risch HA, Dubrow R, et al. Nutrient intake and risk of subtypes of esophageal and gastric cancer. Cancer Epidemiol Biomarkers Prev 2001; 10(10):1055–1062.
81. International Agency for Research on Cancer. Cancer: Causes, Occurrence and Control. IARC Scientific Publications No. 100. Lyon: IARC, 1990.
82. International Agency for Research on Cancer. IARC Monographs on the Evaluation of Carcinogenic Risks to Humans, Vol. 44. Alcohol drinking. Lyon: IARC, 1998.
83. Gammon MD, Schoenberg JB, Ahsan H, et al. Tobacco, alcohol, and socioeconomic status and adenocarcinomas of the esophagus and gastric cardia. J Natl Cancer Inst 1997; 89(17):1277–1284.
84. Zeka A, Gore R, Kriebel D. Effects of alcohol and tobacco on aerodigestive cancer risks: a meta-regression analysis. Cancer Causes Control 2003; 14(9):897–906.
85. Steinmetz KA, Potter JD. Vegetables, fruit and cancer prevention: a review. J Am Diet Assoc 1996; 96(10):1027–1039.
86. Terry P, Lagergren J, Ye W, Wolk A, Nyren O. Inverse association between intake of cereal fiber and risk of gastric cardia cancer. Gastroenterology 2001; 120(2):387–391.
87. Fountoulakis A, Martin IG, White KL, et al. Plasma and esophageal mucosal levels of vitamin C: role in the pathogenesis and neoplastic progression of Barrett's esophagus. Dig Dis Sci 2004; 49(6): 914–919.
88. Blot WJ, Li JY, Taylor PR, et al. Nutrition intervention trials in Linxian, China: supplementation with specific vitamin/mineral combinations, cancer incidence, and disease-specific mortality in the general population. J Natl Cancer Inst 1993; 85(18):1483–1492.
89. Jankowski JA, Anderson M. Review article: management of oesophageal adenocarcinoma—control of acid, bile and inflammation in intervention strategies for Barrett's oesophagus. Aliment Pharmacol Ther 2004; 20(suppl 5):71–80; discussion 95–96.

3 Surgical Treatment of Esophageal Carcinoma

J. D. Hayden and G. G. Jamieson
Department of Surgery, University of Adelaide and Royal Adelaide Hospital, Adelaide, South Australia, Australia

INTRODUCTION

There has been an improvement in the outcome of surgical resection for esophageal carcinoma in recent years (1). In a review of publications of esophagectomy performed during the decade 1990–2000, the overall mortality from surgery was 6.7%, compared with 13% for the period 1980–1988 (2). Overall five-year survival for those undergoing resection currently ranges from 23% for Western series to 30.5% for Eastern patients (2). This may be in part due to better selection of cases through more accurate staging using endoscopic ultrasound (EUS), cross-sectional imaging, and more recently, positron emission tomography (PET) scanning (3).

In the West, neoadjuvant treatment prior to resection (4) is increasingly being made use of, whereas Eastern surgeons favor more radical surgery incorporating extensive lymphadenectomy, involving the abdominal, mediastinal, and cervical nodal dissection (5). Esophagectomy is being performed more safely at increasingly specialized and high-volume centres (6–8). Despite these advances, the overall prognosis for patients remains poor due to the late presentation of this disease in the majority of cases. In this situation, optimization of palliative measures may lead to improved quality of life (9).

Despite optimism for a minority of patients who benefit from a curative resection, a number of controversies exist. First, what are the most appropriate and cost-effective staging investigations? This aspect of care is critical in identifying resectable (and potentially curable) disease. Second, if early stage disease is identified, is radical surgery appropriate, and if so, by which approach? Finally, does surgery have any part to play in advanced disease or should these patients be treated nonsurgically?

PREOPERATIVE STAGING

Endoscopy and Ultrasound

The staging of esophageal carcinoma has become a multimodal process with tests that complement rather than replace one another, in order to improve accuracy. Investigations aim to determine the clinical International Union Against Cancer "tumor node metastases" (TNM) stage that would help determine the prognosis and hence the management plan for each patient. The decision whether to proceed with extensive staging investigations rests with the clinician and depends on the general health and wishes of the patient, and their performance status and fitness for intervention. Preoperative staging results are typically compared with the histopathological stage of those who have undergone a resection in order to determine their sensitivity and specificity.

Conventional endoscopy with or without a barium swallow is usually performed as an initial assessment of the primary tumor to enable a tissue diagnosis. More recently, high-resolution endoscopy has been performed for early esophageal lesions with chromoendoscopy using methylene blue dye for known cases of Barrett's esophagus and Lugol's iodine where squamous-cell carcinomas are common (10). The accuracy of high-resolution endoscopy in the diagnosis of superficial esophageal lesions is in the region of 80% (10).

EUS with fine-needle aspiration offers proven effective discrimination of tumors involving the lamina propria (T1) from those invading the muscularis propria (T2), and of carcinomas invading the adventitia (T3) from those involving adjacent structures (T4) (11). It has an overall reported sensitivity for staging of 71.4% to 100% and specificity of 66.7% to 100%, which is superior to that of conventional computerized tomography (CT) (11). However, there is a drawback in that up to 45% of tumors are nontraversable with the endoscopic probe (the majority of which are T3) (11). The use of fine EUS probes may resolve this problem in the future. From a practical point of view, the addition of EUS has been shown to increase the agreement between surgeons regarding the management of patients with esophageal carcinoma and should play a role in the initial staging of this disease (12). In patients who have undergone neoadjuvant chemoradiotherapy, EUS becomes less accurate in restaging owing to surrounding fibrosis and soft-tissue changes and the results (which have a tendency toward overstaging) should be interpreted with caution (13,14).

Cross-Sectional Imaging

The most commonly used staging investigation for esophageal carcinoma is CT. Magnetic resonance imaging has been shown to be comparable to CT in accuracy, but not as easily available (15). CT has a recognized sensitivity of 40% to 80% and specificity of 14% to 97% for the primary tumor and a sensitivity of 40% to 79% and specificity of 25% to 67% for the lymph node stage (11). The variations in these values reflect the interobserver variability in the interpretation of results (16).

Using more modern and sensitive spiral CT scanners and in a unit where there is a special interest in esophageal cancer, the sensitivity and specificity of staging may be increased to that obtained by EUS (17). If both investigations are used together, there is an increased agreement between clinical stage and pathologic stage, suggesting that CT and EUS should be considered as complementary rather than supplementary investigations (17).

There is some similarity with EUS in that the accuracy of CT in restaging disease after neoadjuvant treatment may be unpredictable. There are reports of overstaging in 36% of cases and understaging in 20% (18) and of difficulty in estimating tracheobronchial invasion (19). Following neoadjuvant treatment, if restaging is required, then a multimodality approach would seem advisable.

Laparoscopy and Thoracoscopy

Direct visualization of either the thoracic or peritoneal cavity is an attractive staging approach. In addition to its diagnostic potential, laparoscopy may provide therapeutic options, such as insertion of a feeding jejunostomy tube for patients with irresectable disease (20). However, there is controversy concerning the balance of risks and benefits of performing these investigations routinely. A staging investigation that can prevent unnecessary surgery and guide more appropriate treatment should be considered.

If laparoscopy and thoracoscopy are combined and added to conventional investigations (CT and EUS), the stage may be altered in over 30% of patients by reducing it in 19% and advancing it in 13% (21). Nguyen et al. used a package of minimally invasive staging modalities (laparoscopy, bronchoscopy, esophagoscopy, and laparoscopic ultrasound) and found that it predicted resectability in 97% of cases, compared with only 61% of those staged by conventional imaging by CT and EUS (22). The treatment plan was altered in 36% of patients by this approach (22).

Others have shown that the inclusion of laparoscopy (with ultrasound) avoided a laparotomy in only 5% of patients with gastroesophageal junction tumors (23). Using laparoscopy with at least five ports and a median operation time of 32 minutes, Menon and Dehn (24) detected incurable disease in 24% of patients deemed resectable on CT criteria. They did not include EUS in their staging investigations. The majority of these studies were performed on Western series of patients with predominantly lower third adenocarcinomas. These results cannot be extrapolated to Eastern patients with squamous-cell carcinoma and a more proximal tumor distribution.

Based on the evidence, it is difficult to justify the routine use of both thoracoscopy and laparoscopy. Performing a laparoscopy alone for carcinomas of the lower third of the esophagus or gastroesophageal junction appears justifiable as it offers additional staging information (including histology) that may alter the management of a number of patients and also enables insertion of a feeding jejunostomy for inoperable cases. The procedure should be performed in a methodical manner with several ports inserted to enable manipulation of the upper abdominal viscera, lymph node sampling where appropriate and routine opening and inspection of the lesser sac (24).

Positron Emission Tomography

There is growing evidence concerning the use of fluorodeoxyglucose PET scanning to stage esophageal cancer. The majority of reports evaluate PET when used in addition to established modalities, such as CT and EUS. A recent study that reviewed the world literature on the diagnostic accuracy of PET reported a sensitivity of 0% to 92% (median of 57%) and specificity of 75% to 100% (median of 90%) for the detection of lymph-node status. The same study identified a sensitivity of 35% to 100% (median of 69%) and specificity of 87% to 100% (median of 93%) for the detection of metastatic disease (3). The variability of results is attributed to heterogeneous groups of selected series of patients, differences in imaging protocols and in the interpretation of results, and the inclusion of patients who have received neoadjuvant treatment.

PET has been shown to detect incurable disease (i.e., upstage the tumor) in 17% of patients who have been deemed resectable using CT and EUS (25). However, when PET was compared with spiral CT, the benefit gained in the prevention of unnecessary explorations was minimal (26). When compared with other staging methods, PET was the only investigation able to independently predict a curative resection in patients who underwent an attempt at surgery (27). There is probably more evidence to recommend the inclusion of PET alongside CT and EUS for staging esophageal carcinoma. This investigation is currently expensive and not yet widely available. When combined with EUS, PET has been shown to be the most cost-effective staging option for esophageal carcinoma (28). Investigations are currently proceeding to evaluate the combination of PET and CT to stage this disease.

Analysis Summary

Based on level Ib evidence, a grade A recommendation can be made that CT and EUS are the imaging modalities of choice for the staging of esophageal carcinoma. PET scanning should be considered in addition if available. A level C recommendation can be made based on level III evidence for the use of a staging laparoscopy for gastroesophageal junction and lower-third esophageal carcinomas.

APPROACH TO SURGICAL RESECTION

Open Esophagectomy

The main modality for cure of esophageal carcinoma is surgical resection. When the tumor is confined to the epithelium, mucosa, or submucosa (Tis, T1a, and T1b, respectively), it may be categorized as early-stage disease (29). There are good prospects for long-term survival in this group of patients, and surgery plays a key role in the management (30). A variety of different operations have been performed, ranging from a limited transthoracic esophagectomy to transhiatal esophagectomy (without a thoracotomy), through to radical esophagectomy with two- or three-field lymphadenectomy and en-bloc esophagectomy. Recently, we have also seen the introduction of minimally invasive esophagectomy (31). These differences in approach and philosophy regarding radicality are in part due to the spectrum of disease encountered in Western populations (a relative paucity of early disease and predominantly lower-third adenocarcinoma) versus eastern centers with a relatively larger proportion of early stage- disease and squamous carcinoma (32).

In considering the optimal approach, the main controversy is whether a thoracotomy is necessary. Transhiatal esophagectomy can be performed safely in patients with stage I disease with a five-year survival of 59% (33). There was an in-hospital mortality rate of 4%, an anastomotic-leak rate of 13%, and incidence of other serious complications, such as recurrent laryngeal nerve injury and chylothorax of less than 1% each (33). These impressive results are from a unit with considerable experience of the transhiatal approach and may not be assumed by other centers. A radical transhiatal subtotal esophagectomy has been performed on patients with early stage disease with a 30-day mortality of 2.4% and five-year survival of 83% (34).

Ivor–Lewis esophagectomy involves a thoracotomy and abdominal incision, and can be performed with an in-hospital mortality rate of 2% to 4%, leak rate of 2% to 3.5%, and complication rate of 29% to 45% (35,36). Five-year survival rates of over 94% have been reported for stage I disease (37). Several studies have directly compared the outcome of transhiatal esophagectomy with the Ivor–Lewis esophagectomy. A prospective randomized clinical trial of 67 patients showed no significant difference in postoperative complications, including anastomotic-leak rate between the two approaches, although the operating time for the Ivor–Lewis operation was significantly longer (38). Two similar randomized clinical trials with smaller numbers of cases showed no significant difference in morbidity (including anastomotic-leak rate), mortality, or median survival between the two operations, although the operating time again was significantly longer with a thoracotomy (39,40).

A meta-analysis that compared the outcome of transhiatal and transthoracic esophagectomy in all studies published up to 2001 showed a significantly higher in-hospital mortality rate of 9.2% for transthoracic versus 5.7% for a transhiatal resection (41). In the same study, the three-year survival rate was 25% for transthoracic versus 26.7% for transhiatal resection (41). There were no significant differences in postoperative complications observed. The majority of studies have been performed on mixed series of cases that include early-stage esophageal cancer, and the evidence suggests that either operative approach is appropriate for this group of patients.

What is becoming clear from the literature is the relationship between outcome and case volume for esophageal resection. An analysis of 10 years of esophagectomy data revealed that units in which over 20 cases are performed per year, the in-hospital mortality can be kept below 5% (7). There is evidence from the United Kingdom that the centralization of cancer services leads to more accurate staging and better 30-day mortality, presumably as a result of increasing case volume (6). It is possible that the increase in the proportion of operations being performed at "high-volume" centers has contributed to the improvement in survival observed following esophagectomy over the past 10 years or more (8).

Minimally Invasive Surgery

There have been several reports of the performance of all or part of an esophagectomy through smaller incisions using thoracoscopic and laparoscopic techniques (31). Initially, a thoracoscopic esophageal mobilization was accompanied by a laparotomy to fashion the gastric conduit (42). This was followed by a laparoscopic version of the transhiatal esophagectomy, where thoracotomy and single-lung ventilation was avoided (43). The total minimally invasive esophagectomy eventually followed with an anastomosis performed in the neck (44–47). More recently, a minimally invasive Ivor-Lewis resection technique has been described (48). Although the literature has confirmed that these approaches are feasible, they are technically demanding and time-consuming operations, and can be associated with substantial intraoperative blood loss (31). Even so, they could be appropriate for early-stage disease where performing a radical lymphadenectomy may not be essential.

Outcomes of minimally invasive esophagectomy from experienced units have been impressive with respect to mortality. The largest published series of 222 cases reported a mortality of 1.4%, leak rate of 11.7%, and conversion rate of 7.2%, and similar stage-specific survival to open procedures (46). Of more concern is that leak rates of over 28% have been reported for the total endoscopic technique, making this approach difficult to recommend after initial reports (45). Recently, Panalivelu et al. reported their excellent results of minimally invasive esophagectomy and lymphadenectomy for squamous carcinoma, with the thoracoscopic component performed with the patient in the prone position (47). Their operative mortality in 130 cases was 1.5% and anastomotic-leak rate was 2.3% with stage-specific survival similar to published series of open cases (47). Experience with a minimally invasive Ivor-Lewis resection is limited to a series of 50 cases from James Luketich with an operative mortality of 6% and anastomotic-leak rate of 6% (48). Further studies, preferably within the context of controlled trials, are required in order to evaluate this technique before it can be accepted as a standard practice.

The Role of Lymphadenectomy

There are contrasting views on the role of radical lymphadenectomy in the management of esophageal carcinoma. Japanese surgeons advocate extended lymphadenectomy involving cervical, mediastinal, and abdominal lymph node groups: three-field lymphadenectomy (5) or an en-bloc resection involving a margin of neighboring structures (5,49). Their experience with predominantly squamous-cell carcinoma and its pattern of lymph-node metastasis has probably influenced their strategy. Japanese patients generally also have less comorbidity, are physically leaner, and have more early-stage disease. These factors have undoubtedly led to a more aggressive approach. The potential advantages include improved locoregional control of the disease and improved prognostic information provided by analysing a larger number of lymph nodes (49). The potential disadvantages relate to the morbidity associated with extensive lymph-node dissection leading to tissue ischaemia, anastomotic and lymphatic leaks, and damage to other important structures.

A recent review of 522 cases of radical three-field esophagectomy, consisting of predominantly Eastern series of squamous carcinomas, reported cervical-node metastases in 16.7% to 35.0% of patients with positive nodes in the recurrent laryngeal nerve region in 35.0% to 48.6% of cases (49). They report an operative mortality of 4% and major morbidity rate of 37.7% to 46.7% that included anastomotic leaks in 96 cases (18.4%), recurrent laryngeal nerve palsies in 139 patients (26.6%), and tracheal injury (owing to ischemia following nodal dissection) occurring in 26 (4.9%). Five-year survival of 30% to 50% is reported, and may rise to 94% for stage I disease (49).

An alternative to three-field lymphadenectomy is a two-field approach with resection of just the mediastinal and abdominal nodal groups and avoiding a neck incision. There have been two studies attempting to compare the three-field with the two-field approach in a randomized fashion. Kato et al. (50) used strict selection criteria, and randomly allocated 150 patients in total. They found a significantly larger lymph-node yield and operating time for the three-field approach (50). However, the more extensive resection had a lower in-hospital mortality of 2.6% for three-field dissection compared with 12.3% for the two-field operation and a five-year survival rate of 49% for the more radical procedure versus 34% for the two-field operation (50).

A smaller trial by Nishihira et al. randomly allocated patients to a three-field or a two-field lymphadenectomy with their esophagectomy, and again identified an unsurprisingly significant difference in lymph-node yield and operating time between the two groups (51). They found a significantly higher incidence of nerve injury (recurrent laryngeal and phrenic) and requirement for a tracheostomy in the three-field approach (51). However, the anastomotic-leak rate for the two-field group was 20% and in-hospital mortality rate was 7% (51). These values were significantly higher than those in the three-field group (6% and 3%, respectively). A possible explanation for this is that a leak from an anastomosis performed in the chest is more dangerous than one completed in the neck. There was a nonsignificant trend toward improved five-year survival for the more radical operation.

These two randomized studies do not enable conclusions to be drawn regarding the justification for a radical (three-field) approach to esophageal resection. This type of surgery has a high morbidity, even in the hands of those units with the most experience. It is impossible to extrapolate the results of a small number of studies of selected groups of patients from specialized centers of excellence to the wider surgical community. Outside the context of a unit with experience in this procedure, radical three-field resection for esophageal cancer cannot be recommended.

Neoadjuvant Strategies

There are several potential oncologic advantages in giving chemoradiotherapy preoperatively in esophageal cancer. First, systemic treatment is delivered with an intact tumor blood supply; second, tumors may be down-staged converting irresectable to resectable disease; and finally, the giving of two concurrent treatments may have a synergistic effect on locoregional control (52).

In recent years, there have been two meta-analyses of randomized controlled trials (RCTs) that compared neoadjuvant chemoradiotherapy followed by surgery with surgical resection alone for esophageal carcinoma (both squamous and adenocarcinoma). Urschel and Vasan identified nine RCTs covering some 1116 patients, and Fiorica et al., analysed six trials containing 764 cases in total (4,52). Chemoradiotherapy regimens typically consisted of two to three weeks of radiotherapy together with cisplatin alone or cisplatin and fluorouracil (52,53). These meta-analyses identified a small but statistically significant advantage of neoadjuvant treatment followed by surgery over surgery alone for rate of complete resection, three-year survival, and locoregional recurrence rate (4,54). The survival benefit was evident when chemotherapy and radiotherapy were given concurrently. The survival advantage was lost if trials containing chemotherapy and radiotherapy given sequentially were considered separately (54). These trials contained predominantly squamous-cell carcinomas. A single RCT of patients with esophageal adenocarcinoma showed a significant difference in three-year survival of 32% for the neoadjuvant group versus 6% for surgery alone (53).

Since these meta-analyses have been published, a moderately large multicenter RCT from Australasia, containing 256 patients, showed no significant survival advantage for neoadjuvant treatment (cisplatin and fluorouracil-based chemotherapy with 35 Gy of concurrent radiotherapy given in 15 fractions) followed by surgery compared with surgery alone for esophageal adenocarcinoma (55). For squamous carcinoma, there was a significant difference in relapse-free survival for the neoadjuvant group compared with surgery alone, but only a nonsignificant trend toward improved overall survival for those patients (55).

Despite the optimism of the results of neoadjuvant treatment, there are several disadvantages. These include a lower rate of resection and a higher postoperative mortality rate (4,54). This treatment may make the operation technically more difficult and lead to more anastomotic leaks and cardiopulmonary complications due to the effects of treatment on local tissues (4,54). Until larger RCTs are performed, it is impossible to recommend the routine use of neoadjuvant chemoradiotherapy prior to resection for adenocarcinoma of the esophagus. Its use in squamous cell carcinoma has a stronger scientific basis.

With respect to the use of neoadjuvant chemotherapy prior to surgery versus surgery alone, a meta-analysis of 1976 patients from 11 RCTs has been performed (56). This showed a significant difference in resection rate favoring the surgery-alone group and a significantly higher rate of R0 resection in the neoadjuvant chemotherapy group. There were no significant differences in operative mortality, leak rate, or three-year survival between the groups (56).

Since this report, an important RCT from the United Kingdom of 390 patients who received an infusion of cisplatin and fluorouracil chemotherapy prior to esophagectomy versus 397 patients who received surgery alone has been performed (57). The patient group was typical of a Western case mix, with two-thirds made up of adenocarcinoma, and a third being squamous. Overall survival, two-year survival, and disease-free survival were significantly better for the neoadjuvant chemotherapy group over the surgery-alone group (57). A very recently published RCT, again from the United Kingdom, compared perioperative chemotherapy using epirubicin, cisplatin, and fluorouracil in 250 patients with surgery alone in 253 patients (58). The case mix included resectable gastric adenocarcinoma as well as lower-third esophageal and junctional carcinomas. Postoperative complication and mortality rates were similar between the groups. The chemotherapy group had a higher chance of overall survival with a five-year survival of 36% versus 23% for surgery-alone group (58). These two RCTs support a role for neoadjuvant chemotherapy for esophageal carcinoma, especially in populations where adenocarcinomas predominate.

Analysis Summary

With respect to the surgical approach to esophagectomy, a grade B recommendation can be made based on level II evidence that both transhiatal and Ivor-Lewis esophagectomy are appropriate procedures for esophageal resection in the absence of proven metastatic disease. These operations should preferably be performed in units performing more than 20 cases per year (grade A recommendation, based on category Ib evidence).

Radical three-field lymphadenectomy may improve survival over two-field lymphadenectomy in experienced Eastern centers that deal with predominantly squamous carcinoma (grade B recommendation based on level IIb evidence), but is associated with increased morbidity. Alternatively, the use of preoperative chemoradiotherapy should be considered prior to surgery for patients with squamous carcinoma (grade A recommendation based on level Ia evidence). The routine use of neoadjuvant chemoradiation prior to surgery for esophageal adenocarcinoma cannot be recommended (based on level IIb evidence). Based on level Ia evidence, a grade A recommendation can be made for the use of neoadjuvant chemotherapy prior to resection for esophageal carcinoma.

There is currently insufficient evidence to support the routine practice of minimally invasive esophagectomy (grade C recommendation based on level III evidence). However, this approach may be safely performed in high-volume centers experienced in advanced laparoscopic esophageal surgery (grade C recommendation based on level III evidence).

PALLIATION

Esophageal Stents

The presence of disseminated disease or the poor physical condition of a patient may prevent surgical resection for esophageal cancer. In this situation, the prognosis is very poor, and palliative measures are appropriate. The aims of palliation are to improve symptoms, such as dysphagia, and possibly to prevent fistula formation. Treatment options include placement of an esophageal stent (metal mesh, plastic, covered or uncovered) and radiotherapy, delivered either by external beam or the intraluminal route (brachytherapy) and laser ablation. Unlike surgery for esophageal cancer, the issue of palliation has been subjected to a considerable number of randomized trials. These studies are usually controlled relative to a reference intervention, as it is considered unethical to offer these patients no treatment.

The earliest stents were plastic tubes, and these have been compared with self-expanding metal stents (Wallstent) in a randomized, controlled manner (59). Both types of stent provided immediate and effective palliation for dysphagia and sealed esophageal fistulae, but Wallstents were associated with fewer serious complications and better patency rate of 90% and 88% at one and three months, respectively. Corresponding patency rates were 66% and 50% for the plastic stent (59). In another randomized trial of covered versus uncovered expandable stents, the covered variety were associated with significantly less problems with tumor ingrowth (requiring further intervention) compared with uncovered ones (60).

Expandable metal esophageal stents are relatively expensive and unsurprisingly, several different products have emerged. When Ultraflex™, Flamingo Wallstent®, and Gianturco-Z stent (all covered) are compared, there are no significant differences in the degree of palliation of dysphagia or complications between the groups (61,62). The use of expandable covered stents is emerging as the "gold standard" for the palliation of esophageal cancer.

Brachytherapy

Other therapies, such as laser or thermal ablation, have had limited success (63,64). A single dose of intraluminal brachytherapy has been compared with the placement of an expandable metal stent. Brachytherapy provided better long-term palliation for dysphagia and quality of life scores, but the stent provided more rapid relief of symptoms after deployment (9). Almost a half of the patients in the brachytherapy group also had a stent inserted, and this may explain some of the differences in outcome.

What is clear from the evidence is that covered metal stents provide effective palliation for dysphagia and treatment of esophageal fistulae. Brachytherapy may provide symptom relief for longer for patients who are fit. A combination of both treatments may prove most effective in this unfortunate group of patients whose median survival is less than six months with treatment (9).

Analysis Summary

There is good evidence (level Ia) supporting the routine use of expandable covered stents for the palliation of dysphagia and treatment of esophageal fistulae in patients who are unfit for surgery or have irresectable esophageal cancer (grade A recommendation). The use of intraluminal brachytherapy may be a suitable alternative treatment modality for patients without a fistula (grade A recommendation based on level Ia evidence).

CONCLUSIONS

The mortality of resection for esophageal carcinoma has been improved in recent decades. This has probably resulted from improved case selection by staging and the use of neoadjuvant treatment prior to resection by Western surgeons and radical lymphadenectomy performed by Eastern surgeons.

The most appropriate staging investigations will identify locally advanced or metastatic disease prior to a major resection so that management can be tailored to the patient. There is substantial evidence that a combination of CT, EUS, and PET scan is an ideal package for preoperative imaging, accompanied by a staging laparoscopy for lower-third or gastroesophageal junction tumours. A staging thoracoscopy should be considered in selected cases.

The ideal approach to esophagectomy is the one that gives the highest chance of a complete (R0) resection and the lowest morbidity and mortality in the hands of the particular surgeon. There is no clear evidence favoring one particular open approach compared with another. Minimally invasive esophagectomy is increasingly being performed, but this should be done in institutions with high-volume experience in laparoscopic esophageal surgery. The debate concerning the use of neoadjuvant treatment and surgery versus more radical surgery will require further RCTs in order to determine whether one or the other offers a clear benefit. Either approach is acceptable in the institutions and population groups where they have been assessed.

With respect to palliation for irresectable or metastatic disease, surgery is not appropriate because the life expectancy of these patients is so short. The use of a covered expandable metal stent provides rapid relief of dysphagia and treatment of an esophageal fistula. The use of intraluminal brachytherapy may provide more prolonged relief of symptoms in appropriate cases.

REFERENCES

1. Stein HJ, Siewert JR. Improved prognosis of resected esophageal cancer. World J Surg 2004; 28(6):520–525.
2. Jamieson GG, Mathew G, Ludemann R, Wayman J, Myers JC, Devitt PG. Postoperative mortality following oesophagectomy and problems in reporting its rate. Br J Surg 2004; 91(8):943–947.
3. Kato H, Miyazaki T, Nakajima M, et al. The incremental effect of positron emission tomography on diagnostic accuracy in the initial staging of esophageal carcinoma. Cancer 2005; 103(1):148–156.
4. Fiorica F, Di Bona D, Schepis F, et al. Preoperative chemoradiotherapy for oesophageal cancer: a systematic review and meta-analysis. Gut 2004; 53(7):925–930.
5. Tachibana M, Kinugasa S, Yoshimura H, et al. En-bloc esophagectomy for esophageal cancer. Am J Surg 2004; 188(3):254–260.
6. Branagan G, Davies N. Early impact of centralization of oesophageal cancer surgery services. Br J Surg 2004; 91(12):1630–1632.
7. Metzger R, Bollschweiler E, Vallbohmer D, Maish M, DeMeester TR, Holscher AH. High volume centers for esophagectomy: what is the number needed to achieve low postoperative mortality? Dis Esophagus 2004; 17(4):310–314.
8. Dimick JB, Wainess RM, Upchurch GR, Jr., Iannettoni MD, Orringer MB. National trends in outcomes for esophageal resection. Ann Thorac Surg 2005; 79(1):212–216; discussion 217–218.
9. Homs MY, Steyerberg EW, Eijkenboom WM, et al. Single-dose brachytherapy versus metal stent placement for the palliation of dysphagia from oesophageal cancer: multicentre randomised trial. Lancet 2004; 364(9444):1497–1504.
10. May A, Gunter E, Roth F, et al. Accuracy of staging in early oesophageal cancer using high resolution endoscopy and high resolution endosonography: a comparative, prospective, and blinded trial. Gut 2004; 53(5):634–640.
11. Kelly S, Harris KM, Berry E, et al. A systematic review of the staging performance of endoscopic ultrasound in gastro-oesophageal carcinoma. Gut 2001; 49(4):534–539.
12. Preston SR, Clark GW, Martin IG, Ling HM, Harris KM. Effect of endoscopic ultrasonography on the management of 100 consecutive patients with oesophageal and junctional carcinoma. Br J Surg 2003; 90(10):1220–1224.
13. Laterza E, de Manzoni G, Guglielmi A, Rodella L, Tedesco P, Cordiano C. Endoscopic ultrasonography in the staging of esophageal carcinoma after preoperative radiotherapy and chemotherapy. Ann Thorac Surg 1999; 67(5):1466–1469.
14. Kalha I, Kaw M, Fukami N, et al. The accuracy of endoscopic ultrasound for restaging esophageal carcinoma after chemoradiation therapy. Cancer 2004; 101(5):940–947.
15. Takashima S, Takeuchi N, Shiozaki H, et al. Carcinoma of the esophagus: CT vs MR imaging in determining resectability. AJR Am J Roentgenol 1991; 156(2):297–302.
16. Goei R, Lamers RJ, Engelshove HA, Oei KT. Computed tomographic staging of esophageal carcinoma: a study on interobserver variation and correlation with pathological findings. Eur J Radiol 1992; 15(1):40–44.
17. Weaver SR, Blackshaw GR, Lewis WG, et al. Comparison of special interest computed tomography, endosonography and histopathological stage of oesophageal cancer. Clin Radiol 2004; 59(6):499–504.

18. Jones DR, Parker LA, Jr., Detterbeck FC, Egan TM. Inadequacy of computed tomography in assessing patients with esophageal carcinoma after induction chemoradiotherapy. Cancer 1999; 85(5):1026–1032.
19. Griffith JF, Chan AC, Chow LT, et al. Assessing chemotherapy response of squamous cell oesophageal carcinoma with spiral CT. Br J Radiol 1999; 72(859):678–684.
20. Heath EI, Kaufman HS, Talamini MA, et al. The role of laparoscopy in preoperative staging of esophageal cancer. Surg Endosc 2000; 14(5):495–499.
21. Luketich JD, Meehan M, Nguyen NT, et al. Minimally invasive surgical staging for esophageal cancer. Surg Endosc 2000; 14(8):700–702.
22. Nguyen NT, Roberts PF, Follette DM, et al. Evaluation of minimally invasive surgical staging for esophageal cancer. Am J Surg 2001; 182(6):702–706.
23. Van Dijkum EJ, de Wit LT, van Delden OM, et al. Staging laparoscopy and laparoscopic ultrasonography in more than 400 patients with upper gastrointestinal carcinoma. J Am Coll Surg 1999; 189(5):459–465.
24. Menon KV, Dehn TC. Multiport staging laparoscopy in esophageal and cardiac carcinoma. Dis Esophagus 2003; 16(4):295–300.
25. Imdahl A, Hentschel M, Kleimaier M, Hopt UT, Brink I. Impact of FDG-PET for staging of oesophageal cancer. Langenbecks Arch Surg 2004; 389(4):283–288.
26. Kneist W, Schreckenberger M, Bartenstein P, Menzel C, Oberholzer K, Junginger T. Prospective evaluation of positron emission tomography in the preoperative staging of esophageal carcinoma. Arch Surg 2004; 139(10):1043–1049.
27. Van Westreenen HL, Heeren PA, van Dullemen HM, et al. Positron emission tomography with F-18-fluorodeoxyglucose in a combined staging strategy of esophageal cancer prevents unnecessary surgical explorations. J Gastrointest Surg 2005; 9(1):54–61.
28. Wallace MB, Nietert PJ, Earle C, et al. An analysis of multiple staging management strategies for carcinoma of the esophagus: computed tomography, endoscopic ultrasound, positron emission tomography, and thoracoscopy/laparoscopy. Ann Thorac Surg 2002; 74(4):1026–1032.
29. Holscher A, Siewert J. Surgical treatment of early esophageal cancer. Dig Surg 1997; 14(2):70–76.
30. Endo M, Yoshino K, Takeshita K, Kawano T. Analysis of 1.125 cases of early esophageal carcinoma in Japan. Dis Esophagus 1991; 4(2):71–76.
31. Nguyen NT, Gelfand D, Stevens CM, et al. Current status of minimally invasive esophagectomy. Minerva Chir 2004; 59(5):437–446.
32. Law S, Wong J. Changing disease burden and management issues for esophageal cancer in the Asia-Pacific region. J Gastroenterol Hepatol 2002; 17(4):374–381.
33. Orringer MB, Marshall B, Iannettoni MD. Transhiatal esophagectomy: clinical experience and refinements. Ann Surg 1999; 230(3):392–400; discussion 400–393.
34. Holscher AH, Bollschweiler E, Schneider PM, Siewert JR. Early adenocarcinoma in Barrett's oesophagus. Br J Surg 1997; 84(10):1470–1473.
35. Griffin SM, Shaw IH, Dresner SM. Early complications after Ivor Lewis subtotal esophagectomy with two-field lymphadenectomy: risk factors and management. J Am Coll Surg 2002; 194(3):285–297.
36. Karl RC, Schreiber R, Boulware D, Baker S, Coppola D. Factors affecting morbidity, mortality, and survival in patients undergoing Ivor Lewis esophagogastrectomy. Ann Surg 2000; 231(5):635–643.
37. Visbal AL, Allen MS, Miller DL, Deschamps C, Trastek VF, Pairolero PC. Ivor Lewis esophagogastrectomy for esophageal cancer. Ann Thorac Surg 2001; 71(6):1803–1808.
38. Goldminc M, Maddern G, Le Prise E, Meunier B, Campion JP, Launois B. Oesophagectomy by a transhiatal approach or thoracotomy: a prospective randomized trial. Br J Surg 1993; 80(3):367–370.
39. Jacobi CA, Zieren HU, Muller JM, Pichlmaier H. Surgical therapy of esophageal carcinoma: the influence of surgical approach and esophageal resection on cardiopulmonary function. Eur J Cardiothorac Surg 1997; 11(1):32–37.
40. Chu KM, Law SY, Fok M, Wong J. A prospective randomized comparison of transhiatal and transthoracic resection for lower-third esophageal carcinoma. Am J Surg 1997; 174(3):320–324.
41. Hulscher JB, Tijssen JG, Obertop H, van Lanschot JJ. Transthoracic versus transhiatal resection for carcinoma of the esophagus: a meta-analysis. Ann Thorac Surg 2001; 72(1):306–313.
42. McAnena OJ, Rogers J, Williams NS. Right thoracoscopically assisted oesophagectomy for cancer. Br J Surg 1994; 81(2):236–238.
43. DePaula AL, Hashiba K, Ferreira EA, de Paula RA, Grecco E. Laparoscopic transhiatal esophagectomy with esophagogastroplasty. Surg Laparosc Endosc 1995; 5(1):1–5.
44. Watson DI, Davies N, Jamieson GG. Totally endoscopic Ivor Lewis esophagectomy. Surg Endosc 1999; 13(3):293–297.
45. Watson DI, Jamieson GG, Devitt PG. Endoscopic cervico-thoraco-abdominal esophagectomy. J Am Coll Surg 2000; 190(3):372–378.
46. Luketich JD, Alvelo-Rivera M, Buenaventura PO, et al. Minimally invasive esophagectomy: outcomes in 222 patients. Ann Surg 2003; 238(4):486–494; discussion 485–494.
47. Palanivelu C, Prakash A, Senthilkumar R, et al. Minimally invasive esophagectomy: thoracoscopic mobilization of the esophagus and mediastinal lymphadenectomy in prone position—experience of 130 patients. J Am Coll Surg 2006; 203(1):7–16.

48. Bizekis C, Kent MS, Luketich JD, et al. Initial experience with minimally invasive Ivor Lewis esophagectomy. Ann Thorac Surg 2006; 82(2):402–406; discussion 406–407.
49. Tachibana M, Kinugasa S, Yoshimura H, Dhar DK, Nagasue N. Extended esophagectomy with 3-field lymph node dissection for esophageal cancer. Arch Surg 2003; 138(12):1383—1389; discussion 1390.
50. Kato H, Watanabe H, Tachimori Y, Iizuka T. Evaluation of neck lymph node dissection for thoracic esophageal carcinoma. Ann Thorac Surg 1991; 51(6):931–935.
51. Nishihira T, Hirayama K, Mori S. A prospective randomized trial of extended cervical and superior mediastinal lymphadenectomy for carcinoma of the thoracic esophagus. Am J Surg 1998; 175(1):47–51.
52. Bosset JF, Gignoux M, Triboulet JP, et al. Chemoradiotherapy followed by surgery compared with surgery alone in squamous-cell cancer of the esophagus. N Engl J Med 1997; 337(3):161–167.
53. Walsh TN, Noonan N, Hollywood D, Kelly A, Keeling N, Hennessy TP. A comparison of multimodal therapy and surgery for esophageal adenocarcinoma. N Engl J Med 1996; 335(7):462–467.
54. Urschel JD, Vasan H. A meta-analysis of randomized controlled trials that compared neoadjuvant chemoradiation and surgery to surgery alone for resectable esophageal cancer. Am J Surg 2003; 185(6):538–543.
55. Burmeister BH, Smithers BM, Gebski V, et al. Surgery alone versus chemoradiotherapy followed by surgery for resectable cancer of the oesophagus: a randomised controlled phase III trial. Lancet Oncol 2005; 6(9):659–668.
56. Urschel JD, Vasan H, Blewett CJ. A meta-analysis of randomized controlled trials that compared neoadjuvant chemotherapy and surgery to surgery alone for resectable esophageal cancer. Am J Surg 2002; 183(3):274–279.
57. Surgical resection with or without preoperative chemotherapy in oesophageal cancer: a randomised controlled trial. Lancet 2002; 359(9319):1727–1733.
58. Cunningham D, Allum WH, Stenning SP, et al. Perioperative chemotherapy versus surgery alone for resectable gastroesophageal cancer. N Engl J Med 2006; 355(1):11–20.
59. Sanyika C, Corr P, Haffejee A. Palliative treatment of oesophageal carcinoma–efficacy of plastic versus self-expandable stents. S Afr Med J 1999; 89(6):640–643.
60. Vakil N, Morris AI, Marcon N, et al. A prospective, randomized, controlled trial of covered expandable metal stents in the palliation of malignant esophageal obstruction at the gastroesophageal junction. Am J Gastroenterol 2001; 96(6):1791–1796.
61. Siersema PD, Hop WC, van Blankenstein M, et al. A comparison of 3 types of covered metal stents for the palliation of patients with dysphagia caused by esophagogastric carcinoma: a prospective, randomized study. Gastrointest Endosc 2001; 54(2):145–153.
62. Sabharwal T, Hamady MS, Chui S, Atkinson S, Mason R, Adam A. A randomised prospective comparison of the Flamingo Wallstent and Ultraflex stent for palliation of dysphagia associated with lower third oesophageal carcinoma. Gut 2003; 52(7):922–926.
63. Dallal HJ, Smith GD, Grieve DC, Ghosh S, Penman ID, Palmer KR. A randomized trial of thermal ablative therapy versus expandable metal stents in the palliative treatment of patients with esophageal carcinoma. Gastrointest Endosc 2001; 54(5):549–557.
64. Spencer GM, Thorpe SM, Blackman GM, et al. Laser augmented by brachytherapy versus laser alone in the palliation of adenocarcinoma of the oesophagus and cardia: a randomised study. Gut 2002; 50(2):224–227.

4 Surgical Treatment of Carcinomas Involving the Esophagogastric Junction

B. H. A. von Rahden, J. R. Siewert, and H. J. Stein
Departments of Surgery, Paracelsus Private Medical University, Salzburg, Austria and Klinikum rechts der Isar, Technical University, Munich, Germany

INTRODUCTION

What are the Indications for Surgical Resection?

Surgical resection is considered the treatment of choice for esophagogastric junction tumors, provided that (*i*) local resectability can be anticipated with high likelihood, (*ii*) there is no evidence of systemic disease, and (*iii*) the patient is fit and willing to undergo a major surgical procedure. In case of local irresectability and manifestations of distant metastases (pM1-disease) according to the tumor node metastases (TNM) staging system by the Union Internationale Contre le Cancer/International Union Against Cancer (UICC) (1), surgical interventions with curative intention are not indicated. Surgery under these circumstances is merely palliative, does not improve the prognosis, and should be reserved for tumor complications, which cannot be managed conservatively (2,3).

An exception to this generally accepted basic oncologic principle is the increasing use of neoadjuvant treatment strategies, which provide—in case of response—the chance of downsizing the tumor or—occasionally—downstaging the disease [evidence level 4, (4,5)]. A previously irresectable tumor may become amenable to surgical resection in this manner, and the patient's prognosis may be significantly improved. Responders to neoadjuvant treatment are the beneficiaries of this strategy—nonresponders derive none (4,5).

All curative approaches to esophagogastric junction carcinomas—either with multimodal/neoadjuvant strategies, or with surgery alone—require a classification of these tumurs. There is plenty of evidence to suggest that the tumors arising within the vicinity of the esophagogastric junction comprise different entities with respect to their tumor biology, pathogenesis, and pattern of lymphatic spread, and consequently require adjustment of therapeutic approaches. An unequivocal classification is therefore mandatory as a basis for distinguishing these tumors, for standardizing decisions on the appropriate therapeutic approach, and for making results from different institutions comparable.

How to Classify Esophagogastric Junction Tumors?

A classification of adenocarcinomas of the esophagogastric junction (AEG) from a surgical viewpoint was introduced approximately 19 years ago (6,7), to aid in tailoring the surgical approach. Since that time, the classification has proved very useful in clinical practice (8), has been recommended by the consensus conference of the International Society for Diseases of the Esophagus (ISDE) (9) and is increasingly used in centers all over the world (10–16) (evidence level 3).

Tumors are distinguished according to the center of the tumor mass in relation to the anatomic cardia: Adenocarcinomas of the distal esophagus (AEG type I) are distinguished from adenocarcinomas arising at the level of the cardia (AEG type II) and subcardiac gastric cancers (AEG type III). The cardia is best defined (from the viewpoint of the endoscopist) as the proximal end of the gastric folds. This definition is superior to defining the cardia according to the squamo-columnar junction (the so-called Z-line), which is inconsistent, being shifted proximally under the pathological condition of Barrett's esophagus (17).

The AEG classification has been proven appropriate for distinguishing esophagogastric junction tumours and for tailoring the surgical approach (8,10–16). Furthermore, new insights into the pathophysiology have suggested that the different AEG tumor types comprise entirely different entities (18,19): The most relevant aspect from the clinical viewpoint is the strong association of AEG I tumors with Barrett's esophagus: The vast majority of these tumors is associated with this precancerous condition. Neoadjuvant chemotherapy frequently "unmasks" Barrett's epithelium, previously 'overgrown' by a locally advanced tumor (20). The presence of Barrett's epithelium may serve as an additional criterion to classify a tumor as AEG type I carcinoma (18,19) and to plan the therapeutic/surgical approach in accordance.

How to Choose the Appropriate Operation?

The appropriate approach to esophagogastric junction tumors (and particularly to cardia carcinomas, AEG type II) is a matter of debate. The controversy concerns

- which operation should be performed, that is, whether an esophagectomy, an extended gastrectomy, or an esophago-gastrectomy is required;
- which length of esophagus should be resected;
- which extent of lymph-node dissection should be performed; and
- which surgical exposure is appropriate?

Most of these questions have not been addressed in randomized trials. Thus, high-quality data in the terms of "evidence-based medicine" are usually lacking. However, there is plenty of indirect evidence—mostly from analysis of surgical series—to support current surgical strategies.

Pattern of Lymphatic Spread: Major Determinant of the Surgical Approach

One major determinant of the surgical approach to esophagogastric junction carcinomas is their pattern of lymphatic spread, because complete nodal clearance (removal of tumor-infiltrated nodes) is regarded as one of the key factors for long-term survival. Infiltration of locoregional lymph nodes [pN1-disease according to the TNM staging system by the UICC; (1)] is a strong negative prognostic factor (21,22).

The recommended extent of lymphadenectomy is determined by the distribution of lymph-node metastases. Study of lymph nodes from the major lymph-node "stations" after surgical resection has clearly revealed, that the primary route of lymphatic spread in AEG type I tumors leads to the mediastinal lymph nodes. Occasionally, lymph nodes of the abdominal compartment are affected. Lymphatic spread from AEG type II and type III tumors, by contrast, predominantly affects the abdominal compartment (8,23–29), and lymph nodes in the lower mediastinum. This concept is also supported by recent data on lymphatic spread determined with the sentinel lymph node method (29,30): The lymphatic drainage leads primarily to one or two locoregional lymph nodes, localized in the immediate neighborhood of the tumor. Occurrence of skip metastases (infiltration of more distant lymph nodes, without infiltration of the sentinel node) has been shown to occur only rarely.

This knowledge of the primary routes of lymphatic spread provides the basis for the current concept of lymphadenectomy and the primary surgical procedure in esophagogastric junction carcinomas.

AEG I tumors (adenocarcinomas of the distal esophagus, mostly Barrett's cancers) are almost universally approached by esophagectomy (8,15,31). However, different approaches to

TABLE 1 Tumor-Infiltrated Lymph Node Stations in AEG II Tumors, in Decreasing Order

The paracardial lymph nodes
The lymph nodes at the lesser and greater curvature
Lymph nodes along the left gastric artery toward the celiac trunk
Lymph nodes along the splenic artery, at the superior margin of the pancreas toward the splenic hilum
Lymph nodes in the lower posterior mediastinum
Lymph nodes close to the left adrenal gland and the left renal vein

Abbreviation: AEGII, adenocarcinomas of the esophagogastric junction arising at the level of the cardia.
Source: From Refs. 23,26–28.

this procedure (transhiatal, abdominothoracic/Ivor-Lewis, thoracoabdominal) are chosen (see subsequently). AEG III tumors (subcardiac gastric cancers) are approached by extended gastrectomy (8,15).

The above considerations lead us to believe that an extended gastrectomy should also be the preferred operation for AEG II tumors (cardia carcinomas). The lower mediastinal lymph nodes, which may be tumor-infiltrated in this entity, can be reached by means of transhiatal dissection. Lymphatic spread towards the upper mediastinum represents advanced disease and can not be cured by surgical resection alone, even when lymphadenectomy is extended toward the upper mediastinum and the neck (31,32). In contrast to these concepts, a large series summarizing the experience from centers from France ($n = 1192$ patients resection for AEG tumors by members of the French Association of Surgery between 1985 and 2000), reports the preferred use of esophagectomy plus proximal gastrectomy in the majority (58%) of AEG type II tumors (15). In our own experience, short-term postoperative results, that is, morbidity and mortality, are better with an extended gastrectomy as compared to esophagectomy (e.g., 5.6% vs. 1.9% mortality in a consecutive patient series), while the more radical procedure provided no long-term survival benefit (8). No high-quality literature evidence currently exists about this question.

Extensive (Three-field) Lymphadenectomy?

A more extended approach to cardia carcinomas is performed and recommended by the group of Lerut in Leuven, Belgium, who perform a three-field lymphadenectomy for esophageal adenocarcinomas (AEG I), esophageal squamous-cell cancers, and cardia carcinomas (AEG II). A large consecutive series, including 192 patients (174 R0 resections), has recently been reported from that institution [evidence level 3, (31)]. Extensive, three-field lymphadenectomy (dissection of thoracic, abdominal, and cervical lymph nodes, in addition) revealed a high percentage of tumor-infiltrated lymph nodes at the neck (25.8% in adenocarcinomas of the distal esophagus and 17.6% in cardia carcinomas). However, the survival figures suggest that these were not curative resections: None of the patients with cardia carcinomas (AEG II) and tumor-infiltrated cervical nodes survived for five years. Furthermore, five year-survival of patients with esophageal adenocarcinomas (AEG I) and involvement of cervical nodes was only 11.9%. Presumably, these patients would have better been chosen as candidates for multimodal treatment, with initial neoadjuvant chemotherapy followed by surgical resection in case of response. Involvement of cervical lymph nodes in these tumors is a big step toward systemic generalization of the disease. This is the reason why it seems justified to address these positive lymph nodes as pM1b disease, as suggested by the TNM staging system by the UICC (1).

In conclusion, the beneficial role of radical lymphadenectomy appears to apply to a defined "therapeutic window," in which only local and locoregional nodes are affected. More distant nodal involvement represents generalized disease for which multimodal treatment is an option.

Transhiatal, Transthoracic, or Thoracoabdominal Resection—What is the Appropriate Approach and Extent of Exposure?

The choice of the approach to esophagectomy is another important issue, with at least three different approaches to exposure route.

1. Transhiatal esophagectomy, without thoracotomy.
2. Abdominothoracic (transthoracic) esophagectomy with laparotomy and right-sided thoracotomy (Ivor-Lewis procedure).
3. Thoracoabdominal esophagectomy with extensive mediastinal and abdominal exposure through a continuous left-sided thoracoabdominal incision.

The choice of either the transhiatal or the transthoracic procedure is one (if not the only) surgical question in this area which has been adequately addressed in randomized controlled trials. The single, large, modern prospective randomized trial [evidence level Ib; (33)] showed a clear trend toward increased survival in patients undergoing transthoracic *en bloc* esophagectomy with lymphadenectomy, compared to patients undergoing transhiatal resection, but statistical significance was not reached. This result can be legitimately interpreted either as showing no difference between the two techniques or as indicating that a difference may exist that could be demonstrated by further trials. Skeptical clinical epidemiologists are likely to prefer the former conclusion, while surgeons with an interest in the tumor biology of the disease tend to favor the latter.

Some authorities have argued that the transhiatal approach is superior because of reductions in postoperative morbidity and mortality by avoiding the thoracotomy. This view has not been supported by another recent prospective multicenter cohort study from the United States (33): In this large-scale investigation, the reported differences between transhiatal and transthoracic approach—in respect to morbidity and mortality—were statistically nonsignificant (evidence level Ib). The only published meta-analysis of comparisons between these approaches (34) is hampered by the tiny number of patients in randomized comparisons. Overall, these analyses found no difference in risk of complications, but there were more vocal-cord palsies and anastomotic leaks in the transhiatal group, while the transthoracic operation had more pulmonary complications, chylous leakage, and wound infection. These results, which mainly came from non-randomized comparisons (evidence level 4) also suggested a higher mortality for transthoracic surgery, but amongst randomized patients no difference was seen. In the randomized trial, pulmonary complications and chyle leak were significantly more frequent after transthoracic surgery, but there was no difference in mortality (evidence level 1b).

A clear superiority of either of the procedures has not been demonstrated by the available evidence. In this circumstance, a more differentiated view and an individualized strategy based on experience and pathophysiological reasoning are permissible. Our current surgical doctrine based on the above is as follows:

- Patients who are likely to benefit from the complete nodal clearance should be approached with *abdominothoracic esophagectomy (Ivor-Lewis procedure)*. These are patients with a high prevalence of lymphatic involvement, young patients (who have more capacities to cope with a more extended surgical trauma), and responders to neoadjuvant therapy.
- The more oncologically limited procedure, *transhiatal esophagectomy*, might be appropriate for earlier tumor stages of distal esophageal adenocarcinomas (with low probability of lymphatic involvement) and patients with substantial comorbidity (who may benefit from avoiding the thoracotomy).
- There is no evidence that the abdominothoracic approach, with extensive mediastinal and abdominal exposure through a continuous thoracoabdominal incision (31), is superior with respect to oncological radicality or extent of lymphadenectomy (but there is no definitive evidence of inferiority either).

Which Length of Esophagus Should be Resected?

Another important issue of surgery for esophagogastric junction tumors is the length of esophagus to be resected. Although this topic has never been addressed in a controlled investigation, sensible recommendations can be made based on analyses of surgical series (15,21,31), despite the formally low evidence level (evidence level 4). Based on the analysis of the recurrence pattern of resected squamous-cell esophageal cancers, it is frequently advocated that esophageal resection margins be at least 10 cm in length (35). But this claim could never be substantiated for adenocarcinoma of the distal esophagus or cardia. Rather, a safe R0-situation without the risk of anastomotic recurrences can be achieved with a much lesser extent of resection. Currently, tumor-free resection margins, proven by intraoperative frozen-sections, are considered adequate. Especially in adenocarcinomas of the distal esophagus (AEG I), intramural tumor spread is of much lesser importance, compared to esophageal squamous-cell cancers (21,36). Recurrence of these tumors mostly does not occur at the proximal or distal resection margins. The greater problem is the third dimension (the circumferential margin).

Preserving as much of the healthy esophagus as possible is important with respect to the patient's quality of life. A good swallowing function depends on a preferably long segment of "healthy esophagus." Problems with the initiation of swallowing are especially closely related to a short cervical esophageal stump. In terms of quality of life and good swallowing function, an intrathoracic anastomosis is thus superior to a cervical anastomosis (Evidence level 4).

One aim of resection for Barrett's cancer, however, must be removal of the entire length of the metaplastic mucosa. Despite the low overall frequency of malignant progression of this precancerous lesion [between 0.5% and 2% in the studies reported in the meta-analysis by (37)], it is not advisable to leave remnants of Barrett's mucosa behind after surgical resection for Barrett's cancer: Barrett's esophagus that has become neoplastic in one area may become neoplastic in another area as well. Although this is not entirely proven, the molecular properties of the epithelium may have changed toward increased malignant potency. Furthermore it is well-known, that carcinomas originating in Barrett's mucosa are often multifocal, and may be associated with areas of high-grade intraepithelial neoplasia or invasive carcinoma with high frequency (38,39).

Is a Limited Approach Justified for Early Cancers?

In early tumor stages, an even more limited procedure has been suggested, and initial results have indicated it to be pathophysiologically and surgically appropriate (19,24): A limited resection of the distal esophagus and the esophagogastric junction is performed through a transabdominal/transhiatal approach. The regional lymphadenectomy includes all nodes of the primary lymphatic drainage and interposition of a pedicled jejunal segment is used for reconstruction. Short- and long-term results have indicated that this approach is a suitable surgical alternative to extensive resections (gastrectomy and/or esophagectomy: evidence level 4). This procedure is also well-suited as an alternative to the currently emerging endoscopic ablation and resection techniques because it allows for an adequate lymphadenectomy, removes the entire Barrett's esophagus, and provides a surgical specimen with adequate tumor-free resection margins. However, current data on limited resection are still scant and require confirmation in larger trials.

CONCLUDING SUMMARY

Surgical resection with lymphadenctomy is the treatment of choice for all adenocarcinomas of the esphagogastric junction prior to generalization of the disease. Multimodal protocols, with neoadjuvant treatment, are an option when the likelihood of achieving an R0-resection is low. Classification of AEG tumors is best performed as suggested by Siewert and collegues: This allows the surgical strategy to be tailored to the oncological problem, the procedures to be standardized, and helps to make results from different institutions comparable. We believe the best approach to AEG I tumors, which are mostly Barrett's cancers, is an abdominothoracic *en bloc* esophagectomy and reconstruction with gastric pull-up and intrathoracic anaostomosis. A prospectively randomized trial from the Netherlands provides some support for this notion. Extended gastrectomy with lymphadenectomy of the abdominal and lower mediastinal compartment is the preferred approach to AEG II and III tumors. Only in case of carcinomas with tumor growth extending far into the esophagus, additional lymphadenectomy through a thoracotomy may be beneficial.

REFERENCES

1. Sobin LH, Wittekind Ch (eds.). UICC. TNM Classification of Malignant Tumors 6th ed. New York: Wiley-Liss, 2002.
2. von Rahden BH, Stein HJ. Therapy of advanced esophageal malignancy. Curr Opin Gastroenterol 2004; 20:391–396.
3. von Rahden BH, Stein HJ. Staging and treatment of advanced esophageal cancer. Curr Opin Gastroenterol 2005; 21:472–477.
4. Siewert JR, Stein HJ, von Rahden BH. Multimodal treatment of gastrointestinal tract tumors: consequences for surgery. World J Surg 2005; 29:940–948.
5. Lordick F, Stein HJ, Peschel C, Siewert JR. Neoadjuvant therapy for oesophagogastric cancer. Br J Surg 2004; 91:540–551.
6. Siewert JR, Hölscher AH, Becker K, Gössner W. Cardia cancer: attempt at a therapeutically relevant classification Chirurg 1987; 58:25–34.

7. Siewert JR, Stein HJ. Classification of carcinoma of the oesophagogastric junction. Br J Surg 1998; 85:1457–1459.
8. Siewert JR, Feith M, Werner M, Stein HJ. Adenocarcinoma of the esophagogastric junction: results of surgical therapy based on anatomical/topographic classification in 1002 consecutive patients. Ann Surg 2000; 232:353–361.
9. Siewert and Stein, 1989
10. Hardwick RH, Williams GT. Staging of oesophageal adenocarcinoma. Br J Surg 2002; 89:1076–1077.
11. Ichikura T, Ogawa T, Kawabata T, Chochi K, Sugasawa H, Mochizuki H. Is adenocarcinoma of the gastric cardia a distinct entity independent of subcardial carcinoma? World J Surg 2003; 27:334–338.
12. de Manzoni G, Pedrazzani C, Pasini F, et al. Results of surgical treatment of adenocarcinoma of the gastric cardia. Ann Thorac Surg 2002; 73:1035–1040.
13. Swisher SG, Pisters PW, Komaki R, Lahoti S, Ajani JA. Gastroesophageal junction adenocarcinoma. Curr Treat Options Oncol 2000; 1:387–398.
14. Mariette C, Castel B, Balon JM, Van Seuningen I, Triboulet JP. Extent of oesophageal resection for adenocarcinoma of the oesophagogastric junction. Eur J Surg Oncol 2003; 29:588–593.
15. Sauvanet A, Mariette C, Thomas P, et al. Mortality and morbidity after resection for adenocarcinoma of the gastroesophageal junction: predictive factors. J Am Coll Surg 2005; 201:253–262.
16. Kodera Y, Yamamura Y, Shimizu Y, et al. Adenocarcinoma of the gastroesophageal junction in Japan: relevance of Siewert's classification applied to 177 cases resected at a single institution. J Am Coll Surg 1999; 189:594–601.
17. Spechler SJ. Clinical practice. Barrett's Esophagus. N Engl J Med 2002; 346:836–842.
18. von Rahden BHA, Feith M, Stein HJ. Carcinoma of the cardia. Classification as esophageal or gastric cancer? Int J Colorectal Dis 2005; 20:89–93.
19. Stein et al., 2002
20. Theisen J, Stein HJ, Dittler HJ, et al. Preoperative chemotherapy unmasks underlying Barrett's mucosa in patients with adenocarcinoma of the distal esophagus. Surg Endosc 2002; 16:671–673.
21. Siewert JR, Stein HJ, Feith M, Brücher BLDM, Bartels H, Fink U. Tumor cell type is an independent prognostic parameter in esophageal cancer: Lessons learned from more than 1000 consecutive resections at a single institution in the Western world. Ann Surg 2001; 234, 360–369.
22. Stein 2001
23. Feith M, Stein HJ, Siewert JR. Pattern of lymphatic spread of Barrett's cancer. World J Surg 2003; 27:1052–1057.
24. Stein HJ, Feith M, Bruecher BL, Naehrig J, Sarbia M, Siewert JR. Early esophageal cancer: pattern of lymphatic spread and prognostic factors for long-term survival after surgical resection. Ann Surg 2005; 242:566–573.
25. Siewert and Stein, 1996
26. de Manzoni G, Morgagni P, Roviello F, et al. Nodal abdominal spread in adenocarcinoma of the cardia. Results of a multicenter prospective study. Gastric Cancer 1998; 1:146–151.
27. Wang LS, Wu CW, Hsieh MJ, Fahn HJ, Huang MH, Chien KY. Lymph node metastasis in patients with adenocarcinoma of gastric cardia. Cancer 1993; 71:1948–1953.
28. Dresner SM, Lamb PJ, Bennett MK, Hayes N, Griffin SM. The pattern of metastatic lymph node dissemination from adenocarcinoma of the esophagogastric junction. Surgery 2001; 129:103–109.
29. Lamb PJ, Griffin SM, Burt AD, Lloyd J, Karat D, Hayes N. Sentinel node biopsy to evaluate the metastatic dissemination of oesophageal adenocarcinoma. Br J Surg 2005; 92:60–67.
30. Burian M, Stein HJ, Sendler A, et al. Sentinel node detection in Barrett's and cardia cancer. Ann Surg Oncol 2004; 11:255–258.
31. Lerut T, Nafteux P, Moons J, et al. Three-field lymphadenectomy for carcinoma of the esophagus and gastroesophageal junction in 174 R0 resections: impact on staging, disease-free survival, and outcome: a plea for adaptation of TNM classification in upper-half esophageal carcinoma. Ann Surg 2004; 240:962–967.
32. Lagarde SM, Cense HA, Hulscher JBF, et al. Prospective analysis of patients with adenocarcinoma of the gastric cardia and lymph node metastasis in the proximal field of the chest. Br J Surg 2005; 92: 1404–1408.
33. Rentz J, Bull D, Harpole D, et al. Transthoracic versus transhiatal esophagectomy: a prospective study of 945 patients. J Thorac Cardiovasc Surg 2003; 125:1114–1120.
34. Hulscher JB, van Sandick JW, de Boer AG, et al. Extended transthoracic resection compared with limited transhiatal resection for adenocarcinoma of the esophagus. N Engl J Med 2002; 347:1662–1669.
35. Tam PC, Siu KF, Cheung HC, Ma L, Wong J. Local recurrences after subtotal esophagectomy for squamous cell carcinoma. Ann Surg 1987; 205:189–194.
36. Stein 2005
37. Shaheen NJ, Crosby MA, Bozymski EM, Sandler RS. Is there publication bias in the reporting of cancer risk in Barrett's esophagus? Gastroenterology 2000; 119:333–338.
38. van Sandick JW, van Lanschot JJ, ten Kate FJ, et al. Pathology of early invasive adenocarcinoma of the esophagus or esophagogastric junction: implications for therapeutic decision making. Cancer 2000; 88:2429–2437.

39. Buttar NS, Wang KK, Sebo TJ, et al. Extent of high-grade dysplasia in Barrett's esophagus correlates with risk of adenocarcinoma. Gastroenterology 2001; 120:1630–1639.
40. Stein HJ, Feith M, Mueller J, Werner M, Siewert JR. Limited resection for early adenocarcinoma in Barrett's esophagus. Ann Surg 2000; 232:733–742.
41. Stein HJ, von Rahden BHA, Höfler H, Siewert JR. Carcinoma of the oesophagogastric junction and Barrett esophagus: an almost clear oncologic model? Chirurg 2003; 74:703–708.
42. Stein HJ, von Rahden BHA. Cancer of the esophagus. In Sobin LH and Wittekind Ch, eds. Prognostic Factors in Cancer, Wiley-Liss Inc, New York, 2006, in press.
43. Stein HJ, von Rahden BHA, Feith M. Surgery for early stage esophageal adenocarcinoma. J Surg Oncol 2005; 92:210–217.

5 The Role of Chemotherapy and Radiotherapy in the Management of Adenocarcinoma of the Gastroesophageal Junction and Lower Esophagus

Stéphanie Laurent, Karin Haustermans, and Eric Van Cutsem
Digestive Oncology Unit, University Hospital Gasthuisberg, Leuven, Belgium

INTRODUCTION

There has been a change in the epidemiology of adenocarcinoma of the lower esophagus and gastroesophageal junction (GEJ) in the developed countries with a significant increase in the incidence for both sexes (1). This growing incidence could be at least partially related to the increasing incidence of Barrett esophagus (2). The prognosis of patients with GEJ cancer is often poor as a result of late presentation, early spread and anatomic proximity to vital organs, making treatment difficult. Dysphagia is a cardinal symptom of these tumors and develops only when obstruction accounts for at least 50% of the esophagus lumen. No reliable correlation, however, can be observed between dysphagia and tumor staging.

Management of adenocarcinoma of the GEJ has been largely controversial and poses specific intellectual and practical challenges because of the confusion about whether it should be regarded as esophageal or gastric cancer. A consensus conference defined adenocarcinoma of the GEJ as tumors that have their center within 5 cm proximal or distal of the anatomic cardia and is further subdivided into three different types: type I, adenocarcinoma of the distal esophagus; type II, true carcinoma of the cardia; and type III, subcardial gastric carcinoma (3).

This classification is purely morphological and is based on the anatomical location of the tumor center or in patients with advanced tumors on the location of the tumor mass. The prognosis is related to the staging (4) and patients can be divided into three distinct groups: patients with resectable tumors, patients with locally advanced disease, and patients with metastatic disease.

Surgical resection remains the only curative treatment for adenocarcinoma of the GEJ and lower esophagus. However, in most randomized studies, surgical resection resulted in three-year survival rate of only 30% to 35% and five-year survival rates of no more than 20% (5–7). The adequacy of surgical resection is an important issue. Extensive surgery (extensive lymphadenectomy) was associated with better survival for locally advanced tumors of the esophagus in nonrandomized studies (8,9) but failed to demonstrate an improvement in five-year overall survival in gastric cancer in two randomized trials (10,11). The nodal dissection remains a subject of serious controversy in surgical oncology.

Several factors may contribute to improved survival in patients undergoing surgery; including complete response to neoadjuvant treatment, completeness of resection (R0 vs. R1 resection), size and location of the tumor, and the experience of the center and surgeon. Many physicians administer combinations of preoperative chemotherapy and radiation to downstage the primary tumor, aiming to increase resectability rate as well as eliminating micrometastases and prolonging survival. Clearly, the poor prognosis among patients whose cancer was resected justifies evaluation of potentially promising neoadjuvant strategies. Therefore, the addition of preoperative therapy (neoadjuvant) or postoperative therapy (adjuvant) in resectable adenocarcinoma has been intensively investigated. One of the difficulties in analyzing the results of these studies is the heterogeneity of the study populations. Experts recognize the lack of specific studies in patients with GEJ adenocarcinomas. Many studies in esophageal cancer include also patients with GEJ cancers and most studies in gastric cancer also include GEJ cancers. The studies in esophageal cancer commonly include patients with both adenocarcinoma and squamous-cell cancer. Moreover, most studies include relatively early or clearly resectable cancers as well as locally advanced cancers. Conclusions can therefore not easily be drawn (12). The data of the trials in esophageal and gastric cancer are therefore discussed separately before conclusions are drawn.

NEOADJUVANT AND ADJUVANT TREATMENT FOR ESOPHAGEAL CANCER

Surgery remains the standard approach in resectable esophageal cancer. Many patients still die from metastases or from locoregional relapse. This has resulted in an interest in combined therapeutic modalities. Attempts to improve cure rates through the use of systemic chemotherapy alone, radiotherapy alone, or the combination chemoradiotherapy have been extensively studied during the last 20 years.

Over the last decade, the use of neoadjuvant (induction) protocols aiming at downsizing or downstaging the disease and trying to improve the survival has been widely tested. Different trials unfortunately have yielded conflicting results. Several literature reviews and meta-analysis studies have been published on this subject.

Preoperative radiotherapy has failed to improve the outcome of patients compared to patients who underwent surgery alone. At least five older randomized trials have compared preoperative radiotherapy followed by surgery with surgery and have shown no improvement in resectability or survival. A meta-analysis of these trials showed a small, nonsignificant difference in survival of 3% at two years and 4% at five years (level 1a evidence) (13).

Several phase II and a few small phase III studies have shown interesting results of preoperative chemotherapy [most often 5-fluorouracil (5-FU)/cisplatin-based] in esophageal cancer: they concluded that preoperative chemotherapy is feasible, does not increase the postoperative morbidity and mortality, leads to lower distant failure rate, but did not influence the local failure rate. The pathological complete response (pCR) rate after neoadjuvant chemotherapy is in the range of 10%. Two large randomized phase III trials led however to conflicting results. The U.S. intergroup study evaluating preoperative chemotherapy followed by surgery compared to surgery alone in 467 patients did not show a difference in median survival or in three-year survival (14.9 vs. 16.1 months and 23% vs. 26%, respectively for the combined modality approach compared with surgery) (14). A U.K. Medical Research Council (MRC) study in 802 patients with esophageal cancer showed a significantly improved median survival (16.8 vs. 13.3 months) and two-year survival (43% vs. 34%) in favor of the combined modality treatment (15). The Cochrane meta-analysis including 11 trials with 2019 patients concludes that preoperative chemotherapy may offer some survival advantage, but that the data are not completely conclusive (level 1a evidence) (16).

More than 50 phase II and several phase III studies evaluating the role of neoadjuvant chemoradiotherapy have been published. The phase II studies concluded that the approach of preoperative chemoradiotherapy is feasible, but leads to slightly higher morbidity and mortality. In many of the trials, the chemotherapy combination was 5-FU/cisplatin-based and there was a wide variety of radiotherapy doses, fractionation, and fields.

The individual randomized phase III trials show conflicting results (17–24). The patient populations studied are often heterogeneous for stage, histological type, and/or site. The treatment regimens have a wide variety of chemotherapy regimens (often 5-FU and cisplatin-based), different radiotherapy schedules (often in the range of 40–45 Gy in fractions of 1.8–2.0 Gy), and both synchronous chemoradiotherapy and sequential chemoradiotherapy are used. Several trials are underpowered.

A meta-analysis of nine randomized trials of preoperative chemoradiotherapy plus surgery versus surgery, comprising 1116 patients, showed a pathologic complete response in 21% of patients, an improved three-year survival [odds ratio (OR) 0.66; $P=0.01$], an improved R0 resection rate (OR 0.53; $P=0.07$), and a lower loco-regional recurrence rate (OR 0.38; $P = 0.0002$) (level 1a evidence). There was a trend toward an increased operative mortality (OR 1.63; $P=0.053$) (25). These findings were confirmed in another meta-analysis (26). Another review stated however that a significant increase in the risk of mortality at three years for the combined arm was detected [risk ratio=0.87; 95% confidence interval (CI) 0.80–0.96; $P=0.004$] (27). Based on these data, the authors concluded that for patients with resectable esophageal cancer for whom surgery was considered appropriate, surgery alone is considered as the standard practice (level 1a evidence). The more recently published trial by Burmeister et al. (24) randomized 256 patients also between preoperative chemoradiotherapy followed by surgery and surgery alone. The dose of the radiotherapy was however lower than in most other studies (35 Gy). Neither overall progression-free survival nor overall survival differed between the two groups. The combined arm group, however, did have more R0 resections (80% vs. 59%; $P=0.002$) and fewer positive lymph nodes (43% vs. 67%; $P=0.003$) as compared with the surgery alone arm (level 1b evidence). Further subgroup analysis showed that patients with squamous-cell carcinoma had better disease-free survival with chemoradiotherapy plus surgery than did those with nonsquamous-cell carcinoma [hazard ratio (HR) 0.47 vs. 1.02]. In this trial as in all other trials, it should be noticed that the overall survival figures at five years are generally well below the survival figures obtained after radical primary surgery and extensive lymphadenectomy, mostly not exceeding 25% at three years. Moreover, postoperative mortality was significantly increased by neoadjuvant chemoradiotherapy. From the meta-analysis by Fiorica (26), the impact of postoperative mortality clearly favors the surgery alone arm (OR 0.53; 95% CI 0.31–0.92; $P=0.03$).

The general conclusion is that preoperative neoadjuvant chemoradiotherapy may improve survival of patients with resectable esophageal cancer, but at significant cost in terms of increased risk of perioperative death. It is however not clear who benefits most from a neoadjuvant chemoradiotherapy. Across the different trials, approximately 20% of patients have a pathological complete response during surgery after a neoadjuvant chemoradiotherapy. The patients who have a complete response at pathological examination seem to benefit in many studies and patients with a partial response benefit possibly, whereas nonresponding patients and patients with progressive disease do not benefit from preoperative chemoradiotherapy. The challenge is therefore to determine which patients will benefit most from the preoperative chemoradiotherapy. There are currently no accurate ways to predict this before the start of the neoadjuvant treatment. No molecular or other markers have been able to predict consistently and adequately for response. The emerging and promising role of ^{18}F-labeled deoxyglucose-positron emission tomography (FDG-PET) in the early response prediction during or after chemoradiotherapy needs further validation. It is now well accepted that both computed tomography (CT) and endoscopic ultrasound (EUS) have a low accuracy in assessing response to neoadjuvant therapy (28,29) (levels 2b, 1b). This is mainly due to the difficulty of discriminating between the morphological aspects of therapy-related inflammation on fibrosis versus residual tumor.

PET scan is now increasingly used as tool for response assessment. Indeed several studies have indicated a close correlation between changes in metabolic activity and pathologic response after induction therapy. The metabolic changes induced by induction chemotherapy are clearly preceding the morphologic ones (30). Trials are now on the way to investigate the value of PET-CT as an early predictor of response to allow setting up of tailored therapeutic strategies for responders (continuing induction therapy) versus nonresponders (discontinuing induction therapy).

In esophageal cancer, the combination of radiotherapy and concurrent chemotherapy with cisplatin and 5-FU has led to long-term survival in approximately 25% of patients, an outcome similar to that associated with surgery alone, or even surgery after preoperative therapy (31). Therefore, a few trials have investigated the role of definitive chemoradiotherapy. In a German trial (32), patients with locally advanced squamous-cell cancer were randomized after chemoradiotherapy into an arm without surgery and an arm with surgery. In the nonsurgical arm, a dose of 60 to 65 Gy was used. Overall survival was equivalent between the two groups ($P < 0.05$) (level 1b). The surgical arm, however, had a significantly better disease-free survival at two years, that is, 64.3% versus 40.7% ($P=0.003$), but at a price of a significantly increased treatment-related mortality (12.8% vs. 3.5%; $P=0.03$). In a French study, patients responding to chemoradiotherapy were randomized between surgery and further completion of chemoradiotherapy (33). There was no difference in survival between the two groups. The major drawback of this study, however, is that only responders were randomized. Prospective determination of responders is at this moment not yet possible.

The data of these two relatively small studies do not yet dismiss the role of surgery in resectable esophageal cancer. In view of the difficulty of determining which patients do have a complete response by conventional imaging (34), surgery is certainly still advocated in patients with resectable esophageal cancer after neoadjuvant chemoradiotherapy.

Data from well-performed trials on adjuvant treatment in esophageal cancer are scarce and do not support the routine use of adjuvant chemo- and or radiotherapy in esophageal cancer. In patients with a locally advanced nonresectable esophageal cancer, a strategy of chemoradiotherapy is clearly the preferred option, if the general condition allows. In case of a response, a reevaluation is warranted to evaluate the appropriateness of a resection.

NEOADJUVANT AND ADJUVANT TREATMENT FOR GASTRIC CANCER

Surgical resection remains the primary curative treatment option in gastric cancer, with five-year survival rates of 58% to 78% and 34% reported for stage I and II disease, respectively (35). Despite this, the overall five-year survival rate for all patients remains poor and ranges between 15% and 38%. Recurrences are frequent after surgery. Recurrence rate and subsequent survival is dependent on the stage at diagnosis.

Prospective randomized trials have evaluated the role of D1 or D2 resection in the management of gastric cancer and they did not show any advantage in terms of overall survival in favor of D2 lymphadenectomy (10,11,36). In an expert consensus report, it has been agreed that at least a D1 resection should be performed and that it is mandatory that at least 15 lymph nodes are removed and recovered (12).

Local or regional recurrence in the gastric or tumor bed, anastomosis, or the regional lymph nodes occurs in 40% to 65% of patients after gastric resection with curative intent (37,38). Metastases occur most often in the liver and the peritoneum. Different strategies have been explored in randomized studies in patients with gastric cancer: adjuvant chemotherapy, adjuvant chemoradiotherapy, and perioperative chemotherapy. In many of the trials, a heterogeneous patient group is studied, including patients with gastric adenocarcinoma and GEJ cancer and patients with less and more advanced stages.

Most of the individual trials studying the effect of postoperative adjuvant chemotherapy do not show a survival advantage compared to surgery alone. These studies often randomized a low number of patients and are clearly underpowered. The trials studied also were predominantly older chemotherapy regimens. Further, the patient populations studied were heterogeneous, including patient populations with both high- and low-risk of recurrence.

Five meta-analyses (or combined analyses) of adjuvant chemotherapy have been published (39–43). Most of the analyses show a small benefit in survival for patients treated with postoperative adjuvant chemotherapy (evidence level 1a). Because of the nature of the data, however, adjuvant chemotherapy is not generally advised for patients who undergo a complete surgical resection of gastric cancer.

A major change in the management of gastric cancer is based on the results of the U.S. GI-Intergroup study, which randomized 556 patients with resected adenocarcinoma of the stomach or GEJ to surgery plus postoperative chemoradiotherapy (bolus 5-FU before, during, and after the irradiation) or surgery alone (44). The median overall survival in the surgery only arm was 27 months, compared to 36 months in the chemoradiotherapy group ($P < 0.05$). The survival at three years was 50% versus 40% in favor of patients treated with postoperative chemoradiotherapy. After a median follow-up of five years, compared with surgery alone, five-year overall survival was improved by 11.6% (40% vs. 28.4%, respectively; $P < 0.001$) and the relapse-free survival was increased from 25% to 31%. Patients treated with postoperative chemoradiotherapy had significant less loco-regional recurrences (level 1b evidence). Most patients did not undergo an extensive surgical resection although the protocol recommended a D2 resection. Fifty-four percent of the patients did not even have a D1 resection (44). So it is possible that the adjuvant therapy was simply making up for inadequate surgery. The chemotherapy used in this study was never considered to be a highly effective combination for stomach cancer. Therefore, better chemotherapeutic options should be investigated in this setting, such as infused regimens of 5-FU, which are currently recommended in this combination regimen. The addition of new cytotoxic agents is under investigation.

The Magic trial compared a strategy of surgery alone with perioperative chemotherapy (three cycles of preoperative 5FU/cisplatin-based chemotherapy followed by surgery followed by three cycles of postoperative chemotherapy) in 503 patients with gastric, GEJ, and distal esophageal adenocarcinoma. The patients treated with perioperative chemotherapy had a significantly better survival: 50% versus 41% were alive at two years and 36% versus 23% at five years compared with patients who were treated with surgery only. The progression survival was also significantly improved for patients treated with perioperative chemotherapy: HR 0.66 (95% CI 0.53–0.81; P=0.0001) (level 1b evidence) (45).

It can be concluded that there is growing evidence that (neo)adjuvant treatment improves the outcome of selected patients with gastric cancer. As a general strategy, there is an agreement to recommend postoperative chemoradiotherapy in fit patients who already underwent inadequate surgery or less than D1 resection (12). The strategy of either postoperative chemoradiotherapy or perioperative chemotherapy can be recommended after multidisciplinary team discussions. For both strategies, the evidence is based on data from a large well-performed randomized trial (level 1b evidence). The evidence supporting postoperative chemotherapy is not so strong because of the nature of the randomized trials included in the combined analyses. Generally, either perioperative chemotherapy or postoperative chemoradiotherapy is recommended for patients who have stage T3, T4, or N+ M0 gastric cancer. There is no general agreement whether patients with stage T2bN0 should be offered an adjuvant treatment. In this setting, other factors should be taken into consideration (e.g., factors presented in nomograms).

A neoadjuvant or adjuvant treatment should be offered only to fit patients without important comorbidities. Crucial in good tolerance, especially for the postoperative chemoradiotherapy, is the ability of the patient to have an adequate calorie intake during the treatment. Adequate measures are therefore necessary, including the administration of enteral nutrition where required.

The strategy of neoadjuvant chemoradiotherapy in gastric cancer has been examined only in relatively small phase II studies. This approach is certainly feasible and promising activity has been suggested. Most patients had in these studies proximal gastric cancers.

GASTROESOPHAGEAL JUNCTION TUMORS: WHAT EVIDENCE EXISTS FOR OR AGAINST A SURVIVAL BENEFIT FROM ADJUVANT OR NEOADJUVANT THERAPY?

Despite a large number of phase II and III trials, the role of multimodality therapy remains unclear in GEJ cancer. Adjuvant or neoadjuvant studies in patients with GEJ cancers alone are not available. There is a large amount of data in literature on the adjuvant or neoadjuvant treatment in esophageal and in gastric cancer. Most of these trials in esophageal and in gastric cancer include patients with GEJ cancers as well. The clinical attitude toward patients with GEJ cancers stems therefore from the evidence in esophageal and gastric cancer. Surgery remains the standard treatment option and the only curative option in the majority of patients with cancer of the esophagus, GEJ, and stomach. In view of the high incidence of recurrent disease after surgery, there is an arguable need of an (neo)adjuvant therapy. Although the data are not conclusive in all trials, the evidence is growing that preoperative chemoradiotherapy improves the outcome in esophageal cancer and might be proposed for fit patients with a locally advanced GEJ cancer (especially Siewert types 1 and 2). However, others advocate a strategy of perioperative chemotherapy or postoperative chemoradiotherapy in patients with GEJ cancer (especially Siewert type 3), based on the evidence that both these strategies clearly improve the outcome of patients with gastric cancer.

An important aspect for the future is the possibility to predict more adequately than with histopathologic staging, the outcome of patients and the likelihood of benefit of a neoadjuvant or adjuvant treatment. Predictive molecular markers as well as different diagnostic modalities (e.g., FDG-PET) that may help in the early response prediction therefore need to be validated in clinical trials.

A multidisciplinary approach in experienced centers is certainly mandatory for adequate staging, for optimal surgery, and for the selection of an adequate (neo)adjuvant strategy (12). Physicians involved in the treatment of patients with GEJ cancers should also be encouraged to participate in well-designed clinical trials, to increase the evidence-based knowledge and to make future progress.

REFERENCES

1. Vizcaino AP, Moreno V, Lambert R, Parkin DM. Time trends incidence of both major histologic types of esophageal carcinomas in selected countries, 1973–1995. Int J Cancer 2002; 99:860–868.
2. Pera M, Pera M. Recent changes in the epidemiology of oesophageal cancer. Surg Oncol 2001; 10:81–90.
3. Siewert JR, Stein HJ. Classification of adenocarcinoma of the oesophagogastric junction. Br J Surg 1998; 85:1457–1459.
4. Hagen JA, DeMeester SR, Peters JH, Chandrasoma P, DeMeester TR. Curative resection for esophageal adenocarcinoma: analysis of 100 en bloc esophagectomies. Ann Surg 2001; 234:520–530.
5. Kelsen DP. Adjuvant and neoadjuvant therapy for gastric cancer. Semin Oncol 1996; 23:379–389.
6. Refaely Y, Krasna MJ. Multimodality therapy for esophageal cancer. Surg Clin N Am 2002; 82:729–746.
7. Enzinger PC, Mayer RJ. Esophageal cancer. N Engl J Med 2003; 349:2241–2252.
8. Akiyama H, Tsurumaru M, Udagawa H, Kajiyama Y. Radical lymph node dissection for cancer of the thoracic oesophagus. Ann Surg 1994; 220:364–372.
9. Lerut T, Coosemans W, Decker G, et al. Extended surgery for cancer of the oesophagus and gastroesophageal junction. J Surg Res 2004; 117:58–63.
10. Bonenkamp JJ, Hermans J, Sasako M, van de Velde CHJ. Extended lymph-node dissection for gastric cancer. N Engl J Med 1999; 340:908–914.
11. Cuschieri A, Weeden S, Fielding J, et al. Patient survival after D1 and D2 resections for gastric cancer: long-term results of the MRC randomized surgical trial. Br J Cancer 1999; 79:1522–1530.
12. Van Cutsem E, Dicato M, Arber N, et al. The neo-adjuvant, surgical and adjuvant treatment of gastric adenocarcinoma. Current expert opinion derived from the seventh World Congress on Gastrointestinal Cancer, Barcelona, 2005. Ann Oncol 2006; 17:VI13–VI18.
13. Arnott SJ, Duncan W, Gignoux M, et al.. Preoperative radiotherapy for oesophageal carcinoma (Cochrane Review). London: The Cochrane Library, 2003 (issue 4).
14. Kelsen D, Ginsberg R, Pajak T, et al. Chemotherapy followed by surgery compared with surgery alone for localized esophageal cancer. N Engl J Med 1998; 339:1979–1984.
15. Medical Research Council (MRC) Oesophageal Working Party. Surgical resection with or without preoperative chemotherapy in oesophageal cancer: a randomised controlled trial. Lancet 2002; 359:1727–1733.
16. Malthaner R, Colin S, Fenlon D. Preoperative chemotherapy for resectable thoracic esophageal cancer. Cochrane Database Syst Rev 2006; 3:CD001556.
17. Nygaard K, Hagen S, Hansen HS, et al. Pre-operative radiotherapy prolongs survival in operable esophageal carcinoma: a randomized, multicenter study of pre-operative radiotherapy and chemotherapy: the second Scandinavian trial in esophageal carcinoma. World J Surg 1992; 16:1104–1110.
18. Le Prise E, Etienne PL, Meunier B, et al. A randomized study of chemotherapy, radiation therapy, and surgery versus surgery for localized squamous-cell carcinoma of the esophagus. Cancer 1994; 73:1179–1184.
19. Apinop C, Puttisak P, Preecha N. A prospective study of combined therapy in esophageal cancer. Hepatogastroenterology 1994; 41:391–393.
20. Walsh T, Noonan N, Hollywood D, Kelly A, Keeling N, Hennessy TPJ. A comparison of multimodal therapy and surgery for esophageal adenocarcinoma. N Engl J Med 1996; 335:462–467.
21. Bosset J-F, Gignoux M, Triboulet J-P, et al. Chemoradiotherapy followed by surgery compared to surgery alone in squamous-cell cancer of the esophagus. N Engl J Med 1997; 337:161–167.
22. Law S, Kwong D, Tung H, et al. Preoperative chemoradiation for squamous-cell esophageal cancer: a prospective randomized trial. Can J Gastroenterol 1998; 12(suppl B):56B (abstract).
23. Urba SG, Orringer RB, Turrisi A, Iannettoni M, Forastiere A, Strawderman M. Randomized trial of preoperative chemoradiation versus surgery alone in patients with locoregional esophageal carcinoma. J Clin Oncol 2001; 19:305–313.
24. Burmeister BH, Smithers BM, Gebski V, et al. Trans-Tasman. Radiation Oncology Group; Australasian Gastro-Intestinal Trials Group. Surgery alone versus chemoradiotherapy followed by surgery for resectable cancer of the oesophagus: a randomised controlled phase III trial. Lancet Oncol 2005; 6:659–668.
25. Urschel JD, Vasan H. A meta-analysis of randomized controlled trials that compared neoadjuvant chemoradiation and surgery to surgery alone for resectable esophageal cancer. Am J Surg 2003; 185:538–543.
26. Fiorica F, Di Bona D, Licata A, et al. Preoperative chemoradiotherapy for oesophageal cancer: a systematic review and meta-analysis. Gut 2004; 53:925–930.
27. Malthaner RA, Wong RK, Rumble RB, Zuraw L. Gastrointestinal Disease Group of Cancer Care Ontario's Program in Evidence-based Care. Neoadjuvant or adjuvant therapy for resectable esophageal cancer: a clinical practice guideline. BMC Cancer 2004; 4:67.

28. Kalha I, Kaw M, Fukami N, et al. The accuracy of endoscopic ultrasound for restaging esophageal carcinoma after chemoradiation therapy. Cancer 2004; 101:940–947.
29. Cerfolio RJ, Bryant AS, Ohja B, et al. The accuracy of endoscopic ultrasonography with fine-needle aspiration, integrated positron emission tomography with computed tomography, and computed tomography in restaging patients with esophageal cancer after neoadjuvant chemoradiotherapy. J Thorac Cardiovascular Surg 2005; 129:1232–1241.
30. Wieder HA, Beer AJ, Lordick F, et al. Comparison of changes in tumor metabolic activity and tumor size during chemotherapy of adenocarcinomas of the esophagogastric junction. J Nucl Med 2005; 46:2029–2034.
31. Herskovic A, Martz K, Al-Sarraf M, et al. Combined chemotherapy and radiotherapy compared with radiotherapy alone in patients with cancer of the esophagus. N Engl J Med 1992; 326:1629–1631.
32. Stahl M, Stuschke M, Lehmann N, et al. Chemoradiation with and without surgery in patients with locally advanced squamous-cell carcinoma of the esophagus. J Clin Oncol 2005; 23:2310–2317.
33. Bedenne L, Michel P, Bouche O, et al. Randomized phase III trial in locally advanced esophageal cancer: radiochemotherapy followed by surgery versus radiochemotherapy alone (FFCD 9102). Proc ASCO 2003; 21:a519.
34. Flamen P, Van Cutsem E, Lerut A, et al. Positron emission tomography for assessment of the response to induction radiochemotherapy in locally advanced oesophageal cancer. Ann Oncol 2002; 13:361–368.
35. Hundahl SA, Phillips JL, Menck HR. The National Cancer Data Base Report on poor survival of U.S. gastric carcinoma patients treated with gastrectomy: Fifth Edition American Joint Committee on cancer staging, proximal disease, and the "different disease" hypothesis. Cancer 2000; 88(4):921–932.
36. McCulloch P, Nita ME, Kazi H, Gama-Rodrigues J. Extended versus limited lymph nodes dissection technique for adenocarcinoma of the stomach. Cochrane Database Syst Rev 2003; 4:CD001964.
37. Landry J, Tepper JE, Wood WC, Moulton EO, Koerner F, Sullinger J. Pattern of failure following curative resection of gastric cancer. Int J Radiat Oncol Biol Phys 1990; 191:1357–1362.
38. Gunderson LL, Sosin H. Adenocarcinoma of the stomach: areas of failure in re-operation series (second or symptomatic look): clinicopathologic correlation and implications for adjuvant therapy. Int J Radiat Oncol Biol Phys 1982; 8:1–11.
39. Hermans J, Bonnenkamp JJ, Boon MC, et al. Adjuvant therapy after curative resection for gastric cancer: meta-analysis of randomized trials. J Clin Oncol 1993; 11:1441–1447.
40. Mari E, Floriani I, Tinazzi A, et al. Efficacy of adjuvant chemotherapy after curative resection for gastric cancer: a meta-analysis of published randomized trials. A study of GISCAD. Ann Oncol 2000; 11:837–843.
41. Earle CC, Maroun JA. Adjuvant chemotherapy after curative resection for gastric cancer in non-Asian patients: revisiting a meta-analysis of randomised trials. Eur J Cancer 1999; 35(7):1059–1064.
42. Gianni L, Panzini I, Tassinari D, et al. Meta-analyses of randomized trials of adjuvant chemotherapy in gastric cancer. Ann Oncol 2001; 12(8):1178–1180.
43. Janunger KG, Hafström L, Nygren P, et al. A systematic overview of chemotherapy effects in gastric cancer. Acta Oncol 2001; 40(2–3):309–326.
44. Macdonald JS, Smalley SR, Benedetti J, et al. Chemotherapy after surgery compared with surgery alone for adenocarcinoma of the stomach or gastroesophageal junction. N Engl J Med 2001; 345:725–730.
45. Cunningham D, Allum WH, Stenning SP, et al. Perioperative chemotherapy versus surgery alone for resectable gastroesophageal cancer. N Engl J Med 2006; 355:11–20.

6 Esophageal Cancer—Chemotherapy and Radiotherapy

Tom Crosby and Somnath Mukherjee
Velindre Cancer Centre, Cardiff, U.K.

INTRODUCTION

Surgery has been the cornerstone of curative therapy for patients with esophageal cancer. However, less than half of patients are suitable for potentially curative surgery, and even in patients who are physiologically fit and whose tumor appears resectable, two-thirds will relapse and die of locally recurrent and/or metastatic disease. Attempts have been made therefore to improve patient survival through the use of adjuvant therapy.

ADJUVANT THERAPY: PREOPERATIVE OR POSTOPERATIVE?

Chemotherapeutic agents are selected for adjuvant therapy trials having first demonstrated significant activity in advanced disease. Given before surgery neoadjuvant therapy can potentially downstage locoregional disease, and thus increase operability, as well as eradicate occult micrometastatic disease. The tumor is still well-vascularized, the patients are more likely to be fit for treatment, and tumor response can be assessed radiologically and histologically. However, it does inevitably delay definitive surgery and, although neoadjuvant chemotherapy may increase the rate of curative (R0) resections, it will seldom lead to a pathologically complete response (1,2).

Postoperative therapy may allow better patient selection based on defined pathological findings, for example, by defining patients with very early disease who already have an excellent prognosis, and those with disseminated disease for whom chemotherapy will not increase the chance of cure. However, it has been shown to be difficult to administer these therapies after major upper gastrointestinal (GI) surgery. In addition, residual tumor is devascularized, making it relatively resistant to chemotherapy or radiotherapy and as there is no visible tumor, benefits can only be measured in the long term as an improvement in disease-free or overall survival (OS).

Radiotherapy, with or without sensitizing chemotherapy treats locoregional disease, such as that in the surgical field. Preoperative chemoradiation certainly yields higher pathological response rates compared to either chemotherapy or radiotherapy alone but is also associated with a greater physiological stress, potentially increasing surgical morbidity and mortality. As with chemotherapy, preoperative therapy tends to be better tolerated than postoperative treatment. The presence of intact tumor vasculature is important, as hypoxic tumor cells are known to be radioresistant and the radiotherapy treatment volumes are easier to define. Once again, however, this approach fails to select patients for therapy based on pathological findings which determine a high chance of locoregional disease relapse.

ADJUVANT CHEMOTHERAPY

Preoperative Chemotherapy

There have been 11 trials that have tested the benefit of neoadjuvant chemotherapy followed by surgery with surgery alone (1–11). Most have used cisplatin and 5-fluorouracil (5-FU)–based regimens but are otherwise heterogeneous in design and outcome (Table 1). A systematic review of 11 of these studies, randomizing a total of 2051 patients, has been published in the Cochrane Library (12) (evidence level 1a). This meta-analysis found a survival advantage for neoadjuvant chemotherapy which becomes apparent from the third year [21% increase in three-year survival;

TABLE 1 Trails of Neoadjuvant Chemotherapy for Esophageal Cancer

Author (year), treatment, trial	*n*	SCC (%)	One year (%)	Two years (%)	Three years (%)	Four years (%)	Five years (%)	MS (months)	Survival difference (*P*)
Nygaard et al. (1992),									
S,	50	100	34	13	9	NR	NR	7	NS
S + CT	56		31	6	3	NR	NR	7	
Schlag et al. (1992),									
S,	24	100	32	NR	NR	NR	NR	7.5	NS
S + CT	22		20	NR	NR	NR	NR	7	
Maipang et al. (1994),									
S,	22	100	85	40	36	NR	NR	17	NS
S + CT	24		58	31	31	NR	NR	17	
Law et al. (1997)									
S	73	100	50	31	14	14	NR	13	NS
S + CT	74		60	44	38	28	NR	16.8	
Kok et al. (1997),									
S,	74	100	NR	NR	NR	NR	NR	11	0.002
S + CT	74		NR	NR	NR	NR	NR	18.5	
Kelsen et al. (1998),									
S,	234	45	60	37	26	21	20	16	NS
S + CT	233		59	35	23	19	18	15	
Ancona et al. (2001),									
S,	47	100	75	55	41	38	22	24	NS
S + CT	47		75	55	44	42	34	25	
MRC OE02 (2002),									
S,	402	33	54	34	27	20	15	13	0.004
S + CT	400		59	43	35	28	26	17	

Abbreviations: CT, computed tomography; MS, median survival; NR, not relevant; S, surgery; SCC, squamous cell carcinoma.

risk ratio (RR) = 1.21; 95% confidence interval (CI) 0.88–1.68; *P* = 0.25] but only becoming statistically significant five years after therapy (44% increase in five-year survival; RR = 1.44; 95% CI 1.05–1.97; *P* = 0.02). Although there was a trend toward reduction in local recurrence (LR) rate (19% reduction; RR = 0.81; 95% CI 0.54–1.22; *P* = 0.3), preoperative therapy did not increase the resection rate and the pathological complete response rate was only 3%. The combined modality therapy was associated with increased surgical morbidity, and these effects appeared independent of the type of chemotherapy used or tumor morphology.

A previous meta-analysis by Bhansali et al. included 11 randomized control studies but these were heterogeneous in design and therapeutic intervention (including radiation therapy) making interpretation inconclusive (13). It should also be emphasized that in both these reviews individual patient data was not analyzed (14).

It is worth considering the two largest individual studies, U.S. Intergroup INT 0113 and U.K. Medical Research Council (MRC) OEO2, in more detail, as these appear to demonstrate contrasting results (Table 2). Kelsen et al. (1) reported a U.S. study of 467 patients comparing three cycles of preoperative cisplatin and 5-FU to surgery alone. The patients were able to receive further two cycles of chemotherapy following surgery if there had been an objective response or stable disease after preoperative therapy. There was no significant survival difference between the trial arms, median survival being 14.9 months in patients receiving preoperative chemotherapy versus 16.1 months for immediate surgery, *P* = 0.53 (two-year survival 35% vs. 37%, *P* = NS) (evidence level 1b). The U.K. MRC study compared 802 patients who were randomized between two cycles of preoperative cisplatin and 5-FU and surgery alone (2). This study found a survival advantage at two years for patients who received preoperative therapy (43% vs. 34%; HR = 0.79; 95% CI 0.67–0.93; *P* = 0.004) (evidence level 1b). It is possible that the greater duration and dose intensity of chemotherapy in the U.S. Intergroup study deferred and ultimately denied patients definitive potentially curative surgery.

More recently, the results of the MRC ST01 (MAGIC) trial have been reported in abstract form only (15). Five hundred and three patients were randomized to receive three cycles of

TABLE 2 Characteristics of U.S. Intergroup 0013 and U.K. OE02 Trials of Neoadjuvant Chemotherapy in Oesophageal Cancer

Parameters	MRC OE02	U.S. Intergroup 0113
No. of patients	802	440
Chemotherapy	Two cycles cisplatin/5-FU preoperatively	Three cycles cisplatin/5-FU preoperatively (+two cycles postoperatively)
Dose of cisplatin	80 mg/m^2	100 mg/m^2
Percentage (%) receiving all cycles	90	71% preoperative, 38% postoperative
Delay to surgery (days)	63	93
SCC (%)	31	47
Radiotherapy given (%)	9	Not published "at discretion of center"
Surgery performed (%)	92	80
Median survival (preoperative chemotherapy)	168	149
Two-year overall survival (%) (preoperative chemotherapy)	43	35

Abbreviations: 5-FU, 5-flourouracil; MRC, Medical Research Council; SCC, squamous-cell carcinoma.

preoperative and postoperative chemotherapy (epirubicin, cisplatin, and infusional 5-FU; ECF) or surgery alone in operable gastric adenocarcinoma. The study accrued patients over eight years, and in the latter stages recruitment was opened to 75 patients with adenocarcinoma of the lower-third of the oesophagus. The results demonstrate a survival advantage for perioperative therapy (five-year survival 36% vs. 23%; HR 0.76; CI 0.6–0.93; $P = 0.009$) with no difference in treatment effects for patients with esophageal and gastric cancer.

In conclusion, preoperative chemotherapy appears to offer a survival advantage, that becomes significant only some years after treatment. This benefit is mitigated somewhat by the additional morbidity associated with chemotherapy. The optimal chemotherapy regimen is yet to be defined. In the ongoing CRUK MRC OE05 study, patients are randomized to receive either four cycles of preoperative epirubicin, cisplatin, and capecitabine or two cycles of cisplatin and 5-FU, as given in the MRC OE02 trial.

Postoperative Chemotherapy

The potential advantage of using postoperative therapy is that one can be relatively selective, based on pathological factors, in the patients who receive treatment, and there is no delay in definitive surgical therapy. However, the selection of only "fit" postoperative patients for clinical studies of postoperative treatment should lead one to be cautious in interpreting the applicability of such treatment to the general population, for example, excluding patients with R1 or R2 resections (microscopic and macroscopic residual disease, respectively) or those with prolonged postoperative complications. This potential bias is not present in trials of pre- or perioperative therapy. Indeed, patients randomized to receive chemotherapy before and after surgery show that less than 50% of the patients are able to receive full doses of chemotherapy following major upper GI surgery (1,15).

The results of three Japanese randomized control trials have failed to show a benefit for postoperative adjuvant chemotherapy (16–18) (level 1b evidence). One study initially published in abstract form suggested a benefit of two cycles of postoperative cisplatin and 5-FU (18). This study was terminated early due to slow accrual rate. In the final publication, there was an improvement in five-year disease-free survival in favor of postoperative therapy (55% vs. 45%, $P = 0.037$). OS was not statistically different (52% vs. 61% in favor of postoperative therapy, $P = 0.13$) although a subgroup of patients with lymph node-positive disease did appear to have a better outcome. The use of such treatment cannot therefore be routinely recommended outside of clinical trials.

ADJUVANT CHEMORADIOTHERAPY

Combining all three treatment modalities (chemotherapy, radiotherapy, and surgery) attempts were made to utilize the benefits of all three single treatment modalities, usually in the form of preoperative chemoradiotherapy (CRT). Such triple modality therapy however represents complicated and physiologically challenging treatment requiring justification in terms of a significant and meaningful survival advantage and mindful of any detrimental effect to quality-of-life (QOL).

A meta-analysis of nine randomized trials tested the value of chemotherapy and radiotherapy prior to surgery (19) (evidence level 1a). This analysis included patients receiving both concurrent and sequential CRT, and concluded that concurrent CRT was more effective than sequential treatment. In an intention to treat review of 1116 patients, 21% achieved complete pathological response in the CRT arm and there was a survival advantage for preoperative CRT, becoming statistically significant three years after surgery [odds ratio (OR) 0.66, CI 0.47, 0.92; $P = 0.416$], an increase in curative (R0) resection (OR 0.53; CI 0.33–0.84; $P = 0.007$) and a reduction in locoregional recurrence (LRR) (OR 0.38; CI 0.23, 0.63; $P = 0.0002$). However, there was a strong trend toward an increase in postoperative mortality (OR 1.72; CI 0.96, 3.07; $P = 0.06$).

Of the nine individual randomized trials of preoperative chemoradiation (20–28) (Table 3), four have included more than 100 patients and these trials are discussed next. However, all have been criticized because of their small size and consequent lack of statistical power, the use of inadequate staging protocols, or suboptimal treatment regimens.

A prospective trial performed in Dublin randomized 113 patients with adenocarcinoma of the esophagus to preoperative CRT (two cycles cisplatin and 5-FU, the first being concurrent with 40 Gy in 15 fractions of radiotherapy) and surgery alone (23). Walsh et al. reported a highly significant difference in favor of combined modality therapy (three-year survival 32% vs. 6%; $P = 0.01$). Inadequate staging and the very poor survival rate of patients in the surgery alone arm of the study raised concerns over case selection and surgical treatment quality.

The study from the University of Michigan, reported by Urba et al., (24) randomized 100 patients with carcinoma of the esophagus of either histological type to preoperative CRT

TABLE 3 Trials of Neoadjuvant Chemoradiation in Esophageal Cancer

			Survival						
Author (year), treatment, trial	*n*	SCC (%)	One year (%)	Two years (%)	Three years (%)	Four years (%)	Five years (%)	MS (months)	Survival difference (*P*)
Law et al. (1998),									
S,	30	100	NR	NR	NR	NR	NR	26	NS
S + CRT	30		NR	NR	NR	NR	NR	27	
Nygaard et al. (1992),									
S,	50	100	34	13	9	NR	NR	7	NS
S + CRT	53		39	23	17	NR	NR	7	
Le Prise et al. (1994),									
S,	45	100	47	33	14	NR	NR	11	NS
S + CRT	41		47	27	19	NR	NR	11	
Apinop et al. (1994),									
S,	34	100	39	23	20	19	10	7.4	NS
S + CRT	35		49	30	26	24	24	9.7	
Bosset et al. (1994),									
S,	139	100	67	43	37	34	32	18.6	NS
S + CRT	143		69	48	39	35	33	18.6	
Walsh et al. (1996),									
S,	55	0	44	26	6	NR	NR	11	0.01
S + CRT	58		52	37	32	NR	NR	16	
Walsh et al. (2000),									
S,	52	100	NR	NR	16	NR	11	8	0.017
S + CRT	46		NR	NR	32	NR	36	12	
Urba et al. (2001),									
S,	50	25	58	38	16	14	10	16.9	NS
S + CRT	50		72	42	30	25	20	17.6	
Burmeister et al. (2002),									
S,	128		NR	NR	NR	NR	NR	27.3	NS
S + CRT	128		NR	NR	NR	NR	NR	28.2	

Abbreviations: CRT, chemoradiotherapy; CT, computed tomography; MS, median survival; NR, not relevant; S, surgery; SCC, squamous-cell carcinoma.

(cisplatin, vinblastine, and 5-FU given concurrently with radiotherapy, 45 Gy in 30 fractions; 1.5 Gy per fraction given twice daily), and surgery alone (24). Despite showing a decrease in LR (three-year LR; 19% vs. 42%) and near doubling of OS, this underpowered study was not able to demonstrate statistical significance (three-year OS; 30% vs. 16%; $P = 0.15$).

In an European Organization for Research and Treatment of Cancer (EORTC) trial of 282 patients with squamous cell carcinoma of the esophagus, preoperative CRT (two split courses two weeks apart; 18.5 Gy in five fractions with cisplatin 80 mg/m^2) was compared to surgery alone. Bosset et al. (25) reported an increased three-year disease-free survival (RR of recurrence or death from cancer 0.6; 95% CI 0.4–0.9; $P = 0.003$) and local control (RR of LR 0.6; 95% CI 0.4–0.9; $P = 0.01$) but this was negated by a higher postoperative mortality in the chemoradiation arm (12% vs. 4%; $P = 0.012$). There was no OS advantage to combined modality therapy. The split-course radiation technique used in this study has subsequently been found to be inferior to a continuous schedule (29).

An Australian multicentered study, reported in abstract only, compared a low-dose preoperative schedule (one cycle cisplatin and 5-FU administered concurrently with 35 Gy in 15 fractions) with surgery alone in patients with adenocarcinoma or squamous cell carcinoma of the esophagus (26). Overall, there was no statistical difference between the trial arms, although a subgroup analysis of patients with squamous cell carcinoma showed an increased disease-free survival.

One of the most important determinants of long-term outcome appears to be pathological response following chemoradiation (30–34). Phase II trials have demonstrated high pathological complete response (PCR) rates with preoperative chemoradiation but interpretation of these results is limited by small sample size, variations in patient selection, and lack of quality assurance procedures in defining key outcome measures (34–36). If PCR rates are to be used as a determining endpoint in future studies, it is vital that pathological reporting of the surgical specimen is standardized. Mandard et al. has described a detailed scoring system based on the relative quantities of fibrosis to viable tumor following CRT (37). This has yet to be validated in prospective multicentered studies. While acknowledging these difficulties, Geh et al. have undertaken a comprehensive review of 26 trials (1335 patients) in an attempt to identify those factors associated with preoperative CRT treatment that correlate with a PCR (38). The overall PCR rate was 26% and the probability of PCR improved with increasing doses of radiotherapy ($P = 0.006$), 5-FU ($P = 0.003$), and cisplatin ($P = 0.018$). Increase in radiotherapy treatment time ($P = 0.035$) and increase in median age of patients ($P = 0.019$) reduced the probability of PCR. The results of completed studies using different dose schedules and the implications for future research work are discussed next.

The overall benefits of preoperative chemoradiation are uncertain and cannot be recommended as standard practice. The higher rates of PCR, a factor associated with improved outcome, and an apparent survival benefit that becomes significant some years after treatment needs to be balanced against the morbidity of therapy and increased surgical mortality. Attempts to improve patient selection and optimize the chemotherapeutic regimen should be made through clinical trials run in specialized esophagogastric units and multidisciplinary teams.

ADJUVANT RADIOTHERAPY

Rates of relapse following surgery occur at similar frequency in both local and distal sites. Radiation therapy has been used both before and after surgery in an attempt to improve local control. There have been six published randomized trials of preoperative therapy (39–44). There is considerable heterogeneity in dose schedules used ranging from 20 Gy in 10 fractions to 52 Gy in 20 fractions. All but one trial (45) was exclusively in squamous-cell carcinoma. None of these trials demonstrated an improvement in survival and a subsequent meta-analysis of updated individual patient data from five of these studies (46) failed to show a survival advantage for this approach (HR 0.89; CI 0.78–1.01; $P = 0.062$) (45) (level 1a evidence).

Postoperative radiotherapy has been compared to surgery alone in five published trials (44,46–49) (level 1b). Two trials showed improved local disease control in patients receiving radiotherapy but this was at the expense of increased morbidity (46,47). None of the studies demonstrated improved survival, indeed in one trial survival was significantly inferior (46).

DEFINITIVE RADIOTHERAPY AND CHEMORADIOTHERAPY

The majority of patients with esophageal cancer are not suitable candidates for surgery at presentation. This may be due to the presence of metastatic disease, infiltration of mediastinal structures, making a complete (R0) resection unlikely, or the presence of comorbidities, which make surgery unacceptably hazardous (50–52). Although improvements in perioperative care and specialization of surgical services have led to significant improvements in outcomes from surgery, the majority of patients still do not survive more than two years (1,2). Furthermore, patients who relapse within two years of surgery never regain their former QOL (53). This, together with evidence that nonsurgical therapy can lead to long-term disease control and survival (54,55) has led to organ-preserving definitive radiation-based therapy becoming a standard of care in the United States (56).

In a carefully selected cohort of 101 patients who were not suitable for surgery, Sykes et al. (54) demonstrated that with single modality radiation therapy alone (45–52.5 Gy in 15 or 16 fractions), 21% were alive five years after therapy (evidence level 2b). Although endoscopic ultrasound (EUS) was not available for staging, the majority of patients had tumors less then 5 cm, which is known to be associated with a lower risk of mediastinal lymph node spread.

A seminal study RTOG 85-01 reported initially by Herskovic et al. (57) and most recently updated by Cooper et al. (55), compared CRT 50 Gy in 25 fractions over five weeks together with four cycles of cisplatin and 5-FU (the first two cycles given concurrently with radiotherapy) with radiotherapy alone (64 Gy in 32 fractions). Nearly 90% of patients had squamous-cell carcinoma and the radiotherapy fields in both arms included the whole of the esophagus and regional lymph nodes. Patient survival was significantly better with combined modality therapy (three-year survival 27% vs. 0%; $P < 0.0001$) and the data monitoring committee stopped the trial following an early planned interim analysis. A further cohort of patients was treated with the same chemoradiation protocol with very similar results. This study not only confirmed the superiority of chemoradiation over radiotherapy alone but also demonstrated similar survival to that seen in surgical series. It should be noted however that combined modality therapy was associated with significant toxicity, 60% of patients had severe [World Health Organization (WHO) grade 3, 46%] or life-threatening (WHO grade 4, 14%) toxicity. There was one treatment-related death and about 30% of patients could not complete all four planned cycles of chemotherapy.

A Cochrane review comparing definitive CRT with radiotherapy alone (without surgery) has been published (58). Fifteen studies were included for this review, nine and six of which used concomitant and sequential chemoradiation, respectively (55,59–72). No benefit, either in LR or in OS, was demonstrated for sequential CRT over radiotherapy alone. There was a significant reduction in LR (OR 0.6; 95% CI 0.39–0.92; $P = 0.02$) and mortality (OR 0.58; CI 0.5–0.98; $P = 0.01$) at two years in patients treated with *concomitant* CRT (Table 4) (evidence level 1a). There was significant heterogeneity between studies reporting three- and four-year survival but when considered alone, the RTOG study showed a 28% (95% CI 16–39%) reduction in mortality at three, four, and five years. The absolute risk reduction of 11% in one-year and 7% in two-year mortality and a 12% reduction in LR favor the use of concomitant CRT in patients with good performance status. In patients with poor performance status, the toxicities of therapy need to be weighed against the potential benefits.

In the United Kingdom, CRT is largely reserved for patients with nonmetastatic disease who either have disease infiltrating into other mediastinal structures or whose comorbidities make surgical resection unacceptably hazardous. Nevertheless, even in this cohort of patients encouraging long-term survival can be achieved. Crosby et al. described a consecutive series of 90 such patients treated with CRT similar to the Herskovic regimen but with some important differences (73). First, two nonconcurrent cycles of cisplatin and 5-FU chemotherapy were given in a neoadjuvant treatment phase. This improves patient's dysphagia prior to chemoradiation while allowing time for careful radiotherapy planning. Second, radiotherapy fields were considerably smaller due to better definition of the gross tumor volume (GTV), that is, the primary tumor and nodal disease, through the use of EUS. Despite the expected poor prognosis of

TABLE 4 Studies of Concomitant Chemoradiation as Definitive Treatment for Esophageal Cancer

Author (year), treatment, trial	*n*	SCC (%)	One year (%)	Two years (%)	Three years (%)	Four years (%)	Five years (%)	MS (months)	*P* value	LRR (%)
Roussel et al. (1994)										
Ph III CRT vs. RT										
CRT	110	100	47	20	NA	8	NA	11	0.17	NA
RT	111		31	16	NA	10	NA			
Cooper et al. (1999)										
Ph III CRT vs. RT										
CRT (rand)	61	85	52	36	30	30	30	14	<0.001	47
CRT (nonrand)	69	80		35	26			17		
RT	62		34	10	0	0	0			
Minsky et al. (2002)										
Ph III CRT vs. High-dose CRT										
CRT	109	84	NA	40	36	NA	NA	18	NS	56
HD CRT	109		NA	31	24	NA	NA	13		
Bedenne et al. (2002)										
Ph III CRT vs CRT + surgery										
CRT	117	90	NA	40	NA	NA	NA	18	0.56	NA
CRT + surgery			NA	34	NA	NA	NA			
Stahl et al. (2003)										
Ph III CRT vs CRT + surgery										
CRT	88	100	NA	35	24	NA	NA	15	0.006	NA
CRT + surgery	89		NA	38	31	NA	NA	16	(equiv)	
Denham et al. (2003)										
Series										
CRT	274	74	NA	36	NA	NA	NA	NA	NR	45
Crosby et al. (2004)										
Series										
CRT	90	48	66	51	44	34	25	26	NR	45

Abbreviations: CRT, chemoradiotherapy; LRR, locoregional recurrence; MS, median survival; NA, not applicable; NR, not relevant; RT, radiotherapy; SCC, squamous-cell carcinoma.

this patient group, the median survival was 26 months [two- and five-year survival 51% (CI 41, 64) and 26% (CI 13, 52), respectively) (level 2b evidence). In this study, 45 patients (50%) suffered WHO grade 3 or 4 toxicities, although there were no treatment-related deaths. There are currently no published data of the impact on QOL of this protracted treatment, although data from patients undergoing concomitant neoadjuvant chemoradiation shows that QOL is diminished during chemotherapy, and it further deteriorates with additional radiotherapy (Blazeby, in press). It would appear, however, that in the absence of progressive disease, QOL returns to baseline values soon after completion of therapy (74).

Studies of chemoradiation consistently demonstrate a relatively high rate of local disease failure, that is,. disease relapse within the mediastinal area treated by radiotherapy fields (Table 4). In an attempt to build on the results of RTOG 85-01, and in particular reduce the rate of local disease failure, Intergroup 0123 compared a regimen similar to the Herskovic regimen (modified with narrower radiotherapy fields, radiotherapy using 1.8 Gy per fraction and an alteration in the chemotherapy schedule to reduce anticipated toxicity) with the same schedule but with a higher dose of radiotherapy (64.8 Gy in 36 fractions) (75). Two hundred and thirty-six patients, once again predominantly with squamous cell cancer, were randomized within this study. The trial had to be closed prematurely due to an excess of treatment-related deaths in the experimental arm, although the majority of these occurred before the higher dose section of the treatment protocol had been received. Although this trial did not show better disease control with higher doses of radiotherapy (56% failure at two years compared to 52% in the standard arm) it did demonstrate remarkably consistent outcomes of approximately 30% survival at three years with definitive CRT (evidence level 1b).

Another unsuccessful attempt to reduce the rate of local disease failure was tested in a phase I/II study where external beam chemoradiation (50 Gy in 25 fractions with two cycles of cisplatin and 5-FU chemotherapy) was followed by an intraluminal brachytherapy boost (15 Gy in three fractions, one week apart), given concurrently with two further cycles of chemotherapy. Once again this led to an unacceptable morbidity of 24% developing life-threatening complications. Twelve percent of patients developed a fistula, three of whom died subsequently. Despite this toxicity, there was still a high rate of local disease failure (76) (evidence level 2b).

Given the initially encouraging results of CRT together with a high rate of local relapse, two trials were designed to test the benefit of surgery following CRT compared to CRT alone (77,78). Both these studies were performed largely in patients with squamous cell carcinoma, and one has been published in abstract form only. Bedenne et al. presented data of FFCD 9102, a randomized control trial in patients with locally advanced but resectable esophageal cancer (77). Patients received 5-FU–cisplatin chemotherapy in conjunction with external beam radiotherapy, either 46 Gy in 2-Gy fractions over 4.5 weeks given continuously or using a split course (2 x 15 Gy, days 1–5 and days 22–26). Those patients with a partial response and fit for surgery or CRT were offered randomization to further chemoradiation (20 Gy in 10 fractions over two weeks or split course 15 Gy, with three cycles of chemotherapy) or surgical therapy. Four hundred and fifty-five patients initially received chemoradiation and 259 were subsequently randomized (level 2b evidence). Two-year survival was not significantly different, 40% versus 34% favoring CRT, $P = 0.56$. Ninety-day mortality was higher in the surgical arm. QOL appeared similar at two years from treatment although a greater proportion of patients required a stent in the chemoradiation arm (27% vs. 13%, $P = 0.005$).

A German study reported by Stahl et al. randomized patients to three cycles of chemotherapy (5-FU, folinic acid, etoposide, and cisplatin) and either 40 Gy radiotherapy with concurrent etoposide and platinum followed by surgery or to a total radiation dose of 66 Gy of the same CRT alone (78). With a median follow-up of six years, analysis of outcome in the 172 eligible patients (86 in each arm) has shown no difference in OS in either arm (log rank for equivalence $P = 0.05$) although local, progression-free survival was superior in patients who underwent surgery (HR 2.1; 95% CI 1.3–3.5; $P = 0.003$) (evidence level 1b). Treatment-related mortality was significantly increased in the surgery group (12.8% vs. 3.5%; P (0.03), and response to induction chemotherapy was the single independent prognostic factor for OS in Cox's regression analysis (HR 0.3; 95% CI 0.19–0.47; $P < 0.001$). This latter finding is of interest for future directions of research as it may be that early assessment of response to induction chemotherapy using positron emission tomography (PET) may be able to select out those patients unlikely to benefit from further CRT (79).

In an attempt to circumvent some of the known mechanisms of radioresistance, different radiotherapy fractionation schedules have been tested. Accelerated schedules are used to counter repopulation which occurs following the start of radiation, and hyperfractionation to reduce sublethal cellular repair. Zhao et al., using radiotherapy alone, treated patients with squamous carcinoma with a conventional fractionation schedule followed by late-course, accelerated, hyperfractionated radiotherapy (80). The three- and five-year OS of 34% and 26% respectively, is similar to that seen with chemoradiation schedules (evidence level 2b). Choi et al. used a chemoradiation schedule containing paclitaxel, cisplatin, and 5-FU (81). In addition to the standard radiotherapy dose of 45 Gy in 25 fractions, a concomitant boost of 13.5 Gy in nine fractions (days 1–5; 29–32) was used. Survival with this protocol was very encouraging, 50% and 37% of patients remaining alive three and five years after therapy, respectively (evidence level 4). Only by testing these protocols in prospective randomized studies will they be established as standard therapeutic approaches.

It is likely that refining the radiation schedule will lead to modest, though important, improvements in outcome. More substantial advances are likely to occur through improvements to the systemic component, initially with more active cytotoxic agents and subsequently through targeted therapy. Drugs such as capecitabine, oxaliplatin, irinotecan, and the taxanes are all known to have activity in esophagogastric cancer, and are all known to be potent radiosensitizers (82–88). In addition, most would involve more convenient schedules for patients, avoiding long hydration schedules with cisplatin and chemotherapy-infuser devices and central lines required for infusional 5-FU.

With the development of targeted therapies, it may be possible to counter some of the cellular mechanisms of radiation resistance. In vitro studies have demonstrated that cells transfected with an EGFR vector demonstrate resistance to radiotherapy proportional to the quantity of EGFR expression and this can be overcome with C225, a monoclonal antibody which competitively inhibits the receptor. When this receptor is bound by ligands such as EGF and transforming growth factor (TGF), autophosphorylation of its intracellular tyrosine kinase domain occurs with subsequent activation of a number of downstream signal pathways leading to cell growth, neoangiogenesis, and reduced apoptosis. Radiation also activates the receptor through homodimerization, an effect which is at least partly responsible for the mechanism of repopulation (89–92). In a study of 400 patients with squamous cell carcinoma of the head and neck, cancers with much in common with squamous cell carcinoma of the esophagus, patients who received the anti-EGFR antibody cetuximab in addition to radiotherapy had an improved three-year survival [44% vs. 57%, doubling the median survival as well (28 vs. 54 months)] (93). Apart from a predictable and manageable skin rash caused by cetuximab there was little other additional toxicity. Studies are required to confirm whether such early, promising data will translate into a real therapeutic improvement for patients with carcinoma of the esophagus.

CONCLUSION

There have been numerous attempts to improve outcomes for patients with esophageal cancer treated with surgery. Conflicting results and different interpretations in the trade-off between modest survival gains and the addition of toxic combined modality therapies has inevitably led to variations in standard practise throughout the world. In patients who are physiologically fit, for the relatively few patients presenting with early disease (T1-2, N0), surgery alone remains the treatment of choice. For patients with more typically locally advanced disease (T3-4 and/or N1), where an R0 resection appears possible, surgery, with or without preoperative chemotherapy, is the preferred therapy in the United Kingdom and Europe. In the United States, patients more commonly receive chemoradiation either as preoperative or definitive treatment (94). Patients with nonmetastatic disease who are unfit for surgery should be considered for definitive chemoradiation.

Refining the optimum schedule and combination of treatments requires further clinical research preferably in the form of prospective randomized studies. Comparing the relative benefits of preoperative chemotherapy with preoperative CRT and definitive CRT and, surgical-based therapy should be a priority. These studies should be performed with adequate assessment of differences in toxicity and QOL so that clinicians and patients can make informed decisions on treatment alternatives.

Future directions of clinical research should lead to earlier diagnosis, improved patient selection, and better assessment of treatment response. Perhaps the most important research will lead us toward selection of therapy based on the genetic phenotype of the patient's tumor. Such predictive testing should lead to optimization of treatment schedules in those patients most likely to benefit and avoid unnecessary toxicities in those that are not.

EVIDENCE SUMMARY

- There is level 1 evidence for a survival benefit from preoperative chemotherapy, although this only becomes significant after five years. Two very similar large recent trials disagree about this outcome.
- There is no good evidence for a survival benefit from postoperative chemotherapy.
- There is level 1 evidence for a survival benefit and reduction of LRR after neoadjuvant chemoradiation. However, there is a strong trend toward increased operative mortality.
- There is no good evidence of survival benefit from preoperative radiotherapy alone.
- There is level 1 evidence that concomitant but not sequential chemoradiation (without surgery) produces better survival than radiotherapy alone, but combined treatment has high toxicity (74% of patients experience WHO grade 3 or 4 effects).
- There is level 2 evidence that chemoradiation without surgery can produce median survival similar to that seen after surgery. Two randomized trials have compared chemoradiation alone with chemoradiation followed by surgery. Neither found a survival difference,

although results of one are not mature. Both found an increased treatment-related mortality with surgery, but the mature trial found that surgery halved the rate of LRR.

REFERENCES

1 Kelsen DP, Ginsberg R, Pajak TF, et al. Chemotherapy followed by surgery compared with surgery alone for localized esophageal cancer. N Engl J Med 1998; 339(27):1979–1984.
2. Medical Research Council Oesophageal Cancer Working Group. Surgical resection with or without preoperative chemotherapy in oesophageal cancer: a randomised controlled trial. Lancet 2002; 359(9319):1727–1733.
3. Wang C, Ding T, Chang L. A randomized clinical study of preoperative chemotherapy for esophageal carcinoma. Zhonghua Zhong Liu Za Zhi 2001; 23(3):254–255.
4. Ancona E, Ruol A, Santi S, et al. Only pathologic complete response to neoadjuvant chemotherapy improves significantly the long term survival of patients with resectable esophageal squamous cell carcinoma: final report of a randomized, controlled trial of preoperative chemotherapy versus surgery alone. Cancer 2001; 91(11):2165–2174.
5. Baba M, Natsugoe S, Shimada M, et al. Prospective evaluation of preoperative chemotherapy in resectable squamous cell carcinoma of the thoracic esophagus. Dis Esophagus 2000; 13(2):136–141.
6. Kok TC, vLanschot J, Siersema PD, vOverhagen H, Tilanus HW. Neoadjuvant chemotherapy in operable esophageal squamous cell cancer: final report of a phase III multicenter randomized controlled trial. Proc Am Soc Clin Oncol 1997; 17:984 (abstr).
7. Law S, Fok M, Chow S, Chu KM, Wong J. Preoperative chemotherapy versus surgical therapy alone for squamous cell carcinoma of the esophagus: a prospective randomized trial. J Thorac Cardiovasc Surg 1997; 114(2):210–217.
8. Maipang T, Vasinanukorn P, Petpichetchian C, et al. Induction chemotherapy in the treatment of patients with carcinoma of the esophagus. J Surg Oncol 1994; 56(3):191–197.
9. Nygaard K, Hagen S, Hansen HS, et al. Pre-operative radiotherapy prolongs survival in operable esophageal carcinoma: a randomized, multicenter study of pre-operative radiotherapy and chemotherapy. The second Scandinavian trial in esophageal cancer. World J Surg 1992; 16(6):1104–1109.
10. Roth JA, Pass HI, Flanagan MM, Graeber GM, Rosenberg JC, Steinberg S. Randomized clinical trial of preoperative and postoperative adjuvant chemotherapy with cisplatin, vindesine, and bleomycin for carcinoma of the esophagus. J Thorac Cardiovasc Surg 1988; 96(2):242–248.
11. Schlag PM. Randomized trial of preoperative chemotherapy for squamous cell cancer of the esophagus. The Chirurgische Arbeitsgemeinschaft Fuer Onkologie der Deutschen Gesellschaft Fuer Chirurgie Study Group. Arch Surg 1992; 127(12):1446–1450.
12. Malthaner R, Fenlon D. Preoperative chemotherapy for respectable thoracic esophageal cancer (Cochrane Review). In: The Cochrane Library, Issue 3. Oxford: Update Software, 2004.
13. Bhansali MS, Vaidya JS, Bhatt RG, Patil PK, Badwe RA, Desai PB. Chemotherapy for carcinoma of the esophagus: a comparison of evidence from meta-analyses of randomized trials and of historical control studies. Ann Oncol 1996; 7(4):355–359.
14. Piedbois P, Buyse M. Meta-analyses based on abstracted data: a step in the right direction, but only a first step. J Clin Oncol 2004; 22(19):3839–3841.
15. Cunningham D, Allum WH, Stenning SP, Weeden S for the NCRI Upper GI Cancer Clinical Studies Group. Perioperative chemotherapy in operable gastric and lower oesophageal cancer: final results of a randomised, controlled trial (the MAGIC trial, ISRCTN 93793971). Proc Am Soc Clin Oncol 2005; 23:308s (abstr).
16. Group JEO. A comparison of chemotherapy and radiotherapy as adjuvant treatment to surgery for esophageal carcinoma. Japanese Esophageal Oncology Group. Chest 1993; 104:203–220.
17. Iizuka T, Isono K, Watanabe H, et al. A randomized trial comparing surgery to surgery plus postoperative chemotherapy for localized squamous carcinoma of the thoracic esophagus: The Japan Clinical Oncology Group (JCOG) Study. Proc Am Soc Clin Oncol 1998; 17:282 (abstr).
18. Ando N, Iizuka T, Ide H, et al. Japan Clinical Oncology Group. Surgery plus chemotherapy compared with surgery alone for localized squamous cell carcinoma of the thoracic esophagus: a Japan Clinical Oncology Group Study—JCOG9204. J Clin Oncol 2003; 21(24):4592–4596.
19. Urschel JD, Vasan H. A meta-analysis of randomised controlled trials that compared neoadjuvant chemoradiation and surgery to surgery alone for resectable esophageal cancer. Am J Surg 2003; 185(6):538–543.
20. Nygaard K, Hagen S, Hansen HS, et al. Pre-operative radiotherapy prolongs survival in operable esophageal carcinoma: a randomized, multicenter study of pre-operative radiotherapy and chemotherapy. The second Scandinavian trial in esophageal cancer. World J Surg 1992; 16:1104–1109.
21. Le Prise E, Etienne PL, Meunier B, et al. A randomized study of chemotherapy, radiation therapy, and surgery versus surgery for localized squamous cell carcinoma of the esophagus. Cancer 1994; 73:1779–1784.

22. Apinop C, Puttisak P, Preecha N. A prospective study of combined therapy in esophageal cancer. Hepatol Gastroenterol 1994; 41:391–393.
23. Walsh TN, Noonan N, Hollywood D, Kelly A, Keeling N, Hennessy TPJ. A comparison of multimodal therapy and surgery for esophageal adenocarcinoma. N Engl J Med 1996; 335:462–467.
24. Urba SG, Orringer MB, Turrisi A, Iannettoni M, Forastiere A, Strawderman M. Randomized trial of preoperative chemoradiation versus surgery alone in patients with locoregional esophageal carcinoma. J Clin Oncol 2001; 19:305–313.
25. Bosset JF, Gignoux M, Triboulet JP, et al. Chemoradiotherapy followed by surgery compared with surgery alone in squamous-cell cancer of the esophagus. N Engl J Med 1997; 337:161–167.
26. Burmeister BH, Smithers BM, Fitzgerald L, et al., Trans Tasman Radiation Oncology Group, Australasian Gastrointestinal Trials Group and Clinical Trials Centre: A randomized phase III trial of preoperative chemoradiation followed by surgery (CR-S) versus surgery alone (S) for localized resectable cancer of the esophagus. Proc Am Soc Clin Oncol 2002; 21:518(abstr).
27. Law S, Kwong DLW, Tung HM, Chu KM, Sham JST, Choy D, Wong J. Preoperative chemoradiation for squamous cell esophageal cancer: A prospective randomised trial. Can J Gantroenterol 1998; 12(suppl 8):56B.
28. Walsh TN, McDonnell CO, Mulligan ED, et al. Multimodal therapy versus surgery alone for squamous cell carcinoma of the esophagus: a prospective randomized trial [abstract]. Gastroenterology 2000; 118(suppl 2):1008.
29. Jacob JH, Seitz JF, Langlois C, et al. Definitive concurrent chemo-radiation therapy (CRT) in squamous cell carcinoma of the Esophagous (SCCE): preliminary results of a French randomized trial comparing standard vs split course irradiation (FNCLCC-FFCD 9305). Proc Am Soc Clin Oncol 1999; 18:1035 (abstr).
30. Forastiere A, Orringer M, Perez-Tamayo C, Urba SG, Zahurak M. Preoperative chemoradiation followed by transhiatal oesophagectomy for carcinoma of the esophagus: final report. J Clin Oncol 1993; 11:1118–1123.
31. Stahl M, Wilke H, Fink U, et al. Combined preoperative chemotherapy and radiotherapy in patients with locally advanced esophageal cancer: interim analysis of phase II trial. J Clin Oncol 1996; 14:829–837.
32. Suntharalingam M, Vines E, Slawson R, et al. Important predictors of response determined by surgical staging prior to triple modality therapy for esophageal cancer. Int J Radiat Oncol Biol Phys 1997; 39(suppl):204 (abstr).
33. Jones DR, Detterbeck FC, Egan TM, Parker LA Jr, Bernard SA, Tepper JE. Induction chemoradiotherapy followed by esophagectomy in patients with carcinoma of the esophagus. Ann Thorac Surg 1997; 64(1):185–192.
34. Forastiere AA, Heitmiller RF, Lee DJ, et al. Intensive chemoradiation followed by esophagectomy for squamous cell and adenocarcinoma of the esophagus. Cancer J Sci Am 1997; 3:144–152.
35. Girvin GW, Matsumoto GH, Bates DM, Garcia JM, Clyde JC, Lin PH. Treating esophageal cancer with a combination of chemotherapy, radiation and excision. Am J Surg 1995; 169:685–695.
36. Adham M, Baulieux J, Gerard JP, Delaroche E, Berthoux N, Ducerf C. Oesophageal epidermoid carcinoma: results of surgery after neoadjuvant radiochemotherapy. Br J Surg 1998; 85(suppl 2):6 (abstr).
37. Mandard AM, Dalibard F, Mandard JC, et al. Pathologic assessment of tumour regression after preoperative chemoradiotherapy of esophageal carcinoma. Cancer 1994; 73:2680–2686.
38. Geh J, Bond S, Bentzen S, Glynne-Jones R. Preoperative chemoradiotherapy in esophageal cancer: evidence of dose response. Proc Am Soc Clin Oncol 2000; 19:958 (abstr).
39. Gignoux M, Roussel A, Paillot B, et al. The value of preoperative radiotherapy in esophageal cancer: results of a study of the E.O.R.T.C. World J Surg 1987; 11(4):426–432.
40. Wang M, Gu XZ, Yin WB, Huang GJ, Wang LJ, Zhang DW. Randomized clinical trial on the combination of preoperative irradiation and surgery in the treatment of esophageal carcinoma: report on 206 patients. Int J Radiat Oncol Biol Phys 1989; 16(2):325–327.
41. Nygaard K, Hagen S, Hansen HS, et al. Pre-operative radiotherapy prolongs survival in operable esophageal carcinoma: a randomized, multicenter study of pre-operative radiotherapy and chemotherapy. The second Scandinavian trial in esophageal cancer. World J Surg 1992; 16(6):1104–1109.
42. Arnott SJ, Duncan W, Kerr GR, et al. Low dose preoperative radiotherapy for carcinoma of the oesophagus: results of a randomized clinical trial. Radiother Oncol 1992; 24(2):108–113.
43. Launois B, Delarue D, Campion JP, Kerbaol M. Preoperative radiotherapy for carcinoma of the esophagus. Surg Gynecol Obstet 1981; 153(5):690–692.
44. Fok M, McShane J, Law SYK, Wong J. Prospective randomised study in the treatment of oesophageal carcinoma. Asian J Surg 1994; 17:223–229.
45. Arnott SJ, Duncan W, Gignoux M, et al. Preoperative radiotherapy in esophageal carcinoma: a meta-analysis using individual patient data (Oesophageal Cancer Collaborative Group). Int J Radiat Oncol Biol Phys 1998; 41(3):579–583.
46. Fok M, Sham JS, Choy D, Cheng SW, Wong J. Postoperative radiotherapy for carcinoma of the esophagus: a prospective, randomized controlled study. Surgery 1993; 113(2):138–147.

47. Teniere P, Hay JM, Fingerhut A, Fagniez PL. Postoperative radiation therapy does not increase survival after curative resection for squamous cell carcinoma of the middle and lower esophagus as shown by a multicenter controlled trial. French University Association for Surgical Research. Surg Gynecol Obstet 1991; 173(2):123–130.
48. Zieren HU, Muller JM, Jacobi CA, Pichlmaier H, Muller RP, Staar S. Adjuvant postoperative radiation therapy after curative resection of squamous cell carcinoma of the thoracic esophagus: a prospective randomized study. World J Surg 1995; 19(3):444–449.
49. Xiao ZF, Yang ZY, Liang J, et al. Value of radiotherapy after radical surgery for esophageal carcinoma: a report of 495 patients. Ann Thorac Surg 2003; 75(2):331–336.
50. Pye JK, Crumlin MK, Charles J, Kerwat R, Foster ME, Biffin A. Hospital clinicians in Wales. One-year survey of carcinoma of the oesophagus and stomach in Wales. Br J Surg 2001; 88:278–285.
51. Muller JM, Erasmi H, Stelzner M, Zieren U, Pichlmaier H. Surgical therapy of oesophageal carcinoma. Br J Surg 1990; 77:845–857.
52. Coia LR. Chemoradiation: a superior alternative for the primary management of oesophageal carcinoma. Semin Radiat Oncol 1994; 4(3):157–164.
53. Blazeby J, Farndon J, Donovan J, Alderson D. A prospective longitudinal study examining the quality of life of patients with esophageal carcinoma. Cancer 2000; 88(8):1781–1787.
54. Sykes AJ, Burt PA, Slevin NJ, Stout R, Marrs JE. Radical radiotherapy for carcinoma of the oesophagus: an effective alternative to surgery. Radiother Oncol 1998; 48(1):15–21.
55. Cooper JS, Guo MD, Herskovic A, et al. Chemotherapy of locally advanced esophageal cancer: long term follow-up of a prospective randomized trial (RTOG 85-01). JAMA 1999; 281:1623–1627.
56. Suntharalingam M, Moughan J, Coia LR, et al. The national practice for patients receiving radiation therapy for carcinoma of the esophagus: results of the 1996–1999 Patterns for Care Study. Int J Radiat Oncol Biol Phys 2003; 56(4):981–987.
57. Herskovic A, Martz K, Al-Sarraf M, et al. Combined chemotherapy and radiotherapy compared with radiotherapy alone in patients with cancer of the esophagus. N Engl J Med 1992; 326(24):1593–1598.
58. Wong R, Malthaner R. Combined chemotherapy and radiotherapy (without surgery) compared with radiotherapy alone in localized carcinoma of the esophagus (Cochrane Review). In: The Cochrane Library, Issue 2. Oxford: Update Software, 2005.
59. Andersen AP, Berdal P, Edsmyr F, et al. Irradiation, chemotherapy and surgery in esophageal cancer: a randomized clinical study. The first Scandinavian trial in esophageal cancer. Radiother Oncol 1984; 2:179–188.
60. Araujo CM, Souhami L, Gil RA, et al. A randomized trial comparing radiation therapy versus concomitant radiation therapy and chemotherapy in carcinoma of the thoracic esophagus. Cancer 1991; 67:2258–2261.
61. Cooper JS, Guo MD, Herskovic A, et al. Chemotherapy of locally advanced esophageal cancer: long term follow-up of a prospective randomized trial (RTOG 85-01). JAMA 1999; 281:1623–1627.
62. Earle JD, Gelber RD, Moertel CG, Hahn RG. A controlled evaluation of combined radiation and bleomycin therapy for squamous cell carcinoma of the esophagus. Int J Rad Onc Biol Phys 1980; 6:821–826.
63. Hatlevoll R, Hagen S, Hansen HS, et al. Bleomycin/cisplatin as neoadjuvant chemotherapy before radical radiotherapy in localized, inoperable carcinoma of the esophagus. A prospective randomized multicenter study: the second Scandinavian trial in esophageal cancer. Radiother Oncol 1992; 24:114–116.
64. Hishikawa Y, Miura T, Oshitani T, et al. A randomized prospective study of adjuvant chemotherapy after radiotherapy in unresectable esophageal carcinoma. Dis Esophagus 1991; 4(2):85–90.
65. Lu XJ, Miao RH, Li XQ. Combination of selective arterial infusion chemotherapy with radiotherapy in the treatment of advanced esophageal carcinoma. Chn J Clin Oncol 1995; 22(4):262–265.
66. Roussel A, Bleiberg H, Dalesio O, et al. Palliative therapy of inoperable oesophageal carcinoma with radiotherapy and methotrexate: final results of a controlled clinical trial. Int J Radiat Oncol Biol Phys 1989; 16:67–72.
67. Roussel A, Haegele P, Paillot B, et al. Results of the EORTC-GTCCT phase III trial of irradiation vs irradiation and CDDP in inoperable esophageal cancer. Proc Am Soc Clin Oncol 1994; 13:199 [abstr].
68. Slabber CF, Nel JS, Schoeman L, Burger W, Falkson G, Falkson Cl. A randomized study of radiotherapy alone versus radiotherapy plus 5-fluorouracil and platinum in patients with inoperable, locally advanced squamous cancer of the esophagus. Am J Clin Oncol 1998; 21:462–465.
69. Wobbes Th, Baron B, Paillot B, et al. Prospective randomised study of split-course radiotherapy versus cisplatin plus split-course radiotherapy in inoperable squamous cell carcinoma of the oesophagus. Eur J Cancer 2001; 37:470–477.
70. Zhang A. Radiation combined with bleomycin for esophageal carcinoma—a randomized study of 99 patients. Chung Hua Chung Liu Tsa Chih 1984; 6(5):372–374.
71. Zhou JC. Randomized trial of combined chemotherapy including high dose cisplatin and radiotherapy for esophageal cancer. Chung Hua Chung Liu Tsa Chih 1991; 13:291–294.

72. Zhu S, Wan J, Zhou D, et al. Combination of external beam and intracavitary radiation and carboplatin chemotherapy in the treatment of esophageal carcinoma. Chn J Clin Oncol 2000; 27(1):5–8.
73. Crosby TD, Brewster AE, Borley A, et al. Definitive chemoradiation in patients with inoperable oesophageal carcinoma. Br J Cancer 2004; 90(1):70–75.
74. Bonnetain F, Bedenne L, Michel P, et al. Definitive results of a comparative longitudinal quality of life study using the Spitzer index in the randomized multicentric phase III trial FFCD 9102 (surgery vs radiochemotherapy in patients with locally advanced esophageal cancer). Proc Am Soc Clin Oncol 2003; 22:1002 (abstr).
75. Minsky BD, Pajak TF, Ginsberg RJ, et al. INT 0123 (Radiation Therapy Oncology Group 94-05) phase III trial of combined-modality therapy for esophageal cancer: high-dose versus standard-dose radiation therapy. J Clin Oncol 2002; 20(5):1167–1174.
76. Gaspar LE, Winter K, Kocha WI, Coia LR, Herskovic A, Graham M. A phase I/II study of external beam radiation, brachytherapy, and concurrent chemotherapy for patients with localized carcinoma of the esophagus (Radiation Therapy Oncology Group Study 9207): final report. Cancer 2000; 88(5):988–995.
77. Bedenne L, Michel P, Bouche O, et al: Randomized phase III trial in locally advanced esophageal cancer: radiochemotherapy followed by surgery versus radiochemotherapy alone (FFCD 9102). Proc Am Soc Clin Oncol 2002; 21:130a (abstr).
78. Stahl M, Stuschke M, Lehmann N, et al. Chemoradiation with and without surgery in patients with locally advanced squamous cell carcinoma of the esophagus. J Clin Oncol 2005; 23(10):2310–2317.
79. Weber WA, Ott K, Becker K, et al. Prediction of response to preoperative chemotherapy in adenocarcinomas of the esophagogastric junction by metabolic imaging. J Clin Oncol 2001; 19:3058–3065.
80. Zhao KL, Shi XH, Jiang GL, Wang Y. Late-course accelerated hyperfractionated radiotherapy for localized esophageal carcinoma. Int J Radiat Oncol Biol Phys 2004; 60(1):123–129.
81. Choi N, Park SD, Lynch T, et al. Twice-daily radiotherapy as concurrent boost technique during two chemotherapy cycles in neoadjuvant chemoradiotherapy for resectable esophageal carcinoma: mature results of phase II study. Int J Radiat Oncol Biol Phys 2004; 60(1):111–122.
82. Chong G, Cunningham D. Can cisplatin and infused 5-fluorouracil be replaced by oxaliplatin and capecitabine in the treatment of advanced oesophagogastric cancer? The REAL 2 trial. Clin Oncol (R Coll Radiol) 2005; 17(2):79–80.
83. Maurel J, Cervantes A, Conill C, et al. Phase I trial of oxaliplatin in combination with cisplatin, protacted-infusion fluorouracil, and radiotherapy in advanced esophageal and gastroesophageal carcinoma. Int J Radiat Oncol Biol Phys 2005; 62(1):91–96.
84. Sumpter KA, et al. Randomised, multicenter phase III study comparing capecitabine with fluorouracil and oxaliplatin with cisplatin in patients with advanced oesophagogastric cancer: confirmation of dose escalation. Proc Am Soc Clin Oncol 2003; 22:1031(abstr).
85. Giovannini M, Conroy T, Francois E, et al. Phase I study of first line radiochemotherapy (RCT) with oxaliplatin (Ox) fluorouracil (FU) and Folinic Acid (FA) in inoperable locally advanced (LA) or metastatic (M) esophageal cancer (EC). Proc Am Soc Clin Oncol 2004; 23:4044 (abstr).
86. Ilson DH, Bains M, Kelsen DP, et al. Phase I trial of escalating-dose irinotecan given weekly with cisplatin and concurrent radiotherapy in locally advanced esophageal cancer. J Clin Oncol 2003; 21:2926–2932.
87. Adelstein DJ, Rice TW, Rybicki LA, et al. Does paclitaxel improve the chemoradiotherapy of locoregionally advanced esophageal cancer? A nonrandomized comparison with fluorouracil-based therapy. J Clin Oncol 2000; 18(10):2032–2039.
88. Meluch A, Greco A, Gray JR, et al. Preoperative therapy with concurrent paclitaxel/carboplatin/infusional 5-FU and radiation therapy in locoregional esophageal cancer: final results of a Minnie Pearl Cancer Research Network Phase II Trial. Cancer J 2003; 9(4):251–260.
89. Liang K, Kian Ang K, Milas L, Hunter N, Fan Z. The epidermal growth factor receptor mediates radioresistance. Int J Rad Onc Biol Phys 2003; 57(1):246–254.
90. Baumann M, Krause M. Targeting the epidermal growth factor receptor in radiotherapy: radiological mechanisms, preclinical and clinical results. Radiother Oncol 2004; 72:257–266.
91. Eriksen JG, Steiniche T, Askaa J, Alsner J, Overgaard J. The prognostic value of epidermal growth factor receptor expression is related to tumour differentiation and the overall treatment time of radiotherapy in squamous cell carcinomas of the head and neck. Int J Radiat Oncol Biol Phys 2004; 58:561–566.
92. Petersen C, Eicheler W, Frommel A, et al. Proliferation and micromilieu during fractionated irradiation of human FaDu squamous cell carcinoma in nude mice. Int J Radiat Biol 2003; 79(7):469–477.
93. Bonner JA, Giralt J, Harari PM, et al. Cetuximab prolongs survival in patients with locoregionally advanced squamous cell carcinoma of head and neck: a phase III study of high dose radiation therapy with or without cetuximab. Proc Am Soc Clin Oncol 2004; 22:5507 (abstr).
94. Coia LR, Minsky BD, John MJ, et al. The evaluation and treatment of patients receiving radiation therapy for carcinoma of the esophagus: results of the 1992–1994 Patterns of Care Study. Cancer 1999; 85:2499–2505.

Search Strategy. OVID version of MEDLINE 1980-2006

1. esophageal neoplasms/
2. [(esophag$ or esophag$) adj3 (cancer$ or carcinomas or neoplas$ or tumo?r$ or malignan$ or adenocarcinoma$ or squamous$ or adenosquamous$ or carcinoid$ or basosquamous$)]jnp.
3. 1 or 2
4. exp chemotherapy, adjuvant/
5. exp radiotherapy, adjuvant/
6. exp drug therapy, combination/
7. exp combined modality therapy/
8. exp multimodal treatment/
9. exp Neoadjuvant Therapy/
10. exp Antineoplastic Combined Chemotherapy Protocols/
11. exp radiotherapy/
12. chemoradiation.mp.
13. (multimod$ or adjuvant or neoadjuvant or adjunct$ or concurrent or combin$ or conjunct$).mp.
14. or/3-13
15. 3 and 14
16. exp Randomized Controlled Trials/
17. randomized controlled trial.pt.
18. (random$ adj3 trial).tw.
19. or/16-18
20. 15 and 19
21. limit 20 to (humans and english language and yr="1980-2006")

The above search strategy identified papers of possible relevance to the chapter. This list of references was then manually reviewed to select the articles that were used as supporting evidence. This was supplemented by cross-references from selected articles, hand searching relevant proceedings from ASCO and authors' own knowledge of the topic.

7 The Role of Surgery in Cancer of the Stomach

Nikhil Misra and R. Hardwick
Addenbrooke's Hospital, Cambridge, U.K.

Peter McCulloch
Nuffield Department of Surgery, University of Oxford, Oxford, U.K.

INTRODUCTION

Gastric cancer remains one of the commonest causes of death from cancer worldwide, despite a decreasing incidence, particularly in Western countries (1). The majority of patients with this disease present at an advanced stage, especially in Western countries, and the chances of a cure for patients with advanced disease remain low. Surgery remains the mainstay of treatment, but because of the poor survival rates, the use of adjuvant and neoadjuvant chemotherapy and radiotherapy have been explored, as have more radical surgical techniques. The latter, in the form of D2 extended lymphadenectomy, has remained highly controversial in the world of gastric surgery over the last three decades. Even more radical surgery (D4 dissection) is still contemplated in Japan. Endoscopic mucosal resection seems now to have a useful and defined role in early cancer. Minimally invasive surgery is now reaching a stage of development where its role needs to be clarified. Surgery has a diminishing role in palliation as other methods have supplanted it in several of its symptom-relieving roles.

EPIDEMIOLOGY

While the overall worldwide incidence of gastric cancer has decreased, there has been a dramatic change in the epidemiology of the disease, especially in western countries. While tumors of the distal and midstomach have declined, there has been a rapid increase in the incidence of proximal gastric tumors (1). Combined with the increasing incidence of adenocarcinoma of the lower esophagus, this has created a new pathological entity—adenocarcinoma of the gastro-esophageal junction, which Siewert and Stein defined as a tumor located 5 cm proximal or distal to the gastro-esophageal junction (2). These junctional tumors now represent the majority of new cases presenting to upper gastrointestinal surgeons in the western world and their surgical management is dealt with in detail by Stein et al. in this volume.

The number of new cases of gastric cancer worldwide was recently estimated as over 600,000 in males and over 330,000 in females (3), giving age-standardized incidence rates of 22.0 and 10.4 per 100,000 population, respectively. Stomach cancer was the second most common cause of cancer mortality in males globally, behind carcinoma of the lung, accounting for around 445,000 male deaths or an age-standardized mortality rate of 16.3 per 100,000. The changing epidemiology of gastric cancer incidence at different anatomical subsites has been well documented in the United States and in Europe (4,5). Newnham et al. (4) examined epidemiological data from England and Wales between 1977 and 1998, and documented an increase in the incidence of gastric cardia tumors, from 2.0 to 5.4 per 100,000 population in males, and from 0.6 to 1.4 per 100,000 in females, in contrast to a decrease in the incidence of noncardial tumors in both sexes, and an overall declining incidence of the disease. Devessa et al. (5) documented a similar rise in the incidence of cardia cancer in white males in the United States between 1974 and 1994, from 2.1 to 3.3 per 100,000 population. Again, there was a decrease in the incidence of tumors arising in other gastric subsites from 5.1 to 3.7 per 100,000. An element of misclassification in the past has been suggested as part of the reason for this trend (6), but the evidence for a real increase seems secure. Data from a register of resected gastric cancer in Japan between 1963 and

1990 in Japan, shows a similar trend but with a much lower magnitude in the rising incidence of cardia cancer. There was an increase in the proportion of resected tumors located within the proximal third of the stomach from 12.2% to 17.3% (7). The records from two major cancer centers also showed an increase in the proportion of proximal gastric cancers resected—from 0.4% to 4.5% between 1962 and 1997 in Tokyo, and from 0.9% to 1.8% in Osaka.

In conclusion, gastric cancer remains one of the biggest causes of cancer mortality worldwide, despite its overall decreasing incidence. The epidemiology of the disease has changed over the last four decades, with an increase in the proportion of tumors of the gastric cardia, a change more pronounced in western countries (evidence level 1).

PATHOLOGY

Malignant tumors of the stomach can be divided into four main pathological types—epithelial, mesenchymal, and neuroendocrine tumors and lymphomas. Mesenchymal tumors can be subdivided into categories as defined by immunohistochemical markers such as desmin (derived from muscle), S100 (from nerve), and c-kit (from the interstitial cells of Cajal). Leiomyomas and leiomyosarcomas are strongly positive for desmin; neurofibromas are positive for S100, and gastrointestinal stromal tumors (GISTs) are positive for the c-kit protein. Neuroendocrine or carcinoid tumors are derived from specialized endocrine cells found within the gastric mucosa, such as enterochromograffin-like cells. Examples of such tumors include the gastrin-producing carcinoid tumors seen in Zollinger-Ellison syndrome.

Gastric lymphoma accounts for around 5% of all tumors of the stomach. The stomach is the commonest site for gastrointestinal lymphomas, the majority of which are B-cell non-Hodgkin's lymphomas. Many low-grade lymphomas are thought to be caused by the interaction of native lymphoid tissue and *Helicobacter pylori* infection [mucosal associated lymphoid tissue (MALT) lymphomas]. These tumor types in the gastrointestinal tract are dealt with generically elsewhere in this volume.

The majority of malignant tumors are of epithelial origin, with over 90% being adenocarcinomas. The pathogenesis of these epithelial cancers is multifactorial. Correa et al. described a stepwise pathological change from normal gastric mucosa to chronic atrophic gastritis leading to intestinal metaplasia, dysplasia, and eventually adenocarcinoma (8). This process is mainly driven by inflammatory damage such as that occurring in chronic bacterial (*H. pylori*) infection, or chemical irritation (duodeno-gastric reflux). The Correa model fits the pattern of endemic, distal, well-differentiated cancer, but does not adequately describe the development of diffuse cancers. The progression from dysplasia to cancer appears to be reversible until a late stage in the process (9). Lauren proposed a classification differentiating between intestinal-type tumors (53%), which form glandular structures microscopically, and diffuse carcinomas (33%), which have no distinct structure and secrete mucin (10). The remaining 14% have features of both types and are defined as unclassified. Despite this drawback, the classification has survived because it correlates with the molecular oncology of the tumors described.

Early gastric cancer is defined as a carcinoma limited to the mucosa or submucosa. The Japanese Endoscopic Society classifies these tumors into three main types—type I (protuberant, polypoidal lesions), type II (superficial lesions, further divided into elevated, flat, and depressed tumors, a, b and c), and type III (depressed) (11). Intramucosal cancer metastasizes to perigastric nodes in less than 5% of cases, but submucosal lesions are associated with lymphatic metastases in up to 20% of cases, probably because an abundant layer of lymphatic plexuses exists in the submucosal layer (12). The prognosis for early gastric cancer is favorable, with five-year survival rates of around 90% being reported after surgery (13), and 15-year survival rates being over 75% (14).

Adenocarcinomas of the stomach spread by four means. First is direct invasion of the tumor into adjacent organs, commonly extension into the esophagus, or invasion into the pancreas, spleen or transverse colon. Second is lymphatic metastasis, the most commonly encountered route of spread for both the diffuse and intestinal types. The probability of lymph-node metastases depends on the depth of penetration of the primary lesion through the layers of the stomach. Detailed retrospective accounts of lymph-node spread in large numbers of Japanese patients provided the basis for our current knowledge of this pathway (15).

Despite the vascular nature of gastric tissue and the rich blood supply of the stomach, hematogenous spread of the stomach, most commonly to the liver, is relatively uncommon and late. Finally, peritoneal spread of malignant cells occurs once the visceral peritoneum of the stomach has been breached. This method of spread is more common with diffuse-type cancers than the intestinal-type (16).

STAGING

The appropriate management of gastric cancer depends on the stage of the disease. This can be quantified using both clinicopathological and histopathological staging methods. In current U.K. practice, staging results are discussed in mandatory multidisciplinary meetings involving surgeons, gastroenterologists, radiologists, pathologists, oncologists, palliative care physicians, and paramedical staff including dieticians and nurse specialists. The end point of this process is to plan appropriate management for each patient with a new diagnosis of stomach cancer.

Clinical staging depends on the anatomical extent of penetration of the lesion, involvement of adjacent organs, the involvement and extent of lymph node spread, hematogenous spread to distant sites, and peritoneal involvement. The internationally unified TNM (tumor node metastases) system was created in 1986 in concordance between the American Joint Committee on Cancer (AJCC), the Japanese Joint Committee (JJC), and the Union International Cancer Centre (UICC). This resulted in a single staging system, most recently updated in 2003 (17).

T-Stage

Tx	Tumor cannot be assessed
T0	No evidence of primary tumor
Tis	Intraepithelial tumor confined to the lamina propria
T1	Tumor extends into but not beyond the submucosa
T2a	Tumor extends into but not beyond the muscularis propria
T2b	Tumor invades the subserosa
T3	Tumor extends into the serosa but not into adjacent organs
T4	Tumor invades into adjacent organs.

N-Stage

Nx	Regional lymph nodes cannot be assessed
N0	No regional lymph nodes involved
N1	Metastases in one to six regional lymph nodes
N2	Metastases in 7 to 15 regional lymph nodes
N3	Metastases in more than 15 lymph nodes.

M-Stage

Mx	Distant metastatic spread cannot be assessed
M0	No evidence of distant metastases
M1	Evidence of distant metastases.

Regional lymph-node groups are defined as perigastric nodes (along both curvatures), regional nodes around the celiac axis and along its main tributaries (left gastric, splenic, and common hepatic arteries), and the nodes in the hepatoduodenal ligament. There is a minimum requirement of 15 analyzed lymph nodes before an N-stage can be assigned. Evidence from Japan indicates that at least 30 nodes should be examined, as patients with equivalent-stage disease who had 20 to 30 negative nodes examined had a more favorable prognosis than those with 10 to 19 negatively examined nodes (18).

The derived TNM categories are assigned to four main stages.

Stage	T	N	M
0	Tis	N0	M0
Ia	T1	N0	M0
Ib	T1	N1	M0
	T2a/b	N0	M0
II	T1	N2	M0

	T2a/b	N1	M0
	T3	N0	M0
IIIa	T2a/b	N2	M0
	T3	N1	M0
	T4	N0	M0
IIIb	T3	N2	M0
IV	T4	N1,2,3	M0
	T1,2,3	N3	M0
	T any	N any	M1

The Japanese Research Society for Gastric Cancer (JRSGC) took a quite different approach to staging and classification, and set out a detailed set of clinical "rules" to accurately describe gastric cancer in 1963. They have published multiple subsequent editions of their initial set of rules, and in 1998 published their second English edition, based on the thirteenth Japanese edition (19). The position within the stomach of the primary tumor is assigned to three locations: C-area—proximal stomach; M-area—body of the stomach; and A-area—distal stomach (Fig. 1).

The Japanese peitoneum, hepatic, nodal, serosal (PHNS) system is created from four clinical factors: peritoneal dissemination; liver metastasis (H); nodal metastasis; and serosal invasion. The N-stage uses a system of anatomical grouping of lymph nodes, divided into "stations" which are themselves separated into groups which are sequentially further and further from the tumor in terms of lymphatic anatomy. The anatomical locations of the particular tiers of nodal drainage (group 1 being the immediately local drainage nodes and group 3 being more distant) differ depending on the location of the tumor in a complex manner determined by anatomical studies of the directions of normal lymph flow. Thus, the European TNM system differs quite significantly from the anatomically based Japanese system. Certain studies have shown that the TNM system provides better prognostic information in terms of N-staging than the PHNS system (20,21), but, as was noted in a large, retrospective, multivariate analysis, both the anatomically and numerically derived N-stage systems were independent prognostic factors for five-year survival (22) (evidence level 2b).

Resection of the local group 1 (perigastric) nodes with the tumor is referred to as a D1 dissection, and the extended dissection to involve group 2 nodes (along the branches of the celiac axis) is referred to as D2 lymphadenectomy.

STAGING METHODS

Staging methods vary with local facilities and expertise, but a computed tomographic (CT) scan of the chest and abdomen is essential. CT is moderately effective at estimating T-stage, and the

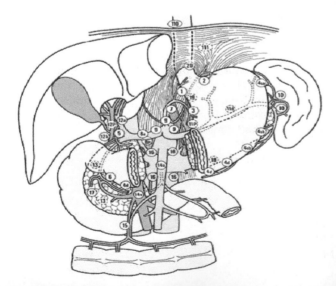

FIGURE 1 Topographical distribution of lymph node stations as defined by the second English edition of the Japanese classification of gastric carcinoma. The numbers indicate the recognized nodal "stations."

involvement of local and regional lymph nodes. It is extremely useful in the detection of lung and liver metastases, where its sensitivity approaches 90% and its specificity 98% (23–25). Endoscopic ultrasound (EUS) is established as a key investigation in esophageal cancer, but is more controversial in gastric cancer. Studies using operative specimen pathology as the "gold standard" indicate that it has an overall accuracy of 80% to 90% for T-stage and 68% to 86% for N-stage (26–30) (evidence level 1). EUS can be particularly useful in demonstrating whether there is direct invasion of the pancreas posteriorly, as this question can be very difficult to determine either by laparoscopy or CT scan, and is very important operatively.

Positron emission tomography (PET) scanning using 5-fluorodeoxy glucose as a probe has proved extremely sensitive in a wide variety of cancers both pre- and post-treatment. Difficulties in defining its exact role have arisen because of its limited availability in many countries, the plethora of other staging tests which predated it, and its relative lack of specificity. As we already have sensitive and specific tests for liver and lung metastases and loco-regional disease, PET (or increasingly PET/CT) currently tends to be used as the arbiter in cases where there is discomfort with the results of other methods. This perhaps reduces its success rate, as these are by definition the most difficult cases. Current evidence suggests that PET/CT has a sensitivity of 98% to 100% and a specificity of up to 89% in detecting lung and liver metastases in gastrointestinal tumors (31–33), but is less effective in detecting peritoneal disease. It appears less effective in gastric than esophageal tumors as the uptake of isotope is usually less avid. There is a considerable need for further research on the appropriate management of patients with very small volume of metastatic disease detected by PET.

Laparoscopy predates the other commonly used staging methods but remains extremely valuable because of its high degree of accuracy for small volume peritoneal disease (34–40). Its sensitivity for peritoneal metastasis is quoted at 96% (41) and its specificity nearly 100%, which compares favorably with the best figures quoted for PET, CT, and other modalities. There is an extensive literature on the use of peritoneal washings for cytology. Using a fairly straightforward lavage and conventional cytological staining, the yield of this technique is fairly low, but the prognostic implications if cancer cells are found are grave (42–45). A recent study has suggested that this may not be so if the tumor is fully staged in other respects, particularly T-stage (46). Most surgeons currently use washings for cytology on a limited basis or not at all. The other benefits of laparoscopy include the ability to pick up small surface liver metastasis missed by CT scanning, and the opportunity for surgeon and anesthetist to assess the response of the patient to a brief anesthetic.

Staging should always include an assessment of fitness for operation, particularly where the surgery may be a significant risk to the patient. The American Society of Anaesthesiologists (ASA) grade and the physiological and operative severity score for enumeration of morbidity and mortality (POSSUM) score component are independent predictors of mortality in large prospective series (47,48), and the Goldman Cardiac Index has been validated in general and vascular surgery, although it seems less predictive than ASA (49–52). An index scoring the preoperative function of multiple organs has been derived by Bartels et al. (53), and has been carefully validated in esophageal cancer patients including many with cancer at the gastro-esophageal junction. Whether this is accurate for gastrectomy patients is unclear. At present, most

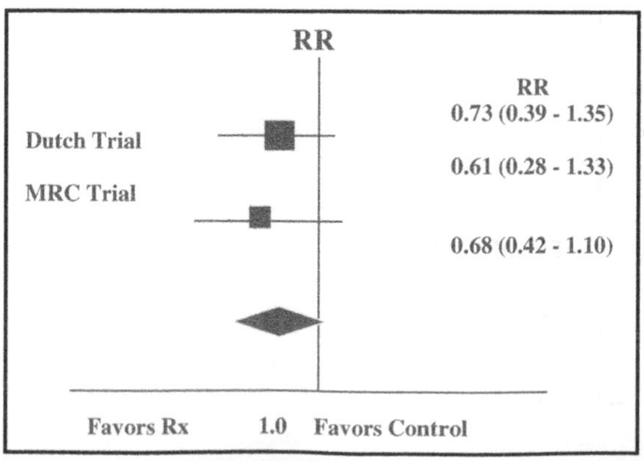

FIGURE 2 Forrest plot of long-term survival after D1 versus D2 gastrectomy for the subgroup of patients with T3 or T4 tumors. *Abbreviations*: RR, risk ratio; MRC, Medical Research Council.

experienced surgeons rely on crude subjective assessment of the patient's overall functional capacity, sometimes assessed slightly more rigorously by climbing stairs with the patient. Cardio-pulmonary exercise testing (CPET) seems to hold promise as a single test of real predictive value, but has so far not been validated in this kind of surgery.

TREATMENT SELECTION

Surgeons dealing with gastric cancer have to make a series of choices in designing the appropriate operation for an individual patient. First, the proximal and distal extent of the resection of the stomach; second, the extent and site of the lymph node dissection required to remove any loco-regional disease; third, the least invasive option combining adequate resection of both the gastrointestinal tube and the lymph nodes; finally, what reconstruction technique should be used. The factors which need to be taken into account include the stage of the disease, the site of the tumor, the fitness of the patient, and the patient's attitude to risk, that is, whether to do a larger and potentially more dangerous operation that might have a better chance of cure or a more limited but safer one. Less radical options include endoscopic mucosal resection for early disease, local, and nonradical dissections.

Nonradical Surgical Treatments

Endoscopic mucosal resection has been developed for early cancers in Japan, and is now well established there. A well-established set of prognostic criteria are used to select suitable patients. Essentially tumors need to be protuberant or flat, without ulceration or deep penetration into the submucosa (54). Most authorities set a diameter limit of about 2 cm (55–58). These criteria are based on large prospective cohorts, but not on randomized trials comparing endoscopic mucosal? (EMR) with open surgery (evidence level 2b). For relatively early tumors in the distal stomach, techniques have been described preserving the vagus nerves and pylorus, to improve gastric emptying and function (59–61). Series have also been reported where small T2 tumors are resected locally with only a cuff of surrounding stomach tissue, together with appropriate lymph node dissection in well-defined areas of maximum risk (62). For disease in the proximal half of the stomach, one attractive solution for relatively small or early tumors is a jejunal interposition with proximal gastrectomy. This was originally described by Merendino as a possible antireflux procedure (63), but Japanese surgeons have reported good results using it for early proximal cancer (64). There are no data comparing these techniques directly with more radical surgery. Laparoscopic or lap-assisted gastrectomy is increasingly performed, again with much of the experience reported being Japanese. Initial evidence from case series suggests that hospital stay, gastrointestinal function, and return to normal quality of life may be improved, while there is no definite evidence of reduced radicality of resection, increase in specific complications, or increase in involved resection margins (65–67). A single randomized controlled trial (RCT), which confirms these findings, is a single surgeon study (68), and further trials are clearly needed (evidence level 2b). It is not yet clear whether it is feasible to perform radical nodal dissection laparoscopically.

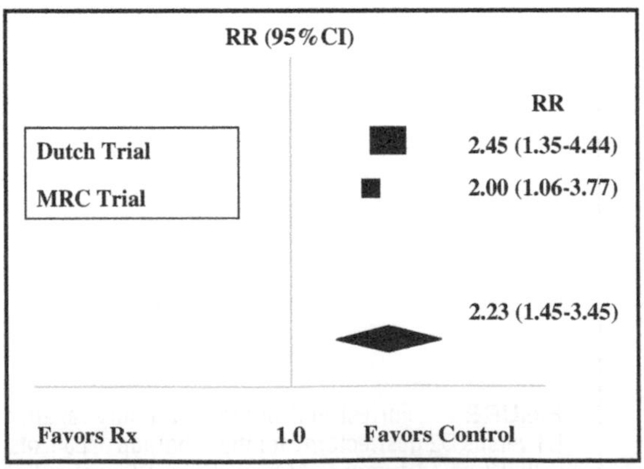

FIGURE 3 Forrest plot of mortality risk meta-analysis for D1 and D2 gastrectomy in randomized trials. Mortality for D2 is approximately double that for D1 in these studies. *Abbreviations*: MRC, Medical Research Council; RR, risk ratio; CI, confidence interval.

Radical Surgery: Gastrectomy with Systematic D2 Lymphadenectomy

The overall poor prognosis for gastric cancer led to a nihilistic approach by Western clinicians, which persisted for many years, but expert Japanese centers began to report much more favorable outcomes in terms of both perioperative mortality, and long-term prognosis in the 1970s, associated with the adoption of radical lymphadenectomy. Subsequently, several Western specialist centers have been able to report similar figures, stimulating great interest in radical surgery (69–71).

Figures for some Japanese centers described five-year survival rates of around 75% for all curative gastric resections. In stage-by-stage analysis, five-year survival was, over 90% for stages 0 and I disease, over 70% for stage II, and over 40% for stage III disease (71) (evidence level 2b). Several confounding factors may have contributed to these impressive figures. There is little evidence that gastric cancer is a different disease in Japan, but a greater proportion of the disease is of the intestinal type in Japan, and a lower proportion is located in the proximal stomach, where the prognosis is worse, than in the west (72). One of the effects of radical lymph node resections is to yield greater numbers of lymph nodes for histopathological examination. This may in turn lead to an apparent improvement in stage-specific survival of patients having undergone the more radical procedure (stage migration). Perioperative mortality reported in Japanese series is considerably lower than that reported in western centers (47,73), probably because of a mix of concentration of expertise (74), and favorable physiological status of Japanese patients, who are on average younger, less likely to have significant cardiovascular morbidity, and less likely to be obese than their Western counterparts.

One systematic review, two high-quality, RCTs, and numerous nonrandomized comparisons, cohort studies and case series comprise the evidence about the effectiveness of D2 dissection. The systematic review from the Cochrane Collaboration (75) meta-analyzed the pooled data from the only contemporaneous RCTs to date—the British Medical Research Council (MRC) gastric cancer STO1 trial (76,77) and the Dutch gastric cancer trial (78,79)—providing a total population of around 1121 patients.

In terms of survival, the meta-analysis showed no statistically significant difference between the D1 and D2 groups—the weighted mean five-year survival was 42.6% for D2 surgery and 41% for D1, giving a risk ratio (RR) of 0.95 [95% confidence interval (CI) 0.83–1.09]. When serosa-positive (T3 and T4 lesions) and negative subgroups were analyzed according to an a priori hypothesis, a risk ratio was produced that favored the D2 group in terms of survival—RR 0.68 (CI 0.42–1.10)—but this was not statistically significant (Fig. 2). In terms of postoperative mortality, there was a clear and significant excessive mortality in the D2 group—RR 2.23 (95% CI 1.45–3.45, Fig. 3). Subgroup analysis showed a very strong independent association between postoperative death and resection of the spleen (RR 5.5) and pancreatic tail (RR 5.8).

Although methodologically sound, areas of systematic bias were noted within these trials. There was a noted inadequacy of pretrial training in the D2 technique for participating surgeons in both trials There was also significant cross-contamination between the treatment groups in terms of number of nodes resected. For example, 36% of D1 cases had additional nodes resected than necessary, and 51% of D2 cases had nodes missing that should have been resected.

The review concluded that the possible risks and the possible benefits of D2 surgery should both be considered unproven. Current evidence was compatible with no benefit from D2 resection or with a substantial benefit in a specific subgroup. The 11-year follow-up results of one of the RCTs was recently published (80). There was no significant overall difference in survival between the D1 and D2 cohorts—30% versus 35% ($P = 0.53$), but subgroup analyses showed that patients with lymph-node stage N2, who had a D2 radical lymphadenectomy exhibited a greater rate of long-term survival, 21% compared with 0% in the D1 group. This result did not reach statistical significance, with the P-value calculated at $P = 0.8$. Patients with TNM stages II and IIIa also exhibited trends to higher rates of 11-year survival after D2 surgery—37% versus 23% ($P = 0.1$) for stage II, and 22% versus 4% ($P = 0.38$) for stage IIIa disease. These results could be viewed as supporting the benefit of the D2 technique in selected subgroups, but this contention requires further validation, possibly by future studies. For patients who did not have a splenectomy, mortality was higher in the D2 group (6.3% vs. 3.8%; $P = 0.19$), as was major morbidity (35% vs. 23%; $P < 0.001$), but long-term survival was significantly higher—43% versus 32% ($P = 0.015$). Similar results were demonstrated for patients who did not have a pancreatic resection (mortality 9.0 vs. 3.8%, $P = 0.004$; morbidity 39% vs. 23%, $P = 0.0001$; long-term survival 42% vs. 31%, $P = 0.2$).

A smaller Italian prospective randomized study, with just over 80 patients in each arm (81) has shown that the major morbidity of D2 surgery can be acceptable with prior training (16.3% mortality 0% in the D2 limb). Survival results should be available shortly. Two more recent RCTs from the East have reported on the morbidity and mortality of even more radical nodal dissection extending to the hepato-duodenal ligament and mesenteric root (D3) or to these areas plus the para-aortic nodes (D4) gastrectomy (82,83). Both studies reported near-zero mortality but increased morbidity for the more extensive surgery (evidence level 1b).

SURGICAL HARMS

Postoperative Complications

The mortality of gastrectomy remains high in nonspecialist settings, and appears to be higher in low-volume units (73), in elderly or unfit patients (47), and perhaps in males. Gastrectomy shares many postoperative complications with other major abdominal operations. In addition to the major complications leading to postoperative mortality, there are a variety of others of importance shown in the following table. Bleeding and wound dehiscence are relatively rare, as are deep vein thrombosis and pulmonary embolus in modern practice, but this remains highly lethal when it does occur. The issue of hospital-acquired infection has grown in importance over the last decade, and the risk of acquiring invasive methycillin-resistant *Staphylococcus aureus* (MRSA) infection or *Clostridium difficile* colitis is now a significant problem in many hospitals.

Postoperative Complications After Gastrectomy
Respiratory tract infection/adult respiratory distress syndrome
Myocardial infarction
Cardiac failure
Atrial fibrillation
Other arrhythmias
Abscess
Wound infection
Anastomotic leakage
Leakage from duodenal stump
Enteric fistula
Pancreatic fistula
Hemorrhage
Wound dehiscence
Hospital-acquired specific infection (MRSA/ *Clostridium difficile*)
Deep vein thrombosis
Pulmonary thromboembolism

Abbreviation: MSRA, methycillin-resistant *Staphylococcus aureus*.

In addition to the complications described, the normal, uncomplicated course of events after a gastrectomy will include a number of expected but undesirable health consequences. The weakness and tiredness associated with any major surgery usually takes several months to resolve completely, and in the case of gastrectomy, this is further added to by the nutritional problems induced by removal of part or all of the stomach. Patients can expect to have a smaller appetite and small capacity, and to lose weight for some time after leaving hospital until they reach a stable metabolic state.

Palliative Surgery

The role of surgery in palliating symptoms of gastric cancer has declined in recent years as the results of nonsurgical treatments have improved. The main problem symptoms in patients with advanced gastric cancer are pain, vomiting, bleeding, and anorexia. Gastrectomy will not correct anorexia, but it can deal with the other three symptoms on occasion. Intractable pain from gastric cancer is relatively rare, and often associated with very widespread unresectable disease. Operation should therefore only be undertaken when there is good evidence that a resection is feasible and nonsurgical measures have failed to relieve the pain. Chronic hemorrhage from gastric cancer commonly leads to anemia, which can often be dealt with by top-up transfusions. As the life expectancy of these patients is extremely limited, surgery is often not required. Persistent vomiting from gastric cancer commonly arises either from pyloric stenosis, paralysis of the gastric tube due to widespread infiltration, or multiple peritoneal and retroperitoneal metastases. Occasionally, patients in good condition can derive benefit from a palliative total gastrectomy for linitis plastica and experience an improved quality-of-life for some time. This is a relatively rare situation but well worth defining since there are no other effective treatments for it. Pyloric obstruction, on the other hand, is now being dealt with successfully by duodenal stenting in the majority of cases (83,84), and this should probably be preferred to surgical bypass if it is technically possible (85).

EVIDENCE SUMMARY AND OPINION

There is moderately good evidence that screening and case-finding programs increase the detection of early gastric cancer in a high-incidence population with a very high level of awareness, but the evidence that these strategies may be useful in other settings is weak, and it seems unlikely that they will be cost effective. There is good evidence of accuracy for CT staging of T- and M-stage and M-staging by CT/PET, P-staging by laparoscopy, and these modalities can all be recommended (recommendation grade B). The evidence for EUS is less clear-cut. EMR appears to be a safe and effective treatment for a specific group of early cancers (recommendation grade B, evidence level 2). Laparoscopic resection is feasible, appears safe, and may have advantages in terms of short-term recovery (evidence level 4). Whether it can accommodate radical nodal dissection remains to be demonstrated. D2 nodal dissection is not of proven survival benefit, but may improve prognosis for patients with intermediate-stage tumors. It is associated with increased morbidity and mortality when practiced in low-volume units without adequate training, and when combined with pancreatico-splenectomy (evidence level 1). More extensive dissections increase morbidity but not mortality in expert Eastern centers.

REFERENCES

1. Coleman MP, Damiecki P, Arslan A, Renard H. Trends in cancer incidence and mortality. IARC Scientific Publications. Vol. 121, Lyon: IARC Scientific Publications, 1993.
2. Siewert JR, Stein HJ. Classification of adenocarcinoma of the oesophago-gastric junction. Br J Surg 1998; 85:1457–1459.
3. Ferlay J, Bray F, Pisani P, Parkin DM. GLOBOCAN 2002: Cancer Incidence, Mortality and Prevalence Worldwide. IARC Cancer Base No. 5. Version 2.0. Lyon: IARC Press, 2004.
4. Newnham A, Quinn MJ, Babb P, Kang JY, Majeed A. Trends in the subsite and morphology of oesophageal and gastric cancer in England and Wales 1971–1998. Aliment Pharmacol Ther 2003; 17:665–676.
5. Devessa SS, Blot DJ, Fraumeni JF Jr. Changing patterns in the incidence of oesophageal and gastric carcinoma in the United States. Cancer 1998; 83:2049–2053.
6. Forman D. Counting cancers at the junction—a problem of routine statistics. Eur J Gastroenterol Hepatol 2002; 14(2):99–101.
7. Blaser MJ, Saito D. Trends in reported adenocarcinomas of the oesophagus and gastric cardia in Japan. Eur J Gastroenterol Hepatol 2002; 14:107–113.
8. Correa P, Chan VW. Gastric cancer. Cancer Sur 1994; 20:55–76.
9. You WZ, Zhao L, Chang YS, Blot DJ, Fraumeni JF Jr. Progression of precancerous gastric lesions. Lancet 1995; 345:866.
10. Lauren P. The two histological main types of gastric carcinoma; diffuse and so called intestinal-type carcinoma. Acta Pathol Microbiol Scand 1965; 64:31–49.
11. Murakami T. Pathomorphological diagnosis. Definition and gross classification in early gastric cancer. GANN Mono 1971; 11:53–55.
12. Kim JP, Hur YS, Yang HK. Lymph node metastases as a significant prognostic factor in early gastric cancer; analysis of 1136 early gastric cancers.Ann Sur Oncol 1995; 2(4):308–313.
13. Saragoni L, Gaudio M, Vio A, Folli S, Nanni O, Saragoni A. Early gastric cancer in the province of Forli: follow up of 337 patients in a high risk region for gastric cancer. Oncol Rep 1998; 5(4):945–948.

14. Tsuchiya A, Kikuchi Y, Ando Y, Yoshida T, Abe R. Lymph node metastases in gastric cancer invading the submucosal layer. Eur J Surg Oncol 1995; 21(3):248–250.
15. Maruyama K, Gunven P, Okabayashi K, Sasako M, Kinoshita T. Lymph node metastases of gastric cancer. General pattern in 1931 patients. Ann Surg 1989; 210:596–602.
16. Averbach AM, Jaquet P. Strategies to decrease the incidence of intra-abdominal recurrence in resectable gastric cancer. Br J Surg 1996; 83:726–733.
17. Sobin LH, Wittekind CH. TNM classification of malignant tumours, 6th ed. New York: Wiley, 2003.
18. Ichikura T, Ogawa T, Chochi K, Kawabata T, Sugasawa H, Mochizuki H. Minimum number of lymph nodes that should be examined for the UICC/AJCC TNM classification of gastric carcinoma. World J Surg 2003; 27:330–333.
19. Japanese Gastric Cancer Association. Japanese Classification of Gastric Carcinoma. 2nd English ed. Gastric Cancer 1998; 1:10–24.
20. Fujii K, Isozaki H, Okajima K, et al. Clinical evaluation of lymph node metastases in gastric cancer as defined by the 5th TNM edition in comparison with the Japanese system. Br J Surg 1999; 86:685–689.
21. D'Ugo D, Pacelli F, Persiani R, et al. Impact of the latest TNM classification of gastric cancer: retrospective analysis of 94 D2 gastrectomies. World J Surg 2002; 26:672–677.
22. Adachi Y, Shiraishi N, Suematsu T, Shiromizu A, Yamaguchi K, Kitano S. Most important lymph node information in gastric cancer; multivariate prognostic study. Ann Surg Oncol 2000; 7:503–507.
23. Adachi Y, Sakino I, Matsumata T, et al. Preoperative assessment of advanced gastric carcinoma using computed tomography. Am J Gastroenterol 1997; 92:872–875.
24. D'Elia F, Zingarelli A, Palli D, Grani M. Hydro-dynamic CT preoperative staging of gastric cancer: correlation with pathological findings. A prospective study of 107 cases. Eur Radiol 2000; 10:1877–1885.
25. Wakelin SJ, Deans C, Crofts TJ, Allan PL, Plevris JN, Paterson-Brown S. A comparison of computerised tomography, laparoscopic ultrasound and endoscopic ultrasound in the preoperative staging of oesophago-gastric carcinoma. Eur J Radiol 2002; 41:161–167.
26. Dittler HJ, Siewert JR. Role of endoscopic ultrasonography in gastric carcinoma. Endoscopy 1993; 25(2):162–166.
27. Smith JW, Brennan MF, Botet JF, Gerdes H, Lightdale CJ. Preoperative endoscopic ultrasound can predict the risk of recurrence after operation for gastric carcinoma. J Clin Oncol 1993; 11(12):2380–2385.
28. Massari M, Cioffi U, De Simone M, et al. Endoscopic ultrasonography for preoperative staging of gastric carcinoma. Hepatogastroenterology 1996; 43(9):542–546.
29. Hunerbein M, Ghadimi BM, Haensch W, Schlag PM. Transendoscopic ultrasound of esophageal and gastric cancer using miniaturized ultrasound catheter probes. Gastrointest Endosc 1998; 48(4):371–375.
30. Kelly S, Harris KM, Berry E, et al. A systematic review of the staging performance of endoscopic ultrasound in gastro-oesophageal carcinoma. Gut 2001; 49(4):534–539.
31. Nakamoto Y, Higashi T, Sakahara H, et al. Contribution of PET in the detection of liver metastases from pancreatic tumours. Clin Radiol 1999; 54:248–252.
32. Rasanen JV, Sihvo EI, Knuuti MJ, et al. Prospective analysis of accuracy of positron emission tomography, computed tomography, and endoscopic ultrasonography in staging of adenocarcinoma of the esophagus and the esophagogastric junction. Ann Surg Oncol 2003; 10:954–960.
33. Zhuang H, Sinha P, Pourdehnad M, Duarte PS, Yamamoto AJ, Alavi A. The role of positron emission tomography with fluorine-18-deoxyglucose in identifying colorectal cancer metastases to liver. Nucl Med Commun 2000; 21:793–798.
34. Possik RA, Franco EL, Pires DR, Wohnrath DR, Ferreira EB. Sensitivity, specificity, and predictive value of laparoscopy for the staging of gastric cancer and for the detection of liver metastases. Cancer 1986; 58(1):1–6.
35. D'Ugo DM, Persiani R, Caracciolo F, Ronconi P, Coco C, Picciocchi A. Selection of locally advanced gastric carcinoma by preoperative staging laparoscopy. Surg Endosc 1997; 11:1159–1162.
36. Lavonius MI, Gullichsen R, Salo S, Sonninen P, Ovaska J. Staging of gastric cancer: a study with spiral computed tomography, ultrasonography, laparoscopy, and laparoscopic ultrasonography. Surg Laparosc Endosc Percutan Tech 2002; 12:77–81.
37. McCulloch P, Johnson M, Jairam R, Fischer W. Laparoscopic staging of gastric cancer is safe and affects treatment strategy. Ann R Coll Surg Engl 1998; 80:400–402.
38. O'Brien MG, Fitzgerald EF, Lee G, Crowley M, Shanahan F, O'Sullivan GC. A prospective comparison of laparoscopy and imaging in the staging of esophagogastric cancer before surgery. Am J Gastroenterol 1995; 90:2191–2194.
39. Blackshaw GR, Barry JD, Edwards P, Allison MC, Thomas GV, Lewis WG. Laparoscopy significantly improves the perceived preoperative stage of gastric cancer. Gastric Cancer 2003; 6(4):225–229.
40. Sotiropoulos GC, Kaiser GM, Lang H, et al. Staging laparoscopy in gastric cancer. Eur J Med Res 2005; 10:88–91.
41. Ozmen MM, Zulfikaroglu B, Ozalp N, Ziraman I, Hengirmen S, Sahin B. Staging laparoscopy for gastric cancer. Surg Laparosc Endosc Percutan Tech 2003; 13:241–244.
42. Bryan RT, Cruickshank NR, Needham SJ, et al. Laparoscopic peritoneal lavage in staging gastric and oesophageal cancer. Eur J Surg Oncol 2001; 27:291–297.

43. Hayes N, Wayman J, Wadehra V, Scott DJ, Raimes SA, Griffin SM. Peritoneal cytology in the surgical evaluation of gastric carcinoma. Br J Cancer 1999; 79:520–524.
44. Ribeiro U Jr, Gama-Rodrigues JJ, Bitelman B, et al. Value of peritoneal lavage cytology during laparoscopic staging of patients with gastric carcinoma. Surg Laparosc Endosc 1998; 8:132–135.
45. Ribeiro U Jr, Safatle-Ribeiro AV, Zilberstein B, et al. Does the intraoperative peritoneal lavage cytology add prognostic information in patients with potentially curative gastric resection? J Gastrointest Surg 2006; 10(2):170–176.
46. de Manzoni G, Verlato G, Di Leo A, et al. Peritoneal cytology does not increase the prognostic information provided by TNM in gastric cancer. World J Surg 2006; 30(4):579–584.
47. McCulloch P, Ward J, Tekkis PP. Mortality and morbidity in gastro-oesophageal cancer surgery: initial results of ASCOT multicentre prospective cohort study. BMJ 2003; 327:1192–1197.
48. Tekkis PP, McCulloch P, Polonieoki J, et al. Risk-adjusted prediction of operative mortality in oesophagogastric surgery with O-POSSUM. Br J Surg 2004; 91:288–295.
49. Goldman L, Caldera DL, Nussbaum SR, et al. Multifactorial index of cardiac risk in noncardiac surgical procedures. N Engl J Med 1977; 297:845–850.
50. Prause G, Ratzenhofer-Comenda B, Pierer G, Smolle-Juttner F, Glanzer H, Smolle J. Can ASA grade or Goldman's Cardiac Risk Index predict peri-operative mortality? A study of 16,227 patients. Anaesthesia 1997; 52:203–206.
51. White GH, Advani SM, Williams RA, Wilson SE. Cardiac risk index as a predictor of long-term survival after repair of abdominal aortic aneurysm. Am J Surg 1988; 156:103–107.
52. Zeldin RA. Assessing cardiac risk in patients who undergo noncardiac surgical procedures. Can J Surg 1984; 27:402–404.
53. Bartels H, Stein HJ, Siewert JR. Preoperative risk analysis and postoperative mortality of oesophagectomy for resectable oesophageal cancer. Br J Surg 1998; 85:840–844.
54. Makuuchi H, Kise Y, Shimada H, Chino O, Tanaka H. Endoscopic mucosal resection for early gastric cancer. Semin Surg Oncol 1999; 17(2):108–116.
55. Ono H, Kondo H, Gotoda T, et al. Endoscopic mucosal resection for treatment of early gastric cancer. Gut 2001; 48(2):151–152.
56. Miyata M, Yokoyama Y, Okoyama N, et al. What are the appropriate indications for endoscopic mucosal resection for early gastric cancer? Analysis of 256 endoscopically resected lesions. Endoscopy 2000; 32(10):773–778.
57. Wang YP, Bennett C, Pan T. Endoscopic mucosal resection for early gastric cancer. Cochrane Database Syst Rev 2006; 1:CD004276.
58. Uedo N, Iishi H, Tatsuta M, et al. Longterm outcomes after endoscopic mucosal resection for early gastric cancer. Gastric Cancer 2006; 9(2):88–92.
59. Imada T, Rino Y, Takahashi M, et al. Gastric emptying after pylorus-preserving gastrectomy in comparison with conventional subtotal gastrectomy for early gastric carcinoma. Surg Today 1998; 28:135–138.
60. Kodama M, Koyama K. Indications for pylorus preserving gastrectomy for early gastric cancer located in the middle third of the stomach. World J Surg 1991; 15:628–633.
61. Shibata C, Shiiba KI, Funayama Y, et al. Outcomes after pylorus-preserving gastrectomy for early gastric cancer: a prospective multicenter trial. World J Surg 2004; 28:857–861.
62. Takahashi S, Maeta M, Mizusawa K, et al. Long-term postoperative analysis of nutritional status after limited gastrectomy for early gastric cancer. Hepatogastroenterology 1998; 45:889–894.
63. Thomas GI, Merendino KA. Jejunal interposition operation; analysis of thirty-three clinical cases. J Am Med Assoc 1958; 168:1759–1766.
64. Katai H, Sano T, Fukagawa T, Shinohara H, Sasako M. Prospective study of proximal gastrectomy for early gastric cancer in the upper third of the stomach. Br J Surg 2003; 90:850–853.
65. Lee SI, Choi YS, Park DJ, Kim HH, Yang HK, Kim MC. Comparative study of laparoscopy-assisted distal gastrectomy and open distal gastrectomy. J Am Coll Surg 2006; 202(6):874–880.
66. Miura S, Kodera Y, Fujiwara M, et al. Laparoscopy-assisted distal gastrectomy with systemic lymph node dissection: a critical reappraisal from the viewpoint of lymph node retrieval. J Am Coll Surg 2004; 198(6):933–938.
67. Adachi Y, Shiraishi N, Shiromizu A, Bandoh T, Aramaki M, Kitano S. Laparoscopy-assisted Billroth I gastrectomy compared with conventional open gastrectomy. Arch Surg 2000; 135(7):806–810.
68. Huscher CG, Mingoli A, Sgarzini G, et al. Laparoscopic versus open subtotal gastrectomy for distal gastric cancer: five-year results of a randomized prospective trial. Ann Surg 2005; 241(2): 232–237.
69. Sue-Ling HM, Johnston D, Martin IG, et al. Gastric cancer: a curable disease in Britain. Br Med J 1993; 71:2918–2925.
70. Roukos D, Lorenz M, Encke A. Evidence of survival benefit of extended (D2) lymphadenectomy in western patients with gastric cancer based on a new concept: a prospective long term follow up study. Surgery 1998; 123:573–578.
71. Maruyama K, Okabayashi K, Kinoshita T. Progress in gastric cancer surgery in Japan and its limits of radicality. World J Surg 1987; 11:418–425.

72. Roder JD, Bonenkamp JJ, Craven J, et al. Lymphadenectomy for gastric cancer in clinical trials: update. World J Surg 1995; 19:546–553.
73. Bachmann MO, Alderson D, Edwards D, et al. Cohort study in south and west England of the influence of specialisation on the management and outcome of patients with oesophageal and gastric cancer. Br J Surg 2002; 89:914–922.
74. Sano T, Katai H, Sasako M, Maruyama K. One thousand consecutive gastrectomies without operative mortality. Br J Surg 2002; 89(1):123.
75. McCulloch P, Nita ME, Kazi H, Gama-Rodrigues J. Extended versus limited lymph nodes dissection technique for adenocarcinoma of the stomach.Cochrane Database Syst Rev 2004; 4:CD001964.
76. Cuschieri A, Fayers P, Fielding J, et al. Postoperative morbidity and mortality after D1 and D2 resections for gastric cancer: preliminary results of the MRC randomised controlled surgical trial. Lancet 1996; 347:995–999.
77. Cuschieri A, Weeden S, Fielding J, et al. Patient survival after D1 and D2 resections for gastric cancer surgery: long term results of the MRC randomized surgical trial. Br J Cancer 2000; 79:1522–1530.
78. Bonenkamp JJ, Songun I, Hermans J, et al. Randomized comparison of morbidity after D1 and D2 dissection for gastric cancer in 996 Dutch patients.Lancet 1995; 345:745–748.
79. Bonenkamp JJ, Hermans J, Sasako M, et al. Dutch Gastric Cancer Group. Extended lymph node dissection for gastric cancer. N Engl J Med 1999; 340:908–958.
80. Hartgrink HH, van de Velde CJ, Putter H, et al. Extended lymph node dissection for gastric cancer: who may benefit? Final results of the randomized Dutch gastric cancer group trial. J Clin Oncol 2004; 22(11):2069–2077.
81. Degiuli M, Sasako M, Calgaro M, et al. Italian Gastric Cancer Study Group. Morbidity and mortality after D1 and D2 gastrectomy for cancer: interim analysis of the Italian Gastric Cancer Study Group (IGCSG) randomised surgical trial. Eur J Surg Oncol 2004; 30(3):303–308.
82. Wu CW, Hsiung CA, Lo SS, Hsieh MC, Shia LT, Whang-Peng J. Randomized clinical trial of morbidity after D1 and D3 surgery for gastric cancer. Br J Surg 2004; 91(3):283–287.
83. Sano T, Sasako M, Yamamoto S, et al. Gastric cancer surgery: morbidity and mortality results from a prospective randomized controlled trial comparing D2 and extended para-aortic lymphadenectomy—Japan Clinical Oncology Group study 9501. J Clin Oncol 2004; 22(14):2767–2773.
84. Kaw M, Singh S, Gagneja H, Azad P. Role of self-expandable metal stents in the palliation of malignant duodenal obstruction. Surg Endosc 2003; 17(4):646–650.
85. Fiori E, Lamazza A, Volpino P, et al. Palliative management of malignant antro-pyloric strictures. Gastroenterostomy vs. endoscopic stenting. A randomized prospective trial. Anticancer Res 2004; 24(1):269–271.

8 Evidence-Based Practice: The Role of Adjuvant Radiotherapy in the Treatment of Gastric Adenocarcinoma

Abigail S. Caudle and Hong Jin Kim
Department of Surgery/Division of Surgical Oncology, University of North Carolina School of Medicine, Chapel Hill, North Carolina, U.S.A.

Joel E. Tepper
Department of Radiation Oncology, University of North Carolina School of Medicine, NC Clinical Cancer Center, Chapel Hill, North Carolina, U.S.A.

INTRODUCTION

The incidence of gastric cancer in the United States is decreasing, but it remains the third most common cancer worldwide (1). Although complete surgical resection is potentially curative in early stages, locoregional recurrence remains a frustrating problem in patients presenting with more advanced stages of disease (T3-4 or N1-2). Numerous factors contribute to the overall dismal survival rates in gastric cancer, including limited public awareness of the disease in Western cultures, a lack of standardization in diagnostic and clinical algorithms, a paucity of multi-institutional prospective randomized trials to help define standards of care, and an overall aggressive underlying tumor biology. The end result is that most patients are not cured by surgery alone, with high rates of relapse that beg for advances in adjuvant therapy to improve overall the outcomes. Complicating the treatment algorithm for aggressive locoregional therapy are controversies regarding the extent of gastric and lymph-node resection (1–5). In addition to refinements in surgical standards, efforts to improve outcomes have centered on earlier detection of disease, more sophisticated staging tools, and combined modality therapies (6–10).

As the role of adjuvant chemotherapy continues to be debated, the effectiveness of locoregional modalities, such as surgery and radiation, continue to take on greater clinical significance. Locoregional failure rates of almost 60% have been reported in patients with tumors extending through the serosa or with lymph-node metastasis (11,12). Surgical approaches alone, regardless of the extent of lymph-node dissection, clearly will not suffice in more advanced disease. The standards of adjuvant therapy after resection in high-risk patients was established by the Intergroup 0116 trial (INT 0116), which demonstrated a significant improvement in disease-free survival (DFS) and overall survival (OS) rates with postoperative chemoradiation over surgery alone (13). Determining the exact timing and nature of the adjuvant radiotherapy is our challenge, in order to optimize clinical standards in the treatment of high-risk gastric cancer.

PATTERNS OF RECURRENCE IN GASTRIC CANCER

Early sites of recurrent gastric cancer are difficult to identify, even with current advances in imaging techniques. Most recurrent disease goes undetected until it is fairly advanced (14–16). Historical autopsy series outline late patterns of recurrence in gastric cancer, but typically demonstrate large volumes of disease obscuring the initial site of treatment failure (17). A valuable addition to our understanding of recurrence patterns was provided by studies from Wangensteen et al. at the University of Minnesota, where they routinely performed "second-look" laparotomies. In 1982, they reported on this reoperative series, finding that locoregional recurrence was at least one component of treatment failure in 88% of patients with relapse and the only component in 29% (18). Of those patients with recurrence, 55% recurred in the gastric bed, 27% at the anastomosis, and 43% in locoregional lymph nodes. In studies from Japan, 67% of a total of 107 patients had evidence of a locoregional recurrence. Caution must be exercised in

TABLE 1 Studies Outlining the Patterns of Failure in Gastric Cancer (Percentage of Total Patients)

Author	Treatment	No. of patients	Locoregional failure only (%)	Locoregional failure as any component (%)	Distant metastasis only (%)	Distant metastasis as any component (%)
Gunderson (Minnesota) (18)	Surgery	105	41	69	5	23
Landry (MGH) (21)	Surgery	130	16	38	30	52
Lim (Korea) (47)	Surgery + adj CRT[a]	291	4	16	23	35
D'Angelica (MSKCC) (51)	Surgery ± adj CRT[a]	367	26[b]	54[b]	28[b]	51[b]

[a]Adjuvant chemoradiation therapy.
[b]Percentage based on the number of patients with known recurrence.
Abbreviations: CRT, chemoradiotherapy; MGH, Massachusetts General Hospital; MSKCC, Memorial Sloan-Kettering Cancer Center.

interpreting this data, however, since 42% of these patients had peritoneal seeding, rendering the stage equivalent to distant metastasis (18). Wisbeck et al. (17) reported similar results in their autopsy study of 85 patients dying of stomach cancer; of those patients with relapse, the first site was local in 22% and regional in 19%. Recent studies have attempted to outline both the patterns and sites of recurrence in high-risk gastric cancer (Tables 1 and 2) (19).

Of course, not all gastric cancers have the same patterns of recurrence. The location of the primary tumor is one factor that the Japanese have shown to be important in considering the areas at risk harboring the disease. They delineated the patterns of nodal spread by dividing lymph nodes into 16 stations, and grouping metastases to each station by region of the primary tumor (proximal, middle, or distal stomach) (20). The tumor depth (T stage) should also be factored into both the therapeutic and prognostic decisions. A recent large series from Korea chronicling the patterns of recurrence following aggressive curative resections found that the incidence of local failure increased when the primary disease extended through the gastric wall or when lymph nodes were involved at the initial surgery (9,10,21). Furthermore, other clinical and pathologic features have been implicated, including histologic differentiation, lymphovascular invasion, and positive peritoneal cytology (5).

Systemic recurrences account for almost a third of all treatment failures, pointing to the obvious need for improvements in chemotherapy in addition to locoregional treatment. One series reported that liver metastases occurred in 30% of patients and peritoneal seeding in 23%. Interestingly, extra-abdominal failure was relatively rare and occurred in only 13% of patients (22). What has become evident is that there are a few opportunities to salvage patients presenting with recurrent disease. Therefore, the quality of the initial locoregional treatment is critical to minimize the risk of recurrence. The radiation treatment field should be tailored around known patterns of recurrence.

THE IMPACT OF RESECTION MARGINS

Given the known patterns of recurrence, it is logical that the extent of surgical resection should vary with the size, depth, and location of the primary tumor, as well as the stage of disease. However, the importance of obtaining negative surgical margins applies to all gastric tumors. Several studies have reported that a positive surgical resection margin is associated with a

TABLE 2 Studies Defining Sites of Locoregional Failures in Patients with Recurrent Gastric Cancer (Percentage of Total Patients)

Author	Stomach/remnant (%)	Anastomosis (%)	Lymph nodes (%)
Gunderson (18)	55	26	43
Landry (23)	21	25	8
Lim (49)	1	5	
D'Angelica (19)	12[a]	18[a]	28[a]

[a]Percentage based on the number of patients with known recurrence.

significant decrease in OS (2,7,8,23). In 1984, the British Stomach Cancer Group reported that stage II/III gastric cancer patients with microscopic resection line disease had similar survival rates to patients with stage IV disease (24). A review of the literature reveals that the incidence of positive surgical resection margins varies from 5% to 20% in most series, and is usually associated with more advanced stage of gastric cancer. Gall et al. reported a rate of microscopically positive proximal margin of 11.5%, but all had undergone palliative resections for advanced disease (three with metastatic disease) (6,25). Similarly, the Dutch Gastric Cancer trial reported a positive microscopic margin rate of 6% (n=41/699); on subset analysis, the predictive value of positive microscopic margins was lost in patients with advanced disease (T3/T4 or stage III/IV) (26).

Earlier studies from Memorial Sloan-Kettering Cancer Center (MSKCC) by Papachristou et al. examined the role of resection margin length and the incidence of histologically positive margins finding the lowest incidence with proximal margins of 6 cm or more. Twenty percent of the 350 patients had positive microscopic proximal resection margins; however, anastomotic recurrence was not a major component of their disease progression since the majority of these patients (predominantly stage III/IV) went on to die of regional and distant metastatic disease (27). In 1999, Kim et al. defined the clinicopathologic features that predicted outcome in stage II/III gastric cancer patients with microscopic disease at the resection margins. In their retrospective analysis, 7.6% of the 619 advanced-stage patients had a positive resection margin which was a significant independent predictor of outcome (p=0.003). The presence of a positive margin lost significance in the subset of patients with >5 positive lymph nodes (n=189), Since this group represented advanced disease with outcomes not determined by locoregional surgical clearance. In patients undergoing adequate staging (>15 lymph nodes examined) with pathology revealing ≤5 positive lymph nodes (n=277), survival was significantly worsened (p=0.03) by the presence of an involved margin (28).

The confirmation of a complete resection with negative margins has important implications for adjuvant radiotherapy. One retrospective review of 63 patients looked at results with postoperative radiotherapy in high-risk patients, including those with complete resection but thought to be at risk for relapse, those with microscopic disease, and 10 with gross disease left after gastrectomy. Eighty-four percent received chemotherapy in addition to external beam radiotherapy (EBRT) with median survival of 19.3 months for patients with no residual disease, 16.7 months for those with residual disease, and 9.2 months after R2 resection (p=0.01). Another important finding was that patients treated with four or more irradiation fields had a significant decrease in grade 4 and 5 toxicity compared with those treated with two fields (29). In patients with positive-margin resections, radiation therapy (RT) and re-resection to obtain negative histologic margins may play a beneficial and critical role. As these studies indicate, an R0 resection with adequate lymph-node dissection is essential to have the best outcome in patients with potentially curable disease. Clinical staging of lymph nodes is notoriously inaccurate; hence, margin status should be assessed at the time of resection whenever the intent of treatment is cure. However, efforts to obtain a negative margin in the gastric cancer patient with bulky nodal metastases and obvious advanced disease must be tempered by the risk of increasing operative morbidity, as survival in this subset of patients will not be substantially altered by aggressive local treatment measures.

GOALS OF RADIATION

Prior to the more recent trials demonstrating the benefits of adjuvant chemoradiation, the role of RT in gastric cancer was limited to palliation for advanced disease, to control bleeding, or to alleviate pain. The use of adjuvant radiation therapy (RT) as a single modality was investigated in several small studies, none of which demonstrated a significant benefit, although there was a suggestion of improved local control (30–34). The INT 0116 trial was the first phase III multi-institutional trial to establish improvements in locoregional control as well as a survival benefit with combined postoperative chemoradiotherapy. Similar to the difficulties seen in establishing surgical standards of care, the goals and delivery of radiotherapy vary widely among radiation oncologists (31). Even in the well-designed Intergroup trial, approximately one-third of the proposed treatment plans had to be modified to conform to the trial protocol. Radiotherapy in this region is limited by the position of the stomach near vital organs, such as spinal cord, kidney, pancreas, bowel, and liver. The stomach itself (or remnant) is a highly radiosensitive organ, which is prone to ulceration and bleeding with high radiation doses. This makes it even more crucial that radiotherapy be tailored for the specific patient. What follows is a critical evaluation of the evidence supporting the role of radiation oncology in the adjuvant care of patients with gastric adenocarcinoma.

NEOADJUVANT AND INTRAOPERATIVE RADIATION THERAPY

A brief overview of neoadjuvant radiation therapy (RT) and intraoperative radiation therapy (IORT) will be outlined, although the focus will remain on the evidence for the role of adjuvant RT in the treatment algorithm for patients with gastric adenocarcinoma. Recently, neoadjuvant RT has been used primarily to downstage patients and to select patients with favorable biology of disease that may be candidates for potentially curative resections. In one study of 32 patients treated preoperatively with docetaxel and cisplatin followed by EBRT, 14 had complete pathologic responses (pCR), whereas an additional 10 had only microscopic residual disease after resection (35). A study examining a preoperative regimen with 5-fluorouracil (5-FU) and EBRT was less encouraging, but still resulted in a complete pathological responses (pCR) in five of 34 patients, and a pathologic partial response (pPR) in 18 patients (36). In addition to potential downstaging, neoadjuvant chemoradiation can be a useful selection tool to identify patients with responsive disease. In a multi-institutional trial using preoperative chemotherapy (5-FU, leucovorin, and cisplatin) followed by 45 Gy of RT with concurrent 5-FU, patients demonstrating a pCR or pPR had longer median survival than those with no response to neoadjuvant therapy (63.9 months vs. 12.6 months, $p=0.03$) (37). In addition, resection rates have also been found to be higher in patients who receive neoadjuvant chemoradiotherapy (38,39).

Unfortunately, the majority of studies examining the role of neoadjuvant RT as a sole modality are single-institution, nonrandomized studies, making the results difficult to extrapolate. Multiple studies show no benefit to neoadjuvant RT, such as the one large study from Russia involving 293 patients which did not show a change in survival (40). In contrast, a randomized trial from China using preoperative EBRT versus surgery alone improved five-year survival from 19% to 30% ($p=0.0094$) and 10-year survival from 13% to 20% (39). Obviously, further studies are needed to determine the role of neoadjuvant RT or chemoradiation in the treatment of gastric cancer, although it will probably be most beneficial in efforts to downstage patients with marginally resectable or unresectable disease.

Intraoperative radiotherapy has been largely limited to investigational approaches; although the approach is intriguing, there are few studies to guide treatment. A phase II study from the Radiation Therapy Oncology Group (RTOG) 85-01 examined outcomes in 27 patients who received IORT [12.5–16.5 Gray (Gy)] in addition to postoperative EBRT (in 23 of the patients), with two-year survival rates of 47% (30). A large study out of Japan randomized 211 patients based on the day of hospitalization, but not stratified for prognostic factors. This study reported improved five-year survival in patients who received IORT versus those who underwent surgery alone (41). Likewise, a study in China randomized patients with stages III and IV gastric cancer to surgery plus IORT (25–40 Gy) versus surgery alone; the survival advantage was only seen in stage III patients (42). In contrast, a randomized trial performed by the National Cancer Institute found no difference in survival rates between groups that received IORT versus those that did not receive IORT, although subset analysis demonstrated an improvement in local recurrence rates in the IORT group (44% vs. 92%, $p < 0.001$) (43). Similar to the evidence outlining the role of neoadjuvant RT, further well-conducted, randomized, prospective studies are needed to define the role of IORT in the treatment of patients with gastric cancer.

EVIDENCE FOR THE ROLE OF POSTOPERATIVE RADIOTHERAPY

The predominance of studies reported in the literature have centered on the adjuvant role of RT in patients with optimal surgical resection (Table 3) (44). Early nonrandomized studies showed

TABLE 3 Summary of Studies Defining the Role of Adjuvant Chemoradiation in Patients with High-Risk, Resectable, Gastric Cancer

Author	(*N*)	Median survival (months)	Five-year survival (%)
Phase II trials			
Gez (Israel) (44)			
Surgery + 5-FU + EBRT (50 Gy)	25	33	40
Regine (Thomas Jefferson Univ) (48)			
Surgery alone	70	10	10
Surgery + 5-FU/FAM + EBRT	20	18	24
Gunderson (MGH) (18)			
Surgery alone	110		38 (4-year)
Surgery + 5-FU + EBRT	14	24	43 (4-year)
Phase III trials			
Hallissey (British Stomach Group) (32)			
Surgery alone	145		20
Surgery + EBRT (45 Gy)	153		12
Moertal (Mayo Clinic) (46)			
Surgery alone	23	15	4
Surgery + 5-FU + EBRT (37.5 Gy)	39	24	23
MacDonald (Intergroup 0116) (13)			
Surgery alone	275	27	41 (3-year)
Surgery + 5-FU/Leu + EBRT (45 Gy)	281	36	50 (3-year)

Abbreviations: 5-FU, 5-fluorouracil; EBRT, external beam radiotherapy; FAM, fluorouracil adriamycin mitomycin ; Leu, leucovorin; MGH, Massachusetts General Hospital.

no survival difference when patients were treated with postoperative chemoradiotherapy (45). The Mayo Clinic performed a randomized prospective study in patients thought to have a poor prognosis due to advanced clinicopathologic features. Patients underwent either gastrectomy alone or gastrectomy with 37.5-Gy EBRT with concurrent 5-FU. These results are complicated by the fact that informed consent was obtained after randomization in only the adjuvant therapy group, resulting in 10 patients in the treatment group declining therapy. In an intent-to-treat analysis, a significant difference in OS rates was found between the two groups (4% vs. 23%, $p < 0.05$). However, when the groups were analyzed more closely, the five-year survival rates were found to be 20% in those who actually received treatment, 30% in those who declined treatment, and 4% in the control group (46).

Two large randomized prospective clinical trials were conducted by the British Stomach Cancer Group, to define the role of adjuvant therapy in gastric cancer. Both trials randomized patients to three arms: surgery alone, surgery plus postoperative EBRT, or surgery and postoperative chemotherapy [either 5-FU, doxorubicin, methotrexate, and mitomycin (47) or 5-FU, doxorubicin, and mitomycin (32)]. Neither trial demonstrated a significant survival benefit attributed to adjuvant treatment. In the first trial, only 68% of the patients in the surgery plus EBRT arm received a dose of 40.5 Gy or higher, and 24% did not receive any EBRT. Another criticism of the trial was that 21% of the patients were noted to have gross residual disease after surgical extirpation. Notable in the British trials is that RT and chemotherapy were studied as single modalities, since later trials demonstrated benefits of combined multimodality therapy. Regine et al. took this additional step by dividing patients who underwent gastrectomy but were deemed to be high risk (T3/4 or N1/2) into four groups: control, chemotherapy alone [5-FU/fluorouracil adriamycin mitomycin (FAM)], postoperative RT alone, or the combination of chemoradiation. There was a statistically significant improvement in survival in the chemoradiotherapy group as compared with the control group, but not when chemotherapy or radiotherapy was administered as a single modality. Locoregional relapse was seen in 45% of the control group versus 19% in the chemoradiotherapy group, although there was no difference in distant relapse pointing to the fact that differences in survival are probably related to improved local control (48).

INTERGROUP 0116 TRIAL

The well-designed INT 0116 study reported by MacDonald in 2001, established postoperative chemoradiotherapy as the standard of care for patients with resectable gastric cancer (13). Patients who underwent a complete resection with negative margins were stratified according to tumor node metastases (TNM) staging and then randomized to surgery alone (275 patients) versus surgery plus adjuvant therapy (281 patients). The treatment protocol in the adjuvant arm consisted of chemotherapy beginning 20 to 40 days after gastrectomy with 5-FU and leucovorin for five days. Twenty-eight days after the start of chemotherapy, patients started EBRT with 45 Gy given in 180-cGy fractions five days a week for five weeks with concurrent 5-FU and leucovorin on the first four and last three days of radiation. They continued with chemotherapy 28 to 35 days after the completion of EBRT with two five-day courses of 5-FU and leucovorin one month apart (schema of INT 0116 in Fig. 1). The design of the radiation field was very strictly delineated, covering the tumor bed, proximal and distal resection margins plus 2 cm, and regional nodes as defined by the stations outlined by the Japanese Research Society for the Study of Gastric Cancer (JRSGC). The tumor bed was determined by preoperative computed tomography (CT) scans, barium studies, and surgical clips. Perigastric, celiac, para-aortic, splenic, hepatoduodenal, porta hepatis, and pancreaticoduodenal lymph nodes were included in all fields; splenic nodes were excluded if the kidney would be affected. Patients with tumors of the gastroesophageal junction also had treatment to paracardiac and paraesophageal nodes, but pancreaticoduodenal nodes were excluded. Radiation treatment plans were checked before initiation of EBRT to ensure standardization with 35% of the plans being modified to fit the radiation protocol.

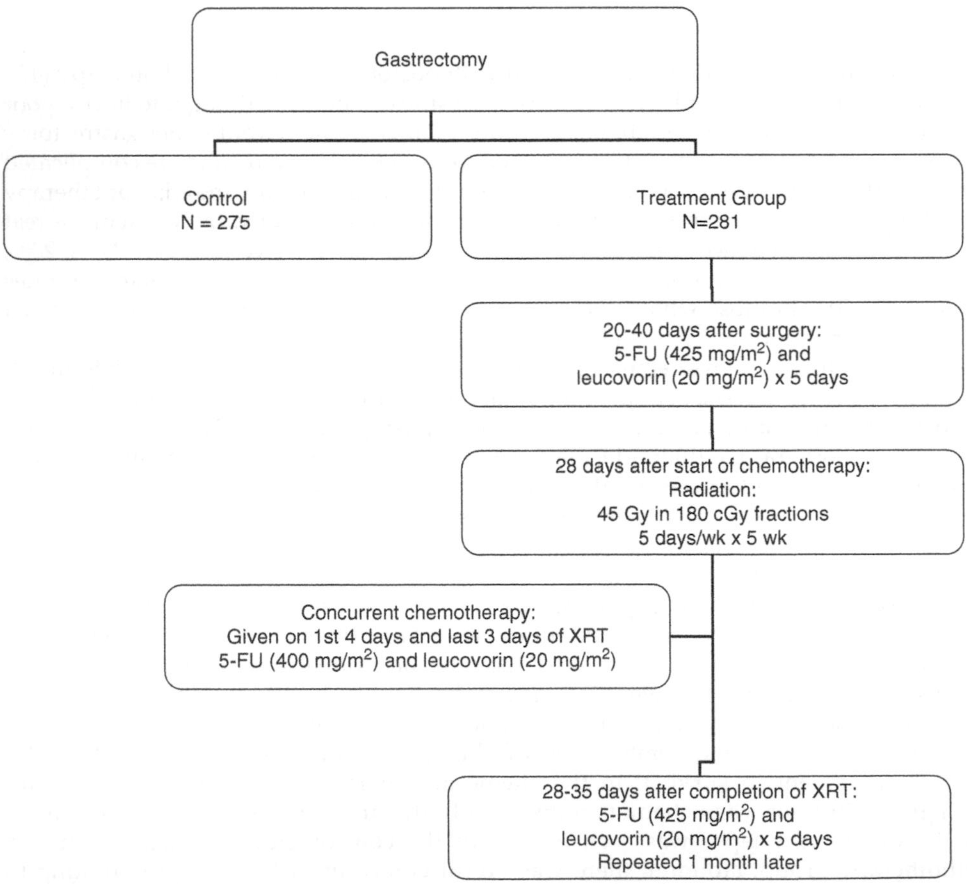

FIGURE 1 Schema of Intergroup 0116 trial (INT 0116). *Abbreviations*: 5-FU, 5-fluorouracil; Gy, Gray; XRT, radiotherapy; N, number.

The median survival was 36 months in the treatment group and 27 months in the control group ($p=0.005$). A benefit of adjuvant therapy was seen in the three-year OS rate (50% vs. 40%, $p=0.005$) and the disease-free survival rate (48% vs. 31%, $p=0.001$). Seventeen percent of patients had to stop therapy secondary to toxicities, and three patients died from complications related to their therapy. Although the study has been criticized for the fact that there was no standardization of surgical technique (only 9% had a full D2 resection), this represented the surgical practice in the institutions where the trials were performed. These data established the benefit of adjuvant combined modality therapy in resectable gastric cancer.

Following the report of INT 0116, a Korean group looked at the patterns of recurrence after a D2 resection and the INT 0116 postoperative regimen, accruing 322 patients into the prospective trial. Seven percent had local recurrence (the majority at the anastomosis), 12% had regional relapse, and 30% had distant failure. Recurrences were found in the original radiation field in 16%, accounting for 35% of all relapses (49). These locoregional failures compare favorably to those reported with surgery alone.

DESIGNING RADIATION FIELDS

Based on the evidence for the role of RT in patients with high risk gastric cancer, the radiation field should be designed with many factors in mind. Surgical clips, preoperative and postoperative imaging studies, knowledge of the location of the primary tumor, extent of tumor by TNM staging criteria, and communication with the surgeon about areas of concern should help guide the radiation oncologist. These patient-specific factors can then be combined with the clinicopathologic prognostic factors and patterns of recurrence described earlier.

The goal is to administer a total dose of 45 to 50 Gy to the stomach or remnant, at the same time as limiting toxicities to the many other vulnerable organs in the upper abdomen, such as intestine, liver, kidneys, and spinal cord (50). Of these, the kidneys are of special concern. At least two-thirds of one functioning kidney should be spared from the radiation fields. In proximal cancers, a part of the left kidney can usually be spared as long as surgical clips in the splenic hilum and porta hepatic are present to guide the creation of the fields (51). The presence of a good quality CT scan which can be registered to the RT treatment planning scan is of major assistance in providing good tumor coverage. Distal cancers are more problematic since the duodenum must usually be included. In these cases, both kidneys will be in the field and must have portions preserved. Proximal tumors should also have 3 to 5 cm of esophagus included; individualized blocks can be used to protect the heart and other structures, particularly in patients treated with the cardiotoxic drug, adriamycin, as a component of the chemotherapy regimen. The left diaphragm may also need to be irradiated in patients with proximal gastric cancers. As mentioned earlier, the use of multiple fields is associated with less toxicity. Therefore, anterior-posterior–posterior-anterior (AP-PA) fields should be combined with lateral or oblique fields (with care to limit liver and kidney exposure) (52). The use of multifield-conformal or intensity-modulated RT can assist in providing good coverage of the tumor while sparing normal tissues.

Tepper et al. (31) used the results of the studies of postoperative radiotherapy in conjunction with what is known about recurrence patterns to design guidelines for therapy based on not only TNM staging, but also the location of the primary tumor and the extent of disease (Table 4). In general, patients with lymph node metastases should be treated with a wide coverage of the tumor bed, the residual stomach, resection margins, and regional nodal stations. Radiation of the nodal basins is optional in patients with node-negative disease, a good surgical resection, pathologic evaluation of greater than 15 lymph nodes, and >5-cm margins. The field should be modified with respect to tolerance levels of the surrounding organs (Table 5).

DISCUSSION

Surgical clearance with negative resection margins, combined with a systematic and pragmatic approach to clinically significant perigastric lymph nodes, is what defines an R0 resection. The quality of initial locoregional treatment is critical to reduce the risk of recurrence, and impact

TABLE 4 Impact of the Site of Primary Lesion and Tumor-Node Stage on Irradiation Treatment Volumes (General Guidelines)

Site of primary and TN stage	Remaining stomach	Tumor-bed volumes	Nodal volumes
Gastroesophageal junction			
GE junction	If allows exclusion of 2/3 R kidney	T-stage dependent	N-stage dependent
T2N0 with invasion in subserosa	Variable	Medial L diaphragm Adjacent body pancreas	None or perigastric, periesophageal[a]
T3N0	Variable	Medial L diaphragm Adjacent body pancreas	None or perigastric, periesophageal, mediastinal, celiac[a]
T4N0	Preferable	As for T3N0 plus sites of adherence with 3- to 5-cm margins	Nodes related to sites of adherence ± as for T3N0
T1-2N(+)	Preferable	Not indicated for T1, as above for T2 into subserosa	Periesophageal, mediastinal, proximal perigastric, celiac
T3-4N(+)	Preferable	As for T3, T4N0	As for T1-2N(+) and T4N0
Cardia/proximal third of stomach			
Cardia/Prox 1/3	Preferred, but spare 2/3 of one kidney (usually R)	Based on T stage	Based on N stage
T2N0 with invasion in subserosa	Variable	Medial L hemidiaphragm, adjacent body of pancreas (±tail)	None or perigastric[a]
T3N0	Variable	Medial L hemidiaphragm, adjacent body of pancreas (±tail)	None or perigastric, optional: periesophageal, mediastinal, celiac[a]
T4N0	Variable	As for T2N0 plus sites of adherence with 3- to 5-cm margins	Nodes related to sites of adherence, ± perigastric, periesophageal, celiac, mediastinal
T1-2N(+)	Preferable	Not indicated for T1, as above for T2 into subserosa	Perigastric, celiac, splenic, suprapancreatic, ± periesophageal, mediastinal, panc-duod, portal
T3-4N(+)	Preferable	As for T3, T4N0	Same as T1-2N(+) and T4N0
Body/mid-third of stomach			
Body/mid 1/3	Yes, spare 2/3 of one kidney	Based on T stage	Based on N stage
T2N0 with invasion in subserosa	Yes	Body of pancreas (±tail)	None or perigastric, optional: celiac, splenic, suprapancreatic panc-duod, portal[a]
T3N0	Yes	Body of pancreas (±tail)	Same as T2N0[a]
T4N0	Yes	As for T3N0	Nodes related to sites of adherence ± perigastric, celiac, splenic, suprapanc, panc-duod, portal
T1-2N(+)	Yes	Not indicated for T1, as above for T2	Perigastric, celiac, splenic, suprapanc, panc-duod, portal
T3-4N(+)	Yes	As for T3, T4N0	Same as T1-2N(+) and T4N0
Pylorus/distal third of stomach			
Pylorus/distal 1/3	Yes, spare 2/3 of one kidney (usually L)	Based on T stage	Based on N stage
T2N0 with invasion in subserosa	Variable	Head of pancreas (±body), 1st and 2nd duodenum	None or perigastric, optional: suprapancreatic panc-duod, celiac, portal[a]
T3N0	Variable	Same as T2N0	Same as T2N0[a]
T4N0	Preferable	As for T2N0 plus sites of adherence with 3- to 5-cm margins	Nodes related to sites of adherence, ± perigastric, panc-duod, celiac, suprapanc, portal
T1-2N(+)	Preferable	Not indicated for T1	Perigastric, panc-duod, celiac, portal, suprapanc, optional: splenic hilum
T3-4N(+)	Preferable	As for T3, T4N0	Same as T1-2N(+) and T4N0

[a]Optional node inclusion for T2-3N0 lesions if there has been an adequate surgical nodal dissection (D2 dissection) or at least 15 nodes examined pathologically.
Abbreviations: GE, gastroesophageal; TN, tumor node; N, node.

TABLE 5 Tolerance Organ Structures by Site of Primary Gastric Tumor

Site of primary tumor	Tolerance organ structures
Gastroesophageal junction (GEJ)	Heart, lung, spinal cord, kidneys
Cardia/proximal 1/3	Heart, lung, spinal cord, kidneys, liver
Body/middle 1/3	Kidneys, spinal cord, liver
Pylorus/distal 1/3	Kidneys, spinal cord, liver

on overall prognosis. Although survival is dictated predominantly by the stage of disease at presentation, the impact of an R0 resection with at least a minimum standard of lymph node dissection takes on a greater significance in the face of limited systemic therapies. It is only when the extent of disease is clear do we begin to understand the biology of the disease, and the impact of adjuvant therapies.

In summary, there are advantages seen in locoregional control and survival with the addition of radiotherapy in the treatment of patients with gastric cancer, especially those at high risk for recurrence. Postoperative chemoradiotherapy is now the standard of care, given the results of INT 0116, whereas the use of intraoperative therapy may play a part in the future pending more investigation. Preoperative therapy can help downstage marginally resectable patients and may yield clues to the biology of the disease, but should not be the standard therapy for all patients.

REFERENCES

1. Greenlee R, Hill-Harmon M, Murray T, et al. Cancer statistics, 2001. CA Cancer J Clin 2001; 51:15–36.
2. Siewert J, Bottcher K, Stein H, et al. Relevant prognostic factors in gastric cancer: ten-year results of the German Gastric Cancer Study. Ann Surg 1998; 228:449–461.
3. Bonenkamp J, Hermans J, Sasako M, et al. Extended lymph-node dissection for gastric cancer. Dutch Gastric Cancer Group. NEJM 1999; 340:908–914.
4. Cuschieri A, Weeden S, Fielding J, et al. Patient survival after D1 and D2 resections fro gastric cancer: long-term results of the MRC randomized surgical trial. Surgical Co-operative Group. Br J Cancer 1999; 79:1522–1530.
5. Karpeh M, Leon L, Klimestra D, et al. Lymph node staging in gastric cancer: is location more important than number? An analysis of 1038 patients. Ann Surg 2000; 232:362–371.
6. Bozzetti F. Rationale for extended lymphadenopathy in gastrectomy for carcinoma. J Am Coll Surg 1995; 180:505–508.
7. Doglietto G, Pacelli F, Caprino P, et al. Surgery: independent prognostic factor in curable and far advanced gastric carcinoma. World J Surg 2000; 24:459–463.
8. Hartgrink H, Bonenkamp H, van de Velde C. Influence of surgery on outcomes in gastric cancer. Surg Oncol Clin N Am 2000; 9:97.
9. Kim J, Kwon O, Oh S, et al. Results of surgery on 6589 gastric cancer patients and immunochemosurgery as the best treatment of advanced gastric cancer. Ann Surg 1992; 216:269–278.
10. Kim J. Surgical results in gastric cancer. Semin Surg Oncol 1999; 17:132–138.
11. Hughes B, Yip D, Chao M, et al. Audit of postoperative chemoradiotherapy as adjuvant therapy for resected gastroesophageal adenocarcinoma: an Australian multicentre experience. ANZ J Surg 2004; 74:951–956.
12. Hundahl S, Phillips J, Menck H. The National Cancer Data Base Report on poor survival of US gastric carcinoma patients treated with gastrectomy. Cancer 2000; 88:921–932.
13. MacDonald J, Smalley S, Benedetti J, et al. Chemoradiotherapy after surgery compared with surgery alone for adenocarcinoma of the stomach or gastroesophageal junction. NEJM 2001; 345:725–730.
14. Yoo C, Noh S, Shin D, et al. Recurrence following curative resection for gastric carcinoma. Br J Cancer 2000; 87:236–242.
15. Maehara Y, Hasuda S, Koga T, et al. Postoperative outcome and sites of recurrence in pateints following curative resection of gastric cancer. Br J Cancer 2000; 87:353–357.
16. Minsky B. The role of radiation therapy in gastric cancer. Semin Oncol 1996; 23:390–396.
17. Wisbeck W, Bevher E, Russell A. Adenocarcinoma of the stomach: autopsy observations with therapeutic implications for the radiation oncologist. Radiother Oncol 1986; 7:13–18.
18. Gunderson L, Sosin H. Adenocarcinoma of the stomach: areas of failure in a reoperation series (second or symptomatic looks): clinicopathologic correlation and implications for adjuvant therapy. Int J Radiat Oncol Biol Phys 1982; 8:1–11.

19. D'Angelica M, Gonen M, Brennan M, et al. Patterns of initial recurrence in completely resected gastric adenocarcinoma. Ann Surg 2004; 240:808–816.
20. Maruyama K, Gunven P, Okabayashi K. Lymph node metastases of gastric cancer. General pattern in 1931 patients. Ann Surg 1989; 210:586–602.
21. Iivonen M, Mattila J, Nordback I, et al. Long-term follow-up of patients with jejunal pouch reconstruction after total gastrectomy. A randomized prospective study. Scand J Gastroenterol 2000; 35:679–685.
22. Landry J, Tepper J, Wood W, et al. Patterns of failure following curative resection of gastric carcinoma. Int J Radiat Oncol Biol Phys 1990; 19:1357–1362.
23. Fujimoto S, Takahashi M, Mutou T, et al. Clinicopathologic characteristics of gastric cancer patients with cancer infiltration at surgical margins at gastrectomy. Anticancer Res 1997; 17:689–694.
24. Group BSC. Resection line disease in stomach cancer. Br Med J 1984; 289:601–603.
25. Gall C, Rieger N, Wattchow D. Positive proximal resection margins after resection for carcinoma of the oesophagus and stomach: effect on survival and symptom recurrence. Aust N Z J Surg 1996; 66:734–737.
26. Songun I, Bonenkamp J, Hermans J, et al. Prognostic value of resection line involvement in patients undergoing curative resection for gastric cancer. Eur J Cancer 1996; 32A:433–437.
27. Papachristou D, Agnanti N, D'Agostino H, et al. Histologically positive esophageal margins in the surgical treatment of gastric cancer. Am J Surg 1980; 139:711–713.
28. Kim S, Karpeh M, Klimestra D, et al. Effect of microscopic resection line disease on gastric cancer survival. J Gatsrointest Surg 1999; 3:24–33.
29. Henning G, Schild S, Stafford S, et al. Results of irradiation or chemoirradiation following resection of gastric adenocarcinoma. Int J Radiat Oncol Biol Phys 2000; 46:589–598.
30. Avizonis V, Buzydlowski J, Lanciano R, et al. Treatment of adenocarcinoma of the stomach with resection, intraoperative radiotherapy, and adjuvant external beam radiation: a phase II study from Radiation Therapy Oncology Group 85-01. Ann Surg Oncol 1995; 2:295–302.
31. Tepper J, Gunderson L. Radiation treatment parameters in the adjuvant postoperative therapy of gastric cancer. Semin Radiat Oncol 2002; 12:187–195.
32. Hallissey M, Dunn J, Ward L, et al. The second British Stomach Cancer Group Trial of adjuvant radiotherapy or chemotherapy in resectable gastric cancer: a five-year follow-up. Lancet 1994; 343:1309–1312.
33. Slot A, Meerwaldt J, van Putten W, et al. Adjuvant post-operative radiotherapy for gastric carcinoma with poor prognostic signs. Radiother Oncol 1989; 16:269–274.
34. Calvo F, Aristy J, Avizonis V, et al. Intraoperative and external radiotherapy in resected gastric cancer: updated report of a phase II trial. Int J Radiat Oncol Biol Phys 1992; 24:729–736.
35. Mauer A, Haraf D, Ferguson M, et al. Docetaxel-based combined modality therapy for locally advanced carcinoma of the esophagus and gastric carcinoma. Proc Am Soc Clin Oncol 2000; 19: A954.
36. Mansfield P, Lowy A, Feig B, et al. Preoperative chemoradiation for potentially respectable gastric cancer. Proc Am Soc Clin Oncol 2000; 19:A955.
37. Ajani J, Mansfield P, Janjan N, et al. Multi-institutional trial of preoperative chemoradiotherapy in patients with potentially resectable gastric carcinoma. JCO 2004; 22:2774–2780.
38. Kosse V. Combined treatment of gastric cancer using hypoxic radiotherapy. Vopr Onkol 1990; 36:1349.
39. Zhang Z, Gu X, Yin W, et al. Randomized clinical trial combinations on the preoperative irradiation and surgery in the treatment of adenocarcinoma of the gastric cardia. (AGC) report on 370 patients. Int J Radiat Oncol Biol Phys 1998; 42:929.
40. Shchepotin I, Evans S, Conry V, et al. Intensive preoperative radiotherapy with local hyperthermia for treatment of gastric carcinoma. Surg Oncol 1994; 3:37.
41. Takahashi M, Abe M. Intraoperative radiotherapy fro carcinoma of the stomach. Eur J Surg Oncol 1986; 12:247.
42. Chen G, Song S. Evaluation of intraoperative radiotherapy for gastric carcinoma analysis of 247 patients. In: Abe M, Takahashi M, eds. Proceedings of the Third International IORT SYmposium, Kyoto, Japan. New York: Pargamon Press, 1991:190.
43. Sindelar W, Kinsella T, Tepper J, et al. Randomized trial of intraoperative radiation in carcinoma of the stomach. Am J Surg 1993; 199165:178–187.
44. Gez E, Sulkes A, Yablonsky-Peretz T, et al. Combined 5-fluorouracil (5-FU) and radiation therapy following resection of locally advanced gastric carcinoma of the stomach. J Surg Oncol 1986; 31:139–142.
45. Dent D, Werner I, Novis B, et al. Prospective randomized trial of combined oncological therapy for gastric carcinoma. Cancer 1979; 44:385–391.
46. Moertel C, Childs D, O'Fallon J, et al. Combined 5-fluorouracil and radiation therapy as a surgical adjuvant for poor prognosis gastric carcinoma. JCO 1984; 2:1249–1254.
47. Allum W, Hallissey M, Ward L, et al. A controlled, prospective, randomized trial of adjuvant chemotherapy or radiotherapy in resectable gastric cancer: interim report. British Stomach Cancer Group. Br J Cancer 1989; 60:739–744.

48. Regine W, Mohiuddin M. Impact of adjuvant therapy on locally advanced adenocarcinoma of the stomach. Int J Radiat Oncol Biol Phys 1992; 24:921–927.
49. Lim D, Kim D, Kang M, Kim Y, Kang Y, et al. Patterns of failure in gastric carcinoma after D2 gastrectomy and chemoradiotherapy: a radiation oncologist's view. Br J Cancer 2004; 91:11–17.
50. Gunderson L, Martenson J. Gastrointestinal tract radiation tolerance. In: Vaeth J, Meyer J, eds. Radiation Tolerance of Normal Tissues. Vol. 23. Basel: Karger, 1989:277.
51. Willett C, Tepper J, Orlow E, Shipley W. Renal complications secondary to radiation treatment of upper abdominal malignancies. Int J Radiat Oncol Biol Phys 1986; 12:1601.
52. Gunderson L, Donohue J, Alberts S. Cancer of the stomach. In: Abeloff M, Armitage J, Niederhuber J, Kastan M, McKenna W, eds. Clinical Oncology. Philadelphia: Elsevier, 2004.

9 The Role of Chemotherapy and Chemoradiation as Adjuvant Treatment for Resected Gastric Adenocarcinoma

John S. Macdonald
Gastrointestinal Oncology Service, Saint Vincent's Comprehensive Cancer Center, New York, New York, U.S.A.

INTRODUCTION

The primary curative treatment of gastric carcinoma and distal esophageal cancer is surgical resection (1–6). In stomach cancer potentially resectable for cure (stages 0–IV M0), the surgical aim should be to perform a tumor resection entailing at least a partial gastrectomy with an en bloc dissection of lymphatic tissue. For at least 20 years (5,6) there has been an international debate regarding the most appropriate surgical procedures to use in cases of potentially curable gastric carcinoma. The value of extended lymph node dissection in increasing the cure rate for respectable gastric cancer is discussed elsewhere in this volume. Whether extended lymph node dissection increases surgical cure rates may still be debatable; however, there is no doubt that extended lymph node dissection improves precision of staging. A report by Bunt et al. (7) in 1995 demonstrated that patients undergoing D2 dissections had significantly more accurate surgical pathological staging than patients undergoing D1 dissections (Table 1). As part of a large randomized comparison of D1 and D2 nodal dissections performed in the Netherlands (1), pathologists were asked to evaluate staging of patients on study who had undergone D2 resections. These pathologic specimens were first evaluated as if only D1 resection (removal of N1 nodes only) had been performed and a pathologic stage was applied. Subsequently, the whole specimen, including the N2 nodes was evaluated and the actual pathologic stage was defined. This study demonstrated that a D1 dissection, when compared to a D2 dissection, understaged 60% to 75% of patients (Table 1). For clinical investigators evaluating the effect of postoperative systemic therapy in gastric cancer, it is important to understand that less than D2 dissections result in a significant risk of understaging.

Irrespective of the surgical procedure used for treatment of gastric cancer, the effectiveness of surgical resection, if increased cure rate is the goal, is poor. Overall survival of resected node-positive patients in the United States and Great Britain is at best 30% to 35% (8–10). The reason patients die is the development of symptomatic metastatic disease arising from unresected microscopic metastases present at the time of surgical resection. Because of the high risk of relapse after gastric resection, there has been a great deal of interest in strategies to prevent relapse and improve survival for patients with stomach cancer. The major approaches that have been explored fall into the categories of preoperative, or neoadjuvant, approaches and postoperative, or adjuvant, therapy strategies.

ADJUVANT CHEMOTHERAPY

Adjuvant cytotoxic chemotherapy for gastric cancer has been studied over the last 40 years. This approach has demonstrated its usefulness in other diseases such as colon and breast cancers. Gastric cancer would seem to be a natural disease to test adjuvant chemotherapy, as there are a number of significantly active advanced disease chemotherapy programs that demonstrated activity in the treatment of disseminated stomach cancer.

A variety of combination chemotherapy regimens have been widely used in the palliative management of patients with gastric cancer (11–19). Over the last decade, there has been interest in the use of prolonged infusion of 5-fluorouracil (FU) as a part of the combination chemotherapy treatment for stomach cancer. Cookes et al. (12) used continuous infusion 5-FU as a major component of a neoadjuvant program and Webb et al. (17) reported important results with a combination regimen designated combination of epirubicin, cisplatin, and 5-fluorouracil

TABLE 1 Gastric Cancer: Stage Migration, D1 Compared to D2 Gastrectomies

D1 TNM		D2 TNM				
		Stage				
Stage	#pts	II	IIIA	IIIB	IV	Change (%)
II	48	30	18			38
IIIA	49		19	21	1	61
IIIB	24			6	18	75

Abbreviation: TNM, tumor node metastases.

(ECF). The ECF regimen uses protracted infusion of 5-FU at a daily rate of 200 mg/m^2 with epirubicin 50 mg/m^2 and cisplatinum 60 mg/m^2 administered every 21 days. Epirubicin is an anthracycline analog available in western Europe for several years and now is commercially available in the United States although its approval indication is for breast cancer, not gastrointestinal cancer in the United States. ECF trial reported by Webb et al. was in gastroesophageal cancer and was a phase III randomized trial (17) reported in 1997. This study compared to ECF with 5-fluorouracil, adriamycin, methotrexate (FAMTX) in patients with locally advanced gastroesophageal adenocarcinoma. In this study, 274 patients with adenocarcinoma or undifferentiated cancer were randomized between FAMTX and ECF. The FAMTX regimen caused significant hematologic toxicity and was inferior with regard to response rate and survival when compared to ECF. The overall response rate for ECF was 45% versus 21% for FAMTX ($P = 0.002$). The median survival for ECF was 8.9 months versus 5.7 months ($P = 0.0009$). At one year, 36% of ECF and 21% of FAMTX patients were alive. Webb et al. (17) also assessed global quality of life scores in their study. The global quality of life was superior for ECF at 24 weeks. This advantage in quality of life however did not persist as patients were followed further on the study. The advanced disease activity of ECF led to its use as neoadjuvant therapy in a clinical trial (20) carried out by the British Medical Research Council (MRC). Epirubicin may not be an essential component of ECF. Ross et al. (21) performed a phase III study of ECF versus a very similar regimen, mitomycin-C, cisplastin, 5-fluorouracil (MCF), that substituted mitomycin-C (7 mg/m^2 every six weeks) for epirubicin and uses somewhat different doses of 5-FU (300 mg/m^2/day × 24 weeks) and cisplatin (50 mg/m^2 every q three weeks). The overall rates of survival were no different between the ECF and MCF regimens. This trial supports the use of MCF if either epirubicin is not available or a clinician would prefer not to use an anthracycline.

Other more recent regimens include the combination of docetaxel–cisplatin (15), and the use of regimen of irinotecan and cisplatin (Table 2). The irinotecan and cisplatin combination (13) has been evaluated and shown to have good activity in gastroesophageal cancers. The response rate for adenocarcinoma with the regimen was 12/23 (57%) with excellent palliation of tumor-related symptoms. Another regimen of interest is the combination of docetaxel and cisplatin (15) (Table 2). In a European study of 85 patients with advanced gastric cancer, the overall response rate was 36% and 7/85 (8%) had complete responses. The median survival in this study was 10 months, and grade IV toxicity was seen in only 4% of cases. In June 2003, the results of a large phase III international clinical trial (Table 2) tested a 5-FU/cisplatin/docetaxel (DCF) versus a control arm of a 5-FU/cisplatin. This study (22) demonstrated that DCF had a superior time to progression (5.5 months) versus that produced by cisplatin plus 5-FU (3.8 months). Survival for DCF, a median of 10.2 months, was superior but not statistically significantly improved compared to the platinum–fluorouracil (CF) therapy (8.5 months). The final results of this study were reported at American Society of Clinical Oncology (ASCO), 2005 (23). Although the median survival for DCF fell from 10.2 months as reported in 2003 (22) to 9.2 months, there was demonstrated a statistical survival benefit for DCF over CF. However, DCF remains quite toxic (23). DCF is clearly a regimen of interest and will undoubtedly be evaluated as adjuvant and neoadjuvant therapy in the future.

The data on therapy of advanced gastric cancer allows one to draw some conclusions with regard to the standard of care for patients with metastatic stomach cancer. It is reasonable to assume that several approaches are appropriate standards of chemotherapeutic management

TABLE 2 Selected Chemoradiation Regimens

Drug	Dose	Day 1	Day 2	Frequency
Irinotecan/cisplatin		1	2	
Irinotecan	65 mg/m^2	X	X	Repeat every 21 days
Cisplatinum	30 mg/m^2	X	X	Repeat every 21 days
Docetaxel/cisplatin	Day 1			
Docetaxel	75 mg/m^2			Repeat every 21 days
Cisplatin	75 mg/m^2			Repeat every 21 days
DCF				
Docetaxel	75 mg/m^2 IV			Every 3 wk
Cisplatin	75 mg/m^2 IV			Every 3 wk
5-FU	750 mg/m^2/day CIV			Every 3 wk

Abbreviations: 5-FU, 5-fluorouracil; CIV, continous intravenous infusion; DCF, docetaxel cisplatin 5-fluorouracil.
Source: From Refs. 13,15,22.

for patients with gastric cancer. FAMTX is well tolerated and can certainly result in some complete responses in patients with gastric cancer, but is no longer considered a front-line regimen for advanced gastric cancer. The more exciting approaches entail the use of continuous infusions of fluorinated pyrimidines. The ECF data in comparison to FAMTX is certainly of interest and ECF or similar regimens using other anthracyclines require further phase II and III evaluation. Finally, taxane- and irinotecan-based regimens such as described previously are also of interest and appropriate for use in patients with advanced gastric cancer. However, it is important that none of these regimens result in long-term control of metastatic adenocarcinoma of the stomach. Although some regimens produce complete response rates as high as 15%, these complete responses are not durable.

Adjuvant therapy of gastric cancer using systemic therapy alone or as part of combined modality therapy with curative intent has also been widely tested within the last three decades. Adjuvant cytotoxic chemotherapy alone has been of minimal benefit. A meta-analysis published by Hermans et al. in 1993 (24) demonstrated no conclusive value for adjuvant chemotherapy. A meta-analysis published in 1999 by Earle et al. (25) showed borderline statistically significant, but clinically insignificant, survival improvement from the use of adjuvant chemotherapy. In the United States, a clinical trial (9) testing 5-fluorouracil, adriamycin, mitomycin-C (FAM) chemotherapy in a cooperative group [Southwest Oncology Group (SWOG)] also did not demonstrate any benefit for adjuvant chemotherapy. In this study, (9), 191 patients were randomized between one year of FAM following surgery or surgery alone. There was no benefit for chemotherapy and the survival curves of treatment and control cases were overlapping. The overall survival at five years demonstrated in the study was approximately 35% for both surgery alone, and for surgery followed by FAM chemotherapy. A recent review article of adjuvant chemotherapy trials and meta-analysis of adjuvant therapy in gastric cancer by Meyerhardt and Fuchs (26) concluded that there was no convincing evidence for adjuvant chemotherapy use in resected gastric cancer and that postoperative chemotherapy should be considered investigational.

POSTOPERATIVE CHEMORADIATION

One of the important therapeutic findings in gastric cancer over the last 20 years has been that, in patients with known residual disease, the combination of radiation therapy plus fluorinated pyrimidine (5-FU) used as a radiation sensitizer, could result in the complete control (apparent cure) of small amounts of residual or recurrent stomach cancer (27). This use of combined modality radiation and chemotherapy has also been demonstrated to be efficacious in esophageal cancer (28) and has resulted in that disease, in a prolonged disease-free survival of patients without the need for surgical resection. Because of the demonstrated benefit for combined radiation and fluorinated pyrimidine in patients with known residual gastric and

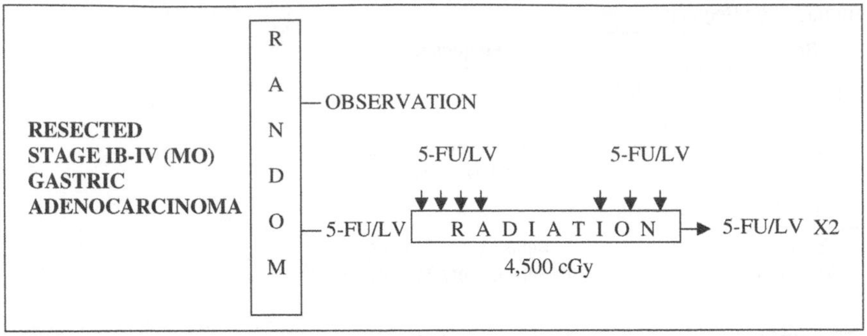

FIGURE 1 Schema for SWOG 9008/INT 0116, patients with resected stage IB-IV (MO) are randomly allocated to either observation or postoperative chemoirradiation. *Abbreviations:* 5-FU, 5-fluorouracil; cGY, centiGray; LV, leucovorin; SWOG, Southwest Oncology Group.

esophageal carcinoma, a U.S. gastrointestinal cancer Intergroup Study was initiated in early 1991 to test whether the combination of 5-FU leucovorin plus radiation therapy after surgical resection would be of value to patients with resected gastric carcinoma (Fig. 1). This study enrolled a total of 603 patients in seven years of accrual and was reported initially at the ASCO in the spring of 2000 (29) and was updated in September 2001 (30) at which time median follow-up was approximately four years. This study included 556 eligible patients, 281 cases receiving 5-FU/leucovorin/radiation and 275 cases in the observation arm. Eighty-five percent of cases in both arms had node-positive carcinoma (stage IIIA, IIIB, or IV). Although the study only mandated that gastric resection with curative intent be performed, the types of surgery performed in this study were carefully analyzed. Results demonstrated that the standard of care in the United States in the 1990s did not include extended lymph node dissections. Fifty-four percent of cases underwent less than a D1 dissection (only partial removal of the N1 nodes), and only 10% of patients were treated with a formal D2 dissection.

As the ultimate goal of adjuvant therapy is prevention of cancer recurrence, improvement in long-term survival, serious long-term toxicities of therapy are unacceptable. The analysis of treatment-related toxicity showed that combined modality therapy as delivered in SWOG 9008/INT-0116 was well tolerated. Although 41% of patients experienced grade III and 32% experienced grade IV toxicities (mainly hematologic toxicity), only three patients (1%) died as a result of treatment. In designing Southwest Oncology Group (SWOG) 9008/INT-0116, it was considered very important to carefully review centrally and verify radiation treatment planning prior to initial treatment to assume the safe and effective delivery of combined modality therapy. When SWOG 9008/INT-0116 radiation treatment plans were reviewed before initiation of therapy, 34% were found to have major deviations. Two-thirds of these deviations would have resulted in undertreatment of patients, while one-third had the potential for delivering severely toxic radiation. Incorrect treatment plans were modified before initiation of therapy.

Disease-free and overall survival (Table 3) was significantly improved by combined modality 5-FU/leucovorin/radiation therapy (30). Median time to relapse was 30 months in the treatment arm versus 19 months in the control arm ($P < 0.0001$, two-sided P value). Overall survival was also improved with a median survival of 35 months in the treatment arm versus 28 months in the control arm ($P = 0.01$, two-sided P value). Although there was a suggestion that local relapse (defined as relapse within the residual stomach or gastric pouch) was decreased by combined modality therapy, this was not statistically significant. The outcome data on SWOG 9008/INT-0116 were updated in January 2004 (31). At this time, median follow-up was seven years. Table 4 compares overall and disease-free survival outcomes from the 2001 and 2004 analyses. As can be seen, results for the major endpoints of disease-free and overall survival did not change. The 2004 analysis confirms that chemoradiation results in prolonged and statistically significant benefit in disease-free and overall survival to patients with resected gastric cancer. Table 4 demonstrates that the improvements in disease-free and overall survival do not deteriorate over time. The 2004 analysis also shows that chemoradiation does not result in late toxic events leading to treatment-related morbidity or mortality in cases on the treatment

TABLE 3 SWOG9008/INT0116 Results

	Chemoradiation	Control
No. of cases	281	275
Disease-free survival median (mo)	30[a]	19
Overall survival median (mo)	35[b]	28

[a]$P < 0.0001$.
[b]$P = 0.01$.
Abbreviations: INT 0116, Intergroup trial 0116; SWOG, Southwest Oncology Group.

arm. Exploratory subset analyses were performed on the INT-0116 data and failed to show any subset (T-stage, N-stage location in the stomach, type of surgery) where chemoradiation could be demonstrated not to be effective. The significant improvements demonstrated in SWOG 9008/INT-0116 in disease-free and overall survival obtained with acceptable toxicity, have made combined modality radiation chemotherapy a standard of care in patients with resected gastric cancer in North America.

The results reported in INT 0116 are provocative and are thought by some experts to result from the fact that in the United States D2 dissections are not a standard of care, but rather lesser nodal dissections are commonly performed. It is a fact (Table 5) that when the extent of surgical procedures was analyzed in INT-0116, it was found that 54% of cases had less than a D1 resection performed. Since the data of Bunt et al. (7) demonstrates that a D1 dissection compared with a D2 dissection understages 60% to 75% of cases, it is highly likely that many of the cases in INT-0116 are understaged and also were left with residual unresected nodal metastases. It is well known that radiation is effective therapy for small volume nodal disease, and therefore one could conclude that the results of INT-0116 are positive as chemoradiation "cleans up" nodal metastases left behind by "inadequate" surgery. Whether this conclusion is valid or not cannot be determined from the data in INT-0116. The ultimate question is the following: Does radical gastrectomy with D2 nodal dissection obviate the need for postoperative chemoradiation? The only way this question may be answered is to perform a phase III trial randomly allocating patients undergoing D2 resections to postoperative chemoradiation or obstruction. Such a study has not been performed. However, there has been an intriguing, although not randomized experience, addressing this question reported by Kim et al. (32) in Korea (Table 6).

TABLE 4 SWOG 9008/INT 0116 Results

	Hazard ratio	95% CI	*P*-value	Median obs	Median RX
Overall survival					
NEJM 2001	1.32	(1.06–1.64)	0.005	27 mo	36 mo
Update 2004	1.31	(1.08–1.61)	0.006	26 mo	35 mo
Disease-free survival					
NEJM 2001	1.52	(1.23–1.86)	<0.001	19 mo	30 mo
Update 2004	1.52	(1.25–1.85)	<0.001	19 mo	30 mo

Abbreviations: CI, confidence interval; INT 0116, Intergroup 0116 trial; SWOG, Southwest Oncology Group; NEJM, the New England Journal of Medicine; obs, observation; RX, treatment .

TABLE 5 SWOG 9008/INT 0116 Results

Surgical procedures (based on 551 cases)
<D1 = 54%
D1 = 36%
D2 = 10%

Abbreviations: INT 0116, Intergroup 0116 trial; SWOG, Southwest Oncology Group.

TABLE 6 Postoperative Chemoradiation Effect in Cases Undergoing D2 Radial Gastrectomy

Gastric cancer			
Postoperative chemoradiation after D2 dissection			
No. of cases	990	CRT: 544	no CRT: 446
Nodes (+)	93%		
>15 nodes resected	98%		
Results			
5yr OS		5yr RFS	
CRT (+)	CRT (−)	CRT (+)	CRT (−)
57.1%	51.0%	54.5%	47.9%
$p=0.019$		$p=0.016$	
Failure	**CRT**	**without CRT**	***P* value**
Locoregional	81/544 (14.9)	97/446 (21.7)	0.0050
Distant	205/544 (37.7)	168/446 (37.7)	0.9962

Abbreviations: CRT, chemoradiation therapy; OS, overall survival; RFS, relapse-free survival. *Source*: From Ref. 32.

These investigators reported on approximately 990 cases of stomach cancer resected with extended radiation (D2 dissections). Five hundred and forty of these cases were treated with the same chemoradiation regimen used in INT-0116. The remaining 440 cases served as only controls. The results for disease-free and overall survival demonstrated statistically significant improvement for cases receiving postoperative chemoradiation; the results from this phase II experience strongly suggests that a phase III study randomizing patients undergoing "ideal surgery" to chemoradiation or observation should be performed.

NEOADJUVANT THERAPY

Neoadjuvant treatment, which typically employs chemotherapy and/or radiation therapy before attempts at surgical resection of gastric cancer, has been an area in which important results have become available in the last several years. It is reasonable to discuss recent phase III results of neoadjuvant chemotherapy as clinicians will be interested in comparing these outcomes with those achieved in SWOG 9008/INT-0116. Until recently, only phase II neoadjuvant studies have been reported. In the spring of 2003, the first well-powered phase III neoadjuvant chemotherapy study was presented at the ASCO meeting (20). This clinical trial named MAGIC, and performed by the British MRC randomly allocated 503 cases of potentially resectable gastric cancer to either preoperative or postoperative ECF chemotherapy versus surgery alone. Because of the general acceptance of postoperative chemoradiation as a result of the reporting of SWOG 9008/INT-0116, clinicians have been interested in comparing the outcomes of the MAGIC study with the results seen with postoperative chemoradiation. The results of the MAGIC study are illustrated in Table 7. Preoperative chemotherapy resulted in statistically significant improvement in disease-free survival. There was an increased rate of overall survival at two years (48% vs. 40%) with preoperative chemotherapy but this improvement was

TABLE 7 Result of Neoadjuvant Therapy: MAGIC Study

Two-year survival	ECF	Surgery only
Progression-free survival	45%	30%[a]
Overall survival	48%	40%[b]

[a] $P = 0.002$ log rank.
[b] $P = 0.063$ log rank.
Abbreviations: ECF, combination of epirubicin, cisplatin, and 5-fluorouracil.

not statistically significant when reported initially in 2003. However, data presented at the ASCO in May 2005 showed statistically significant improved survival with ECF (33). There was no excess in surgical complication rates for neoadjuvant cases versus surgery only cases. Toxicities with preoperative therapy were acceptable and preoperative chemotherapy was delivered as planned in over 91% of cases commencing chemotherapy. However, it was more difficult to deliver postoperative chemotherapy as planned and only 133/250 (53%) of cases commenced postoperative chemotherapy treatment.

There were two other important results of the MAGIC study. First, the curative resection rate appeared to be increased by neoadjuvant therapy. Surgeons were asked to assess whether a curative, "R0," resection had been performed at the time of surgery. Operating surgeons estimated that 69% of surgery only cases were curatively resected versus 79% of patients receiving neoadjuvant therapy ($P = 0.018$) (Table 8). Although the rate of curative resection was increased in the ECF-treated cases, the absolute number of cases resected in this arm was less (212 vs. 232) than in the surgery alone arm. This was because some of the patients randomized to neoadjuvant therapy never came to surgical resection. If the total number of cases randomized to the ECF arm is used as the denominator, rather than those actually resected, the rate of R0 resection would decrease in this arm. Although the increase in R0 resection resulting from neoadjuvant therapy may be questionable, there was a significant (Table 8) downstaging of tumor stage (surgery only T3 = 64%, neoadjuvant therapy T3 = 49%, $P = 0.011$). The results of the MAGIC study including decrease of tumor size, some evidence of an increased rate of R0 resection, and increased overall survival, clearly indicated that there are some potentially important clinical benefits for neoadjuvant chemotherapy. However, it is not yet clear how neoadjuvant therapy may best be incorporated into the multimodality therapy of localized gastric cancer, particularly with regard to how this approach may be combined with postoperative chemoradiation.

In attempting to understand how neoadjuvant chemotherapy and postoperative chemoradiation may best be used in cases with resectable gastric cancer, clinicians have been interested in comparing the outcomes of MAGIC with those obtained in SWOG 9008/INT-0116. In attempting to compare MAGIC and SWOG 9008/INT-0116, it is helpful to compare patient characteristics (Table 9). There are similar numbers of patients in both studies (>500) and an equal frequency of T3/T4 tumors (approximately 65%). The frequency of nodal metastases was greater in INT-0116 (85%) than in MAGIC (72%). Poor prognosis cases with greater than four nodes involved with tumor were more common in INT-0116 (43%) than MAGIC (27%). In general, it appears that the INT-0116 cases were at higher risk for recurrence than MAGIC cases. Although it is not possible to directly compare specific outcomes between the two studies using tests of statistical significance, it is possible to compare general outcomes (Table 10). Cases treated with surgery alone did better in INT-0116 (52% two-year survival) when compared to the surgery only arm of MAGIC (40% two-year survival). When the treatment arms were compared, better two-year survival outcomes for INT-0116 (58%) were seen compared to MAGIC where the two-year survival was 48%. The five-year survival comparisons are also demonstrated in Table 10 and favor INT-0116. It is important to emphasize that validity for these general comparisons would need to be confirmed in prospective studies before any conclusions on relative efficacy may be drawn. However, as it was demonstrated in MAGIC that after preoperative chemotherapy, tumors were down-staged, and resectability increased, both highly desirable results,

TABLE 8 Gastric Cancer—MAGIC Trial Treatment Results: Effects of Neoadjuvant Therapy on Curative Resection and Downstaging of Tumors

	ECF	Surgery only
No. of cases having surgery	212 (85%)	232 (92%)
Median time to surgery	99 days	14 days
Proportion of curative resections	79%[a]	69%[a]
Proportion of T3/T4 tumor	49%	64%[b]

[a]$P = 0.018$.
[b]$P = 0.011$.
Abbreviations: ECF, combination of epirubicin, cisplatin, and 5-fluorouracil.

TABLE 9 Gastric Cancer—Patient Characteristics of INT 0116 and MAGIC Trials

	INT 0116	MAGIC
No. of cases	554	503
T3 /T4	68%	64% (surgery only)
Nodes (–)	15%	28%
Nodes (+)	85%	72%
Nodes>4	43%	27%

Abbreviations: INT 0116, Intergroup 0116 trial.

TABLE 10 Gastric Cancer—Two- and Five-year Survivals: INT 0116 and MAGIC Trials

Study	Surgery (%)	Chemorads or chemo (%)
2-year survival		
INT 0116	52	58
MAGIC	40	48
5-year survival		
INT 0116	25	43
MAGIC	23	36

and because INT-0116 demonstrated that postoperative chemoradiation increased disease-free and overall survival, one could argue that an important strategy in new studies would be to evaluate neoadjuvant therapy combined with postoperative chemoradiation. Such studies would require phase II pilot clinical trials to carefully assess patient tolerance of aggressive pre- and postoperative therapy. Combining neoadjuvant and postoperative chemoradiation may well result in further improvement in outcomes for patients with resectable gastric cancer.

FUTURE PROSPECTS

What future approaches will be used in attempting to improve the survival of patients with stomach cancer? The results of SWOG 9008/INT-0116 demonstrate that for the population of gastric cancer patients undergoing gastrectomy in the United States, postoperative chemoradiation improves survival and future results in clinical trials, and to be considered successful, it must have outcomes equal or superior to the treatment arm of SWOG 9008/INT-0116. The current National Intergroup Adjuvant Therapy Study (Fig. 2) for postgastrectomy cases tests ECF chemotherapy before and after chemoradiation compared to a standard arm, which is essentially the same as the treatment arm of SWOG 9008/INT-0116. Another strategy of interest resulting from the recent evidence of benefit from neoadjuvant chemotherapy would be to combine neoadjuvant chemotherapy with postoperative chemoradiation. To fully understand

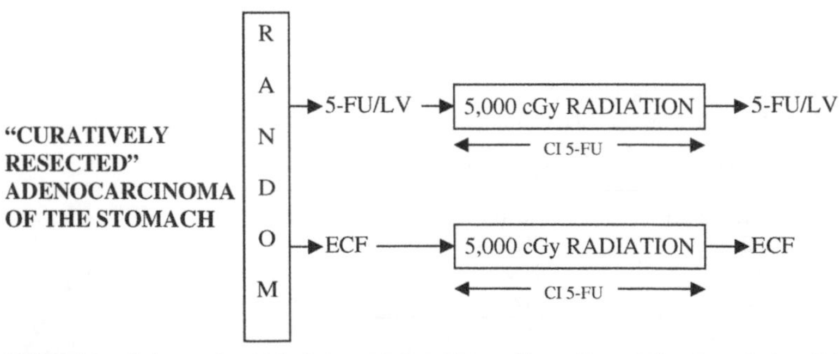

FIGURE 2 Schema for U.S. Intergroup postoperative adjuvant therapy study. *Abbreviations*: 5-FU, 5-fluorouracil; cGY, centiGray; CI, confidence interval; LV, leucovorin; ECF, epirubicin, cisplatin, and 5-fluorouracil.

the potential for combined modality approaches to gastric cancer management, clinical trials need to be mounted to critically evaluate adjuvant and neoadjuvant therapy strategies in appropriate groups of patients. For example, patients identified preoperatively should be candidates for phase III trials testing neoadjuvant therapy followed by surgery versus surgery alone. These preoperative cases also would be candidates for explanatory phase II trials testing the tolerability and efficacy of combined pre- and postoperative modality therapy programs. Patients identified postgastric resection, may be enrolled on the current U.S. Intergroup Study, which evaluates an improved chemoradiation regimen. The specific neoadjuvant and treatment programs of the future may use chemotherapy or chemotherapy plus radiation, as well as newer targeted therapies such as epidermal growth factor receptor (EGFR) (34) and/or vascular endothelial growth factor (VEGF) (35) inhibition.

REFERENCES

1. Bonenkamp JJ, Hermans J, Sasako M, et al. for the Dutch Gastric Cancer Group. Extended lymph node dissection for gastric cancer. N Engl J Med 1999; 340:908–914.
2. Brennan MF. Lymph-node dissection for gastric cancer. N Engl J Med 1999; 340:956–958.
3. Noguchi Y, Imada T, Matsumoto A, Coit DG, Brennan MF. Radical surgery for gastric cancer. A review of the Japanese experience. Cancer 1989; 64(10):2053–2062. Review.
4. Brennan MF, Karpeh MS Jr. Surgery for gastric cancer: the American view. Sem Oncol 1996; 23:352–359.
5. Kodama Y, Sugimachi K, Soejima K. Evaluation of extensive lymph node dissection for carcinoma of the stomach. World J Surg 1981; 5:241–248.
6. Vezerdis MP, Wanebo HJ. Gastric cancer: surgical approach. In: Ahlgren JD, Macdonald JS, eds. Gastrointestinal Oncology. Philadelphia: Lippincott, 1992:159–170.
7. Bunt AM, Hermans J, Smit VT, van de Velde CJ, Fleuren GJ, Bruijn JA. Surgical/pathologic-stage migration confounds comparisons of gastric cancer survival rates between Japan and Western countries. J Clin Oncol 1995; 13(1):19–25.
8. Hermans J, Bonenkamp JJ, Boon MC, et al. Adjuvant therapy after curative resection for gastric cancer: meta-analysis of randomized trials. J Clin Oncol 1993; 11:1441–1447.
9. Macdonald JS, Fleming TR, Peterson RF, et al. Adjuvant chemotherapy with 5-FU, adriamycin, and mitomycin-C (FAM) versus surgery alone for patients with locally advanced gastric adenocarcinoma: a Southwest Oncology Group Study. Ann Surg Oncol 1995; 2(6):488–494.
10. Dent DM, Madden MV, Price SK. Randomized comparison of R_1 and R_2 gastrectomy for gastric carcinoma. Br J Surg 1998; 75:110.
11. Cascinu S, Labianca R, Allesandroni P, et al. Intensive weekly chemotherapy for advanced gastric cancer using fluorouracil, cisplatin, epi-doxorubicin, 6S-leucovorin, glutathione, and filgrastim: a report from the Italian Group for the Study of Digestive Tract Cancer. J Clin Oncol 1997; 15(11):3313–3319.
12. Cookes P, Leichman CG, Leichman L, et al. Systemic chemotherapy for gastric carcinoma followed by postoperative intraperitoneal therapy. Cancer 1997; 79(9):1767–1775.
13. Ilson DH, Saltz L, Enzinger P, et al. Phase II trial of weekly irinotecan plus cisplatin in advanced esophageal cancer. J Clin Oncol 1999; 17:3270–3725.
14. Kelsen D, Atiq OT, Saltz L, et al. FAMTX versus etoposide, doxorubicin, and cisplatin: a random assignment trial in gastric cancer. J Clin Oncol 1992; 10:541–548.
15. Kettner E, Ridwelski K, Keilholz U, et al. Docetaxel and cisplatin combination chemotherapy for advanced gastric cancer: results of two phase II studies. Proc ASCO 2001; 20:165a.
16. Preusser P, Wilke H, Achterrath W, et al. Phase II study with the combination etoposide, doxorubicin, and cisplatin in advanced measurable gastric cancer. J Clin Oncol 1989; 7:1310–1317.
17. Webb A, Cunningham D, Scarffe JH, et al. Randomized trial comparing epirubicin, cisplatin and fluorouracil versus fluorouracil, doxorubicin, and methotrexate in advanced esophagogastric cancer. J Clin Oncol 1997; 15(1):261–267.
18. Wils J, Bleiberg H, Dalesio O, et al. An EORTC gastrointestinal group evaluation of the combination of sequential methotrexate, and 5-fluorouracil combined with adriamycin, in advanced measurable gastric cancer. J Clin Oncol 1986; 4:1799–1803.
19. Wils JA, Klein HO, Wagener DJ, et al. Sequential high-dose methotrexate and fluorouracil combined with doxorubicin: a step ahead in the treatment of advanced gastric cancer: a trial of the European Organization for Research and Treatment of Cancer Gastrointestinal Tract Cooperative Group. J Clin Oncol 1991; 9:827–831.
20. Allum W, Cunningham D, Weeden S for the UK NCRI Upper GI Clinical Studies Group. Perioperative chemotherapy in operable gastric and lower oesophageal cancer: a randomized, controlled trial (the MAGIC trial, ISRCTN 93793971) [Abstract #998]. Proc ASCO 2003; 22:249a.

21. Ross P, Cunningham D, Scarffe H, et al. Results of a randomized trial comparing ECF with MCF in advanced oesophageal gastric cancer. Proc Am Soc Clin Oncol 1999; 8:272a.
22. Ajani JA, Van Cutsem E, Moiseyenko V, et al. Docetaxel (D), cisplatin, 5-fluorouracil compare to cisplatin (C) and 5-fluorouracil (F) for chemotherapy-naïve patients with metastatic or locally recurrent, unresectable gastric carcinoma (MGC): interim results of a randomized phase III trial [Abstract #999]. Proc ASCO 2003; 22:249a.
23. Moiseyenko VM, Ajani J, Tjulandin SA, et al. Final results of a randomized controlled phase III trial (TAX 325) comparing docetaxel (T) combined with cisplatin (C) and 5-fluorouracil (F) to CF in patients (pts) with metastatic gastric adenocarcinoma (MGC). (oral presentation, ASCO 2005, #4002a).
24. Hermans J, Bonenkamp JJ, Boon MC, et al. Adjuvant therapy after curative resection for gastric cancer: meta-analysis of randomized trials. J Clin Oncol 1993; 11:1441.
25. Earle CC, Maroun JA. Adjuvant chemotherapy after curative resection for gastric cancer in non-Asian patients: revisiting a meta-analysis of randomized trials. Eur J Cancer 1999; 35:1059–1064.
26. Meyerhardt JA, Fuchs CS. Adjuvant therapy in gastric cancer: can we prevent recurrences? Oncology 2003; 17:714–728.
27. Gastrointestinal Tumor Study Group. A comparison of combination chemotherapy and combined modality therapy for locally advanced gastric carcinoma. Cancer 1982; 49:1771–1777.
28. Herskovic A, Martz K, Al-Sarraf M, et al. Combined chemotherapy and radiotherapy compared to radiotherapy alone in patients with cancer of the esophagus. N Engl J Med 1992; 326:1593–1598.
29. Macdonald J, Smalley S, Benedetti J, Estes N, Haller DG, Ajani J. Postoperative combined radiation and chemotherapy improves disease-free survival (DFS) and overall survival (OS) in resected adenocarcinoma of the stomach and GE junction. Results of intergroup study INT-0116 (SWOG 9008). [#1] Proc Am Soc Clin Oncol 2000; 19:1a. 2
30. Macdonald JS, Smalley SR, Benedetti J, et al. Chemoradiotherapy after surgery compared with surgery alone for adenocarcinoma of the stomach or gastroesophageal junction. N Engl J Med 2001; 345(10):725–730.
31. Macdonald JS, Smalley S, Benedetti J, et al. SWOG; ECOG; RTOG; CALGB; NCCTG. Postoperative combined radiation and chemotherapy improves disease-free survival (DFS) and overall survival (OS) in resected adenocarcinoma of the stomach and G.E. junction: update of the results of Intergroup Study INT-0116 (SWOG 9008). ASCO 2004.
32. Kim S, Lim DH, Lee J, et al. An observational study suggesting clinical benefit for adjuvant postoperative chemoradiation in a population of over 500 cases after gastric resection with D2 nodal dissection for adenocarcinoma of the stomach (submitted for publication, JCO 2004).
33. Cunningham D, Allum WH, Stenning SP, Weeden S for the NCRI Upper GI Cancer Clinical Studies Group. Perioperative chemotherapy in operable gastric and lower oesophageal cancer: final results of a randomized, controlled trial (the MAGIC trial, ISRCTN 93793971) (oral presentation, ASCO 2005, #4001a).
34. Cunningham D, Humblet Y, Siena S, et al. Cetuximab monotherapy and cetuximab plus irinotecan-refractory metastatic colorectal cancer. N Engl J Med 2004; 351:337–345.
35. Hurwitz H, Fehrenbacher L, Novotny W, et al. Bevacizumab plus irinotecan, fluorouracil, and leucovorin for metastatic colorectal cancer. N Engl J Med 2004; 350:2335–2342.

10 Small Bowel Adenocarcinoma

Kerri A. Nowell and James R. Howe
Department of Surgery, University of Iowa College of Medicine, Iowa City, Iowa, U.S.A.

HISTORY

The small bowel accounts for at least 75% of the total length of the gastrointestinal (GI) tract and over 90% of the mucosal surface, however, less than 25% of all GI tract neoplasms and 2% of all malignant neoplasms arise here (1). The first reported case of a small bowel tumor was a duodenal carcinoma described by Hamburger in 1746 (1,2). The annual incidence of small bowel adenocarcinoma (SBA) in the United States is only 3.9 cases per million persons, with a mean age reported between 60 and 70 years (3).

Our current knowledge of the natural history of small bowel tumors is limited relative to its colorectal counterparts, which are 40 to 60 times more common. However, in the last 10 years, there have been several studies that have added insight into this subject. One of the largest studies published to date reviewed data from the National Cancer Data Base (NCDB) on 4995 SBA (4). This study identified patterns of treatment and prognostic factors that influenced overall survival. More recently, a study summarized the M.D. Anderson Cancer Center's (MDACC) experience in 217 patients with SBA (5). These studies, along with a few others, have been mostly retrospective and descriptive, and therefore the scientific basis for the treatment of SBA has relied in large part from what we have learned in colorectal cancer.

PATHOLOGY

Benign tumors of the small bowel include leiomyomas, adenomas [which are common in the duodenum of familial adenomatous polyposis (FAP) patients], lipomas, hamartomatous polyps (such as those in Peutz-Jeghers and to a lesser degree, juvenile polyposis syndrome), and other miscellaneous lesions (fibroma, ganglioneuromas, neurofibroma, hemangioma, lymphangioma) (1). Surgery is indicated for most symptomatic tumors with simple excision being sufficient treatment. However, villous adenomas of the small intestine have a definite potential for malignant degeneration with estimates ranging from 35% to 58% with the incidence being greatest in those lesions >4 cm (1). These lesions most commonly occur in the duodenum, yet only account for about 1% of all duodenal tumors (1).

The most common malignant lesions of the small bowel are adenocarcinoma, accounting for approximately 35% of cases (4). The next common are carcinoid (28%), lymphoma (21%), and sarcoma/gastrointestinal stromal tumor (10%). Tumors of the ampulla of Vater are typically not included under the heading of adenocarcinoma of the small bowel.

DEMOGRAPHICS

The mean age of patients with SBA is between 55 and 65 years (4,5). There is an almost equal distribution between genders from the NCDB study (52.9% males and 47.1% females, $n = 4995$ patients) while slightly favoring males in the MDACC study (61% males, 39% females, $n = 217$ patients). The breakdown by race/ethnicity was similar to that of the U.S. population, with 80% of SBA seen in whites and 12% in African-Americans. However, only 3% of SBA cases were in Hispanics, as contrasted to their comprising 9% of the U.S. population in 1990 (4). There was a higher proportion of SBA cases in Hispanics seen in the MDACC study at 6% (5), but still below what would be expected.

PRESENTATION

The signs and symptoms of small bowel malignancies are vague and are often present for a number of months or even one to two years before a diagnosis is made (6). A study of 370 Mayo

Clinic patients with malignant small bowel lesions reported that 34% had developed their signs and symptoms less than six months before surgery, 31% within 6 to 12 months of surgery, and 3% more than five years preoperatively (7). These signs and symptoms can be subdivided into chronic and acute (6). Chronic signs are frequently present and include melana, anemia, pain, obstruction, malaise, weight loss, diarrhea, jaundice, and palpable mass. As one may expect, the stomach and colon are usually thoroughly studied when these signs and symptoms are present, often with the small bowel being overlooked, at least initially. Acute symptoms include hemorrhage, pain, obstruction, and perforation. When these are present, the patient is often evaluated by a surgeon, with the diagnosis being made at the time of laparotomy. The most common complaints include abdominal pain and weight loss (7–9). However, up to 14% of patients may have no signs and symptoms and the tumor is first noted at the time of surgery as an incidental finding (10). Incidental tumors tend to be benign; it has been reported that 75% of symptomatic small bowel tumors are found to be malignant (11). Clinical presentation does not appear to differ by primary tumor site, except in a few instances. Obstruction tends to be more common in distally located tumors (5), while jaundice is more likely in patients with duodenal masses because of obstruction of the bile duct (6).

DIAGNOSIS

Diagnosis of SBA is often difficult and delayed because of the vague and nonspecific signs and symptoms. Distal lesions may present with an obstructive pattern that may be seen on plain films. However, this finding is nonspecific. Esophagogastroduodenoscopy (EGD) may sometimes be diagnostic for proximal duodenal lesions, but will obviously miss more distal lesions (9). One advantage of EGD over other diagnostic modalities is the ability to biopsy tumors or excise polyps. On the other end, the ileocecal valve can be intubated with the colonoscope and lesions of the terminal ileum can be visualized and biopsied in 20% to 30% of patients (1). Extended enteroscopy, though not widely available, can allow visualization of up to 70% of the small bowel mucosa (12). Contrast radiography, upper GI series with small bowel follow-through, is commonly employed to visualize luminal defects (1). Subtle abnormalities suggestive of intestinal neoplasia can be detected, as well as mass lesions or intussusception (1). Enteroclysis (selective infusion of contrast through a long tube advanced past the ligament of Treitz) of the small bowel remains the primary radiologic investigational tool (9), demonstrating lesions that were previously missed with routine small bowel follow-through exams (13). In one study, 15/16 duodenal neoplasms were diagnosed with a preoperative barium study (10). Computed tomography (CT) of the abdomen and pelvis is typically performed during the workup of abdominal pain. CT may be useful in detecting extraluminal tumors or extension, staging of disease (especially for lymphomas and carcinoid), or may identify secondary hepatic or mesenteric disease (9). Angiography is helpful only in diagnosing and localizing tumors of vascular origin or those ulcerated lesions that are bleeding at a rate greater than 0.5 to 1.0 mL/min (1). Video capsule endoscopy (VCE) is non-invasive and can be performed in an ambulatory setting. At this time, the primary indication for VCE is locating the site of obscure GI bleeding in adults. However, it is increasingly being used for the diagnosis of small bowel tumors and Crohn's disease. Despite all the available diagnostic modalities, one must remember that diagnosis is often achieved only at the time of surgery.

STAGE

The most commonly used staging system for adenocarcinoma of the small bowel is the tumor node metastases (TNM) system of the American Joint Committee on Cancer (14). In the NCDB series, 2.7% of the tumors were Stage 0, 12.0% were Stage I, 27% were Stage II, 26% were Stage III, and 32% were Stage IV (4). Of patients with Stage IV disease, the liver tends to be the most common site of metastasis (59%), followed by carcinomatosis (25%), the pelvis (9%), and the lungs (3%) (5).

TUMOR CHARACTERISTICS

SBA is most commonly found in the duodenum (57–64%), followed by the jejunum (20–27%) and ileum (14–15%) (4–6). There are several explanations for the observation that such a large percentage of tumors arise in the duodenum. One, the duodenum is the first site exposed to a variety of potentially injurious agents, both those consumed and those produced within the GI tract (bile, pancreatic secretions, stomach acid) (4). Second, duodenal adenocarcinoma may develop in anywhere from 24% to 100% of patients with FAP (15). In fact, patients with FAP have a 331-fold increase in the development of duodenal adenocarcinoma compared to the normal population (16). Third, it can be reached by upper endoscopy. In contrast, patients with Crohn's disease have an 86-fold increase in incidence of SBA (17), but the majority of these lesions occur in the ileum.

Histologic differentiation is performed using the World Health Organization's standard grading system. There are four separate categories of adenocarcinoma, including well differentiated, moderately well differentiated, poorly differentiated, and undifferentiated. In the NCDB series, 15% of the tumors were well differentiated, 50% were moderately differentiated, 34% were poorly differentiated, and less than 2% were undifferentiated (4).

SURVIVAL

The overall five-year survival rate for SBA is 26% to 30.5% (4,5), with 60.2% survival at one year, 44.4% at two years, and 37% at three years (4). The 5-year survival rate for patients with duodenal tumors (28.2%; median survival 16.9 months) is significantly less than for patients with jejunal (37.6%; median survival 28.9 months) and ileal tumors (37.8%; median survival 30.8 months) (4). The difference in survival for patients with duodenal tumors was significant compared with both patients with jejunal and ileal tumors ($P < 0.0001$), but not between those with jejunal and ileal tumors (Fig. 1) (4).

Five-year survival is significantly decreased in patients with poorly differentiated tumors (22.4%, median survival 11.1 months) compared to patients with well-differentiated tumors (39.4%, median survival 28.6 months) and moderately to well-differentiated tumors (33.3%, median survival 23.6 months) (4). There was no survival difference found between the two latter groups.

There is a clear association between pathologic stage and survival (Fig. 2). The disease-specific survival (DSS) for patients with Stage IV disease (4.2% five-year DSS; median survival 9.0 months) is significantly worse than for patients with Stage I to III disease, and the DSS rate for patients with Stage I disease (65% five-year DSS; median survival >5 years) differed significantly compared with patients with Stage III disease (35.4% five-year DSS; median survival 29.8 months) (4).

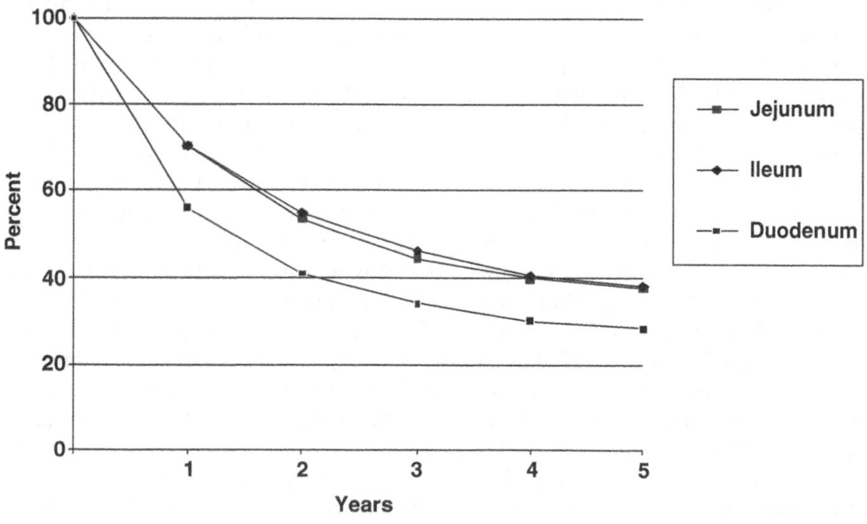

FIGURE 1 Disease-specific survival by site for adenocarcinoma of the small bowel, 1985 to 1990; $P < 0.0001$, duodenum versus jejunum and ileum. *Source*: Adapted from Ref. 4.

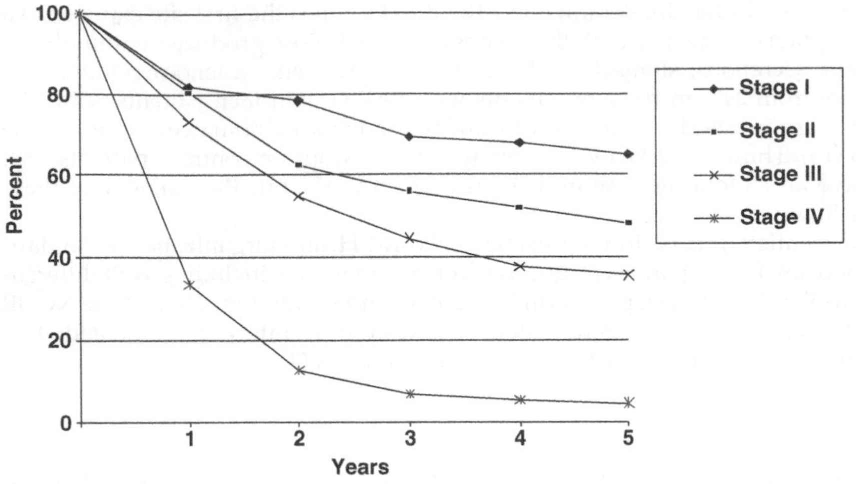

FIGURE 2 Disease-specific survival by AJCC stage for adenocarcinoma of the small bowel, 1985 to 1990; $P < 0.0001$ for stages I, II, III versus IV, $P = 0.0015$ for stage I versus III, $P =$ not significant for stage II versus I and III. *Abbreviation*: AJCC, American Joint Committee on Cancer. *Source*: From Ref. 4.

Gender, race/ethnicity, and income were examined with respect to DSS, and no significant correlation was found (4). However, the age of the patient at presentation was significantly associated with survival (4), with the five-year survival for patients aged over 75 years being 22% compared to 33% for patients aged 60 to 75 years and 34% for those younger than 60 years ($P < 0.0001$).

SURGICAL TREATMENT

Adenocarcinomas of the small bowel are generally treated by segmental resection. While small bowel resection with the lymph node-bearing mesentery (or ileocolectomy for terminal ileal tumors) is the surgical treatment for jejunal or ileal tumors, pancreaticoduodenectomy is often necessary for patients with tumors involving the duodenum, due to anatomic constraints (4). In the NCDB series, 11.9% of patients with SBA underwent no surgical therapy, 20.4% underwent noncancer-directed surgery [including biopsy, exploration, bypass, and unknown/not otherwise specified (NOS) nondisease-directed procedures], and 67.6% underwent cancer-directed surgery (radical or simple excision with or without lymph node dissection, fulguration, cryosurgery, laser ablation, surgery at regional or distant sites only, and unknown/NOS cancer-directed procedures) (4). The therapy for jejunal and ileal tumors were similar, with about 90% of patients undergoing cancer-directed surgery. However, a significantly smaller percentage of patients with duodenal tumors underwent cancer-directed surgery (52%; $P < 0.0001$) and more underwent noncancer-directed surgery (31.6%) (4). This difference in treatment is likely explained by the anatomic location of duodenal masses, which often requires a more extensive pancreaticoduodenectomy for complete resection. The five-year survival rate for patients who underwent cancer-directed surgery (40.3%) was significantly higher than for those who did not (9.3%; $P < 0.0001$) (4). There was no significant difference in the DSS rate between patients who had no surgery (11.7% five-year DSS; $n = 239$ patients) and those who underwent noncancer-directed surgery (7.4% five-year DSS; $n = 333$ patients). Patients who underwent cancer-directed surgery without adjuvant therapy had a longer median survival (47.8 months) compared with those who had surgery, chemotherapy, and radiation (23.6 months), surgery plus chemotherapy (17.2 months), and surgery plus radiation therapy (15.9 months) (4). Because of the low number of patients in these groups, it is difficult to draw inferences from this data, but there is a noticeable trend toward improved survival with surgery alone, which is likely related to the fact that earlier stage tumors do not require adjuvant therapy.

CONCLUSIONS

Primary adenocarcinoma of the small bowel, although rare, continues to challenge current diagnostic and treatment modalities. Studies have shown that patients diagnosed with earlier stage disease have a significantly improved five-year survival rate. However, the nonspecific nature of symptoms contributes to a delay in diagnosis. Once the diagnosis of SBA is made, cancer-directed surgery offers the best prospects for long-term survival.

REFERENCES

1. Ashley SW, Wells SA. Tumors of the small intestine. Semin Oncol 1988; 15:116.
2. Hamburger G. Dr rupture intestine duodeni. Jena Ritterianis, 1746.
3. Delaunoit T, Neczyporenko F, Limburg PJ, Erlichman C. Pathogenesis and risk factors of small bowel adenocarcinoma: a colorectal cancer sibling? Am J Gastroenterol 2005; 100:703–710.
4. Howe JR, Karnell LH, Menck HR, Scott-Conner C. The American College of Surgeons Commission on Cancer and the American Cancer Society. Adenocarcinoma of the small bowel: review of the National Cancer Data Base, 1985–1995. Cancer 1999; 86:2693–2706.
5. Dabaja BS, Suki D, Pro B, Bonnen M, Ajani J. Adenocarcinoma of the small bowel: presentation, prognostic factors, and outcome of 217 patients. Cancer 2004; 101:518.
6. Martin, RG. Malignant tumors of the small intestine. Surg Clin North Am 1986; 66:779.
7. Pagtalunan RDG, Mayo CW, Dockerty MB. Primary malignant tumors of the small intestine. Am J Surg 1964; 108:13.
8. Wilson JM, Melvin DB, Gray GF, Thorbjarnarson B. Primary malignancies of the small bowel: a report of 96 cases and review of the literature. Ann Surg 1974; 180:175.
9. O'Riordan BG, Vilor M, Herrera L. Small bowel tumors: an overview. Dig Dis 1996; 14:245.
10. Darling RC, Welch CE. Tumors of the small intestine. N Engl J Med 1959; 260:397.
11. North JH, Pack MS. Malignant tumors of the small intestine: a review of 144 cases. Am Surg 2000; 66:46.
12. Lewis BS, Kornbluth A, Waye JD. Small bowel tumors: yield of enteroscopy. Gut 1991; 32:763.
13. Maglinte DDT, Hall R, Miller RE, et al. Detection of surgical lesions of the small bowel by enteroclysis. Am J Surg 1984; 197:226.
14. Fleming ID, Cooper JS, Henson DE, et al. (eds). AJCC Handbook for Staging of Cancer. 5th ed. Philadelphia: Lippincott, 1997, p. 78.
15. Campbell WJ, Spence RA, Parks TG. Familial adenomatous polyposis. Br J Surg 1994; 81:1722.
16. Offerhaus GJ, Giardiello FM, Krush AJ, et al. The risk of upper gastrointestinal cancer in familial adenomatous polyposis. Gastroenterology 1992; 102:1980.
17. Greenstein AJ, Sachar DB, Smith H, Janowitz HD, Aufses AH Jr. A comparison of cancer risk in Crohn's disease and ulcerative colitis. Cancer 1981; 48:2742.

11 Surgical Treatments for Colon and Rectal Cancer: A Critical Appraisal of Evidence-Based Data

David E. Rivadeneira
Division of Surgical Oncology and Colon and Rectal Surgery, State University of New York at Stony Brook, Stony Brook, New York, U.S.A.

Alison G. Killelea
State University of New York, Downstate Medical Center, Brooklyn, New York, U.S.A.

Colon and rectal cancer is an extremely prevalent malignancy worldwide. Approximately one million new cases of colorectal cancer are diagnosed yearly and account for nearly 529,000 deaths worldwide (1). In the United States, colorectal cancer represented the third highest ranked malignancy in both incidence and mortality. It represented an estimated 22% of all new cancer cases (with an estimated 147,000 new cases) and an estimated 20% of all cancer deaths (an estimated 56,730 deaths) (2). The mainstay curative treatment for both colon and rectal cancer is surgical resection. We will review evidence-based data regarding surgical applications to both disease processes including recent studies relating to the laparoscopic techniques, extent of resection, preoperative radiation/chemotherapy treatment, total mesorectal excision (TME), types of anastomoses, and follow-up regimens.

LAPAROSCOPIC/MINIMALLY INVASIVE VS. OPEN/CONVENTIONAL SURGICAL RESECTION FOR COLON CANCER

In recent years, extensive discussions have been made of minimally invasive or laparoscopic techniques in addressing colon cancers. Initial concerns surrounded such issues as the appropriateness of the surgical margins, number of harvested lymph nodes, and port site recurrences, that is, tumor recurrence at the site of laparoscopic trocar insertion areas or specimen removal sites. Several large studies have addressed these concerns. A prospective but nonrandomized study reported by Franklin et al. (3) compared 191 patients undergoing laparoscopic resection versus 224 patients with open techniques. They found that the laparoscopic method was able to accomplish equal or greater lymph node retrieval, length of resection and distal margins than the open method. Benefits to the laparoscopic method included shorter hospital stay (5.7 vs. 9.7 days), less blood loss, fewer wound complications and a quicker return to bowel function, and in addition there were no trochar implants in the laparoscopic group. Survival, recurrence and death rates were similar between the two groups.

In a prospective, randomized trial from the Cleveland Clinic, Milsom et al. (4) looked at 42 patients undergoing laparoscopic versus 38 patients with open techniques for colon cancer. They demonstrated improved postoperative pulmonary function with overall recovery of 80% of forced expiratory volume in one second, and a median recovery of forced vital capacity in three days for laparoscopy and six days for the conventional open group ($P=0.01$). In addition, patients in the laparoscopic group used significantly less morphine in the first 48 hours postoperatively than the open group (0.78 ± 0.32 vs. 0.92 ± 0.34 mg/kg/day, respectively, $P=0.02$) and flatus returned significantly earlier in the laparoscopic versus open (median three days vs. four days, $P=0.006$). Tumor margins were clear in all patients and there were no port site recurrences after short-term follow-up (median of 1.5 years in laparoscopic and 1.7 years in the open group). Seven cancer-related deaths occurred, three in the laparoscopic group and four in the open group.

In a larger prospective, randomized study, Lacy et al. from Barcelona (5) reported their experience with 111 patients undergoing laparoscopic and 108 patients with open surgical resection for colon cancer. Patients in the laparoscopic group had a shorter recovery time with earlier return to bowel function ($P=0.001$), shorter oral intake times ($P=0.001$) and hospital stay ($P=0.005$) and in addition patients in this group had lower morbidity than in open ($P=0.001$) but a laparoscopic approach did not influence perioperative mortality. Probability of cancer-related survival was higher in the laparoscopic group ($P=0.02$) and was independently associated with reduced risk of tumor relapse, death from any cause, and death from a cancer-related cause compared with open. The increase in survival was only observed in patients with stage III tumors that underwent laparoscopic resection. This reported difference is possibly due to the less traumatic effects of laparoscopy on the immune response. These findings have not been reproduced in any other study to date.

Lezoche et al. (6) reported similar results from Italy with a prospective, nonrandomized study in 310 patients. Of these, 150 patients (75% with malignant lesions) underwent laparoscopic surgery, whereas 160 patients (73% with malignant lesions) were treated by open surgery. Mean operative time for laparoscopic surgery was longer than for open surgery (251 vs. 175 minutes) ($P<0.001$), but mean postoperative hospital stay was shorter after laparoscopic surgery (10.5 days, as compared to 13.3 days, $P<0.05$). In the laparoscopic surgery group, the rate of minor complications (strictures, wound infection and urinary retention) was 3.6% as compared to the 7.5% observed after open surgery ($P=0.261$). No statistically significant difference was observed in the rate of major complications (leakage, fistula, hemoperitoneum, and ileus), which was 9.4% after laparoscopic surgery and 6.8% after open surgery, or in operative mortality (1.4% for laparoscopic surgery and 0.6% for open surgery). The local recurrence rate was lower after laparoscopic surgery (3% vs. 9.2% in open $P=0.152$). Mean follow-up was 34.2 months during which time two cases of port site recurrence were observed. Distant site metastases occurred in 11% in both groups. At 36 months, cumulative survival probability in laparoscopic surgery for malignant cases was 0.74 versus 0.66 for open surgery; this difference was not statistically significant.

Longer follow-ups have been reported. Patankar et al. (7) reported their 10-year experience with laparoscopic resections for colon cancer. This was a prospective, nonrandomized longitudinal cohort study. Each group consisted of 172 patients and the mean follow-up was 52 months. Thirty-day mortality was 1.2% (two deaths) in the laparoscopic resection group and 2.4% (four deaths) in the open resection group ($P>0.05$). Early and late complication incidences were comparable. The incidence of local recurrence (including tumors with a primary in the colon or rectum) was 3.5% (six patients) in the laparoscopic group and 2.9% (five patients) in the open group. One of the local recurrences in the laparoscopy group occurred in the port/extraction site (incidence of 0.6%). Metastasis occurred in 18 patients (10.5%) in the open group and in 21 (12.2%) in the laparoscopy group. Stage-for-stage overall five-year survival rates were similar in both groups.

The results from three large, randomized, multicenter studies, one from the United Kingdom, another from a collaborative European effort, and the third from the United States were eagerly anticipated in the surgical community. The multicenter COLOR (Colon Cancer Laparoscopic or Open Resection) (8) trial was done to compare the safety and benefit of laparoscopic resection compared with open resection for curative treatment of colon cancer. Six hundred and twenty-seven patients were randomly assigned to laparoscopic surgery and 621 patients to open surgery. Patients assigned laparoscopic resection had less blood loss compared to open resection [median 100 mL (range 0–2700) vs. 175 mL (0–2000], $P<0.0001$], although laparoscopic surgery lasted 30 minutes longer than did open surgery ($P<0.0001$). Conversion to open surgery was needed for 91 (17%) patients undergoing the laparoscopic procedure. Radicality of resection (assessed by number of lymph nodes removed and length of resected bowel) did not differ between groups. Laparoscopic colectomy was associated with earlier recovery of bowel function ($P<0.0001$), need for fewer analgesics, and shorter hospital stay ($P<0.0001$) as compared to open colectomy. Morbidity and mortality 28 days after colectomy was similar for both groups.

The Medical Research Council (MRC) Conventional versus Laparoscopic-Assisted Surgery In Colorectal Cancer (CLASICC) trial (9) was a multicenter, randomized clinical trial of

794 patients with colorectal cancer from 27 UK centers. Two hundred and fifty-three and 484 patients received open and laparoscopic-assisted treatment, respectively. One hundred and forty-three (29%) patients underwent conversion from laparoscopic to open surgery and these patients had higher complication rates. Proportion of Duke's C2 tumors did not differ between the two groups [18 patients (7%) open vs. 34 (6%) in laparoscopic, $P=0.89$], and in-hospital mortality was also similar [13 patients (5%) vs. 21 (4%), $P=0.57$]. Positive resection margins were similar between treatment groups except among patients undergoing laparoscopic anterior resection for rectal cancer.

In the United States, the Clinical Outcomes of Surgical Therapy Study group (COST) (10,11) sponsored by the National Cancer Institute reported its results in 2004. This was a randomized, prospective, multicenter noninferiority trial which randomly assigned 872 patients with adenocarcinoma of the colon to undergo open- or laparoscopically assisted colectomy. The median follow-up was 4.4 years. At three years, the rates of recurrence were similar in the two groups: 16% among patients in the laparoscopically assisted group and 18% among patients in the open colectomy group ($P=0.32$). Recurrence rates in surgical wounds were less than 1% in both groups ($P=0.50$). The overall survival rate at three years was also very similar in the two groups (86% in the laparoscopic surgery group and 85% in the open colectomy group; $P=0.51$) with no significant difference between groups in the time to recurrence or overall survival for patients with any stage of cancer. Perioperative recovery was faster in the laparoscopic surgery group than in the open colectomy group, with a shorter median hospital stay (five vs. six days, $P<0.001$) and shorter use of both parenteral and oral analgesics (three days vs. four days, $P<0.001$) and (one vs. two days, $P=0.02$), respectively. The rates of intraoperative complications, 30-day postoperative mortality, complications at discharge and at 60 days, hospital readmission, and reoperation were very similar between groups. This study has caused an increase in the adoption of laparoscopic colon resection for cancer in the United States.

The significant concerns and reservations about the oncologic appropriateness of laparoscopic techniques for curative colon resections have been addressed. It appears that for qualified surgeons, laparoscopic approaches have similar cancer outcomes in terms of recurrence and survival to open surgery. Laparoscopic surgery may provide an advantage to open procedures in providing less postoperative pain, quicker recovery of bowel function, and lessened hospital course. However, it does come at an increased operative time and cost.

Extent of Resection: Hemicolectomy Vs. Segmental Resection

The extent of surgical resection for tumors located in the left side of the colon was evaluated by a prospective, randomized study conducted by Rouffet et al. (12) from the French Association for Surgical Research. They compared left hemicolectomy with left segmental colectomy in 270 consecutive patients with colonic carcinoma located from the left third of the transverse colon up to the colorectal junction. Patients were randomly assigned to undergo either left hemicolectomy, where the entire left colon along with the origin of the inferior mesenteric artery (IMA) and dependent lymphatic territory were removed, or left segmental colectomy, where a more limited segment of the colon was removed and the inferior mesenteric artery left in situ. Preoperative risk factors, pathology findings (including size, differentiation, stage, and lymph node invasion), and associated lesions were all similar between both groups. One hundred and thirty-one patients were analyzed in the left hemicolectomy group, and 129 in the left segmental colectomy group. The authors found that early postoperative abdominal and extra-abdominal complications were similar in both groups, and the only significant operative difference was in the length of the tumor-free margins of colon removed, which was significantly greater in the left hemicolectomy group. Early postoperative mortality was higher among patients undergoing a left hemicolectomy procedure (eight deaths, representing 6%) versus a left segmental colectomy (three deaths, 2%), but this 4% difference was not significant. Median survival was ten years and very similar in the two groups, as were the two actuarial survival curves. A significant difference was found in frequency of bowel movements, which remained significantly increased in the in the left hemicolectomy group during the first postoperative year.

PROCEDURE FOR OBSTRUCTED LEFT-SIDED COLON CANCER

The operation of choice is not clear with an obstructing left-sided colon cancer. There are several options, including resection with colostomy, also known as the Hartman's procedure, subtotal colectomy with or without an anastomosis, resection with on-table lavage, and followed by an anastomosis. Several studies have addressed each.

A report by the Subtotal Colectomy versus On-table Irrigation and Anastomosis (SCOTIA) Study Group (13), was the first prospective randomized, multicenter trial to compare subtotal colectomy with segmental resection and primary anastomosis following intraoperative irrigation for the management of malignant left-sided colonic obstruction. Forty-seven patients were randomized to subtotal colectomy, and 44 to on-table irrigation and segmental colectomy. Hospital mortality and complication rates did not differ significantly, but increased bowel frequency (three or more bowel movements per day) was significantly more common in the subtotal colectomy group after four months (14 of 35 vs. 4 of 35, $P=0.01$). More patients from the subtotal colectomy group had consulted their general practitioner with bowel problems than in the segmental resection group (15 of 37 vs. 3 of 35, $P=0.004$). They concluded that segmental resection following intraoperative irrigation is the preferred option except in cases of cecal perforation or if synchronous neoplasms are present in the colon, when subtotal colectomy is more appropriate.

In a prospective, nonrandomized study by Torralba et al. (14) 35 patients underwent subtotal colectomy with ileorectal anastomosis versus 31 patients with intraoperative colonic irrigation and segmental resection with immediate anastomosis. The mortality rate was similar in groups, 8.5% in the subtotal colectomy group and 3.2 % in the intraoperative colonic irrigation group. Surgical complications were more common in the intraoperative colonic irrigation (ICI) group (41.9%) than in the subtotal colectomy group (14.2%; $P<0.05$), and operating time was shorter in the subtotal colectomy group as well ($P<0.05$). Mean length of hospital stay was similar for both groups. Diarrhea was present in the immediate postoperative period in 10 patients having undergone subtotal colectomy (31.2%) and disappeared spontaneously or with medication in all but two cases (6.2%). The authors concluded that subtotal colectomy is the treatment of choice for obstructed left-sided colonic carcinoma.

Segmental resection with intraoperative colonic irrigation is more appropriate than subtotal colectomy only in patients with carcinomas of the rectosigmoid junction or with previous anal incontinence to avoid the advent of postoperative diarrhea.

STAPLED VS. MANUALLY SUTURED ANASTOMOSIS

One multicenter, prospective, randomized study looked at the difference in tumor recurrence following two methods of reconstructing the anastomosis, either stapled or manually sewn. Docherty et al. (15) from the West of Scotland and Highland Anastomosis Study Group randomized 321 patients to undergo manually sewn colonic anastomosis and 331patients to receive a stapled anastomosis. Patients in the sutured group had a significantly higher radiologic leakage rate than in the stapled group (14.4% vs. 5.2%; $P<0.05$), but clinical anastomotic leak rates, morbidity, or postoperative mortality were not significantly different between groups. Tumor recurrence and cancer-specific mortality were higher (7.5% and 6.7% higher, respectively) but not statistically significant in the sutured patients and in patients with anastomotic leaks. Although the construction of the anastomosis appears to have no significant effect on tumor recurrence, it seems that the presence of an anastomotic leak portends a poor prognosis with an increase in local recurrence.

Investigating an anastomosis intraoperatively for leakage was the focus of a prospective randomized study by Beard et al. (16). A total of 145 consecutive patients receiving colorectal anastomosis were randomized to "test" (74 patients) or "no test" (71) after completion of the anastomosis. Anastomotic testing was performed with the pelvis filled with saline and the rectum distended by sigmoidoscopic insufflation of air. Any leaks as demonstrated by bubbling were oversewn. A water-soluble contrast enema was performed on the tenth postoperative day. Eighteen (25%) air leaks were detected and repaired in the "test" group. After operation both clinical and radiological leaks were less common in the test group; clinical leaks were present in

4% of patients in the test versus 14% no test ($P=0.043$) and radiologic leaks were present in 11% of patients in the "test" group and 29% of the "no test" group ($P=0.006$). Intraoperative air testing and repair of colorectal anastomoses significantly reduces the risk of postoperative clinical and radiological leaks.

FOLLOW-UP AFTER SURGICAL RESECTION FOR COLON CANCER

A number of recent studies have investigated the follow-up of colorectal cancer patients after surgery (17–20). Among the studies on the subject, there is a great variation between procedures, duration, intensity, and types of follow-up testing; as a result, there is no consistent pattern of follow-up that seems to impact overall and cancer-related survival and no recommendations have been made. One Norwegian study looked into detection of asymptomatic curable recurrence, compliance, and cost of follow-up as compared between two groups, one following a standard follow-up program and the other receiving no follow-up care (17). Although patients in this trial were not randomized into the follow-up or no follow-up group (patients were placed based on guidelines by the Norwegian Gastro-Intestinal Cancer Group, NGICC), there were significant differences in survival: crude survival rate was higher in the follow-up group (73%) than in the no follow-up group (52%), $P<0.0001$. Cancer-specific survival was similar in the two groups with 79% survival in the follow-up group and 86% in the no follow-up group, $P=0.7$, and median time to discovery of local recurrence or distant spread was similar between both groups. However, a second large trial from the United Kingdom (18) demonstrated a benefit to intense follow-up. They investigated the mode of discovery of relapse after adjuvant chemotherapy and how well the recurrence can be eliminated by follow-up surgery. This study supported the hypothesis that using computed tomographic (CT) scan and measuring levels of serum carcinoembyronic antigen (CEA) allowed physicians to detect recurrences sooner and at a time when more could be done surgically to cure patients rather than with the delay of discovering relapses by symptoms alone. Patients with resected stage II and III colorectal cancer (CRC) were randomly assigned to bolus fluorouracil (FU)/leucovorin (LV) or protracted venous infusion FU. Following completion of chemotherapy, patients were seen in clinic at regular intervals for five years. CEA was measured at each clinic visit, and CT of thorax, abdomen, and pelvis was performed at 12 and 24 months after commencement of chemotherapy. The median follow-up was 5.6 years. Disease relapses were observed in 154 of the 530 patients that were recruited. Relapses were detected by symptoms ($n=65$), CEA ($n=45$), CT ($n=49$), and others ($n=9$). The CT-detected group had a better survival after the discovery of relapse as compared with the symptomatic group ($P=0.0046$). Thirty-three patients (21%) proceeded to potentially curative surgery for relapse and enjoyed a better survival than those who did not ($P<0.00001$). For patients who underwent hepatic or pulmonary metastatic resection, thirteen (26.5%) were in the CT group, eight (17.8%) in the CEA group, and two (3.1%) had been discovered by symptomatic recurrence (CT vs. symptomatic, $P<0.001$; CEA vs. symptomatic, $P=0.015$). Similarly, a third prospective study (19) on the subject of follow-up found that in a more intense follow-up group (check-ups every three months for two years, then every six months for three years, as compared to every six months for one year, then yearly) local recurrences were detected significantly earlier (approximately 5–12 months) and curative re-resection was possible in more patients. The investigators also found that the five-year survival rate was significantly higher in the intense follow-up group (73.1% in the intense follow-up group vs. 58.3% with standard follow-up, $P<0.02$) (19). Borie et al. (20) from France examined the effectiveness of the follow-up tests used during the first five years after surgical resection for colorectal cancer. A total of 247 patients were analyzed in regards to the effectiveness of frequent follow-up testing in patients who received either follow-up with CEA monitoring (standard follow-up) or a more minimal follow-up schedule. The five-year survival rates were statistically similar in the standard and minimal follow-up groups and were 85% and 79%, respectively ($P=0.25$).

NEOADJUVANT THERAPY IN RECTAL CANCER

The goals for surgical approaches to rectal cancer should be to develop improved local control and overall survival, while maintaining quality of life and preserving sphincter, genitourinary, and sexual function. Much has been made of neoadjuvant therapy and its application for mid- to lower-lying rectal tumors. The effects of downstaging possibly enhance the rate of curative surgery and may increase sphincter preservation. The Swedish rectal trial reported its five-year follow-up data on a randomized, prospective trial looking at the role of preoperative radiation in resectable rectal cancer (21,22). The study randomly assigned 1168 patients younger than 80 years of age who had resectable rectal cancer to undergo preoperative irradiation [25 Gray (Gy) delivered in five fractions in one week] followed by surgery within one week or to have surgery alone. No chemotherapy was given either pre- or postoperatively. Irradiation did not increase postoperative mortality. After five years of follow-up, the rate of local recurrence was 11% (63 of 553 patients) in the group that received radiotherapy before surgery and 27% (150 of 557) in the group treated with surgery alone ($P<0.001$). Recently, Folkesson et al. (23) reported more recent data with a longer follow-up. A total of 908 patients, 454 patients in each arm, underwent an R0 resection with a 13-year median follow-up. The overall survival was 38% in the group receiving preoperative radiation and surgery versus 30% in that receiving surgery alone ($P=0.008$). The cancer-specific survival was 72% versus 62%, respectively ($P=0.03$). Local recurrence rates were 9% in the preoperative radiation and surgery group and 26% for the surgery alone group ($P<0.001$). This decreased local recurrence was seen in all stages. Stage I (321 patients) had a 4.5% local recurrence in patients with preoperative radiation versus 23% with surgery alone. Stage II (307 patients) had a 6% versus 22% recurrence with surgery alone and stage III (280 patients) had 23% versus 46%, respectively.

The National Surgical Adjuvant Breast and Bowel Project Protocol R-03 (24) was designed to determine the value of preoperative chemotherapy and radiation therapy in the management of operable rectal cancer. All patients received seven cycles of 5-FU/LV chemotherapy. Cycles 1 and 4 through 7 used a high-dose weekly FU regimen. In cycles 2 and 3, FU and low dose LV chemotherapy was given during the first and fifth weeks of radiation therapy (5040 cGy). The preoperative arm (group 1) received the first three cycles of chemotherapy and all radiation therapy before surgery. The postoperative arm (group 2) received all radiation and chemotherapy after surgery. Primary-study end points included disease-free survival and overall survival. Secondary end points included local recurrence, primary tumor response to combination therapy, tumor downstaging, and sphincter preservation. Overall treatment-related toxicity was similar in both groups. However, due to poor accrual of only 267 patients of the expected 900, no long-term data is available.

A population-based prospective, randomized trial on preoperative radiotherapy (RT) in operable rectal cancer, conducted in Stockholm, Sweden (25), included 557 patients; 272 patients were randomized to receive preoperative irradiation with 25 Gy in five cycles during five to seven days to the rectum and pararectal tissues (RT+ group) and 285 patients were allocated to surgery alone (RT− group). The median follow-up time was 50 months. Surgery was considered curative in 479 patients (86%). *Local* recurrence occurred in 10% of the patients in the RT+ group versus 21% in the RT− group ($P<0.01$). Among patients receiving curative surgery, distant metastases occurred in 19% in the RT+ group versus 26% in the RT− group ($P=0.02$). In addition to decreased local and distant recurrence, the overall survival was also improved in the irradiated patients ($P=0.02$). Postoperative complications were more common after irradiation but were usually mild (41% in RT+ vs. 28% in surgery only, $P<0.01$). The postoperative mortality (2% in the RT+ group vs. 1% in the RT- group, $P=0.289$) was low in both groups. These studies support the view that treatment with radiation therapy prior to surgery could reduce local and distant recurrence rates, and thus potentially overall and cancer-related mortality rates with only a small increase in morbidity.

The more recent German Rectal Cancer Study group (26) addressed the issue of neoadjuvant versus adjuvant chemoradiation when they reported randomly assigned patients with clinical stage T3 or T4 or node-positive disease who received either preoperative or postoperative chemoradiotherapy. Four hundred and twenty-one patients were randomized to preoperative chemoradiotherapy which consisted of 5040 cGy and FU, given in a 120-hour continuous infusion at 1000 mg per square meter of body surface area per day during the first and fifth weeks of radiotherapy. Surgery was performed six weeks after the completion of chemoradiotherapy. One month after surgery, four five-day cycles of FU (500 mg per square meter per day) were given. Four hundred and two patients were allotted to receive postoperative chemoradiotherapy which was similar to the preoperative regimen but had in addition a boost of 540 Gy. The overall five-year survival rates were 76% in the preoperative chemoradiotherapy group and 74% in the postoperative group (P=0.80). The five-year cumulative incidence of local relapse was 6% for patients assigned to preoperative chemoradiotherapy versus 13% in the postoperative group (P=0.006). Grade 3 or 4 acute toxic effects occurred in 27% versus 40%, respectively (P=0.001); the corresponding rates of long-term toxic effects were 14% and 24%, respectively (P=0.01).

The addition of intraoperative radiation therapy has also been reported. A retrospective study made a further comparison between patients who had received preoperative radiotherapy or chemoradiotherapy treatment plus intraoperative radiation therapy (IORT) and patients who received surgery only (27). The study comprised 99 patients with clinical T3-4NxM0 adenocarcinoma of the rectum who had received preoperative radio-/chemoradiotherapy, radical surgery, and IORT (group 1) and 68 patients who were treated with surgery alone (group 2). The investigators found that there was a lower local recurrence rate in patients with the combination of preoperative chemoradiotherapy and IORT (2% vs. 16% in the surgery only group, P=0.002) and that patients in the combination group also had a higher disease-free and overall survival rate compared to the surgery only group (five-year disease free rate 71% vs. 54%, P=0.04 and overall survival 79% vs. 58%, P=0.02). Additionally, they found a greater rate of sphincter preservation in the preoperative chemoradiotherapy subgroup than in the preoperative radiotherapy subgroup (78% vs. 42%, P=0.002). The optimal time interval between neoadjuvant radiation and surgery was examined by the Lyon trial (28). This prospective trial compared a short interval (two weeks) between radiation therapy and surgery to a longer interval (six to eight weeks). Two hundred and one patients with T2-T3 tumors in the lower rectum were included. The long interval was associated with a significantly better clinical response and pathologic downstaging (53% vs. 72%, P=0.007) and (10% vs. 26%, P=0.005), respectively. In addition, there was a trend for increased sphincter preservation with the longer time interval (76% vs. 68%, P=0.27). Although the surgery was not standardized in the trial they had a similar morbidity and two-month mortality between the two groups, similar overall five-year survival, similar local recurrence rates of 13% for the short interval group and 10% in the long interval group, and a similar percentage of patients who died from distant metastasis (18% in the short group and 20% in the long group), leading the authors to conclude that waiting longer between radiation therapy and surgical intervention, at least until eight weeks, is not harmful to the patient in terms of local and distant recurrence, mortality, morbidity, and overall survival. The findings in these studies would seem to imply that preoperative chemotherapy or radiation therapy or a combination of the two might help to decrease tumor size and rate of future recurrence, and increase sphincter preservation.

TOTAL MESORECTAL EXCISION

TME involves removal of the entire rectal mesentery, including that distal to the tumor, as an intact unit. It is a precise dissection in an areolar plane between the visceral fascia that envelops the rectum and mesorectum and the parietal fascia overlying pelvic wall structures. Heald (29) and others (30–32) demonstrated that maintaining this meticulous dissection of the rectum yields local recurrence rates of 5% to 10% with surgery alone. The importance of TME has been demonstrated by several prospective studies.

The Dutch Colorectal Cancer Group TME trial (32), the largest of these studies (1861 randomized patients), investigating preoperative radiotherapy with TME surgery versus TME surgery alone, found that patients in the experimental group that received preoperative radiotherapy of 5 Gy for five days before a TME procedure had a considerably lower local recurrence rate of 2.4%, as opposed to patients receiving no radiotherapy (surgery only) who had a local recurrence rate of 8.2% (P<0.001). In addition, there were no significant differences in postoperative morbidity and mortality; overall survival and local and distant recurrence rates were similar as well. Several advocates of TME contend therefore that radiation therapy is not necessary in patients who undergo resection utilizing this technique. However, instead of considering TME as a competitor to adjuvant therapy, this meticulous surgical technique should be considered central to the successful management of rectal cancer and a crucial component of the ultimate therapy.

Although there is a robust body of evidence-based data to support laparoscopic techniques for colectomy in patients with colon cancer, little evidence exists in laparoscopic approaches to rectal cancer (33,34). A prospective, observational study by Kockerling et al. (33) in Germany and Austria, reported the results of patients undergoing laparoscopic abdominoperineal resections. In 116 patients who underwent laparoscopic abdominoperineal resections, 98 (84.5%) were performed with curative intent. The mean operating time was 226 minutes. Seven patients (6%) experienced an intraoperative complication, which in more than one-half of the cases was a vascular injury involving the presacral venous plexus; the conversion rate was 3.4%. The recurrence-free survival rate was 71%, postoperative mortality rate was 1.7%, and morbidity rate was 34.4% (33).

A smaller, but randomized prospective study from Brazil, Araujo et al. (35) reported results in 28 patients. Thirteen underwent laparoscopic abdominoperineal resection and 15 a conventional approach. There was no significant difference between the two studied groups regarding: intra- and postoperative complications, need for blood transfusion, hospital stay after surgery, length of resected segment, or pathological staging. Mean operation time was shorter in the laparoscopic abdominoperineal resection (228 minutes vs. 284 minutes for the conventional approach, $P=0.04$); mean anesthesia duration was also shorter for the laparoscopic procedure (304 vs. 362 minutes, respectively, $P=0.03$). There was no need for conversion to open approach in this series. After a mean follow-up of 47.2 months, local recurrence was observed in two patients in the conventional group and in none in the laparoscopic group. In a retrospective review of three institutions, Fleshman et al. (36) reported results of 194 patients who underwent laparoscopic abdominoperineal resection (42 patients) or open abdominoperineal resection (152 patients). Laparoscopic abdominoperineal resection was converted to open abdominoperineal resection in 21% most often due to vessel injury, poor exposure, and adhesions. Perineal infections occurred more frequently in the laparoscopic abdominoperineal resection group (24% vs. 8%; $P=0.02$). Late stromal complications were similar. Mean hospital stay was shorter after laparoscopic abdominoperineal resection (7 vs. 12 days). Radial margins were positive in 12% of laparoscopic abdominoperineal resection and 12.5% of open abdominoperineal resection specimens. Tumor recurrence was similar for both local (19% in the laparoscopic and 14% in the open group) and distant (38% and 26%, respectively) recurrence. Survival rates were similar with median follow-up of 19 and 24 months, respectively.

Leroy et al. (37) in Rasbourg, France reported their experience in 102 consecutive unselected patients undergoing laparoscopic TME for rectal cancer. Laparoscopic TME was completed successfully in 99 patients, whereas conversion to an open approach was required in three cases (3%). The overall morbidity and mortality rates were 27% and 2%, respectively, with an overall anastomotic leak rate of 17%. The resection was considered curative in 91.8% of the patients, while the remainder had a palliative resection due to synchronous metastatic disease or locally advanced disease. Mean follow-up was 36 months (range, 6–96). There were no trocar site recurrences. The local recurrence rate was 6%, and the cancer-specific survival of all curatively resected patients was 75% at five years. The overall survival rate of all curatively resected patients was 65% at five years; mean survival time was 6.23 years.

Recently, Barlehner et al. (38) reported their experience in 194 unselected patients resected laparoscopically for rectal carcinoma. The most common procedures were low anterior resection with total mesorectum excision, in 65.5% of patients, and high anterior resection, in 25.3%. Average operative time was 174 minutes. Average number of lymph nodes removed was 25.4, and length of specimen resected was 27.6 cm. Resection was curative in 145 patients and palliative in 49 cases. Intraoperarive complications were <1%. The most common postoperative complication was anastomotic leakage, in 13.5% of patients. There was no postoperative mortality. Mean follow-up evaluation was 46.1 months (range 1 to 128 months). The most common late complication was incisional hernia in 3.6% of patients. Port-site metastases occurred in one patient (0.5%). Tumor recurrence developed in 23 of the 145 curative resected patients (11.7% distant metastases and 4.1% local recurrence). Overall local recurrence rate was 6.7% (4.1% after curative resection and 14.3% after palliative resection). Overall survival rate was 90.6% at one year and 66.3% at five years and overall five-year survival rate after curative resection was 76.9% and after palliative resection was 31.8%. Cancer-related survival rate was

94% at one year and 78.9% at five years. At five years, it was 87.7% after curative resection and 48.5% after palliative resection. When analyzed according to stage the five year survival rate was 100% for stage I, 94.4% for stage II, 66.6% for stage III, and 44.6% for stage IV. Although most of these studies report promising data with regard to laparoscopic approaches for rectal cancer; further randomized, prospective trials are needed to determine the long-term outcome of cancer treatment.

Another important consideration in surgical resection of the rectum is the type of anastomosis used to reconnect the remaining colon to the distal margin in a way that maximizes patient quality of life while minimizing risk of neoplasm recurrence, anastomotic leak, morbidity, and mortality. Studies have compared various techniques while considering factors such as fecal continence, frequency, or difficulty of bowel movements, and rate of anastomotic leaks and tumor reoccurrences at the margins. Several small studies have recently investigated the use of a J-pouch technique versus straight or side-to-end anastomosis to decrease frequency and urgency of defecation by increasing reservoir volume or decreasing bowel motility. Three of those studies that compared J-pouch with side-to-end anastomosis found no significant difference in bowel function between the groups (34,39,40).

One recent paper has examined the difference between closure techniques: the hand-sewn anastomosis approach or the stapling technique. Laurent (41) found no difference in morbidity between patients randomized to the hand-sewn or the stapled groups, although the investigators did find, as could be expected, a significantly shorter operating time for the stapled group (261V40 minutes in stapled vs. 314V46 minutes hand-sewn, P=0.0008). Similarities also existed between the groups in the number of stools per day, frequency, urgency, incontinence, and requirements for protective pads or medications. The only difference in bowel function between the groups was the development of anastomotic stricture in three of the hand-sewn patients, but this was not statistically significant.

REFERENCES

1. Parkin DM, Bray F, Ferlay J, Pisani P. Global Cancer Statistics, 2002. CA Cancer J Clin 2005; 55:74–108.
2. Jemal A, Tiwari R, Murray T, et al. Cancer statistics. CA et al. Cancer J Clin 2004; 54:8–29.
3. Franklin ME Jr, Rosetithal D, Abrego-Medina D, et al. Prospective comparison of open vs. laparoscopic colon surgery for carcinoma. Five-year results. Dis Colon Rectum 1996; 39(10 suppl):S35–S46.
4. Milsom JW, Bohm B, Hammerhofer KA, Fazio V, Steieer E, Elson P. A prospective, randomized trial comparing laparoscopic versus conventional techniques in colorectal cancer surgery: a preliminary report. J Am Coll Surg 1998; 187(1):46–54.
5. Lacy A, Garcia-Valdecasas J, Delgado S, et al. Laparoscopy-assisted colectomy versus open colectomy for treatment of non-metastatic colon cancer: a randomized trial. Lancet 2002; 359:2224–2229.
6. Lezoche E, Feliciotti F, Paganini AM, Guemeri M, Campagnacci R, De Sanctis A. Laparoscopic colonic resections versus open surgery: a prospective non-randomized study on 310 unselected cases. Hepatogastroenterology 2000; 47:697–708.
7. Patankar S, Larach S, Ferrara A, et al. Prospective comparison of laparoscopic vs. open resections for colorectal adenocarcinoma over a ten-year period. Dis Colon Rectum 2003; 46:601–611.
8. Veldkamp R, Kuhrv E, HOP WC, et al. COlon cancer Laparoscopic_or Open Resection Study Group? (COLOR). Laparoscopic surgery versus open surgery for colon cancer: short-term outcomes of a randomised trial. Lancet Oncol 2005; 6(7):477–484.
9. Guillou P, Quirke P, Thorpe H, et al. (The MRC CLASICC trial group). Short-term endpoints of conventional versus laparoscopic-assisted surgery in patients with colorectal cancer (MRC CLASICC trial): multicenter, randomized controlled trial. Lancet 2005; 365:1718–1726.
10. The Clinical Outcomes of Surgical Therapy Study Group. A comparison of laparoscopically assisted and open colectomy for colon cancer. New Engl J Med 2004; 350:2050–2059.
11. Weeks JC, Nelson H, Gelber S, Sargent D, Schroeder G. Short-term quality of life outcomes following laparoscopic-assisted colectomy vs. open colectomy for colon cancer: a randomized trial. JAMA 2002; 287:321–328.
12. Rouffet F, Hay JM, Vacher B, et al. Curative resection for left colonic carcinoma: hemicolectomy vs. segmental colectomy: a prospective, controlled, multicenter trial. Dis Colon Rectum 1994; 37:651–659.
13. Single-stage treatment for malignant left-sided colonic obstruction: a prospective randomized clinical trial comparing subtotal colectomy with segmental resection following intraoperative irrigation. The SCOTIA Study Group. Subtotal Colectomy versus On-table Irrigation and Anastomosis. Br J Surg 1995; 82(1 2):1622–1627.

14. Torralba J, Robles R, Parilla P, et al. Subtotal colectomy vs. intraoperative colonic irrigation in the management of obstructed left colon carcinoma. Dis Colon Rectum 1998; 41:18–22.
15. Docherty JG, McGregor JR, Akyol AM, Murray GD, Galloway DJ. Comparison of manually constructed and stapled anastomoses in colorectal surgery. West of Scotland and Highland Anastomosis Study Group. Ann Surg 1995; 221:176–184.
16. Beard JD, Nicholson ML, Sayers RD, Lloyd D, Everson NW. Intraoperative air testing of colorectal anastomoses: a prospective, randomized trial. Br J Surg 1990; 77:1095–1097.
17. Korner H, Soreide K, Stokkeland P, Soreide JA. Systematic follow-up after curative surgery for colorectal cancer in Norway: a population-based audit of effectiveness, costs and compliance. J Gastrointest Surg 2005; 9:320–328.
18. Chau I, Alien M, Cunningham D, et al. The value of routine serum carcino-embryonic antigen measurement and computed tomography in the surveillance of patients after adjuvant chemotherapy for colon cancer. J Clin Oncol 2004; 22:1420–1429.
19. Pietra N, Sarli L, Costi R, Ouchemi C, Grattarola M, Peracchia A. Role of follow-up in management of local recurrences of colorectal cancer: a prospective, randomized study. Dis Colon Rectum 1998; 41:1127–1133.
20. Bone F, Daures JP, Millat B, Tretarre B. Cost and effectiveness of follow-up examinations in patients with colorectal cancer resected for cure in a French population-based study. J Gastrointest Surg 2004; 8:552–558.
21. Improved survival with preoperative radiotherapy in resectable rectal cancer. Swedish Rectal Cancer Trial. N Engl J Med 1997; 336(14):980–987. Erratum in: N Engl J Med 1997; 336(21):1539.
22. Local recurrence rate in a randomised multicenter trial of preoperative radiotherapy compared with operation alone in resectable rectal carcinoma. Swedish Rectal Cancer Trial. Eur J Surg 1996; 162(5):397–402.
23. Folkesson J, Birgisson H. Pahlman L, Cedermark B, Glimelius B, Gunnarsson U. Swedish Rectal Cancer Trial: long lasting benefits from radiotherapy on survival and local recurrence rate. J Clin Oncol 2005; 23(24):5644–5650.
24. Wolmark N, Fisher B. An analysis of survival and treatment failure following abdominoperineal and sphincter-saving resection in Dukes' B and C rectal carcinoma: a report of the NSABP clinical trials. Ann Surg 1986; 204:480–489.
25. Randomized study on preoperative radiotherapy in rectal carcinoma. Stockholm Colorectal Cancer Study Group. Ann Surg Oncol 1996; 3(5):423–430.
26. Sauer R, Becker H, Hohenbergcr W, et al. German Rectal Cancer Study Group. Preoperative versus postoperative chemoradiotherapy for rectal cancer. N Engl J Med 2004; 351(17):1731–1740.
27. Sadahiro S, Suzuki T, Ishikawa K, et al. Preoperative radio/chemo-radiotherapy in combination with intraoperative radiotherapy for T3-4Nx rectal cancer. EJSO 2004; 30:750–758.
28. Glehen O, Chapet O, Adham M, Nemoz J, Gerard J, Lyons Oncology Group. Long-term results of the Lyons R90-01 randomized trial of preoperative radiotherapy with delayed surgery and its effect on sphincter-saving surgery in rectal cancer. Br J Surg 2003; 90:996–998.
29. Heald RJ, Rvall RD. Recurrence and survival after total mesorectal excision for rectal cancer. Lancet 1986; 1(8496):1479–1482.
30. Havenga K, Enker WE, Norstein J, et al. Improved survival and local control after total mesorectal excision or D3 lymphadenectomy in the treatment of primary rectal cancer: an international analysis of 1411 patients. Eur J Surg Oncol 1999; 25:368–374.
31. Merchant NB, Guillem JG, Paty PB, et al. T3NO rectal cancer: results following sharp mesorectal excision and no adjuvant therapy. J Gastrointest Surg 1999; 3(6):642–647.
32. Kapiteijn E, Marijnen CA, Nagtegaal ID, et al. Dutch Colorectal Cancer Group. Preoperative radiotherapy combined with total mesorectal excision for resectable rectal cancer. N Engl J Med 2001; 345(9):638–646.
33. Kockerling F, Sheidback H, Schneider C, et al. The Laparoscopic Colorectal Surgery Study Group. Laparoscopic abdominoperineal resection: early postoperative results of a prospective study involving 116 patients. Dis Colon Rectum 2000; 43:1503–1511.
34. Machado M, Nygren J, Goldman S, Ljungqvist O. Similar outcome after colonic pouch and sidc-to-end anastomosis in low anterior resection for rectal cancer: a prospective randomized trial. Ann Surg 2003; 238:214–220.
35. Araujo SE, da Silva eSousa AH Jr, de Campos FG, et al. Conventional approach x laparoscopic abdominoperineal resection for rectal cancer treatment after neoadjuvant chemoradiation: results of a prospective randomized trial. Rev Hosp Clin Fac Med Sao Paulo 2003; 58(3):133–140.
36. Fleshman JW, Wexner SD, Anvari M, et al. Laparoscopic vs. open abdominoperineal resection for cancer. Dis Colon Rectum 1999; 42(7):930–939.
37. Leroy J, Jamali F, Forbes L, et al. Laparoscopic total mesorectal excision (TME) for rectal cancer surgery: long-term outcomes. Surg Endosc 2004; 18(2):281–289. E-pub: Dec 29, 2003. Review.
38. Barlchner E, Benhidieb T, Anders S, Schicke B. Laparoscopic resection for rectal cancer: outcomes in 194 patients and review of the literature. Surg Endosc 2005; 19(6):757–766.

39. Jiang JK, Yang SH, Lin JK. Transabdominal anastomosis after low anterior resection: a prospective, randomized, controlled trial comparing long-term results between side-to-end anastomosis and colonic J-pouch. Dis Colon Rectum 2005; 48(11):2100–2108.
40. Machado M, Nygren J, Goldman S, Ljungqvist O. Functional and physiologic assessment of the colonic reservoir or side-to-end anastomosis after low anterior resection for rectal cancer: a two-year follow-up. Dis Colon Rectum 2005; 48(1):29–36.
41. Laurent A, Pare Y, McNamara D, Pare R, Tiret E. Colonic J-pouch-anal anastomosis for rectal cancer: a prospective, randomized study comparing handsewn vs. stapled anastomosis. Dis Colon Rectum 2005; 48(4):729.

12 Adjuvant Therapy for Colorectal Cancer

Catherine R. Jephcott
Department of Oncology, Churchill Hospital, Oxford, U.K.

David J. Kerr
Department of Clinical Pharmacology, Radcliffe Infirmary, University of Oxford, Oxford, U.K.

RATIONALE FOR TREATMENT

Colorectal cancer is a common malignancy. In the United Kingdom, it is the third most frequently occurring cancer in men, with over 18,700 cases diagnosed per year, and in women, it is the second, with 16,800 cases each year (1). Worldwide, it has an annual incidence of approximately 700,000 new cases with 500,000 deaths (2).

Approximately 80% of the patients will have early resectable disease at presentation. The primary treatment for these patients will be surgery. In addition, in the case of some rectal carcinomas, locally directed, neoadjuvant radiotherapy or chemoradiotherapy may also be given. However, despite complete local macroscopic resection, over half of these patients will relapse and may subsequently die of their disease. This is thought to be the result of the early, distant spread of microscopic disease that is not removed at initial surgery, and is not detectable by standard radiologic techniques. Adjuvant treatment is designed to eradicate this potential early spread of tumor cells. Accordingly, chemotherapy (CT) aimed at systemic treatment of distant microscopic metastastic spread is given to patients with apparently localized disease as soon as is practicable after their surgery.

EVIDENCE OF A SURVIVAL BENEFIT FOR ADJUVANT CHEMOTHERAPY IN COLORECTAL CANCER

The efficacy of adjuvant therapy for carcinoma of the colon is now well established. Drugs known to be effective in treating metastatic disease (see Chapter 17) have been used in the adjuvant setting to seek improved survival.

The first large, prospective randomized trial to demonstrate a survival benefit was the National Adjuvant Breast and Bowel Project (NSABP) study protocol C-01 (3). This compared the combination of 5-fluorouracil (5-FU), semustine, and vincristine all given postoperatively for eight, 10-weekly cycles; Bacillus Calmette Guerin (BCG) treatment; and surgery alone; in patients in Dukes' B and C categories. This revealed a small improvement in overall survival (OS) with the 5-FU combination; 1166 patients entered this trial between 1977 and 1983—379 were in the arm receiving CT, 394 were in the observation arm, and 393 patients received BCG therapy. There was an overall improvement of disease free survival (DFS) (p=0.02) and survival (67% vs. 59%; p=0.05) in favor of the CT-treated group. At five years of follow up, patients treated with surgery alone were at 1.29 times the risk of developing treatment failure and 1.31 times the likelihood of dying as were those patients treated with combination adjuvant CT.

A subsequent Intergroup study 0035 established the efficacy of adjuvant 5-FU-based CT. This trial therefore assessed 1296 patients with resected Dukes' B or C colon cancer, randomizing them to no further treatment or to treatment with 5-FU plus levamisole (an antihelminthic drug with poorly described "immunomodulating" properties) for 12 months. The regime used was fluorouracil, 450 mg/m^2/day × 5 then weekly, and levamisole 50 mg tid po, days 1–3 every week for one year. Some of those patients with Dukes' C cancer were also randomized to a further arm of treatment with levamisole alone for 12 months. Nine hundred and twenty-nine eligible patients were followed for five years or more. The initial report was published in 1990 (4) and the results for Dukes' C (stage III) patients were later confirmed in a 1995 publication (5). These showed that treatment with surgery and the combination of 5-FU and levamisole to those

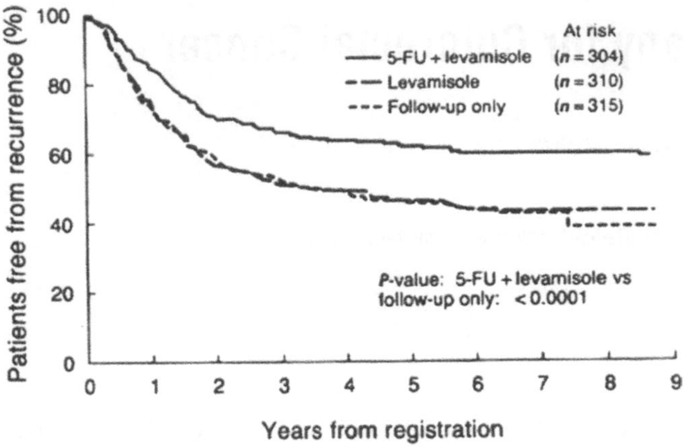

FIGURE 1 Recurrence-free interval according to treatment arm. Patients who died without recurrence have been censored. *Abbreviation*: 5-FU, fluorouracil. *Source*: From Ref. 5.

patients with stage III disease decreased the risk of cancer recurrence by 41% ($p < 0.0001$) after a median follow up of three years, and the overall death rate was decreased by 33% (p=0.006). The five-year DFS with fluorouracil and levamisole was 61% and OS was 60% compared with 44% DFS and 47% OS with observation only (Figs. 1, 2). In retrospect, a trial arm with fluorouracil alone will have been helpful for interpretation of the data.

Patients with Dukes' B (stage II) disease showed a trend toward reduction in the rate of disease recurrence in the 5-FU plus levamisole arm compared to the surgery-alone arm, but there was no difference in OS at a median follow up of seven years. Levamisole therapy alone had no impact on DFS or OS. The overall results of The Intergroup 0035 study (INT0035) therefore established the role of postoperative CT for stage III patients, and following National Institute of Health's (NIH) consensus statement in 1990, this became the standard of care for such patients in America.

A number of studies at about this time demonstrated the combination of 5-FU and folinic acid (FA) to be superior to fluorouracil alone in treating patients with advanced colorectal carcinoma (6), and this combination was subsequently taken into the adjuvant arena. The NSABP protocol C-03 (7) demonstrated that a 5-FU/FA combination (a treatment schedule of eight cycles of a high-dose leucovorin (LV), weekly regime given for six of eight weeks) was superior to methyl-CCNU, vincristine, and 5-FU (MOF, five, 10-weekly cycles) in Dukes' B and C colon cancer patients, providing three-year DFS and OS advantages of 73% versus 64% (P=0.0004) and 84% versus 77% (P=0.003), respectively. (Adjuvant MOF therapy had previously been shown to have a slight advantage over surgery alone.)

Large studies comparing CT to a control group who received no postsurgery treatment were also performed by the North Central Cancer Treatment Group (NCCTG) (8) and

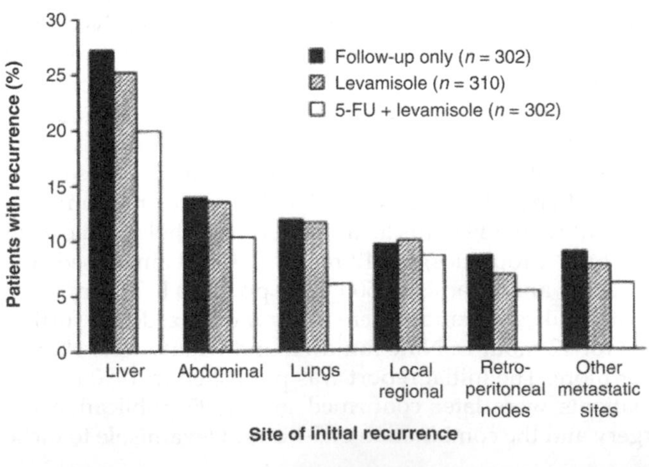

FIGURE 2 Survival according to treatment arm. *Abbreviation*: 5-FU, fluorouracil. *Source*: From Ref. 5.

the International Multicenter Pooled Analysis of Colorectal Cancer Trials (IMPACT) Collaborative Group (9).

The IMPACT study was a pooled analysis of three randomized trials [GIVIO, National Cancer Institute of Canada-Cancer Treatment Group (NCIC-CTG), and FFCD] comparing postoperative treatment with high-dose 5-FU and FA (370- to 400-mg/m^2 5-FU and FA 200 mg/m^2 daily for five days, every 28 days for six cycles) with surgery alone. One thousand five hundred and twenty-six patients with Dukes' B (56%) and C (44%) disease were entered with 1493 eligible for analysis. Chemotherapy was seen to reduce mortality and recurrences, increasing the three-year, event-free survival from 62% to 71% (P=0.0001) and OS from 78% to 83% (P=0.018).

The NCCTG study was performed to compare the classical Mayo regimen of 5-FU (425 mg/m^2) and LV (20 mg/m^2) to observation alone after surgery in patients with Dukes' B and C disease. Due to the emergence of the results of the INT0035 study, this trial was stopped prematurely. Only 309 patients were enrolled—290 of these patients had Dukes' C disease, and their five-year survival was increased from 63% to 74%. These studies therefore gave evidence that adjuvant therapy following primary surgical treatment offers benefits compared to observation alone.

It will seem on theoretical grounds that the earlier the treatment is commenced after surgery, the more likely it is to be successful. However, there is no evidence to support this, and although oncologists recommend it, there may be a window of up to three months after surgery to introduce adjuvant therapy. In practice, it is usual to aim to commence treatment within four to six weeks of surgery. Appropriate candidates are identified by close cooperation between surgeons, oncologists, and other members of the multidisciplinary team.

COMPARISON OF TREATMENT REGIMES

Once the importance of adjuvant therapy was established, studies were devised to determine optimal drug combinations.

5-Fluorouracil with Leucovorin and Levamisole

The INT0035 study encouraged the use of fluorouracil with levamisole as standard adjuvant treatment, as stated earlier, following its demonstration of increased survival over surgery alone and lack of any benefit of levamisole when given without the 5-FU. Two subsequent studies compared the role of levamisole.

The NSABP C-04 trial (10) recruited 2151 patients with Dukes' B or C carcinoma of the colon randomizing them to receive one of three different treatments: (*i*) the Roswell Park regime [5-FU and LV (Chapter 17)]; (*ii*) weekly 5-FU plus levamisole as per the Intergroup 0035 study; (*iii*) the Roswell Park regime plus levamisole. Treatment was for a year. There was no significant difference between the effectiveness of 5-FU/LV and 5-FU/LV plus levamisole. However, comparing 5-FU/LV versus 5-FU/levamisole groups revealed that 5-FU/LV improved five-year DFS from 60% to 65% (P = 0.04) and OS from 70% to 74% (P = 0.07).

The QUASAR study (11) was a large, two-by-two factorial study that aimed to compare high- and low-dose FA and levamisole versus placebo in combination with fluorouracil. Four thousand nine hundred and twenty-seven patients, with mainly Dukes' B (28%) and Dukes' C (72%) disease (and Dukes' A 0.2%), were randomized. 5-FU (370 mg/m^2) was given either daily for five days on a 28-day cycle for 24 weeks or weekly for 30 weeks, together with L-FA 25 mg versus 175 mg. In addition, either active or placebo levamisole (50 mg) was given three times daily for three days, and repeated every two weeks for 12 courses. The study confirmed that levamisole was unhelpful, with results being marginally worse than those for placebo. The three-year OS (69.4% vs. 71.5%; P=0.06) and recurrence rate (37.0% vs. 34.9%; P=0.16) were similar. Survival rates were virtually identical, with high- and low-dose FA (70.1% vs. 71.0% at three years; P=0.43) as were three-year recurrence rates (36% vs. 35.8%; P=0.94). There was no difference between results of the weekly and monthly regimes of 5-FU/FA (although this comparison was not randomized).

Duration of Treatment

The original norm for duration of adjuvant treatment with 5-FU and levamisole for colorectal cancer was a 12-month schedule. However, it has emerged that six months of treatment with these agents is sufficient to obtain similar survival rates.

In a large, randomized study by the NCCTG and NCIC (12), it was shown that there was no additional benefit in the administration of 12 compared to six months of CT. They randomized 915 Dukes' B and C patients to receive 5-FU and levamisole, or 5-FU/LV and levamisole, further randomizing to either six or 12 months of treatment. There was no significant advantage in DFS or OS for either time-duration with either regimen.

The Intergroup 0089 trial, reported at ASCO in 1998 (13) compared: (*i*) levamisole and 5-FU for 12 months; (*ii*) high-dose LV and 5-FU for 32 weeks; (*iii*) low-dose LV and 5-FU for 28 weeks; and (*iv*) levamisole plus low-dose LV and 5-FU for 28 weeks. The shorter duration treatments with 5-FU/FA were seen to be as beneficial as 12 months of 5-FU/levamisole at a median follow-up of five years. Although this was not the primary aim of the trial, it is generally held to validate shorter-term courses of treatment, given the associated improvement in quality of life.

Leading on from this, the SAFFA trial (14) investigated yet shorter treatment duration by administrating 5-FU as a continuous infusion. Seven hundred and fifteen patients with curatively resected Dukes' B or C colorectal cancer were randomized to receive 5-FU/FA (5-FU 425 mg/m^2 iv and FA 20 mg/m^2 iv bolus days one to five every 28 days for six months) or a protracted venous infusion (PVI) of 5-FU alone (300 mg/m^2 per day for 12 weeks). At a median follow-up of 19.8 months, OS was not significantly different between the two groups (three-year survival 83.2% 5-FU/FA vs. 87.9% PVI 5-FU). In fact, relapse-free survival, quality of life, and toxicity were all seen to be improved with the shorter PVI regimen. However, this was a rather small trial when compared with most contemporary studies, and did not directly address the question of duration of therapy, as two quite different CT regimes were employed.

Newer Chemotherapy Agents

The advent of agents that offer easier administration or improved response rates for patients with advanced colorectal cancer has led to assessments of their role in the adjuvant setting. The standard adjuvant treatment has been fluorouracil and FA and several studies are under way to assess the role of combining the new agents with these or with replacing fluorouracil with an oral equivalent.

Capecitabine

Capecitabine is an oral 5-FU analog. It is easier to administer and has a moderate toxicity profile, with less mucositis and neutropenia than 5-FU but more hand/foot syndrome. This has generated interest in its efficacy as an adjuvant agent. The X-ACT study results have recently been made available (15). This study compared capecitabine with bolus 5-FU/LV (Mayo regimen) in patients with surgically resected Dukes' C carcinomas. One thousand nine hundred and eighty-seven patients were randomized to receive oral capecitabine (1250 mg/m^2 twice daily on days 1–14, every three weeks) or IV 5-FU/LV (LV 20 mg/m^2 + 5-FU 425 mg/m^2 on days 1–5 every four weeks) for 24-weeks' treatment. At a median follow up of 3.8 years, results showed that capecitabine was at least equivalent to 5-FU/LV with respect to DFS in the per protocol population [DFS; HR 0.89 95% confidence interval (CI) 0.76–1.04], and in the intention-to-treat-analysis (ITT) showed a trend toward being superior (DFS; HR 0.87; 95% CI 0.75–1.0; P=0.0528) and also showed a trend toward superiority for OS (OS, ITT, HR 0.84, 95% CI 0.69–1.01, P=0.0706). Relapse-free survival was superior with capecitabine versus 5-FU/LV (ITT 0.86; 95% CI 0.74–0.99; P=0.041). Toxicity data had previously been presented, revealing decreased grade 3/4 mucositis and neutropenia but an increase in hand/foot syndrome in patients receiving capecitabine. The authors conclude that these results suggest that capecitabine should replace 5-FU/LV as the standard adjuvant therapy for colorectal cancer. Indeed, the ease of administration makes this treatment option preferable to many clinicians and patients, and on the strength of this X-ACT data, capecitabine treatment will be employed as the standard arm of the QUASAR2 survey.

Oxaliplatin

Oxaliplatin is a third-generation platinum CT agent that has been demonstrated to offer good response rates and valuable improvements in life expectancy in patients with metastatic colorectal cancer (Chapter 17). Interest is now growing in using this agent in the adjuvant setting.

The Multicentre International Study of Oxaliplatin/5-Fluorouracil/Leucovorin in the Adjuvant Treatment of Colon Cancer (MOSAIC) investigators have recently published their findings (16). A large trial randomizing 2246 patients who had undergone curative resection for stage II (899 patients) or III (1347 patients) colon cancer to receive fluorouracil and LV (FL) alone or with oxaliplatin for six months was carried out. The FL regime consisted of a two-hour infusion of 200-mg leucovorin per m^2 followed by a bolus of 400 mg/m^2, and then a 22-hour infusion of 600 mg/m^2 of fluorouracil given on two consecutive days every 14 days, for 12 cycles. Those patients receiving oxaliplatin also were administered the same 5-FU regimen plus a two-hour infusion of 85-mg/m^2 oxaliplatin per m^2 on day one given simultaneously with the LV. The primary end point of the trial was DFS. At three years, this was seen to be 78.2% (95% CI 75.6–80.7%) for the FL + oxaliplatin group and 72.9% (95% CI 70.2–75.7%) in the FL alone group (P=0.002). The authors therefore concluded that the addition of oxaliplatin to 5-FU/FA was beneficial. The main safety concern regarding the use of oxaliplatin is of an induced distal sensory neuropathy. Grade 3 peripheral neuropathy was observed in 12.4% of patients who received oxaliplatin, but this had decreased to 1.1% at one year. This remains a potential concern. Neutropenic fever was documented in 1.8% of patients with the combined therapy, which exceeded than in the FL arm, but was still judged to be reasonably low. The OS data is awaited as the follow-up data matures. These results augur well, and this agent may become very attractive to patients and clinicians.

Irinotecan

Irinotecan is similarly being developed for adjuvant use, having been shown to be active in metastatic colorectal disease both alone and in combination with 5-FU. It is a topoisomerase I inhibitor. (This enzyme is involved in DNA supercoiling.) The advantage over oxaliplatin is a relative lack of long-term side effects, although short-term side effects include diarrhea, myelosuppression, and alopecia.

Saltz et al. (17) recently reported a phase III randomized study, which assessed the role of irinotecan after curative resection for stage III colon cancer. One thousand two hundred and sixty-four patients were randomized between the years 1999 and 2001 to receive either irinotecan plus fluorouracil/LV (IFL), first-line irinotecan 125 mg/m^2 over 90 minutes followed by LV 20 mg/m^2 iv bolus and then fluorouracil 500 mg/m^2 iv bolus, given four weeks on two weeks off, ×5 cycles (30 weeks total), or the Roswell Park schedule of FL [LV 500 mg/m^2 iv over two hours plus fluorouracil 500 mg/m^2 at one hour after start of LV, given six weeks on, two weeks off, ×4 cycles (32 weeks total)]. At a median follow up of 2.6 years, IFL showed no improvement over FL in terms of either OS (P=0.88) or failure-free survival (FFS) (P=0.84). Irinotecan plus fluorouracil/LV, as compared to FL, was associated with a greater degree of grade 3/4 neutropenia (31% vs. 5%), febrile neutropenia (4% vs. 1%) and death on treatment (2.8% vs. 1.0%). They concluded that weekly bolus IFL should not be used in the management of stage III colon cancer. However, further trials are currently in progress to evaluate the role of irinotecan in the adjuvant setting.

The results of the European PETACC-3-EORTC trial are awaited. Stage III colon cancer patients were randomized following surgery to receive either 5-FU/LV alone or in combination with irinotecan. This was either given as the de Gramont LV5FU2 schedule (FA 200 mg/m^2 given over two hours followed by 5-FU iv 600 mg/m^2 over 22 hours days one and two, with irinotecan 180 mg/m^2 given over 60 minutes concurrently with the FA on day 1) or as the German AIO schedule (Arbeitsgemeinschaft internische Oncologie) (FA 500 mg/m^2 over two hours with 60-minute infusion irinotecan 80 mg/m^2 followed by 5-FU 2000 mg/m^2 over 24 hours weekly). Treatment was given for six months. The primary end point of the study was three-year DFS. Recruitment ended in April 2002 with 2333 patients enrolled. The French FNCLCC/FFCD trial (ACCORD-02) randomized high-risk stage III patients (N2 disease with greater than three nodes positive and N1 patients with obstruction or perforation) to LV5FU2 or LV5FU2 + irinotecan. The primary end point is three-year DFS and data are awaited with interest.

The French AERO/GERCOR group is undertaking a study of adjuvant irinotecan in rectal cancer patients. They will be randomizing to irinotecan + LV5FU2 or to 5FU/FA alone (de Gramont or Mayo regimes).

PETACC-4 has been designed to attempt to resolve issues surrounding the adjuvant treatment of patients with stage II disease. Patients with colon cancer (including the rectosigmoid junction) are randomized to surgery alone or surgery followed by irinotecan + 5-FU/FA given according to the de Gramont, AIO, or TTD regimes. Results from these studies are eagerly awaited.

Non-Cytotoxic Therapy

As the potential role of noncytotoxic therapy in fighting colorectal cancer has become evident, increasing numbers of studies assessing the role of these novel strategies have been set up.

The VICTOR trial aims to assess the role of the nonsteroidal anti-inflammatory drug (NSAID) rofecoxib [a potent orally active cyclo-oxygenase (COX)-2 selective inhibitor] in its role as an antiangiogenic agent. Previous epidemiologic, clinical, and laboratory studies have revealed that NSAIDs can grant some protection against colorectal cancer. This trial randomizes patients following their surgical and adjuvant CT treatment to receive either placebo or rofecoxib for either two or five years, with a primary hypothesis that the active agent will provide a greater OS as compared to placebo. If this hypothesis proves correct, then this agent would be a useful and relatively nontoxic addition to our armamentarium of adjuvant therapy agents.

CONTROVERSIAL AREAS

Stage II Disease

There has been considerable controversy as to whether adjuvant therapy for Dukes' B (stage II) colorectal carcinoma patients offers real benefit. Such patients will generally have a better prognosis than those with Dukes' C (stage III) disease (80% vs. 50% five-year survival), and in consequence, in these, the risk benefit ratio of adjuvant therapy becomes more marginal.

The recent release of the uncertain arm data from QUASAR1 (18) has clarified matters, but prior to this, there had been two large retrospective studies which yielded conflicting results. The NSABP reviewed 3820 patients from their trials NSABP C-01, C-02, C-03, and C-04 (19) to determine the benefit of CT in stage II (Dukes' B) versus stage III (Dukes' C) patients. They compared various CT regimes with each other or with surgery alone (i.e., C-01 surgery alone vs. postoperative semustine, vincristine, and 5-FU vs. postoperative BCG; C-02 surgery alone vs. postoperative 5-FU and heparin via PVI; C-03 lomustine, vincristine, and 5-FU vs. 5-FU and FA; C-04 5-FU and levamisole vs. 5-FU and FA vs. 5-FU, FA, and levamisole). This evaluation of 3820 patients (1565 being staged as Dukes' B) revealed that in all the studies, there was an increase in relative OS, DFS, and recurrence-free survival in both Dukes' B and C patients. The mortality reduction was 30% for Dukes' B patients and 18% for Dukes' C patients. However, the absolute reduction in mortality was less in the Dukes' B patients because of the greater likelihood of survival of this group following surgical treatment alone. This was taken as evidence that CT could be recommended to decrease the recurrence rate and improve survival in both these categories of patients.

The IMPACT group also investigated the benefit of therapy specifically in these earlier stage patients (20). They reviewed the results of five different studies with 1016 Dukes' B colon cancer patients randomized to receive fluorouracil and LV or no postsurgery treatment. It was found that the five-year OS increased from 80% to 82%, and with CT treatment, the five-year event-free survival increased from 73% (control) to 76% (CT). The hazard ratio at five years was 0.83 (90% CI 0.72–1.07) for event-free survival and 0.86 (90% CI 0.68–1.07) for OS. It was felt that these small improvements should not encourage the routine use of adjuvant therapy in such patients.

In view of these differing findings, it has become commonplace for physicians to select a subpopulation of Dukes' B patients, offering treatment to those patients with a higher degree of risk of recurrence, such as those with T4 tumors, poor differentiation, or histologic evidence of vascular invasion, and like. However, most of these prognostic factors have been garnered from retrospective studies and entered into multivariate statistical models, and have not been subjected to prospective validation. Accordingly, these prognostic markers or indices are more arbitrary than, is often assumed. The role of CT has recently become clearer, however, with the presentation of the uncertain arm of QUASAR data at ASCO 2004.

This large, randomized study included patients with apparently curative resections of colon or rectal cancer receiving either adjuvant fluorouracil/folinic acid (FUFA) CT or observation alone. Chemotherapy consisted of either six five-day, four-weekly or 30 once-weekly courses of iv fluorouracil (370 mg/m^2) with either high-dose (175 mg) or low-dose (25 mg) L-FA, and with either levamisole or placebo. The primary outcome measured was all-cause mortality. Three thousand two hundred and thirty-eight patients were studied between 1994 and 2003 of which 91% were Dukes' B stage and 71% were colonic cancers. The five-year survival was 80.3% with CT compared to 77.4% in the observation group (P=0.02); there were no CT-associated deaths and the CT was well-tolerated, with little grade 3/4 toxicity (5%). This advantage was felt to be sufficient to outweigh the morbidity and costs of adjuvant treatment, particularly for younger and high-risk patients. The risk of death, at a median follow up of 4.2 years, with CT versus control, was 0.83 (95% CI 0.71–0.97, P=0.02) and recurrence 0.78 (0.67–0.91; P=0.001). (Direct randomized comparisons found no advantage for high-dose FA or levamisole.)

This large study is likely to make physicians feel more comfortable in offering adjuvant treatment to stage II patients by providing a much clearer sense of potential benefits. Clearly, the final arbiter of whether adjuvant therapy should be taken up is the patient, but QUASAR gives a truer description of the size of the benefit.

Rectal Carcinoma

Rectal cancers show a different pattern of disease behavior from that of colonic tumors. This has been generally held to be due to their anatomical position impairing optimal surgical resection, but there is also evidence that these two tumor types may show some biological differences at the molecular level. Thus, there may be differing pathways of tumorigenesis with varying importance of P53 and APC (adenomatous polyposis coli protein).

There is much current interest in refining the treatment of rectal cancer. Newer surgical techniques include the use of total mesorectal excision, and studies on neoadjuvant preoperative and adjuvant postoperative chemoradiation are ongoing. Much effort has been concentrated on local treatment in view of the high risk of local recurrence, and the "down staging" in the patients' disease achieved prior to surgery has indeed improved results by facilitating optimal resection. Nevertheless, it is still likely that those patients with node-positive disease at operation or with tumor-positive resection margins will remain at a significant risk of systemic or local relapse in a similar manner to those patients with metastatic nodal disease from colon carcinoma. Systemic relapse remains a major concern for these patients and CT has been shown to offer a survival advantage. Indeed, many would see it as reasonable to extrapolate the accepted colon adjuvant CT data to apply to rectal cancer, although some studies suggest that rectal cancer patients do not benefit to the same extent as colon cancer patients.

Clearly, adequate efforts must be made to ensure optimal surgical outcome for locoregional disease, but adjuvant therapy following this initial treatment should also be considered. Chemotherapy given as a part of a preoperative chemoradiation regime may be taken into account, but further postoperative adjuvant treatment should also be considered to counter potential systemic relapse, and the current United Kingdom National Institute of Clinical Excellence (NICE) guidance (21) suggests that systemic therapy should be offered to all patients with Dukes' stage C colon or rectal cancer who are fit enough to tolerate it.

The majority of the adjuvant CT studies to date have been performed on patients with colon cancer, but several trials have included rectal cancer patients. Thus, the QUASAR1 randomized a significant number of patients with rectal carcinoma (29% of the total 3238, i.e., 939 patients).

There have also been early studies of rectal cancer patients alone, and these include those of Krook et al. (22) and the NSABP R01 study (23). In this last, Fisher et al. studied 555 postoperative patients with Dukes' B and C rectal cancer and randomized them to no further treatment or to postoperative adjuvant CT with 5-FU, semustine, and vincristine (187 patients) or postoperative radiotherapy (184 patients). Comparing no further treatment with CT revealed an improved survival in the CT arm (DFS improvement, $P=0.006$ and OS improvement, $P=0.05$). Krook et al. studied 204 patients. These received either postoperative radiotherapy alone, or postoperative chemoradiotherapy (with 5-FU), which was both preceded and followed by a cycle of systemic therapy with 5-FU and methyl CCNU (semustine) CT. After a median follow-up period of >7 years, combined therapy was seen to decrease the recurrence rate by 34% ($P=0.0016$; 95% CI 12–50%) and to decrease the rate of cancer-related deaths by 30% ($P=0.0071$; 95% CI 14–53%) and overall death rate by 29% ($P=0.025$; 95% CI 7–45%). The role of chemoradiation in rectal cancer is covered elsewhere in this edition (Chapter 29).

THE NEXT GENERATION OF TRIALS

New issues now coming to the fore are likely to spawn the next generation of trials. The importance of defining those patients who will really benefit from adjuvant therapy is now recognized. Exploitation of molecular markers to determine if it can be established which patients have been cured by their surgery alone, and for which adjuvant therapy would be helpful, is urgently required. The individual responsiveness of a patient to particular CT regimes may also become predictable.

Novel agents will need further investigation as adjuvant treatments in the immediate postoperative period, and also as longer-term adjuvant maintenance treatments. The roles of the novel monoclonal antibodies bevacizumab and cetuximab have recently been established in the metastatic setting, and their adjuvant role needs further investigation. Cost implications and morbidity will be important issues. Two U.S. cooperative group trials will evaluate the addition of antiangiogenesis therapy with bevacizumab (avastin) to CT. QUASAR 2 will assess the role of avastin in combination with capecitabine and irinotecan. One thousand two hundred and fifty patients with stage III or high-risk stage II disease will be randomized to each of three arms (capecitabine for six months; capecitabine + irinotecan for six months; capecitabine + irinotecan for six months + avastin for 12 months). Translational research will be worked into this trial. This will incorporate phamacogenetics with DNA genotyping of up to 3510 patients. Its aim is to determine the population distribution of single nucleotide polymorphisms (SNPs) in enzymes involved in the metabolism of fluorouracil, capecitabine, and irinotecan in colorectal cancer patients receiving adjuvant CT, and to determine the relationship of these SNPs to clinical outcome in terms of toxicity and recurrence rates. Population genetics will also be studied with application of microarrays, aiming to optimize their use to detect somatic mutations in cancer, and hence enable correlation of gain or loss of genetic material with clinical outcome. Immunocytochemical studies are also planned to determine whether a number of tumor markers (p53, TS, dUTP, COX-2, histone proteins, epidermal growth factor receptor, and like) are associated with risk of recurrence from stage II/III colorectal cancer. The trialists hypothesize that patients with mutated p53, low levels of TS, and high levels of dUTPase will have a poorer prognosis, and these factors will be individual adverse prognostic factors.

This may enable, in the future, a more "individualized medicine" approach to cancer care. It may become possible to offer patients treatment appropriate to their particular level of risk of recurrence, and specific chemotherapeutic or other agents that are most likely to achieve an optimal response in that particular individual.

Investigation of the role of cancer vaccines is still in an early stage. Early trials of vaccines constructed from vaccinia virus or fowlpox virus with inserted tumor-associated antigen genes (e.g., *CEA* and *MUC-1*) have been performed. These revealed disease stabilization with acceptable toxicity. Studies in the adjuvant setting are now planned in the United Kingdom and may prove fruitful.

ADJUVANT THERAPY FOR THE INDIVIDUAL PATIENT

Adjuvant therapies now available and currently being investigated have been described in this chapter. For the individual patient assessed in the clinic, a decision must be made by the multidisciplinary team as to whether the patient is fit to receive any of these therapies. All treatments administered are likely to induce some toxic reaction, and these must be weighed against the benefits likely to be achieved. The different regimes with different drugs have their own individual side-effect profiles. These have been detailed in this text and in Chapter 17 when the drugs have been discussed in the metastatic colorectal setting. The risks of infection and thrombophlebitis associated with prolonged venous access, and the likelihood of inducing neutropenic incidents, as well as risks of other physical harm, must be assessed by the physician and presented to the patient. Patients would also have their own views as to which side effects are acceptable to them. Some may find the alopecia associated with irinotecan particularly unpleasant, whereas patients requiring great manual dexterity may find the prospect of potential oxaliplatin-induced peripheral neuropathy untenable; others may find the likelihood of diarrhea from 5-FU and hand/foot syndrome from capecitabine too much of a burden to outweigh possible benefits. All of these side effects are very tangible for a patient, and the potential survival benefit may be insufficient to encourage some to undertake the commitment of several months of treatment. Further, some patients will have considerable comorbidity and will not be fit enough for treatment, and involved staff may be concerned that the social circumstances or understanding of a particular patient would not be conducive to the rapid management of a potentially serious side effect, such as a myelosuppressive episode in the community. It is the responsibility of the physician to ensure that the patient is physically and psychologically equipped to be able to take on adjuvant therapy.

The current picture in this field is one of rapid evolution and hope. Improvements in the range of agents available, in their appropriate deployment, and in their toleration by patients have been achieved. These, together with the future potential to assess which patients would benefit most from treatment, must encourage the view that adjuvant therapy can and should be offered to appropriate patients with colorectal carcinoma in the expectation of offering an improved prognosis.

REFERENCES

1. http://www.cancerresearchuk.org (accessed 31.7.04).
2. Pisani P, Parkin DM, Bray F, Ferlay J. Estimates of the worldwide mortality of 25 cancers in 1990. Int J Cancer 1999; 83(1):18–29.
3. Wolmark N, Fisgher B, Rockette H, et al. Postoperative adjuvant chemotherapy or BCG for colon cancer: results from NSABP protocol C-01. J Natl Cancer Inst 1988; 80(1):30–36.
4. Moertel CG, Fleming TR, MacDonald JS, et al. Levamisole and fluorouracil for adjuvant therapy of resected colon carcinoma. N Engl J Med. 1990; 322(6):352–358.
5. Moertal CG, Fleming TR, MacDonald JS, et al. Fluorouracil plus levamisole as effective adjuvant therapy after resection of stage III colon carcinoma: a final report. Ann Intern Med 1995; 122(5):321–326.
6. Advanced Colorectal Cancer Meta-Analysis Project. Modulation of fluorouracil by leucovorin in patients with advanced colorectal cancer: evidence in terms of response rate. J Clin Oncol 1992; 10(6);382–383.
7. Wolmark N, Rockette H, Fisher B, et al. The benefit of leucovorin modulated fluorouracil as postoperative adjuvant therapy for primary colon cancer: results from National Surgical Adjuvant Breast and Bowel Project protocol C-03. J Clin Oncol 1993; 11(10):1879–1887.
8. O'Connell MJ, Mailliard JA, Kahn MJ, et al. Controlled trial of fluorouracil and low-dose leucovorin given for 6 months as postoperative adjuvant therapy for colon cancer. J Clin Oncol 1997; 15(1):246–250.
9. International Multicentre Pooled Analysis of Colorectal Cancer Trials (IMPACT) investigators. Efficacy of adjuvant fluorouracil and folinic acid in colon cancer. Lancet 1995; 345(8955):939–944.
10. Wolmark N, Rockette H, Mamounas E, et al. Clinical trial to assess the relative efficacy of fluorouracil and leucovorin, fluorouracil and levamisole, and fluorouracil, leucovorin and levamisole in patients with Dukes' B and C carcinoma of the colon: results from National Surgical Adjuvant Breast and Bowel Project C-04. J Clin Oncol 1999; 17(11):3553–3559.
11. Gray RG, Kerr DJ, Mc Conkey CC, et al. On behalf of QUASAR Collaborative Group. Comparison of fluorouracil with additional levamisole, higher-dose folinic acid, or both, as adjuvant therapy for colorectal cancer: a randomised trial Lancet 2000; 355(9215):1588–1596.

12. O'Connell MJ, Laurie JA, Kahn M, et al. Prospectively randomised trial of postoperative adjuvant chemotherapy in patients with high-risk colon cancer. J Clin Oncol 1988; 16(1):295–300.
13. Haller DG, Catalano PJ, MacDonald JS, Mayer RJ. Fluorouracil (FU), leucovorin (LV) and levamisole LEV adjuvant therapy for colon cancer: five year final report of INT-0089. American Society of Clinical Oncology Annual Meeting. 1998; Abstract No.982.
14. Saini A, Norman AR, Cunningham D, et al. Twelve weeks of protracted venous infusion of flurouracil (5 FU) is as effective as 6 months of bolus 5-FU and folinic acid as adjuvant treatment in colorectal cancer. Br J Cancer 2003; 88(12):1859–1865.
15 Scheithauer J, McKendrick J, Kroning H, et al. Capecitabine (X) vs bolus 5-FU/leucovorin (LV) as adjuvant therapy for colon cancer (the X-ACT study): efficacy results of a phase III trial. American Society of Clinical Oncology Annual Meeting. 2004; Abstract No.3509.
16. Andre T, Boni C, Mounedji-Boudiaf L, et al. Multicenter International Study of Oxaliplatin/5Fluorouracil/Leucovorin in the Adjuvant Treatment of Colon Cancer (MOSAIC) Investigators. Oxaliplatin, fluorouracil, and leucovorin as adjuvant treatment for colon cancer. N Engl J Med 2004; 350(23):2343–2351.
17. Saltz LB, Niedzwiecki D, Hollis D, et al. Irinotecan plus fluorouracil/leucovorin (IFL) versus fluorouracil/leucovorin alone (FL) in stage III colon cancer (intergroup trial CALBG C89803). American Society of Clinical Oncology Annual Meeting 2004 Abstact No.3500.
18. Gray RG, Barnwell J, Hills R, McConkey C, Williams N, Kerr D. For the QUASAR collaborative group. QUASAR: a randomized study of adjuvant chemotherapy (CT) vs observation including 3238 colorectal cancer patients. American Society of Clinical Oncology Annual Meeting. 2004; Abstract No.3501.
19. Mamounas E, Weiand S, Wolmark N, et al. Comparative efficacy of adjuvant chemotherapy in patients with Dukes'B vs Dukes'C colon cancer: results from four NSABP studies (C-01,C-02, C-03, C-04). J Clin Oncol 1999; 17(5):1349–1355.
20. International Multicentre Pooled Analysis of B2 Colon Cancer Trials (IMPACT B2) Investigators. Efficacy of adjuvant fluorouracil and folinic acid in B2 colon cancer. J Clin Oncol 1999; 17(5): 1356–1363.
21. National institute of Clinical Excellence. Improving Outcomes in Colorectal Cancers. Guidance on Cancer Services. Manual Update. London: National institute of Clinical Excellence (Pub) May 2004:83.
22. Krook JE, Moertal CG, Gunderson LL, et al. Effective surgical adjuvant therapy for high-risk rectal carcinoma. N Engl J Med 1991; 324(11):709–715.
23. Fisher B, Wolmark N, Rockette H, et al. Postoperative adjuvant chemotherapy or radiation therapy for rectal cancer: results from NSABP protocol R-01. J Natl Cancer Inst 1988; 80(1):21–29.

13 Chemotherapy for Metastatic Colorectal Cancer

Catherine R. Jephcott
Department of Oncology, Churchill Hospital, Oxford, U.K.

David J. Kerr
Department of Clinical Pharmacology, Radcliffe Infirmary, University of Oxford, Oxford, U.K.

INTRODUCTION

Recent years have seen an increase in the range of treatment options available for patients with metastatic colorectal carcinoma, and aggressive management has lead to improvements in survival at a stage in the disease process hitherto deemed incurable.

Fluorouracil (5-FU) has been the mainstay of treatment for patients with colorectal disease for almost five decades. It has been extensively studied to elucidate the most effective treatment regimen with the most acceptable toxicity profile.

During the last few years, several newer agents with promising therapeutic activity and tolerable toxicity profiles have come into use. Oxaliplatin and irinotecan have been shown to be active, especially in combination with 5-FU. The ease of administration of the oral agent capecitabine has encouraged its substitution for more cumbersome infusional 5-FU regimes, and novel agents such as vascular endothelial growth factor (VEG-F) inhibitors and monoclonal antibodies (e.g., cetuximab, bevacizumab, and edrecolomab) have also been found a place in systemic management.

PATTERNS OF METASTASES

Disease dissemination can occur from the primary tumor either by local infiltration, lymphatic spread, or via the bloodstream. The most common site of spread of disease is to the liver, and approximately 80% of patients will have hepatic involvement at the time of death. The liver has a dual blood supply from the hepatic portal circulation, along which most metastases are thought to spread, as well as from the hepatic artery. Isolated lesions confined to anatomic segments can frequently be identified in the liver before further spread elsewhere. Aggressive surgical management at this stage can have a significant impact on the patient's prognosis. However cure is by no means assured and reported five-year survival rates (5YS) post hepatectomy are usually approximately 25% (1,2), while a very recent reviewer has quoted a figure of 40% (3).

The lungs are the next most common site of spread of metastatic disease. This is often asymptomatic and found on routine imaging, but patients can present with symptoms of local pain or cough, or with haemoptysis and dyspnoea due to localized lesions, or, less commonly, with dyspnoea resulting from lymphangitis. Spread to other distant sites occurs less commonly, but as patients live longer following chemotherapy, bone, and, less frequently, brain, adrenals, skin, and other sites may be involved.

In view of the pattern of metastatic spread of this cancer it is important that patients are monitored carefully and relapsed disease is identified at an early stage as there is some trial evidence to suggest that earlier intervention with chemotherapy on recurrence may be more beneficial.

CHEMOTHERAPY IN PRACTICE

For many years it was felt that advanced and metastatic colon cancer would not respond to active treatment, and palliative care was all that could be offered. However, with the widespread use of 5-FU in various modes of administration, increasing evidence of evaluable benefits gained from chemotherapy has emerged in terms of disease progression, overall survival, and quality of life. Several randomized trials have revealed chemotherapy to be valuable when compared to best supportive care (BSC) or delayed chemotherapy (4,5). In 2000, the Colorectal Cancer Collaborative Group (6) reported on a meta-analysis examining individual patient data (866 patients) and published summary statistics from 13 randomized controlled trials comparing palliative chemotherapy with supportive care reported between 1983 and 1998 (total patients 1365). They examined survival, disease progression, quality of life, and toxicity. They found that palliative chemotherapy was associated with a 35% reduction in the risk of death (95% Confidence Intervals (CIs) 24–44%) translating into an absolute survival benefit of 16% at 6 and 12 months, and an improvement in median survival of 3.7 months. Similarly, a systematic review of results of chemotherapy in colorectal cancer was performed by the Swedish Council of Technology Assessment in Health Care (SBU) (7). They based their data collection on 208 scientific articles, including eight meta-analyses and 162 randomized studies of adjuvant and palliative chemotherapy involving approximately 126,800 patients. They concluded that palliative chemotherapy gained a five- to six-month improvement in median survival.

Patient Selection

The question of which patients should be offered chemotherapy is important. The marked improvements found in quality of life, as well as in slowing of disease progression and improvement in survival, make it reasonable to encourage any patient with good performance status (0,1) and a metastatic burden involving 50% or less hepatic replacement by cancer to undergo treatment.

Elder et al. (8) performed a multivariate analysis on potentially adverse prognostic factors in metastatic colorectal cancer and found that performance status, rather than age, proved to be the most significant factor. Similarly while older patients are generally under-represented in clinical trials, there have been a number of studies that investigated chemotherapy effectiveness and toxicity particularly in older patients.

Beretta et al. (9) specifically took elderly patients (>70 years) as a subgroup randomization, comparing leucovorin + fluourouracil to supportive care only. The results of their study showed a statistically significant overall survival benefit ($P < 0.002$) for chemotherapy over supportive care. Hence the authors concluded that elderly, as well as younger patients, benefited from palliative chemotherapy. The Eastern Oncology Group (ECOG) reported on toxicity and survival in 19 trials for advanced cancer (10). A review of 1210 cases detected no differences in toxicity experienced for those 174 patients aged over 70 years compared to the younger patients.

Chemotherapeutic Agent Choice

Over the last decade, time-to-progression, survival benefit, and quality-of-life have all gradually increased while the oncological community has sought to find treatment regimes that combine the most effective disease control, the best tolerated toxicity profile, and simplicity of administration. Drugs have been used either singly or in combination, and new agents as they have become available.

Fluorouracil

Bolus single-agent fluorouracil (5-FU) has modest activity in advanced colorectal cancer. Dose-limiting toxicities include myelosuppression, nausea, and diarrhoea. Continuous infusion treatment is theoretically to be preferred (vide infra) and indeed does offer improved response rates. It has a different side-effect profile with lower levels of myelosuppression, but induces more diarrhoea, mucositis, and palmar-plantar erythrodysesthesia (hand-foot syndrome).

5-FU was developed as a chemotherapeutic agent acting as a pyrimidine antimetabolite. The hydrogen atom in position five in uracil is replaced with a fluorine atom. This converts uracil into cytotoxic agent. 5-FU is a pro-drug that requires metabolic activation. It is handled in same transport system and activation pathways as is uracil, and once activated it can alter cellular function resulting in cell death. 5-FU is converted intracellularly to various metabolites that inhibit the synthesis of DNA, and RNA. There are three active metabolites:

1. FdUMP (5 fluro 2 deoxyuridine 5 monophosphate), which inhibits thymidylate synthase (TS). This enzyme is provides a rate limiting step in DNA synthesis.

2. FUTP (5 flurouridine 5 triphosphate) which becomes incorporated into RNA causing critical alterations in processing and function.
3. FdUTP (5 fluro 2 deoxyuridine 5 triphosphate) which may be incorporated into DNA, disrupting synthesis.

The understanding of this complex metabolic process has led to strategies to enhance the cytotoxic effects of the drug. 5-FU is cycle and phase specific and is most effective against cells dividing in S phase. It has a brief serum half-life (10–20 minutes) so protracted infusions can be predicted to be more effective than intermittent bolus dosage.

5-FU may be given in a variety of clinical schedules, influenced by the pharmacokinetics of the drug, which impact on toxicity and effectiveness. The drug can be given as a weekly bolus, as five daily boluses each month, as a 24- or 48- hour infusion every two weeks, or as a prolonged continuous infusion. Investigations aiming to improve the outcome for palliative chemotherapy patients compared various methods of administration of 5-FU, and many studies have searched for the optimal regimen. No particular schedule has demonstrated a major survival advantage, and so anticipated toxicities and convenience of administration acceptable for patient and the clinic become paramount.

Leucovorin/Fluorouracil Combination Therapy

Folinic acid (also referred to as leucovorin or calcium folinate) Leucovorin (LV), acts synergistically when administered concurrently with 5-FU, increasing the degree of inhibition of TS, and further depleting the cellular levels of thymidine and increasing apoptosis.

The early Machover regime, and its successors the Mayo Clinic and Roswell Park regimens, employed LV with 5-FU and clearly gave survival benefits over 5-FU given alone. The Machover regime consisted of high-dose leucovorin at 200 mg/m^2/day given prior to 5-FU at a dose of 370 mg/m^2/day, both drugs being given for five consecutive days. A modified regime was devised by the Mayo Clinic. It replaced the high-dose LV with a lower dose of 20 mg/m^2/day (this would be cheaper) with the same 5-FU dose. The dose of 5-FU was increased to 425 mg/m^2/day during their initial study of the regimen (11) which compared a 5-FU alone arm with arms given 5-FU and high-dose LV and arms given 5-FU and low-dose LV. This study of their 208 subjects revealed that overall response rates were 10% for 5-FU alone, 26% for the high-dose LV Machover regimen, and 43% for the lower dose LV Mayo regime. Survival was also significantly longer for the two LV-modulated regimes at 12.2 months for high-dose LV, 12 months for low-dose LV, and 7.7 months for 5-FU alone—$P=0.037$ and 0.05, respectively.

Bolus Fluorouracil Vs. Infusional Dosage

Infusional chemotherapy is used more extensively in Europe than in America, being influenced by a randomized Phase III trial (12) of infusion versus bolus 5-FU administration in which the Mayo/NCCTG regime was compared to a bimonthly program of two consecutive days of high-dose 2-hour infusion of LV (200 mg/m^2) followed by bolus 5-FU (400 mg/m^2) followed by a 22-hour 5-FU infusion (600 mg/m^2) (LV5-FU2). The response rates in 348 randomized patients with measurable disease were 14% for the Mayo/NCCTG regimen versus 33% for the infusion regimen ($P = 0.0004$). However the median survivals were not statistically different at 57 versus 62 weeks ($P = 0.07$). The bimonthly regime was associated with more acceptable toxicity with World Health Organization (WHO) Grade 3–4 toxicities occurring in 11.1% patients receiving LV5-FU2 compared with 23.9% for the Mayo regime ($P = 0.0004$), including a decrease in Grade 3 or 4 granulocytopaenia at 1.9% versus 7.3%, in diarrhoea at 2.9% versus 7.3% and in mucositis at 1.9% versus 12.7%.

A simplified bimonthly regimen has recently been evaluated (13). This allowed patients to attend hospital only once every two weeks. Regimen was administered as an outpatient procedure with disposable pumps and involved a 2-hour infusion of the LV l-isomer 200 mg/m^2 on day one, followed by a 5-FU bolus 400 mg/m^2, and a 46-hour infusion of 2400 mg/m^2 to 3600 mg/m^2 repeated every two weeks. A feasibility study demonstrated acceptable antitumor efficacy combined with low toxicity, demonstrating it to be a favorable schedule. Forty-six patients were treated and showed a response rate of 41.3% (95% CI 27.5–55.9%). Median progression-free survival (PFS) was 8.7 months. This regime has a reasonable toxicity profile and appears to have even more activity than other similar regimes.

The Meta-Analysis Group in Cancer (14) reviewed individual data from 1219 patients, determined benefit in terms of tumor response and survival, and compared toxicity profiles. They found that tumor response rates were significantly higher in patients assigned to continuous infusion than in those assigned to 5-FU bolus (22% vs. 14%, overall response odds ratio 0.55; 95% CI 0.41–0.75; $P = 0.0002$). In their analysis overall survival was also significantly higher in patients assigned to 5-FU continuous infusion (overall hazard ratio 0.88, 95% CI 0.78–0.99; $P = 0.04$), although the median survival times were close. Grade 3 or 4 hematological toxicity was more frequent in patients assigned to 5-FU bolus (31% vs. 4%; $P < 10$ (–16) whereas hand-foot syndrome was more frequent in the 5-FU continuous infusion group (34% vs. 13%; $P < 10^{-7}$).

Irinotecan

Irinotecan is a semisynthetic derivative of the plant alkaloid camptothecin. It is an inhibitor of topoisomerase I, an enzyme which facilitates DNA unwinding by the passage of single-stranded DNA through a transient single-strand break in the complementary strand. Inhibition of this process inhibits cell replication and causes breakages in single strand DNA. Irinotecan is metabolized to 7-ethyl-10-hydrocamptothecin (SN-38) that is 40 to 200 times more potent than the parent drug.

For patients requiring second line chemotherapy, having failed with first line 5-FU, studies have revealed a clinically useful activity for irinotecan. An overall response rate of 13% (95% CI 11.5–14.5%) and a tumor growth control rate (complete or partial response or no change) of 50% (95% CI 48–52%) were achieved in more than 1800 patients treated in 20 studies (15). The median response duration ranged from six to eight months and the median survival time from 7 to 13 months.

Two randomized studies then compared irinotecan with either BSC or with the best estimated infusional 5-FU regimen in patients resistant to then conventional 5-FU regimens. Cunningham et al. (16) looked at patients with metastatic colon cancer which had progressed within six months of treatment with 5-FU, allocating 189 patients of performance status zero to two to irinotecan therapy (300–350 mg/m^2 every three weeks) with supportive care, and 90 to supportive care alone. They found that there was an increase in overall survival in the irinotecan group (36.2% with irinotecan, 13.8% for best supportive care, $P = 0.0001$). Quality-of-life scores were improved with irinotecan also (although there was 22% Grade 3 or 4 diarrhoea rate). Similarly Rougier et al. (17) investigated 267 patients who had failed to respond to first-line flurouracil or who had progressed following such treatment. These were allocated to irinotecan 300 mg/m^2 to 350 mg/m^2 once every three weeks (133 patients) or to fluorouracil by continuous infusion (134 patients). Treatment was continued until disease progression, unacceptable toxicity, or patient refusal. They found that survival was increased in the irinotecan arm ($P = 0.035$) with a one-year survival of 45% versus 32% in the 5-FU group. Median survival was 10.8 months in the irinotecan group and 8.5 months in the 5-FU group. Quality-of-life was similar in both groups.

Single-agent irinotecan therefore has found a useful role in second-line treatment of metastatic disease in many countries.

Fluorouracil and Irinotecan

Following success as a second-line agent, studies were undertaken investigating the role of irinotecan in combination therapy for first-line disease. Saltz et al. (18) performed a large, multicenter, three-group trial to compare effect of a combination of irinotecan, fluorouracil and leucovorin to that of bolus doses of 5-FU and leucovorin, and to that of irinotecan alone as first-line treatment. 231 patients were randomized to receive irinotecan (124 mg/m^2 IV), 5-FU (500 mg/m^2 IV bolus) and leucovorin (20 mg/m^2 IV bolus) weekly for four weeks every six weeks; 226 randomized to receive 5-FU (425 mg/m^2 IV bolus) and leucovorin (20 mg/m^2 IV bolus) daily for five consecutive days every four weeks; and 226 patients were allocated to receive irinotecan alone (125 mg/m^2 IV) weekly for four weeks every six weeks.

Combination treatment with irinotecan, 5-FU, and LV compared to only 5-FU plus LV resulted in a significantly longer PFS (median 7.0 months vs. 4.3 months, $p=0.004$) and longer overall survival (median 14.8 months vs. 12.6 months, $p=0.04$). Results for irinotecan alone were comparable to those for 5-FU and leucovorin. Grade 3 diarrhoea was more common during treatment with irinotecan, 5-FU and leucovorin than with 5-FU/FA alone, but the incidence of Grade 4 diarrhoea was similar in the two groups at less than 8%. In fact toxicity in the form of Grade 3 or 4 mucositis, Grade 4 neutropaenia, and neutropaenic fever were less frequent during irinotecan/5-FU/FA combination treatment, and quality-of-life was not worsened with the addition of irinotecan to 5-FU.

Another major study was that of Douillard et al. (19) comparing combination irinotecan and 5-FU with 5-FU alone in the first-line metastatic setting. They randomized 199 of a total of 387 patients to receive irinotecan plus flurouracil plus calcium folinate and 188 to receive 5-FU and calcium folinate alone. Infusion schedules were either once weekly or once every two weeks, as chosen by the treating center. They found that the response rates (RRs) were significantly higher in patients in the irinotecan group than in those in the group not receiving irinotecan (49% vs. 31%, $P < 0.001$ for evaluable patients, 35% vs. 22%, $P < 0.005$ by intention-to-treat). Time-to-progression was significantly longer in the irinotecan group than in the no-irinotecan group (median 6.7 vs. 4.4 months, $P < 0.001$) and overall survival was longer (median 17.4 vs. 14.1 months, $P = 0.031$). There was an increase in toxicity in the irinotecan group with more Grade 3 or 4 diarrhea (13.1% vs. 5.6%), alopecia (56.6% vs. 16.8%), and neutropaenia (46.2% vs. 13.4%) but these were reported as being manageable.

As a result of these surveys this combination was considered by many at the time to be a reference first line treatment for metastatic disease.

Oxaliplatin

Oxaliplatin is a third generation platinum analogue, belonging to the diaminocyclohexane (DACH) platinum family. It is metabolized by nonenzymatic degradation to active metabolites that bind to DNA to form damaging inter- and intrastrand cross-linkage, so causing apoptotic cell death. Oxaliplatin-DNA adducts appear to prevent the binding of mismatch repair protein complexes and, subsequently, the repair of platinum-induced lesions in DNA.

RRs of approximately 10% in second-line patients and 24% in first-line patients were obtained when this drug was initially used (20–22).

Oxaliplatin with Fluorouracil

Combination therapy with oxaliplatin and 5-FU has been studied in the Phase III setting and results reveal improved response rates and progression-free survival. De Gramont et al. (23) investigated the effect of combining oxaliplatin with LV5-FU, comparing it with LV5-FU given alone. The 5-FU was given as a bolus and as an infusion every two weeks, with progression-free survival taken as the primary end point. A total of 420 patients were randomized to receive a two-hour infusion of LV (200 $mg/m^2/d$) followed by a 5-FU bolus (400 $mg/m^2/d$) and 22-hour infusion of 5-FU (600 $mg/m^2/day$) for two consecutive days every two weeks, either alone or in combination with oxaliplatin 85 mg/m^2 as a 2-hour infusion on day one. They found that patients allocated to oxaliplatin plus LV/5-FU had significantly longer PFS (median 9.0 vs. 6.2 months; $P = 0.0003$) and a better response rate (50.7 vs. 22.3%; $P = 0.001$) when compared with the control arm. However the improvement in overall survival did not reach significance (median 16.2 vs. 14.7 months, $P = 0.12$). Toxicity was greater in the oxaliplatin group with more Grade 3 or 4 neutropaenia (41.7% vs. 5.3% of patients), Grade 3 or 4 diarrhoea (11.9% vs. 5.3%), and Grade 3 neurosensory toxicity (18.2% vs. 0%) but these did not worsen quality-of-life.

Another trial has shown oxaliplatin to give a survival advantage. Goldberg et al. (24) reported a multicenter Phase III trial comparing oxaliplatin plus LV/5-FU (FOLFOX4) with bolus irinotecan and LV/5-FU regime irinotecan, bolus flurouracil, and leucovorin (IFL) and found that oxaliplatin and LV/5-FU had a significantly higher response rate than irinotecan and LV/5-FU (45 vs. 31%; $P = 0.002$). Oxaliplatin and LV/5-FU significantly prolonged PFS compared to irinotecan + LV/5-FU (8.7 vs. 6.9 months). Overall survival was also prolonged as compared to that obtained with irinotecan (19.5 vs. 14.8 months).

Capecitabine

Capecitabine is a third generation oral fluropyrimidine prodrug that is metabolized in the liver to 5′-deoxy-5-flurocytidine (DFCR). This is then converted to 5′-deoxy-5-fluorouridine (DFUR) by cytidine deaminase, in the liver and in the tumor. DFUR is then converted to 5-FU by thymidine phosphorylase, which is overexpressed in tumor cells, thus providing a degree of tumor selectivity. Peak plasma concentrations of capecitabine occur 90 minutes after administration and peak levels of 5-FU occur 30 minutes later. The elimination half-life is 45 minutes and greater than 90% of capecitabine and its metabolites are excreted into the urine.

Capecitabine has been studied as a single agent and has proved an acceptable alternative to intravenous 5-FU. Twelves et al. (25) studied 602 patients with advanced colorectal cancer, randomizing them to capecitabine (2500 mg/m^2/d 1–14, every three weeks) or to bolus 5-FU/LV(Mayo regime—5-FU 450 mg/m^2 and LV 20 mg/m^2 d 1–5 every four weeks) until disease progression or unacceptable toxicity. The overall RR was 18.9% for capecitabine and 15.0% for 5-FU/LV. Patients receiving capecitabine experienced significantly less ($P < 0.00001$) stomatitis and alopecia, but more hand-foot syndrome ($P < 0.00001$) and more uncomplicated Grade 3 or 4 hyperbilirubinaemia ($P < 0.0001$). Capecitabine also resulted in lower incidences ($P < 0.00001$) of Grade 3 or 4 stomatitis and neutropaenia, and a lower incidence of Grade 3 or 4 neutropaenic fever and sepsis.

Cox et al. (26) confirmed that capecitabine offered similar clinical efficacy to 5-FU with an improved toxicity profile (26). They prospectively randomized 605 patients to either with oral capecitabine for 14 days every three weeks or IV bolus 5-FU/LV daily for five days in 4-week cycles. The overall objective tumor RR among all randomized patients was significantly higher in the capecitabine group (24.8%) than in the 5-FU/LV group (15.5%; $P = 0.005$). Capecitabine caused less ($P < 0.0002$) diarrhea, stomatitis, nausea, and alopecia, including less Grade 3 or 4 stomatitis and Grade 3 or 4 neutropenia ($P < 0.0001$) leading to significantly less neutropenic fever sepsis. Grade 3 hand-foot syndrome ($P < 0.00001$) and Grade 3 or 4 hyperbilirubinemia were the only toxicities more frequently associated with capecitabine than with 5-FU/LV treatment. It was therefore concluded that oral capecitabine was more active than 5-FU/LV in the induction of objective tumor responses with similar times-to-disease-progression and survival compared with the 5-FU/LV arm and tolerability was improved.

Integrated data from these two large trials (27) has shown that oral capecitabine procured superior response rates, equivalent times-to-disease-progression and overall survival, an improved safety profile, and improved convenience when compared with IV 5-FU/LV as first-line treatment for metastatic colorectal cancer.

Trial results have also shown that capecitabine has the potential to replace intravenous 5-FU as a convenient and effective partner for oxaliplatin or for irinotecan.

Capecitabine Plus Oxaliplatin

Capecitabine plus oxaliplatin (XELOX) was shown to be highly active as first-line combination therapy in metastatic colorectal cancer in an international Phase II trial involving 96 patients (28). The regimen was oxaliplatin given as a 130 mg/m^2 2-hour infusion on day 1 with oral capecitabine 1000 mg/m^2 twice per day on days 1 to 14 with seven days rest before repeating the cycle on day 22 (XELOX). RRs of greater than 50% were seen in all subgroups, and stable disease was prolonged, lasting for over three months in all patients in which this was achieved. There was also a good safety profile with XELOX compared to that of FOLFOX [as discussed above, (23)]. Grade 3 or 4 adverse events occurred in manageable numbers of patients—neutropenia 5%, neurosensory toxicity 14%, diarrhea 15%, nausea and vomiting 13%, stomatitis 6%, and hand-foot syndrome 3%.

Capecitabine with Irinotecan

In the same manner, capecitabine has been investigated in combination with irinotecan in the metastatic setting, and this also has been found to be an active and convenient regimen. Kerr et al. (29) reported on Phase I study results with a regime of irinotecan 250 mg/m^2 as a 30 minute intravenous infusion on day one with oral capecitabine 1000 mg/m^2 bd po on days 1 to 14 given on a 3-weekly cycle. An overall response rate of 52% was achieved ($n = 36$).

A Phase III randomized trial is planned (EORTC 40015) comparing capecitabine 1000 mg/m^2 days 1 to 14 + irinotecan 250 mg/m^2 d1 q21 versus biweekly infused 5-FU/LV) + irinotecan 180 mg/m^2 d1 q14 with a second randomization with or without celecoxib 400 mg/m^2 daily. It is planned to recruit 693 patients. It is hoped that this will provide further evidence.

Sequential Chemotherapy

A GERCOR study (30) investigated two sequences of treatments involving irinotecan and oxaliplatin. These were FA, 5-FU, and irinotecan (FOLFIRI), followed by FA, 5-FU, and oxaliplatin (FOLFOX6) (arm A) and the reverse—FOLFOX6 followed by FOLFIRI (arm B). From December 1997 to Septemper 1999, 226 previously untreated patients with assessable disease were randomly assigned to receive a 2-hour infusion of l-LV 200 mg/m^2 or dl-LV 400 mg/m^2 followed by a 5-FU bolus 400 mg/m^2 and 46-hour infusion 2400 mg/m^2 to 3000 mg/m^2 every two weeks, either with irinotecan 180 mg/m^2 or with oxaliplatin 100 mg/m^2 as a 2-hour infusion on day one. At progression, irinotecan was replaced by oxaliplatin (arm A) or oxaliplatin by irinotecan (arm B).

Both sequences achieved a prolonged survival and similar efficacy but had differing toxicity profiles, as expected. Comparing arm A with arm B, median survival was 21.5 months versus 20.6 months ($P = 0.99$), median second-line PFS was 14.2 months in arm A versus 10.9 months in arm B ($P = 0.64$). In first-line therapy FOLFIRI achieved a 56% RR and 8.5 month PFS versus FOLFOX6 54% RR, 8 months median PFS ($P = 0.26$). Second line FOLFIRI achieved a 4% RR and 2.5 months median PFS versus FOLFOX6 which achieved 15% RR and 4.2 months PFS. With respect to toxicity, Grade 3 or 4 mucositis, nausea or vomiting, and Grade 2 alopecia were more common with FOLFIRI, and Grade 3 or 4 neutropenia and neurosensory toxicity were more common with FOLFOX6. The authors concluded that both sequences were similar and achieved promising survival rates.

Cetuximab

Cetuximab (IMC-C225) is a chimaeric IgG1 monoclonal antibody (Mab) that binds competitively to the extracellular domain of Epidermal Growth Factor Receptor (EGFR), inhibiting Epidermal Growth Factor (EGF) binding and subsequent activation of the receptor with receptor autophosphorylation, and inducing its internalization and degradation. The EGFR is a member of the ErbB family of tyrosine kinase cell-surface receptors that are dysregulated in many tumor types. The EGFR starts intracellular signalling and causes cellular proliferation when it is activated. Cetuximab blocks the production of proangiogenic factors such as VEG-F, interleukin-8 and basic fibroblast growth factor (bFGF).

It is well-tolerated, its main side effect being an acneiform rash, but can also cause asthenia, fever, nausea, elevation of aminotransferases, and allergic reactions. Cetuximab has shown single-agent antitumor activity, unlike the EGFR–tyrosine kinase inhibitors.

Cetuximab has been shown to improve the antitumor activity of irinotecan in preclinical studies (31). The mechanism of this enhancement is not clear but is thought to be due to pro-apoptotic effects or separate antiangiogenic effects caused by the inhibition of EGFR signalling inhibition.

This agent has been studied in patients with advanced disease that is refractory to irinotecan. It has been shown in such cases that the objective response rate with cetuximab alone is approximately 10% and in combination with irinotecan this rises to 22% (32). Cunningham's large randomized trial recently investigated the effect of single agent cetuximab compared with combination cetuximab and irinotecan in 329 patients with advanced, irinotecan-refractory disease (32). This allocated 218 patients who had progressed during or within three months after treatment with irinotecan based chemotherapy to the combination arm and 111 to monotherapy. Amongst other entry criteria patients required immunohistochemical evidence of EGFR expression. A clinically significant activity of cetuximab in both groups was revealed, but there was a higher rate of response in the combination therapy group compared to the cetuximab monotherapy group [22.9% (95% CI, 17.5–18.1%) vs. 10.8% (95% CI 5.7–18.1%) $P = 0.007$]. The median time to progression was greater in the combination-therapy group (4.1 vs. 1.5 months, $P < 0.001$ by log-rank test). The median survival time was 8.6 months in the monotherapy group and 6.9 in the combination arm ($P = 0.48$). The trial organizers felt that the effectiveness of the combination treatment suggested that EGFR inhibition by cetuximab may overcome irinotecan resistance, perhaps by annulling drug efflux, restoring apoptosis or impairing DNA-repair activity. They state that cetuximab may therefore be helpful for patients once the three usual chemotherapy options of 5-FU, oxaliplatin, and irinotecan have been used, by providing a 22.9% tumor response rate in the combination setting described above.

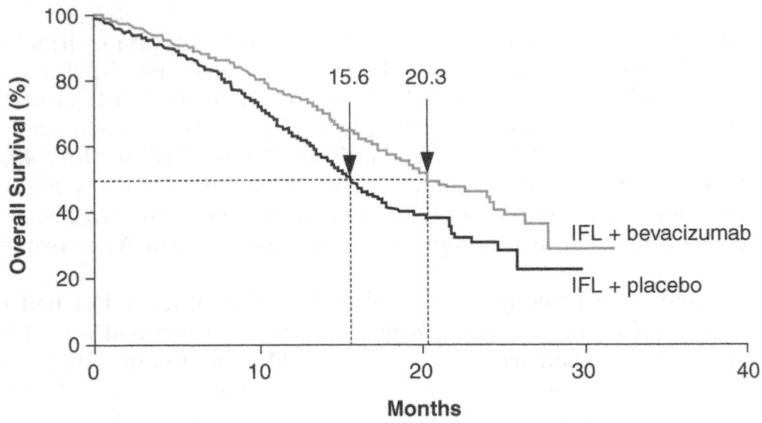

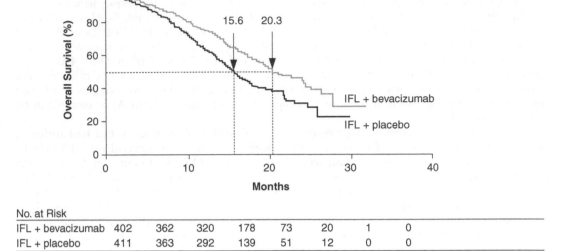

No. at Risk								
IFL + bevacizumab	402	362	320	178	73	20	1	0
IFL + placebo	411	363	292	139	51	12	0	0

FIGURE 1 Kaplan-Meier estimates of survival. *Abbreviation*: IFL, irinotecan, bolus flurouracil, leucovorin. *Source*: From Ref. 35.

Bevacizumab

Bevacizumab (Avastin) is a recombinant humanized Mab with selectivity against VEG-F. This is one of several growth factors that play a vital role in the development of normal and tumor-associated blood vessels; it is a diffusible glycoprotein and is being evaluated in a number of clinical trials as a treatment for several different cancer types. It has direct antiangiogenic effects, but it is thought that it may also have a more indirect role by altering the tumor vasculature (and so decreasing the elevated interstitial pressure in tumors) and hence improving the delivery of chemotherapeutic agents to the tumors (33). It has been shown to have clearly identifiable antivascular effects in human rectal cancer (34). The main toxicities found have been bleeding, headache, fever, asthenia, nausea and vomiting, arthralgia, dyspnoea, and rash.

A large randomized Phase III trial has recently been published which has revealed a statistically significant and clinically meaningful improvement in survival with bevacizumab (35). A total of 813 patients with previously untreated metastatic colorectal cancer were randomly assigned to receive IFL plus bevacizumab (5 mg/kg every 2 weeks) and 411 were allocated to receive IFL and placebo. The median duration of survival was seen to be 20.3 months in the IFL plus bevacizumab group and 15.6 months in the placebo group (hazard ratio for death 0.66, $P < 0.001$) (Fig. 1). The median duration of PFS was 10.6 months versus 6.2 months (hazard ratio for disease progression, 0.54; $P < 0.001$) in the IFL + bevacizumab versus IFL + placebo groups, respectively (Fig. 2). The response rates were 44.8% versus 34.8 % ($P = 0.004$) with median duration of responses 10.4 months (bevacizumab group) versus 7.1 months (placebo group) (hazard ratio for progression, 0.62; $P = 0.001$) (Figs. 1 and 2). The major side effects of note were an increase in Grade 3 hypertension in the bevacizumab arm (11 vs. 2.3 % in the placebo arm) but this was reported to have been manageable. This trial has lead to FDA approval of bevacizumab in patients with colorectal cancer.

The newer agents have the disadvantage of high costs, and this may, at least initially, cause problems in their widescale usage.

DISEASE CONFINED TO THE LIVER: A SPECIAL CASE

In recent years, there have been considerable advances in the treatment of disease confined to the liver. This is a common site for metastatic disease, and, if treated aggressively and early enough, a subpopulation of patients can now be cured.

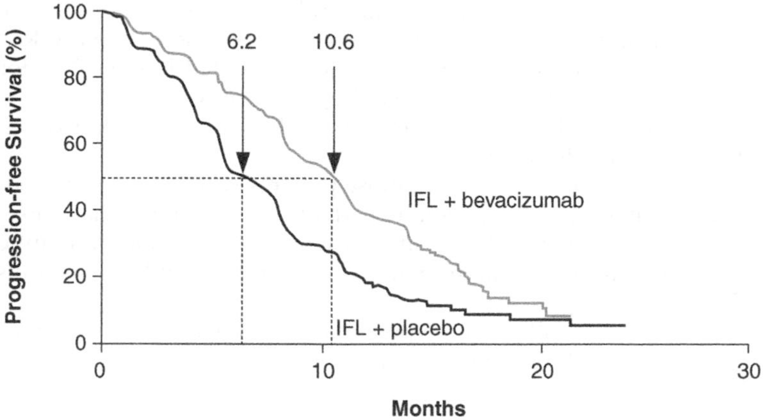

No. at Risk

IFL+bevacizumab	402	269	143	36	6	0
IFL+placebo	411	225	73	17	8	0

FIGURE 2 Kaplan-Meier estimates of progression-free survival. *Abbreviation*: IFL, irinotecan, bolus flurouracil, leucovorin. *Source*: From Ref. 35.

Surgical Excision

Once metastatic disease has been diagnosed as isolated to the liver a decision should be made by the multidisciplinary team on whether the disease is resectable. As surgical expertise increases the extent of disease deemed operable increases. Moreover the positions within the liver and the bulk of disease will be important criteria determining operability rather than only the actual number of metastases. Close collaboration of the surgical and oncological teams is essential in identifying the appropriate treatment pathway for each individual patient.

Adequate preoperative staging is essential. This must include appropriate imaging of the liver and other likely sites of disease spread, such as the lung. The more widespread use of routine magnetic resonance imaging (MRI) and whole body ^{18}F-fluoroxyglucose positron-emission tomography (PET) scanning enables more accurate staging and more accurate preoperative information for the multidisciplinary team. Generally patients are considered for resection when disease is confined to the liver only. However patients with colonic recurrence or limited lung metastases can also be considered for operative, potentially curative, management.

Surgery to resect metastatic disease has been shown to give five-year survival rates ranging from 25% to 38% overall (2,36) and from 18% to 60% for particular stages of disease at time of treatment (36,37).

Neoadjuvant Chemotherapy

Disease that is felt to be inoperable initially may still be rendered potentially operable by the use of the newer chemotherapy agents with their improved rates of response.

One of the first reports (38) investigated chronomodulated chemotherapy in unresectable liver metastases. They reported a trial in which 53 of 330 patients initially deemed to have unresectable liver disease (due to location, large size, multinodular lesions, or extrahepatic disease) were downstaged with systemic, chronomodulated chemotherapy using 5-flurorouracil, folinic acid, and oxaliplatin to the point at which operation could be performed. The cumulative three- and five-year survival rates were 54% and 40%. In 15 cases, hepatic recurrence amenable to repeat surgery occurred.

A larger series reported by the same group (37) revealed a 13.5% rate of conversion from inoperable to operable with a potential for cure by the use of neoadjuvant therapy. Adam and coworkers treated 701 patients with unresectable colorectal liver metastases (as defined by large size, ill location, multinodularity, and extrahepatic disease) with neoadjuvant chemotherapy.

A total of 95 patients, or 13.5%, then underwent resection and the overall five-year survival rate was 35% from the time of resection and 39% from the time of onset of chemotherapy. Respective five-year survival rates were 60% for large tumors, 49% for ill-located lesions, 34% for multinodular disease, and 18% for liver metastases and extrahepatic disease.

It must be borne in mind that these are nonrandom studies, and regardless of size, must be considered subject to potential selection bias.

In the above studies, it became apparent that those patients whose disease was rendered resectable with neoadjuvant chemotherapy generally had a better prognosis than those whose disease remained inoperable. In general, those patients with single tumors initially deemed inoperable due to their size had the best long-term outcome, and those with disease outside the liver did least well (37).

Patients must be assessed carefully and the potential use of neoadjuvant chemotherapy considered in the context of the multidisciplinary team.

Intrahepatic Chemotherapy

The rationale for administering intrahepatic arterial chemotherapy is that by delivering chemotherapy directly to the target organ, high levels of drug will reach the metastatic lesions. As 5-FU undergoes arterial extraction at first pass the concentrations will be far greater (up to 100 times) than that obtained with intravenous administration. This will be of particular benefit due to the steep dose-response curve seen with cytotoxic drugs. However, the procedure is complex and potentially dangerous, requiring insertion of an intra-arterial catheter.

The meta-analysis Group in Cancer carried out a meta-analysis of early trials of intrahepatic arterial (IHA) chemotherapy, using data from individual patients, reviewing response rates and survival rates (39). Their report revealed that IHA treatment gave improved objective tumor response rates when compared to intravenous therapy (IHA 41 vs. 14% IV or 0.25, 95% CI 0.16–0.40, $p < 0.0001$) but a statistically significant survival advantage was only found when the two of the seven included trials comparing IHA with physicians' choice of treatment were combined. In the other five trials comparing IHA with intravenous treatment no significant survival advantage was seen.

A more recent multicenter randomized trial (40) has been undertaken to investigate this further. A total of 290 patients were involved and were allocated to receive either intravenous chemotherapy (folinic acid 200 mg/m^2, fluorouracil bolus 400 mg/m^2 and 22-hour infusion 600 mg/m^2, days 1 and 2, repeated every 14 days) or IHA designed to be equitoxic (folinic acid 200 mg/m^2, fluorouracil 400 mg/m^2 over 15 minutes and 22-hour infusion 1600 mg/m^2, days 1 and 2, repeated every 14 days). The authors found that 50 (37%) of the patients allocated to IHA did not start their treatment and a further 39 (29%) had to stop before completing six cycles of treatment due to catheter failure (thrombosis, etc.). Median overall survival was 14.7 months for the IHA group and 14.8 months for the intravenous group (hazard ratio 1.04, 95% CI 0.80–1.33; log rank test $P=0.79$). There was no significant difference in PFS. The authors concluded that the IHA regimen could not be recommended outside the clinical trial setting.

There may also be no advantage for this route of administration for the newer agents in view of their differing pharmacodynamics. Irinotecan is a prodrug requiring activation to SN-38, hence HIA may not be appropriate. The role of oxaliplatin in this setting has yet to be established.

SUMMARY

In summary, therefore, it is clear that there have been significant gains in terms of improved mortality, with most recent trials reporting median survivals of around 20 months. The next decade will see two parallel advances, the introduction of more novel agents designed to inhibit molecular pathways which drive some aspects of carcinogenesis (proliferation, metastasis, or angiogenesis), and, secondly, the use of molecular diagnostics to determine which patients are likely to most benefit from chemotherapy or who may be at risk of unacceptable toxicity. This implies a significant step towards a more individualized practice of medical oncology.

LEVELS OF EVIDENCE

The levels of evidence supporting the statements in this chapter are as follows:

- Chemotherapy increases survival and quality of life in patients with metastatic disease compared with best supportive care *Level 1a*
- 5-FU/leucovorin regimes produce longer progression free survival and survival than 5-FU alone *Level 1b*
- Response rate and overall survival is superior with infusional 5-FU/leucovorin therapy than with bolus therapy in patients with metastatic disease *Level 1a*
- Irinotecan improves survival over both infusional 5-FU and placebo in patients receiving second line chemotherapy for metastatic disease *Level 1b*
- Response rate, time to progression, and overall survival are all better after combined irinotecan/5-FU for metastatic disease than after infusional 5-FU alone *Level 1b*
- Capecitabine produces a superior response rate, equivalent time to disease progression and overall survival and less GI side effects when compared with i.v. 5-FU/LV as first-line treatment for metastatic colorectal cancer. *Level 1b*
- Cetuximab plus irinotecan procures better response rates and times to progression (but not better survival) than Cetuximab alone as 2nd line therapy for metastatic disease *Level 1b*
- Bevacizumab plus 5-FU/irinotecan results in longer survival than 5-FU/irinotecan alone in patients with metastatic disease *Level 1b*
- Oxaliplatin based downstaging followed by resection renders 15% of inoperable cases of liver metastasis operable, with outcomes equivalent to average liver resection for metastatic disease *Level 4*

REFERENCES

1. Adson MA. Hepatic metastases in perspective. Am J Roentgenol 1983; 140(4):695–700.
2. Adson MA, van Heerden JA, Adson MH, Wagner JS and Ilstrup DM. Resection of hepatic metastases from colorectal cancer. Arch Surg 1984; 119(6):647–651.
3. Bentrem DJ, DeMatteo RP, Blumgart LH. Surgical therapy for metastatic disease to the liver. Ann Rev Med 2004; 56:139–156.
4. Nordic Gastrointestinal Tumour Adjuvant Therapy Group. Expectancy or primary chemotherapy in patients with advanced asymptomatic colorectal cancer: A randomised trial. J Clin Oncol 1992; 10(6):904–911.
5. Scheithauer W, Rosen H, Kornek GV, Sebesta C, Depisch D. Randomised comparison of combination therapy plus supportive care with supportive care alone in patients with metastatic colorectal cancer. BMJ 1993; 306(6880):752–755.
6. Colorectal Cancer Collaborative Group. Palliative chemotherapy for advanced colorectal cancer: Systematic review and meta-analysis. BMJ 2000; 321:531–535.
7. Ragnhammer P, Hafstrom L, Nygren P, Glimelius B, SBU-Group. Swedish Council of Technology Assessment in Health Care. A systematic overview of chemotherapy effects in colorectal cancer. Acta Oncol 2001; 40(2/3):282–308.
8. Edler L, Heim MN, Quintero C, Brummer T, Queisser W. Prognostic factors of advanced colorectal cancer patients. Eur J Cancer Clin Oncol 1986; (10):1231–1237.
9. Beretta G, Bollina R, Martignoni G, Morabito M, Tancini G, Villa E. Flurouracil and folates (FUFO) as Standard Treatment for Advanced/Metastaic Gastrointestinal carcinomas (AGC). Annals of Oncology 1994; 5(suppl 8):P239:48.
10. Begg CB, Carbonne PP. Clinical trials and drug toxicity in the elderly. The experience of the Eastern Cooperative Oncology Group. Cancer. 1983; 52(11):1986–1992.
11. O'Connell MJ. A phase III trial of 5-fluorouracil and leucovorin in the treatment of advanced colorectal cancer: A Mayo Clinic/North Central Cancer Treatment Group Study. Cancer 1989; 63(suppl 6): 1026–1030.
12. de Gramont A, Bosset J-F, Milan C, et al. Randomised trial comparing monthly low-dose leucovorin and fluorouracil bolus with bimonthly high-dose leucovorin and fluorouracil bolus plus continuous infusion for advanced colorectal cancer: A French Intergroup Study. J ClinOncol 1997; 15(2): 808–815.
13. Tournigand C, Gramont AD, Louvet C, et al. A simplified bi-monthly regimen with leucovorin (LV) and 5-fluorouracil (5-FU) for metastatic colorectal cancer (MCRC). Abstract No. 1052. American Society of ClinicalOncology Annual Meeting 1998.

14. Meta-analysis Group in Cancer. Efficacy of intravenous continuous infusion of fluorouracil compared with bolus administration in advanced colorectal cancer. Meta-analysis Group in Cancer. J Clin Oncol 1998; 16(1):301–308.
15. Wilke H, Vanhoefer U, Achterrath W. Irinotecan: Combination chemotherapy. In: Bleiberg H, Kemeney N, Rougier P, Wilke H, eds. Colorectal Cancer: A Clinical Guide to Therapy. United Kingdom: Martin Dunitz, 2002.
16. Cunningham D, Pyrhonen S, James RD, et al. Randomised trial of irinotecan plus supportive care versus supportive care alone after fluorouracil failure for patients with metastatic colorectal cancer. Lancet 1998; 352(9138):1413–1418.
17. Rougier P, Van Cutsem E, Bajetta E, et al. Randomised trial of irinotecan versus fluorouracil by continuous infusion after fluorouracil failure in patients with metastatic colorectal cancer. Lancet 1998; 352(9138):1407–1412.
18. Salz LB, Cox JV, Blanke C, et al. Irinotecan plus fluorouracil and leucovorin for metastatic colorectal cancer. Irinotecan Study Group. N Engl J Med 2000; 343(13):905–914.
19. Douillard JY, Cunningham D, Roth AD, et al. Irinotecan combined with fluorouracil compared with fluorouracil alone as first-line treatment for metastatic colorectal cancer: A multicentre randomised trial. Lancet 2000; 355(9209):1041–1047.
20. Machover D, Diaz-Rubio E, de Gramont A, et al. Two consecutive phase two studies of oxaliplatin (L-OHP) for treatment of patients with advanced colorectal carcinoma who were resistant to previous treatment with fluoropyrimidines. Ann Oncol 1996; 7(1):95–98.
21. Diaz-Rubio E, Sastre J, Labianca R, et al. Oxaliplatin as single agent in previously untreated colorectal carcinoma patients: A phase II multicentric study. Ann Oncol 1998; 9(1):105–108.
22. Becouarn Y, Ychou M, Ducreux M, et al. Phase II trial of oxaliplatin as first-line chemotherapy in metastatic colorectal cancer patients. Digestive Group of French Federation of Cancer Centers. J Clin Oncol 1998; 16(8):2739–2744.
23. de Gramont A, Figer A, Seymour M, et al. Leucovorin and fluorouracil with or without oxaliplatin as first-line treatment in advanced colorectal cancer. J Clin Oncol 2000; 18(16):2938–2947.
24. Goldberg RM, Morton RF, Sargent DJ, et al. N9741:oxaliplatin(Oxal) or CPT-11 + 5-fluorouracil (5-FU)/leucovorin(LV) or oxal + CPT-11 in advanced colorectal cancer (CRC). Updated efficacy and quality of life (QOL) data from an intergroup study. Abstract No. 1009. Proc Am Soc Clin Oncol 2003; 22:252.
25. Van Cutsem E, Twelves C, Cassidy J, et al. Xeloda Colorectal Cancer Study Group. Oral capecitabine compared with intravenous fluorouracil plus leucovorin in patients in patients with metastatic colorectal cancer: Results of a large phase III study. J Clin Oncol 2001; 19(21):4097–4106.
26. Hoff PM, Ansari R, Batist G, et al. Comparison of oral capecitabine versus intravenous fluorouracil plus leucovorin as first-line treatment in 605 patients with metastatic colorectal cancer: Results of a randomised phase III study. J Clin Oncol 2001; 19(8):2282–2292.
27. Van Cutsem E, Hoff PM, Harper P, et al. Oral capecitabine vs intravenous 5-fluorouracil and leucovorin: integrated efficacy data and novel analyses from two large, randomised, phase III trials. Br J Cancer 2004; 90(6):1190–1197.
28. Tabernero J, Butts CA, Cassidy J, et al. Capecitabine and oxaliplatin in combination (Xelox) as first-line therapy for patients (pts) with metastatic colorectal cancer (MCRC): Results of an international multicenter phase II trial. Abstract No. 531. American Society of Clinical Oncology Annual Meeting, 2002.
29. Kerr DJ, Ten Bokkel Huinink WW, Ferry DR, et al. A phase I/II study of CP-11 in combination with capecitabine as first line chemotherapy for metastatic colorectal cancer (MCRC).Abstract No. 643 American Society of Clinical Oncology Annual Meeting, 2002.
30. Tournigand C, Andre T, Achille E, et al. FOLFIRI followed by FOLFOX6 or the reverse sequence in advanced colorectal cancer: A randomised GERCOR study. J Clin Oncol 2004; 22(2):229–237.
31. Prewett MC, Hooper AT, Bassi R, Ellis LM, Waksal HW, Hicklin DJ. Enhanced anti-tumour activity of anti-epidermal growth factor receptor monoclonal antibody IMC-C225 in combination with irinotecan (CPT-11) against human colorectal tumour xenografts. Clin Cancer Res 2002; 8:994–1003.
32. Cunningham D, Humblet Y, Siena S, et al. Cetuximab monotherapy and cetuximab plus irinotecan in irinotecan-refractory metastatic colorectal cancer. N Engl J Med 2004; 351(4):337–345.
33. Jain RK. Normalizing tumor vasculature with anti-angiogenic therapy: A new paradigm for combination therapy Nat Med 2001; 7(9):987–989.
34. Willett CG, Boucher Y, di Tomaso E, et al. Direct evidence that the VEGF-specific antibody bevacizumab has antivascular effects in human rectal cancer. Nat Med 2004; 10(6):145–147.
35. Hurwitz H, Fehrenbacher L, Novotny W, et al. Bevacizumab plus irinotecan, flurouracil, and leucovorin for metastatic colorectal cancer. N Engl J Med 2004; 350(23):2335–2342.
36. Fong Y, Cohen AM, Fortner JG, et al. Liver resection for colorectal metastases. J Clin Oncol 1997; 15(3):938–946.
37. Adam R, Avisar E, Ariche A, et al. Five-year survival following hepatic resection after neoadjuvant therapy for non-resectable colorectal (liver) metastases. Ann Surg Oncol 2001; 8(4):347–353.

38. Bismuth H, Adam R, Levi F, et al. Resection of nonresectable liver metastases from colorectal cancer after neoadjuvant chemotherapy. Ann Surg 1996; 224(4):509–520.
39. Meta-analysis Group in Cancer. Reappraisal of hepatic arterial infusion in the treatment of nonresectable liver metastases from colorectal cancer. Meta-analysis Group in Cancer. J Natl Cancer Inst 1996; 88:252–258.
40. Kerr DJ, McArdle CS, Ledermenn DJ, et al. Medical Research Council's Colorectal Cancer Study Group. European Organisation for Research and Treatment of Cancer Colorectal Study Group. Intrahepatic arterial versus intravenous fluorouracil and folinic acid for colorectal cancer liver metastases: a multicentre randomised trial. Lancet 2003; 361(9355):368–373.

14 The Role of Radiotherapy in the Management of Rectal Carcinoma

Andrew Hartley and David Peake
Cancer Centre, University Hospital Birmingham, Birmingham, U.K.

WHAT IS THE ROLE OF RADIOTHERAPY IN THE TREATMENT OF RECTAL CANCER, AND HOW IS THIS ROLE INFLUENCED WHEN TOTAL MESORECTAL EXCISION SURGERY IS EMPLOYED?

The investigation of the potential role of radiotherapy in rectal cancer was prompted by the unacceptable risk of local recurrence following conventional surgery when total excision of the mesorectum was not performed. This risk varied between 15% and 50% (1). In addition, when local recurrence occurred, it was associated with significant morbidity and was almost always fatal (1,2).

Prior to the Dutch Total Mesorectal Excision (TME) trial which examined the role of short-course preoperative radiotherapy (SCPRT) (25 Gy in five fractions over five to seven days), in addition to TME, many studies examining the role of preoperative radiotherapy in addition to conventional surgery had already been performed and in excess of 6500 patients were randomized into such studies (3).

Early trials employed an anterior- and posterior-field arrangement intended to treat the primary tumor, internal and common iliac, inferior mesenteric, and para-aortic lymph nodes up to the vertebral level L1/2. First described by Kligerman in 1972, the Yale, Veterians Administration Surgical Oncology Study Group (VASOG) 2, University of Bergen, European Organization for Research and Treatment of Cancer (EORTC), and Stockholm I trials all used variants of this technique known as the chimney or the inverted T (4–8). Of these studies, only the Stockholm I ($n = 272$) (25 Gy in five fractions over five to seven days) and the EORTC ($n = 410$) (34.5 Gy in 15 fractions over 19 days) trials used biologically equivalent doses of 30 Gy or more and showed a significant reduction in the rate of local recurrence [relative hazard 0.49; 95% confidence interval (CI) 0.36–0.69; $P < 0.01$ for Stockholm I and five-year local recurrence 15% vs. 35%; $P = 0.001$ for the EORTC] (level 1b evidence). The Stockholm I study also demonstrated the potential toxicity of wide-field irradiation with both a higher postoperative complication (26% vs. 19%; $P < 0.01$) and 30-day mortality rate (8% vs. 2%; $P < 0.01$) in irradiated patients (9).

A second group of trials including the VASOG 1, Medical Research Council (MRC) 1 and 2, Toronto, and International Cancer Research Fund (ICRF) trials used a rectangular pair of parallel-opposed fields to treat the pelvis with no "chimney" component (10–14). Again the VASOG 1, MRC 1, and Toronto studies used biologically effective doses of less than 30 Gy and failed to show a significant reduction in local recurrence. The MRC 2 trial ($n = 279$) (40 Gy in 20 fractions over four weeks) showed a reduction in local recurrence in the irradiated arm (36% vs. 46%; $P = 0.04$) but there was no difference in either postoperative or late complications (12). The International Cancer Research Fund (ICRF) trial ($n = 468$) (15 Gy in three fractions over five days) is the only trial of preoperative radiotherapy to show a significant reduction in local recurrence using a biologically equivalent dose of less than 30 Gy (17% vs. 24%; $P = 0.04$). Postoperative mortality was however, increased in the irradiated arm (9% vs. 4%; $P < 0.05$). Thromboembolic and cardiovascular complications were also more common in irradiated patients (13% vs. 3%; $P < 0.001$). The occurrence of both reduced local recurrence and increased complications at a lower equivalent dose than used in the either MRC 2 or the EORTC trial is difficult to explain, particularly as irradiated volume used is smaller than that used in the EORTC trial. However, the median age of patients was five years older than those in the EORTC trial. The importance of patient selection for preoperative radiotherapy strategies will be discussed next.

The North West England Trial ($n = 284$) (20 Gy in four fractions) employed a unique clinical target volume comprising solely of the primary tumor and the mesorectal lymph nodes (15).

Overall, there was no significant difference in the rate of recurrence between the two arms; however, despite the use of the smallest clinical target volume in any reported randomized trial to date, there was a reduction in local recurrence in the 143 patients (53%) who had a curative resection following radiotherapy (12.8% vs. 36.5%; $P = 0.0001$).

The Stockholm II ($n = 557$) and Swedish Rectal Cancer ($n = 1168$) trials form a final group (8,16). These trials used a three- or four-field technique to treat the posterior pelvis and randomized to surgery preceded by 25 Gy in five fractions over five days or surgery alone. Both studies demonstrated reduced local recurrence at five years (0% vs. 21%; $P < 0.01$ and 11% vs. 27%; $P < 0.001$ respectively) without increased postoperative mortality. In addition, patients receiving radiotherapy in the Swedish Rectal Cancer trial had an overall survival improvement at five years (58% vs. 48%; $P = 0.004$).

Two recent meta-analyses of randomized, controlled trials including the most significant trials described before have been published. One of these analyses included trials of both preoperative and postoperative radiotherapy and identified 28 trials with a total of 8000 patients (3) (evidence level 1a). This demonstrated a highly significant reduction in local recurrence for both preoperative ($P = 0.00001$) and postoperative radiotherapy ($P = 0.002$). There was no statistically significant overall survival advantage for radiotherapy, but there was a reduction in the numbers of patients dying of rectal cancer for patients receiving preoperative radiotherapy (45% vs. 50%; $P = 0.0003$). This was counterbalanced by an excess number of preoperatively irradiated patients dying within one year of treatment (8% vs. 4%; $P < 0.0001$) the excess being mainly due to cardiovascular events. The second analysis was restricted to studies of preoperative radiotherapy and did not have access to individual patient data (17). A similar advantage for the addition of preoperative radiotherapy to surgery was demonstrated in terms of local recurrence ($P < 0.01$), cancer-related mortality ($P < 0.01$) and in addition overall survival at five years ($P = 0.03$).

As evident in the previous discussion of preoperative studies, both meta-analyses support the use of a biologically equivalent dose in excess of 30 Gy in order to impact on the rate of local recurrence. In addition, an analysis of the radiotherapy dose and fractionations employed in trials of both of pre- and postoperative radiotherapy has revealed that a dose of 15 to 20 Gy higher is likely to be required in the postoperative setting to achieve a reduction in the rate of local recurrence of similar magnitude to that achieved by preoperative treatment (18).

Postoperative chemoradiotherapy has been widely employed in North America on the basis of two studies. In a four-arm study, the Gastrointestinal Study Group randomized 227 patients to surgery only, postoperative radiotherapy (4000–4800 Gy over 4.5–5.5 weeks), postoperative chemotherapy (5-fluorouracil and methyl-CCNU), and postoperative chemotherapy and radiotherapy. There was a significant prolongation in the time to tumor recurrence with combination therapy ($P < 0.009$) (19). The second study randomized 204 patients to either postoperative radiotherapy (45–50.4 Gy in 25–28 fractions over 5–5.5 weeks) or to both postoperative radiotherapy and chemotherapy (5-fluorouracil and methyl-CCNU). Both local recurrence (13.5% vs. 25%; $P = 0.036$) and distant recurrence (28.8% vs. 46%; $P = 0.011$) occurred less frequently with combined treatment (20) (evidence level 1b). Radiotherapy was delivered in both these studies with an anterior and posterior field technique to the pelvis only and significantly in the combined arm further adjuvant chemotherapy was administered in addition to 5-fluorouracil given during chemoradiation.

Two randomized studies have specifically examined the question of the optimal timing of radiotherapy. In the Uppsala study, 471 patients were randomized to either SCPRT (25.5 Gy in five fractions over one week) or postoperative radiotherapy (60 Gy over seven to eight weeks). SCPRT was associated with a lower rate of local recurrence (13% vs. 22%, $P = 0.02$) (21). In a more recent German study, 421 patients with resectable rectal cancer were randomized to preoperative chemoradiation (50.4 Gy/28 fractions with continuous 5-fluorouracil infusion in the first and final weeks of radiotherapy) or postoperative chemoradiation (55.4 Gy/31 fractions with identical chemotherapy). The superiority of the preoperative approach was again suggested with improved local recurrence rates (6% vs. 13%; $P = 0.006$) and late toxicity (12% vs. 24%; $P = 0.01$) (22) (evidence level 1b).

TME has become a standard practice in the United Kingdom following recognition of the importance of achieving wide circumferential resection margins (CRM) around the tumor to reduce the risk of local recurrence (23,24). Despite the survival advantage seen with SCPRT in the Swedish Rectal Cancer trial, the local recurrence rates associated with TME in single-center series (3–6%), prompted questioning of the additional benefit of SCPRT (25,26).

To resolve whether SCPRT was still justified prior to TME surgery, the Dutch Colorectal Cancer Group randomized 1861 patients to TME with or without SCPRT. Early results of this trial showed that the addition of radiotherapy significantly reduced the risk of local recurrence at two years (2.4% vs. 8.2%; $P < 0.001$) (27) (level 1b evidence). Although this benefit was achieved without an increase in perioperative mortality (4.0% vs. 3.3%), patients receiving radiotherapy had more frequent perineal complications following abdominoperineal resection (29% vs. 18%; $P = 0.008$) (28). In addition, irradiated patients were significantly slower to recover from defecation problems ($P = 0.006$) and experienced more sexual problems ($P = 0.04$ male; $P < 0.001$ female) than patients with TME only in the two years following surgery (29).

Subgroup analysis of the Dutch TME trial suggests a statistically significant benefit in terms of local recurrence at two years from SCPRT in patients with midrectal tumours (5–10 cm from the anal margin) (1.0 vs. 10.1%; $P < 0.001$), patients whose CRM is greater than 1 mm (0% vs. 14.9%; $P = 0.02$ for CRM of 1–2 mm and 0.9% vs. 5.8%; $P < 0.0001$ for CRM >2 mm) and patients with lymph node involvement (4.3% vs. 15%; $P < 0.001$) (27,30). Conversely, there was no significant benefit from either SCPRT or postoperative radiotherapy if the CRM was 1 mm or less (9.3% vs. 16.4%; $P = 0.08$). The relative reduction in local recurrence for patients undergoing abdominoperineal resection was not as great as for those undergoing anterior resection [4.9% vs. 10.1% for abdominoperineal resection ($n = 248$); 1.2% vs. 7.3% for anterior resection ($n = 577$)]. However, such subgroup analysis should be interpreted with caution until both long-term efficacy data from the Dutch trial is published and further data are available from the MRC CR07 trial that randomizes patients to SCPRT or selective postoperative chemoradiation in the presence of an involved CRM.

In summary, radiotherapy for rectal cancer has evolved considerably since the 1960s. The superiority of a three- to four-field irradiation technique confined to the posterior pelvis to a biologically equivalent dose of greater than 30 Gy prior to surgery is suggested by the available evidence. However, surgery for rectal cancer has also evolved, and despite the use of modern techniques, SCPRT is still associated with increased postoperative and late complications, and relatively small benefits may be restricted to certain subgroups. Individualized treatment protocols based on the preoperative stage would therefore seem attractive.

WHAT EVIDENCE SUPPORTS THE USE OF DIFFERENT RADIOTHERAPY REGIMENS PROPOSED FOR RECTAL CANCER, AND IN WHAT CIRCUMSTANCES SHOULD EACH BE USED?

The ability of staging modalities, such as endorectal ultrasound and magnetic resonance imaging (MRI), to identify early and more locally advanced tumors respectively, and the apparent lack of benefit from SCPRT in some subgroups in the Dutch TME study have led to a trend away from blanket SCPRT for all patients (31,32). At the early end of the disease spectrum, patients predicted by endorectal ultrasound to have Dukes' A tumors could be spared the additional toxicity of SCPRT and proceed straight to total mesorectal excision. Conversely, patients felt to have threatened CRM on MRI may be offered chemoradiation, as SCPRT did not appear to significantly impact on the rate of local recurrence when the CRM was involved. Similarly, patients who are felt to require an abdominoperineal resection may be offered chemoradiation due to the smaller benefit of SCPRT and the high rates of local recurrence following such surgery (33). SCPRT may be reserved for patients with tumors between 5 and 10 cm staged at least T3 but clear of the CRM.

The evidence in support of such a strategy is limited. Assumptions about a lack of an effect of SCPRT based on subgroup analysis are not fully evidence-based, as has already been highlighted. The evidence to support the use of chemoradiation for more advanced disease is contradictory. In the German study described before, there was no difference in the rates of complete resection between patients undergoing preoperative chemoradiation radiotherapy and those preceding straight to surgery followed by postoperative chemoradiation (91% vs. 90%; $P = 0.69$) (22). However, in a Polish randomized trial of 316 patients preoperative chemoradiation (CRT) resulted in a lower risk of circumferential resection margin involvement when compared with SCPRT (4% vs. 13%; $P = 0.017$) (34). The published results of an EORTC study comparing a 45 Gy/25 fraction course of radiotherapy with or without synchronous chemotherapy are awaited. However, preliminary results that have been presented show no significant difference in the rate of CRM involvement suggesting that it is unlikely that there will be a difference in local recurrence rates. Furthermore, with a median follow-up of five years there is no significant difference in overall survival between the two groups (35). It must be remembered, however, that these three studies are examining the role of chemoradiation in resectable disease and not a population defined by MRI as inoperable or to have threatened CRM. Therefore, chemoradiation is often being employed for a more advanced stage of disease than that which has been studied in randomized trials.

The basis for such use may be the responses seen to chemoradiation in advanced disease in nonrandomized studies. All three of the randomized trials discussed before used the single agent, 5-fluorouracil, in chemotherapy given synchronously with radiotherapy. However, there have been multiple chemoradiation trials either employing different methods of administering 5-fluorouracil (e.g., bolus 5-fluorouracil, intermittent or continuous infusion 5-fluorouracil, or oral 5-fluorouracil prodrugs) or adding an additional chemotherapy drug with the radiotherapy (36). There are however difficulties in interpreting such studies. The majority are single-center series reporting early efficacy end-points, and neither postoperative complications nor long-term results in terms of efficacy are commonly reported. There have been no large randomized trials comparing various CRT regimens.

The most commonly reported early end point 2 words is the rate of pathological complete response (pCR). This is defined as the complete absence of intact tumor cells in the resected specimen. It appears to be associated in some nonrandomized studies with improvement in disease-free survival (37,38). However, any attempt in comparing the relative efficacy of CRT regimens using the observed pCR rate is subject to multiple confounding factors. These include the interstudy variability in: the rigor of pathological examination; the radiotherapy volume encompassed; the indications for CRT (resectable tumours vs. locally advanced tumours); the different imaging modalities used for defining the study group; and the time interval between radiotherapy and surgery. One such attempt concluded that higher rates of pCR appear to occur in studies using a two-drug CRT regimen and/or when 5-flurouracil is administered as a continuous infusion or the oral prodrug capecitabine. In addition, radiation dose only appeared to be a significant factor when doses less than 45 Gy were used when lower rates of pCR were encountered (36) (evidence level literature based meta-analysis).

In conclusion, the evidence base for specific treatment protocols as described previously is limited. In particular, there is a lack of randomized evidence for both the superiority of chemoradiation over radiotherapy and the use of chemoradiotherapy in an MRI-defined population. Although, phase II studies may report higher rates of pathological complete response when two drugs are employed during chemoradiation such combinations need examination under randomized conditions.

HOW CAN MORBIDITY BE MINIMIZED WHEN DELIVERING RADIOTHERAPY TO A PATIENT WITH RECTAL CANCER?

The small benefits from the addition of SCPRT to TME surgery necessitate that additional toxicity from radiotherapy is minimized if the therapeutic ratio favors such treatment. In locally advanced and inoperable rectal cancer, it is also important to minimize the toxicity of combined chemoradiotherapy followed by surgery. Patient selection and the radiotherapy technique employed are likely to be important factors in reducing acute and late radiation toxicity. A review of the toxicity seen in previous randomized studies of preoperative radiotherapy reveals how the radiation technique for preoperative radiotherapy has evolved and patient variables have emerged which may facilitate selection.

The Stockholm group modified their radiotherapy technique between the first and second Stockholm trials. This was based on the observation that an increase in postoperative mortality was seen (8% vs. 2%; $P < 0.01$) with the two-field chimney technique used in the first trial, and such an effect was absent in the preoperative arm of the Uppsala trial, which was running concurrently (9). This trial employed either a three- or four-field technique to a smaller volume. When the results of the two Stockholm trials were combined (total of 1399 patients), the increase in risk of postoperative death relative to surgery alone in patients treated with a parallel opposed technique was 4.2 (95% CI 2.3–7.8) (39,40). On changing to a four-field technique, this increase in risk was no longer statistically significant 1.8 (95% CI 0.8–4.2).

Postoperative morbidity was increased in the Swedish Rectal Cancer trial, with 44% of patients in the irradiated arm compared with 34% in the surgery alone arm experiencing complications ($P = 0.001$) (41). This difference was due to an increase in the incidence of perineal wound infection. Despite the fact that the trial protocol specified a three- or four-field technique, 48 patients were treated with parallel opposed fields. In this group, there was an increase in postoperative mortality (15% vs. 3%; $P < 0.001$) (16). The combined data from the SRCT and Stockholm I trials strongly suggest that the use of a two-field technique with 5 Gy per fraction is associated with an increased risk of postoperative mortality.

Late bowel function was also affected by radiotherapy in the Swedish Rectal Cancer trial. Frequency ($P < 0.001$), incontinence ($P < 0.001$), and urgency ($P < 0.001$) were significantly worse when compared to nonirradiated patients (42). However, the routine inclusion of the entire anal canal in the treatment volume (regardless of the distance of the tumor from the anal canal) might partially account for this and therefore should be avoided.

Late effects in the Stockholm studies were again studied by combining patients from the two trials (40). The incidence of venous thromboembolism ($P = 0.01$), femoral neck and pelvic fractures ($P = 0.03$), intestinal obstruction ($P = 0.02$), and postoperative fistulas ($P = 0.01$) were all significantly increased when compared with patients who underwent surgery alone. When the two trials were examined separately, statistical significance persisted only for the rate of fistula formation in the Stockholm II trial. Examination of long-term cardiovascular deaths revealed significantly higher rates of cardiovascular death in both the Stockholm I (RR 4.4; 95% CI 2.1–9.5; $P = 0.0001$) and II trials (RR 3.9; 95% CI 1.1–11.9; $P = 0.02$). Therefore, while the benefit of a three- or a four-field technique in terms of postoperative death is clear, the risks of late complications with this technique are significant.

To reduce the late toxicity seen in the Swedish Rectal Cancer study, particularly with respect to incontinence, the Dutch TME trial defined the lower border of the target volume at 3 cm above the anal verge in patients due to undergo anterior resection thus sparing the anal canal. It also employed what was considered to be the optimal technique for SCPRT of a three- to four-field volume with a full bladder and prone positioning to reduce irradiation of small bowel. Despite this, the overall postoperative complication rate in the Dutch TME trial was higher in patients receiving radiotherapy (48% vs. 41%; $P = 0.008$) (28). Again, this difference is accounted for by delayed perineal wound healing. In addition, as described before, despite the attempt to partially exclude the sphincters from the volume in patients undergoing anterior resection, irradiated patients were slower to recover from difficulties related to defecation (29). Data on bowel function beyond two years in irradiated patients from the Dutch TME study is awaited.

A syndrome of acute neurogenic pain has been reported in 4% of the patients treated in the Swedish Rectal Cancer and Uppsala trials. Typically, this pain was limited to the preoperative period, but in some patients it persisted for years after radiotherapy and surgery. This effect was considered to be due to an effect on the nerves of the lower lumbar region and was characterized by pain in the gluteal region, back, or legs (43,44). In a review of patients treated in Uppsala, the authors concluded that errors in dosimetry or shielding were not responsible for this phenomenon and a radiosensitizing effect of concurrent drugs or diseases (e.g., diabetes) might be implicated. Shielding of the lordotic area of the sacrum was recommended in the Dutch TME trial. Despite this, 53 of 517 patients treated with radiotherapy experienced transient neurological symptoms. Thirteen had sufficiently serious pain in the gluteal region or legs to warrant treatment interruption. The value of such shielding thus remains unproven (28).

In terms of patient selection, particularly for SCPRT, avoidance of such additional treatment in subgroups unlikely to benefit, outlined before, may prove important. In the two Stockholm studies, patients aged over 80 years had a relative risk of postoperative death of 4.4 when compared with patients between the ages of 60 and 69. While it may be possible to select younger patients who may have less toxicity for SCPRT and thus have a favorable therapeutic ratio, further modification of the radiotherapy volume may be necessary in patients with inoperable disease being considered for chemoradiation. The trend in the preoperative trials described before was to reduce the target volume to the extreme of the North West study where a therapeutic effect was still seen despite the use of a much reduced target volume (15).

Many chemoradiation protocols do not employ the optimal SCPRT volume as used in the Dutch TME study but define a clinical target volume (CTV) to include only the primary tumor and mesorectum. It may be that some of the benefit from SCPRT in reducing local recurrence rates is related to the treatment of microscopic deposits in lateral pelvis nodes. However, in the scenario of inoperable disease where tumor shrinkage is required to permit removal, some groups have been sacrificed the potential benefits of irradiating obturator and internal iliac nodes for the ability to intensify chemoradiation schedules to a smaller volume. The rationale for this lies not only in the therapeutic effect seen in the North West trial but also in studies which have measured the amount of small bowel treated in irradiation volumes and examined the relationship with toxicity. This was initially done using the administration of bowel contrast at conventional simulation but more recently using three-dimensional planning systems. In a study based on patients treated in four consecutive phase I chemoradiation trials, a significantly higher volume of irradiated small bowel was reported in preoperative patients experiencing grade 3 versus grade 0–2 toxicity (731 cm^3 vs. 145 cm^3; $P = 0.005$) (45). Initial data from a phase I/II trial of three-dimensionally planned concurrent boost radiotherapy and protracted venous infusion 5-fluorouracil therapy suggests that small bowel volume should be limited to 150 cm^3 when a maximum of 54 Gy in 25 fractions (pelvic volume 45 Gy in 25 fractions with a concurrent boost of 9 Gy) with 1500 mg/m^2 of 5-fluorouracil per week is delivered (46). A similar study of small bowel volume again found a threshold value of 150 cm^3 below which no CTC grade 3 toxicity was seen. In addition, the V_{15}, the volume of small bowel receiving at least 15 Gy was strongly associated with the grade of toxicity seen (47).

In summary, the optimal selection of patients both, in terms of tumor location and stage and patient factors such as age, is important for SCPRT, where the balance between benefit and side effects is fine. A target volume used in the Dutch TME trial and the ongoing MRC CR07 study which has evolved over the series of preoperative trials since the 1960s should be used when SCPRT is to be administered. In inoperable disease, where chemoradiation is to be employed, conformal randomized trial may offer a reduction in small bowel treated and thus provide a reduction in acute and possibly late small-bowel toxicity. This may be particularly important with the increasingly complex concomitant schedules involving multiple drugs. However, the introduction of further reduced CTVs with conformal radiotherapy should be monitored carefully and local recurrences and persistent disease should be carefully studied to ensure that efficacy is not compromised.

EVIDENCE SUMMARY

- There is excellent evidence that preoperative radiotherapy reduces local recurrence in addition to rectal cancer surgery. Most studies show a significant effect with usage of biologically equivalent dose over 30 Gy.
- There was evidence for increased postoperative mortality with this treatment, mostly from cardiovascular/thromboembolic causes in early studies.
- One meta-analysis shows improved survival using this treatment, but this is not a common finding in individual trials.
- There is excellent evidence for reduced local recurrence from postoperative radiotherapy, but higher doses are required.
- There is reasonably good evidence that postoperative chemoradiation delays or prevents both local and distant recurrence after surgery.
- There is good evidence that preoperative radiation or chemoradiation is more effective and less toxic than postoperative therapy.
- Preoperative radiotherapy still reduces local recurrence rates after TME, but the absolute risk reduction is small because the local recurrence rate with TME is low, and

radiotherapy increases local complications. The risk/benefit ratio therefore needs to be weighed carefully.

- The evidence for superiority of chemoradiation over radiation in patients at high risk of local recurrence is limited and conflicting.

REFERENCES

1. McCall J, Cox M, Wattchow D. Analysis of local recurrence rates after surgery alone for rectal cancer. Int J Colorectal Dis 1995; 10:126–132.
2. Kapiteijn E, Marijnen C, Nagetaal I, et al. Preoperative radiotherapy combined with total mesorectal excision for resectable rectal cancer. N Engl J Med 2001; 345:638–646.
3. Colorectal Cancer Collaborative Group Adjuvant Radiotherapy for rectal cancer: a systematic overview of 8507 patients from 22 randomised trials. Lancet 2001; 358:1291–1304.
4. Kligerman M, Urdaneta N, Knowlton A, Vidone R, Hartman P, Vera R. Preoperative irradiation of rectosigmoid carcinoma including its regional lymph nodes. Am J Roentgenol 1972; 114:498–503.
5. Higgins G, Humphrey E, Dwight R, et al. Preoperative radiation and surgery for cancer of the Rectum Veterans Administration Surgery Oncology Group Trial II. Cancer 1986; 58:352–359.
6. Horn A, Halvorsen J, Dahl O. Preoperative radiotherapy in operable rectal cancer. Dis Colon Rectum 1990; 33:823–828.
7. Gerard A, Buyse M, Nordlinger B, et al. Preoperative radiotherapy as adjuvant treatment in rectal cancer final results of a Randomised Study of the European Organisation for Research and Treatment of Cancer (EORTC). Ann Surg 1988; 208(5):606–614.
8. Stockholm Colorectal Cancer Study Group. Randomised study on preoperative radiotherapy in rectal cancer. Ann Surg Oncol 1996; 3(5):423–430.
9. Stockholm Rectal Cancer Study Group. Preoperative short-term radiation therapy in operable rectal carcinoma. Cancer 1990; 66:49–55.
10. Roswit B, Higgins G, Humphrey E, Robinette C. Preoperative irradiation of operable adenocarcinoma of the rectum and rectosigmoid colon. Radiology 1973; 108:389–395.
11. Medical Research Council Working Party. A trial of preoperative radiotherapy in the management of operable rectal cancer. Br J Surg 1982; 69:513–519.
12. Medical Research Council Rectal Cancer Working Party. Randomised trial of surgery alone versus radiotherapy followed by surgery for potentially operable locally advanced rectal cancer. Lancet 1996; 358:1605–1610.
13. Rider W, Palmer J, Mahoney L, Robertson C. Preoperative irradiation in operable cancer of the rectum: report of the Toronto trial. Can J Surg 1997; 20:335–338.
14. Goldberg P, Nicholls R, Porter N, et al. Long term results of a randomised trial of short-course low-dose adjuvant pre-operative radiotherapy for rectal cancer: reduction in local treatment failure. Eur J Cancer 1994; 30A(11):1602–1606.
15. Marsh P, James R, Schofield S. Adjuvant preoperative radiotherapy for locally advanced rectal cancer: results of a prospective randomised trial. Dis Colon Rectum 1994; 37:1205–1214.
16. Swedish Rectal Cancer Trial. Improved survival with preoperative radiotherapy in resectable rectal cancer. N Engl J Med 1997; 336:980–987.
17. Camma C, Giunta M, Fiorica F, Pagliaro L, Craxi A, Cottone M. Preoperative radiotherapy for resectable rectal cancer: a meta-analysis. JAMA 2000; 284:1008–1015.
18. Glimelius B, Isacsson U, Jung B, Pahlman L. Radiotherapy in addition to radical surgery in rectal cancer: evidence for a dose–response effect favoring preoperative treatment. Int J Radiat Oncol Biol Phys 1997; 37(2):281–287.
19. Gastrointestinal Study Group. Prolongation of the disease-free interval in surgically treated rectal carcinoma. N Engl J Med 1985; 312:1465–1472.
20. Krook J, Moertel C, Gunderson L, et al. Effective surgical adjuvant therapy for high risk rectal cancer. N Engl J Med 1991; 324(11):709–715.
21 Frykholm G, Glimelius B, Pahlman L. Preoperative or postoperative irradiation in adenocarcinoma of the rectum: final treatment results of a randomised trial and an evaluation of late secondary effects. Dis Colon Rectum 1993; 36(6):564–572.
22. Sauer R, Becker H, Hohenberger W, et al. Preoperative versus postoperative chemoradiotherapy for rectal cancer. N Engl J Med 2004; 351:1731–1740.
23. Quirke P, Durdey P, Dixon MF, Williams NS. Local recurrence of rectal adenocarcinoma due to inadequate surgical resection: histopathological study of lateral tumour spread and surgical excision. Lancet 1986; 2(8514):996–999.
24. Dahlberg M, Glimelius B, Graf W, Pahlman L. Preoperative irradiation affects functional results after surgery for rectal cancer. Dis Colon Rectum 1998; 41:543–551.
25. Heald R, Ryall R. Recurrence and survival after total mesorectal excision for rectal cancer. Lancet 1986; 1(8496):1479–1482.

26. Martling A, Holm T, Rutquist L, Moran B, Heald R, Cedermark B. Effect of surgical training programme on outcome of rectal cancer in the county of Stockholm. Lancet 2000; 356:93–96.
27. Kapiteijn E, Marijnen C, Colenbrander A, et al. Local recurrence in patients with rectal cancer diagnosed between 1988–1992. Eur J Surg Oncol 1998; 24:528–535.
28. Marijnen C, Kapiteijn E, Van de Velde C, et al. Acute side-effects and complications after short-term preoperative radiotherapy combined with total mesorectal excision in primary rectal cancer: report of a multicenter trial. J Clin Oncol 2002; 20:817–825.
29. Marijnen C, van de Velde C, Putter H, et al. Impact of short-term preoperative radiotherapy on health-related quality of life and sexual functioning in primary rectal cancer: report of a multicentre trial. J Clin Oncol 2005; 23:1847–1858.
30. Marijnen C, Nagtegaal I, Kapiteijn E, et al. Radiotherapy does not compensate for positive resection margins in rectal cancer patients: report of a multicenter randomised trial. Int J Radiat Oncol Biol Phys 2003; 5:1311–1320.
31. Brown G, Radcliffe A, Newcombe R, Dallimore N, Bourne M. Preoperative assessment of prognostic factors in rectal cancer using high resolution magnetic resonance imaging. Br J Surg 2003; 90:355–364.
32. Heriot A, Grundy A, Kumar D. Preoperative staging of rectal cancer. Br J Surg 1999; 86:17–28.
33. Heald R, Smedh R, Kald A, Sexton R, Moran B. Abdominoperineal excision of the rectum—an endangered operation. Dis Colon Rectum 1997; 40:747–751.
34. Bujko K, Nowaki M, Nasierowska-Guttmejer A, et al. Sphincter preservation following preoperative chemoradiotherapy for rectal cancer: report of a randomised trial comparing short-term preoperative radiotherapy vs. conventionally fractionated radiochemotherapy. Radiother Oncol 2004; 72:15–24.
35. Bosset J, Calais G, Mineur L, et al. Preoperative radiotherapy in prostate cancer: role and place of fluorouracil-based chemotherapy. Final results of the EORTC 22921 phase III trial. ASCO 2005 Gastrointestinal Cancers Symposium Miami 27–29 Jan 2005.
36. Hartley A, Ho K, McConkey C, Geh JI. Pathological complete response following chemoradiation in rectal cancer: analysis of phase II/III trials. Br J Radiol 2005; 78(934):934–938.
37. Janjan N, Crane C, Feig B, et al. Improved overall survival among responders to preoperative chemoradiation for locally advanced rectal cancer. Am J Clin Oncol 2001; 24:107–112.
38. Valentini V, Coco C, Picciocchi A, et al. Does downstaging predict improved outcome after preoperative chemoradiation for extraperitoneal locally advanced rectal cancer? A long term analysis of 165 patients. Int J Radiat Oncol Biol Phys 2002; 53:664–674.
39. Holm T, Rutquist L, Johansson H, Cedarmark B. Postoperative mortality in rectal cancer treated with or without preoperative radiotherapy: causes and risk factors. Br J Surg 1996; 83:964–968.
40. Holm T, Singnomklao T, Rutqvist L, Cedarmark B. Adjuvant preoperative radiotherapy in patients with rectal carcinoma: adverse effects during long term follow up of two randomised trials. Cancer 1996; 78:968–976.
41. Swedish Rectal Cancer Trial. Initial report from a Swedish Multicentre Study examining the role of preoperative irradiation in the treatment of patients with rectal carcinoma. Br J Surg 1993; 80:1333–1336.
42. Dahlberg M, Glimelius B, Pahlman L. Changing strategy for rectal cancer is associated with improved outcome. Br J Surg 1999; 86:379–384.
43. Pahlman L, Glimelius B, Graffman S. Pre versus postoperative radiotherapy in rectal carcinoma: an interim report from a randomized multicentre trial. Br J Surg 1985; 72:961–966.
44. Jansson-Frykholm G, Sintorn K, Montelius A, Jung B, Pahlman L, Glimelius B. Acute lumbosacral plexopathy after preoperative radiotherapy in rectal carcinoma. Radiother Oncol 1996; 38:121–130.
45. Minsky B, Conti J, Huang Y, Knopf K. Relationship of acute gastrointestinal toxicity and the volume of irradiated small bowel in patients receiving combined modality treatment. J Clin Oncol 1995; 13:1409–1416.
46. Myerson R, Valentini V, Birnbaum E, et al. A phase I/II trial of three-dimensionally planned concurrent boost radiotherapy and protracted venous infusion of 5-FU chemotherapy for locally advanced rectal carcinoma. Int J Radiat Oncol Biol Phys 2001; 50:1299–1308.
47. Baglan K, Frazier R, Yan D, Huang R, Martinez A, Robertson J. The dose-volume relationship of acute small bowel toxicity from the concurrent 5-FU-based chemotherapy and radiation therapy for rectal cancer. Int J Radiat Oncol Biol. Phys 2002; 52(1):176–183.

15 Metastatic Liver Tumors—Surgical

Paramjeet Singh
Department of Surgery, Memorial Sloan-Kettering Cancer Center, New York, New York, U.S.A.

Yuman Fong
Department of Surgery, Memorial Sloan-Kettering Cancer Center and Weill Cornell Medical College, New York, New York, U.S.A.

INTRODUCTION

The liver is a prime site of hematogenous metastases. Metastatic disease accounts for over 95% of all liver tumors (1,2). Due to high blood flow and unique anatomic location, the liver acts as major repository for cancer cells, particularly of gastrointestinal origin (3). Historically, most patients with liver metastases were considered incurable and not offered surgical interventions (4). However, considerable data have accumulated over the last two decades that have proved surgical treatment for hepatic colorectal metastases to be rational and potentially curative.

There are major biologic reasons to believe hepatic colorectal metastases to be different from other liver metastases and amenable to resection for potential cure. The venous blood carrying tumor cells from colorectal cancer drain via the portal vein and exclusively pass through the liver. The liver is a highly efficient filter, often trapping all tumor cells, preventing systemic spread (4). Not all tumors that arrive at the liver grow into tumor deposits. The process of cancer metastases is a dynamic process (5), which is regulated by interactions between the tumor cells and the host (5–7). Even with millions of tumor cells arriving at the liver, many times, only a limited number of clinically evident tumor deposits form. The timing and pattern of liver tumor presentation are highly predictive for outcome. In this chapter, we will review data justifying partial hepatectomy as treatment for this disease, as well as current practice of staging and patient evaluation for surgery.

INCIDENCE AND EPIDEMIOLOGY

Each year, there are approximately 150,000 new cases of primary colorectal cancer in the United States. This disease accounts for approximately 60,000 deaths per year (8). Recurrences after primary surgery are common, and most occur within the first few years (80% within two years) (9). Almost 50% of colorectal cancers develop liver metastases. Fifteen to 25% of patients present with liver metastases at the time of detection of primary tumor (10). Another 20% to 30% will develop metachronous lesions (11,12). In 30% of patients, the liver is the only site of metastasis, and represents the primary determinant of survival in these patients (13,14). The natural history of untreated hepatic colorectal metastases is that of early mortality (median survival on the order of six months), with virtually no survival beyond five years (15–18).

Two studies have attempted to identify patients with limited liver metastases to define the natural history of the patients who could be considered candidates for resection. In these studies, patients with limited, but untreated, disease, had a one-year survival rate of 77%, a three-year survival rate of 14% to 23%, and a five-year survival rate of 2% to 8% (18,19). Although patients with solitary lesions or unilobar disease appear to have better prognoses than patients with diffuse disease, five-year survival for any untreated patient is unusual. This is the reason that resection is considered a standard treatment for this disease even without a randomized trial, as resection can result in five-year survival in over one-third of patients.

HOW DOES ONE SELECT PATIENTS WITH COLORECTAL CANCER OF THE LIVER WHO WILL BENEFIT FROM SURGICAL RESECTION?

The criteria for the selection of patients have evolved in last two decades. Ekberg et al. (20) proposed three general contraindications to liver resection for metastatic colorectal cancer (CRC) in their landmark article in 1986—the presence of four or more lesions, presence of additional extrahepatic disease, and resection margin of <1 cm. In recent decades, as safety of hepatectomy has improved and long-term follow-up data have matured, surgeons have adopted a more aggressive approach toward liver resection (21–24).

In general, patients are offered resection if (*i*) they are deemed candidates for major surgery from a medical standpoint; (*ii*) there is no extrahepatic disease; and (*iii*) adequate residual liver will remain after resection to allow complete recovery. The contraindications to liver resections are listed in Table 1.

Medical Fitness

Safety from a cardiopulmonary standpoint is as for any major upper abdominal surgery. Patients with any history of coronary artery disease or symptoms should have a cardiac stress test. Most major centers perform hepatectomies under low central venous pressure anesthesia. Therefore, patients may experience relative hypotension that may lead to myocardial hypoperfusion for anyone with significant coronary disease. The major fluid shifts that happen in these individuals postoperatively may also lead to myocardial stress or congestive heart failure in susceptible individuals. Any history, symptoms, or signs of chronic obstructive pulmonary disease (COPD) or other pulmonary ailments should prompt pulmonary function tests. After surgery, patients will experience right pleural effusions and discomfort from the high subcostal incision that combine to produce relative pulmonary dysfunction. Any patient with significant underlying pulmonary disease may then suffer pulmonary failure.

Disease Staging

Staging to ensure no extrahepatic disease is essential. The radiologic workup for a patient being considered for liver resection will be discussed later in this chapter. Usual required preoperative staging should include (*i*) helical computed tomography (CT) of the chest abdomen and pelvis, (*ii*) fluorodeoxyglucose positron emission tomography (PET), and (*iii*) colonoscopy within 12 months. In general, any extrahepatic disease except for tumor in the colorectal regional site is considered a contraindication. However, there is indication that limited metachronous lung metastases may have sufficiently favorable behavior as to warrant liver and lung resections as a part of a multimodality treatment plan. There is also emerging evidence that limited extrahepatic disease that responds to systemic treatment and remains anatomically confined and resectable may be treated surgically with good results.

Hepatic Reserve

In general, patients considered for hepatic resection for colorectal metastases do not have viral hepatitis or cirrhosis. Thus, a good rule of thumb is that such resections can be performed safely if two segments of functional liver can be preserved. Some clinicians will rely on volumetric assessment radiologically for patient selection (25). It is generally accepted that if greater than 20% functional residual liver can be preserved, a liver resection can be performed safely. The only

TABLE 1 Contraindications for Liver Resection

Exclusion criteria
Uncontrolled primary disease
Extrahepatic disease (except for limited lung metastases)
Widespread hepatic involvement such that residual liver function after resection would be inadequate
Lymph node metastases distal to the hepatoduodenal ligament
Inability to obtain tumor-free margin

TABLE 2 Triad of Clinical Findings That Should Alert the Oncologist to Development of Chemotherapy-Associated Steatohepatitis

Fatty infiltration of liver as seen on CT or MRI (on CT, the liver is seen to be darker than the spleen)
Splenomegaly
Refractory thrombocytopenia

Abbreviations: CT, computed tomography; MRI, magnetic resonance imaging.

caveat with respect to the patient with colorectal metastases is that systemic treatment, given as neoadjuvant treatment, may produce liver damage, portal hypertension, and at times cirrhosis (26). Thus, assessment of adequate residual liver should take into account radiologic and serum markers of liver damage. The triad of fatty liver infiltration on CT scan, splenomegaly, and refractory thrombocytopenia should raise suspicion of advanced liver damage (Table 2).

WHAT IS THE EVIDENCE ON THE RELATIVE MERITS OF SURGICAL RESECTION AND OTHER TREATMENT MODALITIES FOR PATIENTS WITH LIVER METASTASES?

Much data has been produced that demonstrate partial hepatectomy to be definitely efficacious in the treatment of hepatic colorectal metastases. These data will be summarized for primary and repeat liver resections. We will then discuss two controversial areas of daily practical importance—outcome of resections according to institutional volume, and simultaneous resections of the liver and colon.

Justification of Liver Resection with Survival Outcomes

Despite the skepticism of the past few decades (27) regarding hepatic resection for metastatic disease, many retrospective studies with matched historical controls have established the role of liver resection in the treatment of patients with colorectal metastases (Table 3). Overall five-year survival rates following liver resections range from 18% to 46% (median survival between 28 and 40 months) (28–32). Data from series with sufficiently long follow-up indicate that 20% of patients are expected to survive beyond 10 years (31,33). Many of these patients will have been subjected to repeated liver resections. With the increasing use of chemotherapy and aggressive salvage surgical therapy, results are expected to further improve (34). Not only will initially resectable patients have improved outcome due to effective adjuvant treatment of microscopic residual disease, many patients not considered to be resectable will be downstaged to become candidates for resection. Adam et al. (35) recently reports on such downstaging. Ten percent of their unresectable patients were downstaged by chemotherapy to become candidates for resection. Furthermore, after subsequent resection, these patients were found to have a 33% five-year survival (Fig. 1). Other long-term studies are maturing that will likely justify an increasingly aggressive surgical approach to this disease. As patients with no therapy have a median survival of six months, and even with the most aggressive systemic therapy, patients have a median survival of 18 months, the median survival of over 40 months for patients after surgery justifies hepatectomy as a standard therapy for patients with disease isolated to the liver.

TABLE 3 Results of Liver Resection for Colorectal Metastases

Author	Number	Mortality	Median (months)	One-year survival	Five-year survival
Hughes et al. (1986)	607	—	—	—	3
Gayowski et al. (1994)	204	0	33	91	3
Scheele et al. (1995)	469	4	40	83	39
Fong et al. (1995)	577	4	40	85	35
Jenkins et al. (1997)	131	4	33	81	25
Jamison et al. (1997)	280	4	33	84	27
Fong et al. (1999)	1001	3	42	—	3
Scheele et al. (2001)	516	3	—	—	38
Choti et al. (2002)	226	1	46	96	40

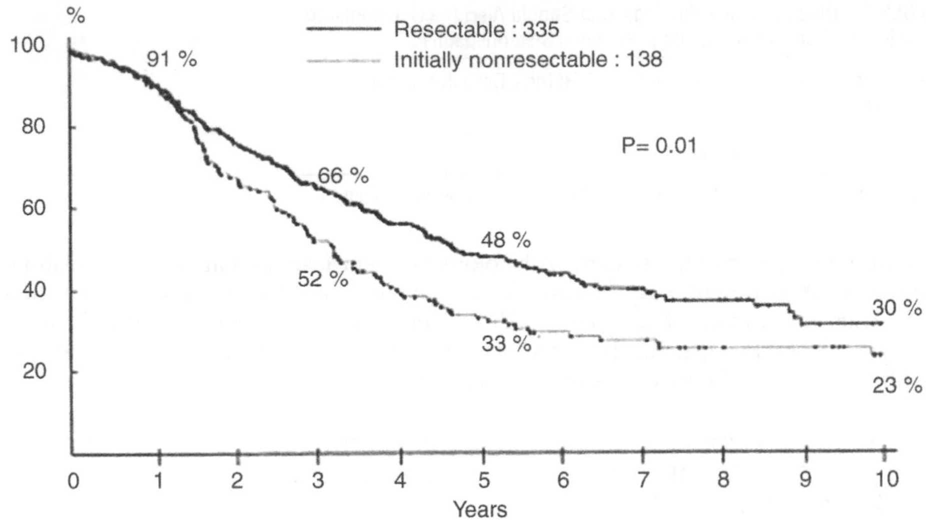

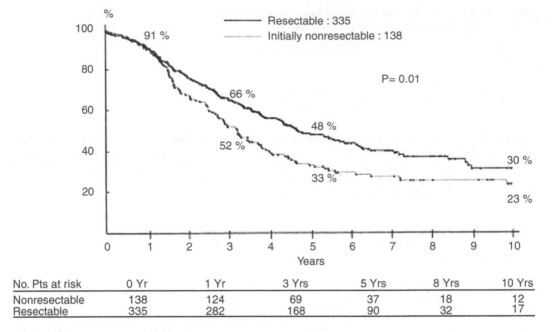

No. Pts at risk	0 Yr	1 Yr	3 Yrs	5 Yrs	8 Yrs	10 Yrs
Nonresectable	138	124	69	37	18	12
Resectable	335	282	168	90	32	17

FIGURE 1 Survival of patients after resection for hepatic colorectal metastases (*thick line*) compared to initially unresectable patients resected after successful downstaging with chemotherapy (*thin line*). *Source*: From Ref. 35.

Repeat Liver Resections

Many studies have documented favorable long-term survival in highly selected patients undergoing a second resection for recurrent colorectal liver metastases, with five-year survival rates of approximately 41% (36–40). Repeat hepatectomy is technically challenging because of the presence of adhesions, the altered morphology of the liver, and the change in position of the vasculature and biliary system. This is the reason that only a few large series have been published reporting results of repeat hepatectomy. Data from centers with extensive experience report similar operative morbidity (19–32%) and mortality rates to those reported for initial hepatectomy (40).

Various studies have looked at the predictors of outcome after repeat liver resection (39,41). Petrowsky et al. (40) identified the number (1 vs. >1) and largest tumor size (>5 vs. <5 cm) of the hepatic tumors as independent risk factors related to the second liver resection. Interestingly, no tumor factor related to the first resection predicted outcome after repeat resection. Thus, in selecting patients for repeat resection, medical fitness, ability to remove all diseases, and long disease-free interval are the most important criteria for consideration.

Outcomes and Institutional Surgical Volume

Fong et al. recently compared survival rates of patients undergoing hepatectomies in high-volume centers (defined as >25 cases/year) and other institutions (42). Superior long-term survival of complex visceral resections for cancer performed at high-volume centers was discovered providing further support for regionalization of such procedures at centers with more experience (42). Outcome seems to be related both to institutional and individual surgeon volume.

Simultaneous Vs. Staged Resection of the Hepatic Metastases

For patients who present with synchronous liver metastases at the time of discovery of primary colonic or rectal tumor, there is great controversy with regard to timing of the liver and large bowel surgery. Advocates of the "watch and wait" approach suggest that observation of the liver metastases for a few months may allow delineation of the biologic behavior of the metastases before choosing a potentially morbid resection (43,44). There is also a worry that an early resection may lead to missed tumors that are smaller than those detected by modern imaging modalities (45). Clinicians may also be challenged by the technical difficulties of combining a major liver resection with a colonic or rectal resection. The result is that for many years, the operation on the liver and the operation on the large bowel were staged, with only the most minor of hepatectomies performed at the time of the colorectal surgery.

Increasingly at major centers, synchronous hepatic colorectal metastases are being treated by combined colorectal–liver resections. This is partly based on the known risk that delayed surgery may allow new metastases to develop from established metastatic sites (46). It is also clear that disease missed at initial liver resection may be effectively treated by repeat liver resections for potential cure (47). In addition, there is a growing literature on the safety and advantages of simultaneous resection. Such combined resections may in fact have fewer overall complication rates and faster recovery than staged resections (48).

Asbun and Hughes (49) had proposed five prerequisites for simultaneous resections: (*i*) solitary lesion that can be removed by limited liver resection, (*ii*) minimal blood loss and an uncomplicated bowel resection, (*iii*) an incision that is also suitable for resection of the liver, (*iv*) a patient who is fit enough to undergo both procedures, and (*v*) a surgeon who is comfortable in proceeding with the liver metastasectomy. We believe that only the last two are essential. In expert hands, even the largest of liver resections can be performed safely with a colonic or rectal resection. Also, a long midline incision can accommodate major liver resections along with low pouch reconstructions in the pelvis. Therefore, in centers where hepatectomies are performed frequently, simultaneous resection is an acceptable treatment strategy in suitable patients with synchronous hepatic metastases, as it allows for prompt completion of surgical therapy and earlier initiation of the adjuvant therapy.

WHAT FACTORS DETERMINE THE PROBABILITY OF CURE OR LONG-TERM SURVIVAL AFTER AN R0 LIVER RESECTION FOR METASTATIC COLORECTAL CANCER?

Choice of invasive and potentially morbid treatments must necessarily take into account patient prognosis after treatment. Many studies have therefore attempted to examine clinical factors which govern outcome after hepatic resection for colorectal metastases (22,30,50). Following is a synthesis of the literature.

Patient Characteristics

1. *Demographics*: Gender (23,31,51,52) and age (22,23,53) have not been consistently found to influence the long-term outcome of the patients, although age may be a factor for increased operative risk.
2. *Primary tumor characteristics*: Several studies have found rectal carcinoma (24,54,55) to have slightly worse outcome compared to colon cancer. The stage of primary tumor (serosal involvement, nodal stage, differentiation, and grade) have a major impact on long-term outcome (23,31,51). Of these, nodal status appears to be most influential.
3. *Disease-free interval*: Hepatic tumors, found synchronously with the colorectal primary, have a poorer outcome compared to metachronous lesions (56). Liver metastases found within 12 months of the primary have also been found to have poor prognosis (57).
4. *Tumor burden*: Larger lesions are associated with a worse prognosis (31). However, the presence of larger lesions should not be a strict contraindication if resection can be performed with free margins. Even for tumors greater than 10 cm, Fong et al. (22) reports a survival rate of 14% and Gayowski et al. (58) found a five-year survival rate of 22%. Reports have described resecting up to 10 or more tumors routinely (23), but the chances of performing radical procedures decrease as the number of lesions increase. Minagawa et al. (23) found a 10-year survival rate of 29% for patients with four or more lesions. Similarly, another study by Imamura et al. (47) found that a liver resection is clearly warranted in

patients between four and nine nodules. Imamura et al. (47) also suggested that for patients with 10 or more lesions, surgery should not be an absolute contraindication especially in high-volume centers where surgical mortality is nearly zero. It has been shown that hepatic micrometastases and therefore the risk of intrahepatic recurrence significantly correlated with the number of gross tumors (59). Logically, as the number of metastases increases, complete resection and negative margins become more difficult (31,60). In the Imamura series (47), almost 40% of patients with >10 nodules had positive resection margins.

5. *Extrahepatic metastases*: Extrahepatic metastases is associated with worse prognosis (58,61,62), and should be considered relative contraindications for resection. A few exceptions should be made. Direct tumor invasion of adjacent structure by liver lesions is to be differentiated from other types of extrahepatic disease as complete resection is still possible with adjacent extrahepatic lesions (31). Limited lung metastases also may be salvageable by lung and liver resections (63,64). In particular, patients with metachronous lung liver metastases have been proven to be curable by surgical therapy. Finally, some studies have suggested that extended survival is possible with limited peritoneal carcinomatosis and intraperitoneal chemotherapy (65,66). This population has such a high probability of tumor recurrence that surgery should be considered only if the tumor is shown to be responsive to treatment with systemic therapy.
6. *Satellite metastases*: Poorer outcome is associated with satellite metastases (53,61,67).
7. *Tumor markers*: Carcinoembryonic antigen (CEA) is a marker of tumor burden and aggressiveness (68). Bakalakos et al. (69) showed that median survival with CEA levels <30 was 25 months compared to 17 months for levels >30. Molecular markers, such as DNA ploidy and p53 mutation may predict poor prognosis and help in patient selection for systemic therapeutic strategies (70).
8. *Treatment Factors*: Resection margin: Most studies indicate that a positive macroscopic or microscopic margin is highly predictive of poor outcome, and long-term survival is most often associated with a R0 resection (58,71,72). However, there are no uniformly accepted criteria in the literature as to what constitutes a safe margin. Kokudo et al. (73) have shown through genetic analysis that liver micrometastases are generally uncommon, and most of them occur within a short distance from tumor edge (5 mm). Current data supports resection when a negative surgical margin of any size could be achieved. Most surgeons strive to obtain at least a 1 cm margin if technically feasible. Diligently staying at a distance from the tumor margin gives the greatest likelihood of pathologic clearance. Anatomical versus nonanatomical resections: Scheele et al. (54) reported an association between shorter survival and nonanatomic resections. Similarly, Liau et al. (74) and Yasui et al. (75) found superior survival after anatomic segmental resections. These associations of anatomic resections with superior outcome are likely due to lower rates of positive margins (64). Relationship of outcome with perioperative complications: There is emerging data proving that intraoperative blood loss (53), hypotension and need for blood (76,77), and administration of fresh frozen plasma (71), to be adversely related to long-term outcome.

Clinical Risk Score

It is now clear that a number of clinical factors greatly affect long-term outcome. The most influential are: the presence of extrahepatic disease, and involvement of resection margins by tumor. These are therefore considered contraindications to hepatectomy.

The other factors described earlier are all taken into account when a clinician attempts to select patients for hepatectomy. The decision to operate depends on these factors tempered by the aggressiveness of the surgeon and the patient. No individual factor should be taken in isolation to be a strict contraindication, as survival following hepatic resection is clearly multifactorial. In order to better classify patients with hepatic colorectal metastases, investigators have attempted to formulate prognostic scoring systems based on factors known to be

TABLE 4 The Prognostic Scale Known as the CRS is Based on Five Factors. One Point is Assigned to Each Positive Criterion. Sum of the Points is the Patient's CRS

Nodal metastases in primary cancer
Short (<12 months) disease-free interval between primary cancer and liver metastases
More than one liver metastases
Largest liver tumor >5 cm
CEA >200 ng/ml

Abbreviations: CEA, carcinoembryonic antigen; CRS, clinical risk score.

influential for outcome (30,50,78–80). The ideal scoring system should be simple to use, and is composed of criteria that is easy to obtain preoperatively.

The most widely utilized of such prognostic scales is that published by Fong et al. (31). This prognostic scale known as the clinical risk score (CRS) is based on five factors: (*i*) nodal metastases in primary cancer, (*ii*) short (<12 months) disease-free interval between primary cancer and liver metastases, (*iii*) more than one liver metastases, (*iv*) largest tumor >5 cm, and (*v*) CEA >200 ng/ml (Table 4). Each criterion was assigned one point, and the sum of the points was proposed as a score for assessment of prognosis. Such a prognostic scoring system has the potential to improve the patient selection for surgery and to select patients for adjuvant treatment. The ability to stratify patients' prognosis preoperatively potentially has the following benefits: (*i*) improve patient information when obtaining informed consent, (*ii*) assess the likely need for adjunctive chemotherapy, and (*iii*) facilitate comparative studies and clinical trials. The success of this CRS derived from data at a single center is evident as it has been validated in many unrelated international centers (81,82) (Table 5).

Utility of Clinical Risk Score

Most surgeons agree that resection alone should not be offered to patients with high CRSs (19,31,33,83). Patients with high prognostic scores should be considered for surgery together with an adjuvant or neoadjuvant treatment protocol (84–87). The extent of preoperative workup can also be tailored to the CRS. Investigators have shown that use of extensive and expensive preoperative staging involving PET, magnetic resonance imaging (MRI), and laparoscopy results in the highest yield in patients who have high scores, but who are otherwise suitable for major liver resection (88–92). Similarly, intensities of follow-up may be organized according to individual CRS.

Schindl et al. (79) recently developed a different scoring system that considered Dukes stage, site of primary tumor, diameter of the largest liver lesion, serum concentration of CEA, alkaline phosphatase, and albumin, which showed significant prognostic value for hepatic resection (79). The prognostic score = ([4Xdukecode] + [6Xmetcode3] + [6XLn Alkphos] + [2XLn CEA] − albumin) (79). In daily clinical practice, prognostic scores calculated from a mathematical equation may not be as practicable as scores derived by giving 1 point for each risk factor (31).

TABLE 5 Validation of CRS

CRS	Fong et al. (31)	Mala et al. (81)	Mann et al. (82)
0	60% (74 mo)	0–2; 40% (40 mo)	0–1; 72%
1	44% (51 mo)	(39 mo)	
2	40% (47 mo)	(30 mo)	2–3; 31%
3	20% (33 mo)	3–4; 12% (20 mo)	
4	25% (20 mo)	(37 mo)	4–5; 0%
5	14% (22 mo)	No patients	

Outcomes of three studies based on CRS proposed by Fong et al. (31). Results are listed as five-year actuarial survival in percent (median survival in months).
Abbreviation: CRS, clinical risk score.

WHICH STAGING INVESTIGATIONS ARE OF MOST VALUE IN IDENTIFYING EXTRAHEPATIC DISEASE?

Preoperative selection of patients with colorectal metastases who are most likely to benefit from surgery has evolved greatly due to improving preoperative radiologic imaging. Findings on imaging provide information to rule out surgery for patients with unresectable disease and to plan a complete resection to eradicate detectable disease. Thus, in addition to reducing the incidence of unnecessary surgical exploration, many believe that advances in preoperative imaging contribute to improvements in long-term outcome by optimizing surgical therapy (34,89,93,94).

The last 10 years have seen great advances of imaging modalities (95). Extensive research has been performed for improving the imaging modalities for the detection of colorectal liver metastases. Despite improved sensitivity and advances seen in the last decade, use of imaging clearly has not been optimized. Several studies still report unresectable disease at the time of laparotomy in 40% to 70% of patients brought to the operating room for liver resection (96,97). The abundance of imaging test available also makes preoperative workup complicated and often expensive. Following is an overview of each major modality and suggestions for optimizing use of these imaging techniques.

Transcutaneous Ultrasound

Because of the noninvasive character, low cost, and widespread availability, ultrasound (US) is a valuable screening tool for the imaging of liver metastases. In skilled hands, it remains one of the most useful exams for identification of liver metastases and for delineation of the relative position of tumors to vasculature. In expert hands, US may be as accurate as CT or MRI in determining the number and size of tumors (98). Ultrasound can also detect lesions too small to be detected by CT. Tumors appear either as hyperechoic or hypoechoic lesions with a surrounding halo. Ultrasound has two relative disadvantages: it is highly operator dependent and parts of the liver can be difficult to evaluate. Its use is limited by overlying air-filled structures, such as the bowel and lungs. Thus, the top of the liver is a particularly difficult place to be evaluated by US.

In daily practice, US is mainly used to define the relationship of tumor to major vessels and to determine if the small lesions seen on other modalities may represent benign cysts. Because US cannot make an accurate survey of the entire abdomen, it has given way to CT, MRI, and ^{18}F- fluorodeoxyglucose positron emission tomography (FDG-PET) as a whole body evaluation and follow-up modality (95).

Computerized Tomography Scan

The most widely used imaging modality for evaluation of the patient with liver metastasis is a CT scan, because it is relatively inexpensive and widely available, and allows both the evaluation of the hepatic and extrahepatic sites of disease. With both oral and intravenous contrast, dynamic CT is particularly helpful for detecting the classically hypovascular hepatic metastases of colorectal cancers. Substantial improvements have been made in CT scanning in recent decades with the introduction of helical CT and multidetector CT. Although CT arterial portography (CTAP) remains the most sensitive preoperative imaging modality for the depiction of focal liver lesions (99,100), it is an expensive and invasive procedure. Therefore, it is gradually being replaced by other imaging modalities like MRI and dual-phase CT scans, which when used in conjunction with intraoperative ultrasound (IOUS), can detect the number of lesions with high sensitivity (101).

Unless the patient has medical contraindications to intravenous contrast, all patients being evaluated for liver resection should have a helical CT of the chest, abdomen, and pelvis. If small lesions are found, or if a patient has a high CEA and no hepatic lesions, CTAP should be considered as this variation of the CT scan is particularly sensitive in the depiction of small lesions (101,102).

Magnetic Resonance Imaging

MRI has improved markedly with the introduction of liver-specific agents and widespread use of higher magnetic field strength (103,104). It is outstanding at visualizing vascular structures, such as hepatic veins and the vena cava. It is also well suited for identifying and characterizing liver lesions (105). Recent studies have shown MRI with superparamagnetic iron oxide (SPIO) enhancement to be more sensitive than dual-phase CT and unenhanced MRI (106), and as accurate as CT hepatic arteriography (CTHA) (107) in the depiction of liver lesions. Gadolinium-enhanced MRI and SPIO-enhanced MRI, however, are significantly better compared to nonenhanced MRI (95). However, these techniques are much more expensive than US or CT.

In practice, MRI should be reserved for patients with lesions that cannot be diagnosed on CT with confidence. In particular, patients with very fatty livers either from obesity, diabetes, or chemotherapy-related liver damage would particularly benefit from MRI evaluation. MRI should also be used if CT and US cannot delineate with certainty the proximity of cancerous deposits to major vasculature.

Positron Emission Tomography Scanning

Unlike conventional diagnostic modalities, such as CT and US, which provide mainly anatomic information on malignancies, FDG-PET provides information on tumor metabolism. In this technique, a radioactive glucose analog is administered, and the glucose-avid nature of tumors is used to visualize cancers. The first reports on the clinical application of FDG-PET in colorectal cancer concentrated on differentiating scar tissue from local recurrence in rectal cancer, which often shows a similar appearance on CT (108,109). Recent studies concentrated on the added value of FDG-PET in staging patients with liver metastases of colorectal carcinoma (110–112).

One recent report addressed the potential role of improved patient selection through better preoperative staging by evaluating the role of preoperative PET scan for improving prognosis (89). Further trials have shown that use of FDG-PET can change the management in significant number of patients and lead to clinically relevant extrahepatic findings different from conventional imaging (111,113). When compared to CT, FDG-PET is more sensitive in the detection of extrahepatic disease (114).

Sensitivity of FDG-PET for colorectal liver metastases is directly related to tumor size (111,113). In a series by Fong et al. (111), only 25% of hepatic lesions <1 cm were detected by a PET scan, compared to the detection of 85% of lesions >1 cm. In a meta-analysis by Bipat et al. (95), FDG-PET was more accurate (94.6%) and had a significantly higher sensitivity estimate on a per-patient basis (95). When compared to CT and MRI for the detection of colorectal liver metastases on a per-lesion basis, helical CT, MRI, and FDG-PET were comparable (95). One study shows that integration of FDG-PET into the presurgical evaluation of patients with hepatic metastases could actually reduce overall costs and patients' morbidity (115).

CT scanning is currently regarded as the best method for evaluating the anatomy and resectability of colorectal liver metastases. FDG-PET scanning should be reserved for patients with a high risk of extrahepatic disease after initial conventional workup has demonstrated resectability of liver metastases. Resectability of liver metastases is generally determined by the extent of liver involvement and the specific relation of metastases to anatomic structures. As the anatomic information provided by FDG-PET is limited, it will not become a substitute for the excellent anatomic imaging provided by helical CT. False positives are common with PET because this scanning technique identifies all tissues that are glucose-avid; therefore, surgeons should carefully evaluate and biopsy extrahepatic positive sites.

Current deployment of combined CT and PET imaging—presenting overlays of anatomic (CT) and functional (PET) information—may lead to significant improvements of preoperative liver staging and preoperative judgment on resectability (116). The yield of FDG-PET is also shown to be related to the CRS (117). In practice, all patients with a CRS>1 should have a PET prior to exploration for potential liver resection.

Laparoscopy

Surgical exploration continues to be a highly accurate method for staging cancer, but open exploration results in significant morbidity that may not be justified if the procedure is not therapeutic. Laparoscopic evaluation also allows highly accurate staging, but reduces procedural morbidity (118–120). The literature documents that staging laparoscopy for colorectal liver metastases reduces the rate of nontherapeutic laparotomy (121,122). Preventing laparotomy with laparoscopy has advantages including decreased length of hospital stay (123), reduced hospital charges, lower morbidity (124,125), and earlier initiation of postoperative chemotherapy (126). However, recent data also show that laparoscopy should be used selectively. In a study by Grobmyer et al. (126), it was found that prior to hepatic resection for colorectal cancer metastasis, diagnostic laparoscopy can be selectively performed to optimize patient outcome. Laparoscopy was found to be unnecessary in patients with a CRS of 0 or 1 due to the low yield (122,126). The yield of laparoscopy increases with increasing CRS (125).

Disease identified at laparoscopy that precludes laparotomy includes additional, unsuspected hepatic tumors and extrahepatic metastases (perihepatic lymph nodes and peritoneal disease). Laparoscopy has the ability to sample and biopsy tissue from multiple areas and confirms resectability of hepatic lesions based on direct visualization of the liver and surrounding tissues. Visualization of small metastases (as small as 1 mm) on the surface of the liver, peritoneum, or omentum can be identified with 80% to 90% accuracy with laparoscopy and biopsied, unlike CT which detects rarely lesion <1 cm (127).

Any patient who requires laparotomy regardless of the laparoscopic findings should not undergo laparoscopy. Such cases include the patient who requires laparotomy for surgical palliation of associated problems or for insertion of a hepatic artery infusion device for chemotherapy administration.

Intraoperative Ultrasound

Several studies have shown that IOUS often reveals important new information not seen on preoperative imaging and that these additional, unsuspected findings change the operative plan in up to 50% of patients (128–131). Consequently, IOUS is now routinely used to evaluate the liver before resection to assess for additional hepatic tumors and to evaluate the relationship of tumors to major vascular structures.

Even though IOUS reveals new findings different from preoperative imaging in a large number of patients, these findings result in unresectability in a minority of patients (129). In the majority, the new intraoperative findings either do not change the planned resection or only produce a modification of the planned resection. This is largely the result of advances in imaging technology that have greatly improved patient selection. Intraoperative ultrasound confirms the preoperative impression in many patients and is the only means of evaluating intraoperatively the relationship between the tumor(s) and the hepatic vascular structures and major bile ducts. In patients with additional tumors identified by palpation, IOUS can further assess the lesions and can be used to guide the resection (132,133). For these reasons, IOUS remains an important component of hepatic resection surgery.

During laparoscopic staging, IOUS is more useful, because the liver cannot be palpated (126,129). The routine addition of laparoscopic US has improved the results over diagnostic laparoscopy alone, especially in detecting nodal disease (122,124,126,134). Staging laparoscopy/IOUS can also influence the nature of planned procedures despite preoperative PET scan (122).

Newer treatment modalities can be applied as an alternative or as an adjunct to resection. There is a definite overlap in patients who would benefit from resection, tumor ablation, and/or regional chemotherapy. Staging laparoscopy/IOUS provides a key step toward making a well-informed treatment selection, prior to performing a laparotomy, and may avoid an unnecessary laparotomy all together.

CONCLUSION

Liver metastases from colorectal cancers are relatively common. Liver resection remains the only form of treatment that is potentially curable. Current evidence does not support replacement of surgery by chemotherapy and other nonresection modalities. These other treatment options are best used as an adjunct to resection.

Most surgeons agree that resection should not be offered to patients with extrahepatic disease or where there is no chance to obtain a tumor-free margin. Regionalization of complex surgical procedures to high-volume centers can further improve the results of liver resection, especially in patients with high CRS who should ideally be treated in the settings of clinical trials.

Finding extrahepatic disease is crucial as it precludes curative surgery. Computed tomography scan is the most widely used noninvasive investigation, but it is not very sensitive to detect extrahepatic disease. PET scan has emerged as the single most important modality to detect extrahepatic disease in preoperative setting. Routine use of staging laparoscopy with IOUS can further bring down the rates of nontherapeutic laparotomies by detecting extrahepatic disease. However, selection of patients for staging by PET scanning and staging laparoscopy can be guided by clinical risk of extrahepatic disease as defined by clinical staging systems, such as the CRS.

REFERENCES

1. Cooperman A, Grace WR, Van Heertum R, Geiss A. The problem of liver metastasis. Surg Annu 1984; 16:151–175.
2. Giarelli L, Melato M, Zanconati F, et al. Primary liver cancer in non-cirrhotic liver. Epidemiological study based on autopsies performed in Trieste, Italy and Kurume, Japan. J Gastroenterol Hepatol 1991; 6(3):278–282.
3. Kavolius J, Fong Y, Blumgart LH. Surgical resection of metastatic liver tumors. Surg Oncol Clin North Am 1996; 5(2):337–352.
4. Cady B. Natural history of primary and secondary tumors of the liver. Sem Oncol 1995; 10(2):127–134.
5. Fidler IJ. The organ microenvironment and cancer metastasis. Differentiation 2002; 70(9,10):498–505.
6. Fidler IJ. Critical determinants of metastasis. Semin Cancer Biol 2002; 12(2):89–96.
7. Fidler IJ. Tumor heterogeneity and the biology of cancer invasion and metastasis. Cancer Res 1978; 38(9):2651–2660.
8. Jemal A, Murray T, Ward E, et al. Cancer statistics, 2005. CA Cancer J Clin 2005; 55(1):10–30.
9. Asbun HJ, Tsao JI, Hughes KS. Resection of hepatic metastases from colorectal carcinoma. The registry data. Cancer Treat Res 1994; 69:33–41.
10. Charnley RM, Morris DL, Dennison AR, Amar SS, Hardcastle JD. Detection of colorectal liver metastases using intraoperative ultrasonography. Br J Surg 1991; 78(1):45–48.
11. Bengmark S, Hafstrom L. The natural history of primary and secondary malignant tumors of the liver. Cancer 1969; 23:198–202.
12. Adson MA, Van Heerden JA, Adson MH. Resection of hepatic metastases from colorectal cancer. Arch Surg 1984; 119:647–651.
13. Weiss L, Grundmann E, Torhorst J, et al. Haematogenous metastatic patterns in colonic carcinoma: an analysis of 1541 necropsies. J Pathol 1986; 150(3):195–203.
14. Steele G Jr, Osteen RT, Wilson RE, et al. Patterns of failure after surgical cure of large liver tumors. A change in the proximate cause of death and a need for effective systemic adjuvant therapy. Am J Surg 1984; 147(4):554–559.
15. Bengmark S, Hafstrom L, Jeppsson B, Jonsson PE, Ryden S, Sundqvist K. Metastatic disease in the liver from colorectal cancer: An appraisal of liver surgery. World J Surg 1982; 6:61–65.
16. Jaffe BM, Donegan WL, Watson F, et al. Factors influencing survival in patients with untreated hepatic metastases. Surg Gynecol Obstet 1968; 127:1–11.
17. Pestana C, Reitemeir RJ, Moertel CG, Judd ES, Dockerty MB. The natural history of carcinoma of the colon and rectum. Am J Surg 1964; 108:826–829.
18. Wood CB, Gillis CR, Blumgart LH. A retrospective study of the natural history of patients with liver metastases from colorectal cancer. Clin Oncol 1976; 2:285–288.
19. Wagner JS, Adson MA, Van Heerden JA, Adson MH, Ilstrup DM. The natural history of hepatic metastases from colorectal cancer. A comparison with resective treatment. Ann Surg 1984; 199:502–508.
20. Ekberg H, Tranberg K.-G, Anderson R, et al. Determinants of survival in liver resection for colorectal secondaries. Br J Surg 1986; 73:727–731.
21. Nordlinger B, Quilichini MA, Parc R, Hannoun L, Delva E, Huguet C. Surgical resection of liver metastases from colorectal cancer. Int Surg 1987; 72:70.
22. Fong Y, Cohen AM, Fortner JG, et al. Liver resection for colorectal metastases. J Clin Oncol 1997; 15(3):938–946.
23. Minagawa M, Makuuchi M, Torzilli G, et al. Extension of the frontiers of surgical indications in the treatment of liver metastases from colorectal cancer: long-term results. Ann Surg 2000; 231(4):487–499.
24. Altendorf-Hofmann A, Scheele J. A critical review of the major indicators of prognosis after resection of hepatic metastases from colorectal carcinoma. Surg Oncol Clin North Am 2003; 12(1):165–192.

25. Vauthey JN, Chaoui A, Do KA, et al. Standardized measurement of the future liver remnant prior to extended liver resection: methodology and clinical associations. Surgery 2000; 127(5):512–519.
26. Fong Y, Bentrem DJ. CASH (Chemotherapy-Associated Steatohepatitis) costs. Ann Surg 2006; 243(1):8–9.
27. Silen W. Hepatic resection for metastases from colorectal carcinoma is of dubious value. Arch Surg 1989; 124:1021–1024.
28. Scheele J, Stang R, Altendorf-Hofmann A, Paul M. Resection of colorectal liver metastases. World J Surg 1995; 19:59–71.
29. Fuhrman GM, Curley SA, Hohn DC, Roh MS. Improved survival after resection of colorectal liver metastases. Ann Surg Oncol 1995; 2(6):537–541.
30. Nordlinger B, Guiguet M, Vaillant JC, et al. Surgical resection of colorectal carcinoma metastases to the liver. A prognostic scoring system to improve case selection, based on 1568 patients. Association Francaise de Chirurgie. Cancer 1996; 77(7):1254–1262.
31. Fong Y, Fortner J, Sun RL, Brennan MF, Blumgart LH. Clinical score for predicting recurrence after hepatic resection for metastatic colorectal cancer: analysis of 1001 consecutive cases. Ann Surg 1999; 230(3):309–318.
32. Bradley AL, Chapman WC, Wright JK, et al. Surgical experience with hepatic colorectal metastasis. Am Surg 1999; 65(6):560–566.
33. Scheele J, Tendorf-Hofmann A, Grube T, Hohenberger W, Stangl R, Schmidt K. Resection of colorectal liver metastases. What prognostic factors determine patient selection? Chirurgia 2001; 72(5):547–560.
34. Choti MA, Sitzmann JV, Tiburi MF, et al. Trends in long-term survival following liver resection for hepatic colorectal metastases. Ann Surg 2002; 235(6):759–766.
35. Adam R, Delvart V, Pascal G, et al. Rescue surgery for unresectable colorectal liver metastases downstaged by chemotherapy: a model to predict long-term survival. Ann Surg 2004; 240(4):644–657.
36. Fernandez-Trigo V, Shamsa F, Sugarbaker PH. Repeat liver resections from colorectal metastasis. Repeat Hepatic Metastases Registry. Surgery 1995; 117:296–304.
37. Tuttle TM, Curley SA, Roh MS. Repeat hepatic resection as effective treatment for recurrent colorectal liver metastases. Ann Surg Oncol 1997; 4(2):125–130.
38. Nordlinger B, Vaillant JC, Guiguet M, et al. Survival benefit of repeat liver resections for recurrent colorectal metastases: 143 cases. J Clin Oncol 1994; 12(7):1491–1496.
39. Adam R, Bismuth H, Castaing D, et al. Repeat hepatectomy for colorectal liver metastases. Ann Surg 1997; 225(1):51–62.
40. Petrowsky H, Gonen M, Jarnagin W, et al. Second liver resections are safe and effective treatment for recurrent hepatic metastases from colorectal cancer: a bi-institutional analysis. Ann Surg 2002; 235(6):863–871.
41. Yamamoto J, Kosuge T, Shimada K, Yamasaki S, Moriya Y, Sugihara K. Repeat liver resection for recurrent colorectal liver metastases. Am J Surg 1999; 178(4):275–281.
42. Fong Y, Gonen M, Rubin D, Radzyner D, Brennan MF. Long-term survival is superior after resection for cancer in high volume centers. Ann Surg 2005; 242(4):540–547.
43. Pinson CW, Wright JK, Chapman WC, Garrard CL, Blair TK, Sawyers JL. Repeat hepatic surgery for colorectal cancer metastases to the liver. Ann Surg 1996; 223(6):765–776.
44. Fong Y, Blumgart LH, Cohen A, Fortner J, Brennan MF. Repeat hepatic resections for metastatic colorectal cancer. Ann Surg 1994; 220(5):657–662.
45. Imamura H, Seyama Y, Kokudo N, et al. One thousand fifty-six hepatectomies without mortality in 8 years. Arch Surg 2003; 138(11):1198–1206.
46. August DA, Sugarbaker PH, Schneider PD. Lymphatic dissemination of hepatic metastases: implications for the follow-up and treatment of patients with colorectal cancer. Cancer 1985; 55:1490–1494.
47. Imamura H, Seyama Y, Kokudo N, et al. Single and multiple resections of multiple hepatic metastases of colorectal origin. Surgery 2004; 135(5):508–517.
48. Martin R, Paty P, Fong Y, et al. Simultaneous liver and colorectal resections are safe for synchronous colorectal liver metastasis. J Am Coll Surg 2003; 197(2):233–241.
49. Asbun HJ, Hughes KS. Management of recurrent and metastatic colorectal carcinoma. Surg Clin North Am 1993; 73(1):145–166.
50. Chafai N, Chan CL, Bokey EL, Dent OF, Sinclair G, Chapuis PH. What factors influence survival in patients with unresected synchronous liver metastases after resection of colorectal cancer? Colorectal Dis 2005; 7(2):176–181.
51. Lise M, Bacchetti S, Da Pian P, Nitti D, Pilati P. Patterns of recurrence after resection of colorectal liver metastases: prediction by models of outcome analysis. World J Surg 2001; 25(5):638–644.
52. Ringe B, Bechstein WO, Raab R, Meyer HJ, Pichlmayr R. Liver resection in 157 patients with colorectal metastases [German]. Chirurgia 1990; 61(4):272–279.
53. Ohlsson B, Stenram U, Tranberg KG. Resection of colorectal liver metastases: 25-year experience. World J Surg 1998; 22(3):268–276.
54. Scheele J, Stangl R, Altendorf-Hofmann A, Gall FP. Indicators of prognosis after hepatic resection for colorectal secondaries. Surgery 1991; 110:13–29.

55. Elias D, Ducreux M, Rougier P, et al. What are the real indications for hepatectomies in metastases of colorectal origin? [French]. Gastroenterologie Clinique et Biologique 1998; 22(12):1048–1055.
56. Ballantyne GH, Quin J. Surgical treatment of liver metastases in patients with colorectal cancer. Cancer 1993; 71(S12):4252–4266.
57. Bentrem DJ, DeMatteo RP, Blumgart LH. Surgical therapy for metastatic disease to the liver. Annu Rev Med 2005; 56:139–156.
58. Gayowski TJ, Iwatsuki S, Madariaga JR, et al. Experience in hepatic resection for metastatic colorectal cancer: analysis of clinical and pathologic risk factors. Surgery 1994; 116:703–711.
59. Yokoyama N, Shirai Y, Ajioka Y, Nagakura S, Suda T, Hatakeyama K. Immunohistochemically detected hepatic micrometastases predict a high risk of intrahepatic recurrence after resection of colorectal carcinoma liver metastases. Cancer 2002; 94(6):1642–1647.
60. Imamura H, Shimada R, Kubota M, et al. Preoperative portal vein embolization: an audit of 84 patients. Hepatology 1999; 29(4):1099–1105.
61. Rosen CB, Nagorney DM, Taswell HF, et al. Perioperative blood transfusion and determinants of survival after liver resection for metastatic colorectal carcinoma. Ann Surg 1992; 216:492–505.
62. Van Ooijen B, Wiggers T, Meijer S, et al. Hepatic resections for colorectal metastases in the Netherlands: a multiinstitutional 10-year study. Cancer 1992; 70:28–34.
63. Bolton JS, Fuhrman GM. Survival after resection of multiple bilobar hepatic metastases from colorectal carcinoma. Ann Surg 2000; 231(5):743–751.
64. Jarnagin WR, Gonen M, Fong Y, et al. Improvement in perioperative outcome after hepatic resection: analysis of 1,803 consecutive cases over the past decade. Ann Surg 2002; 236(4):397–406.
65. Sugarbaker PH, Chang D, Koslowe P. Prognostic features for peritoneal carcinomatosis in colorectal and appendiceal cancer patients when treated by cytoreductive surgery and intraperitoneal chemotherapy. Cancer Treat Res 1996; 81:89–104.
66. Elias D, Dube P, Bonvalot S, et al. Treatment of liver metastases with moderate peritoneal carcinomatosis by hepatectomy and cytoreductive surgery followed by immediate post-operative intraperitoneal chemotherapy: feasibility and preliminary results. Hepato-Gastroenterology 1999; 46(25):360–363.
67. Doci R, Bignami P, Montalto F, Gennari L. Prognostic factors for survival and disease-free survival in hepatic metastases from colorectal cancer treated by resection. Tumori 1995; 81(suppl 3):143–146.
68. Takahashi S, Inoue K, Konishi M, Nakagouri T, Kinoshita T. Prognostic factors for poor survival after repeat hepatectomy in patients with colorectal liver metastases. Surgery 2003; 133(6):627–634.
69. Bakalakos EA, Burak WE Jr, Young DC, et al. Is carcino-embryonic antigen useful in the follow-up management of patients with colorectal liver metastases? Immunohistochemically detected hepatic micrometastases predict a high risk of intrahepatic recurrence after resection of colorectal carcinoma liver metastases. Am J Surg 1999; 177(1):2–6.
70. Crowe P, Yang J, Berney C, et al. Genetic markers of survival and liver recurrence after resection of liver metastases from colorectal cancer. World J Surg 2001; 25(8):996–1001.
71. Beckurts KTE, Holscher AH, Thorban ST, Bollschweiler E, Siewert JR. Significance of lymph node involvement at the hepatic hilum in the resection of colorectal liver metastases. Br J Surg 1997; 84:1081–1084.
72. Jenkins LT, Millikan KW, Bines SD, Staren ED, Doolas A. Hepatic resection for metastatic colorectal cancer. Am Surg 1997; 63:605–610.
73. Kokudo N, Miki Y, Sugai S, et al. Genetic and histological assessment of surgical margins in resected liver metastases from colorectal carcinoma: minimum surgical margins for successful resection. Arch Surg 2002; 137(7):833–840.
74. Liau KH, Blumgart LH, DeMatteo RP. Segment-oriented approach to liver resection. Surg Clin North Am 2004; 84(2):543–561.
75. Yasui K, Shimizu Y. Surgical treatment for metastatic malignancies. Anatomical resection of liver metastasis: indications and outcomes. Int J Clin Oncol 2005; 10(2):86–96.
76. Stephenson KR, Steinberg SM, Hughes KS, Vetto J, Sugarbaker PH. Perioperative blood transfusions are associated with decreased time to recurrence and decreased survival after resection of colorectal liver metastasis. Ann Surg 1988; 208:679–687.
77. Kooby DA, Stockman J, Ben Porat L, et al. Influence of transfusions on perioperative and long-term outcome in patients following hepatic resection for colorectal metastases. Ann Surg 2003; 237(6):860–869.
78. Cady B, Stone MD, McDermott WV Jr, et al. Technical and biological factors in disease-free survival after hepatic resection for colorectal cancer metastases. Arch Surg 1992; 127:561–569.
79. Schindl M, Wigmore SJ, Currie EJ, Laengle F, Garden OJ. Prognostic scoring in colorectal cancer liver metastases: development and validation. Arch Surg 2005; 140(2):183–189.
80. Nagashima I, Takada T, Matsuda K, et al. A new scoring system to classify patients with colorectal liver metastases: proposal of criteria to select candidates for hepatic resection. J Hepatobiliary Pancreat Surg 2004; 11(2):79–83.
81. Mala T, Bohler G, Mathisen O, Bergan A, Soreide O. Hepatic resection for colorectal metastases: can preoperative scoring predict patient outcome? World J Surg 2002; 26(11):1348–1353.

82. Mann CD, Metcalfe MS, Leopardi LN, Maddern GJ. The clinical risk score: emerging as a reliable preoperative prognostic index in hepatectomy for colorectal metastases. Arch Surg 2004; 139(11): 1168–1172.
83. Hughes KS, Simons R, Songhorabodi S, et al. Resection of the liver for colorectal carcinoma metastases: a multi-institutional study of indications for resection. Surgery 1988; 103:278–288.
84. Kemeny MM, Adak S, Gray B, et al. Combined-modality treatment for resectable metastatic colorectal carcinoma to the liver: surgical resection of hepatic metastases in combination with continuous infusion of chemotherapy—an intergroup study. J Clin Oncol 2002; 20(6):1499–1505.
85. Goldberg RM, Sargent DJ, Morton RF, et al. A randomized controlled trial of fluorouracil plus leucovorin, irinotecan, and oxaliplatin combinations in patients with previously untreated metastatic colorectal cancer. J Clin Oncol 2004; 22(1):23–30.
86. Kohne CH, Cunningham D, Di CF, et al. Clinical determinants of survival in patients with 5-fluorouracil-based treatment for metastatic colorectal cancer: results of a multivariate analysis of 3825 patients. Ann Oncol 2002; 13(2):308–317.
87. Giacchetti S. Chronotherapy of colorectal cancer. Chronobiol Int 2002; 19(1):207–219.
88. Strasberg SM, Dehdashti F, Siegel BA, Drebin JA, Linehan D. Survival of patients evaluated by FDG-PET before hepatic resection for metastatic colorectal carcinoma: a prospective database study. Ann Surg 2001; 233(3):293–299.
89. Strasberg SM, Siegal BA. Survival of patients staged by FDG-PET before resection of hepatic metastases from colorectal cancer. Ann Surg 2002; 235(2):308.
90. Zealley IA, Skehan SJ, Rawlinson J, Coates G, Nahmias C, Somers S. Selection of patients for resection of hepatic metastases: improved detection of extrahepatic disease with FDG pet. Radiographics 2001; 21(Spec No):S55–S69.
91. Rohren EM, Paulson EK, Hagge R, et al. The role of F-18 FDG positron emission tomography in preoperative assessment of the liver in patients being considered for curative resection of hepatic metastases from colorectal cancer. Clin Nucl Med 2002; 27(8):550–555.
92. Halkar RK, Toro JR, Lim EH, et al. Role of FDG-PET in the pre-operative evaluation of surgical resection of hepatic metastases from colorectal cancer. Clin Positron Imaging 1999; 2(6):335.
93. Valls C, Andia E, Sanchez A, et al. Hepatic metastases from colorectal cancer: preoperative detection and assessment of resectability with helical CT. Radiology 2001; 218(1):55–60.
94. Cervone A, Sardi A, Conaway GL. Intraoperative ultrasound (IOUS) is essential in the management of metastatic colorectal liver lesions. Am Surg 2000; 66(7):611–615.
95. Bipat S, van Leewen MS, Comans EF, et al. Colorectal liver metastases: CT, MR imaging and PET for diagnosis—meta-analysis. Radiology 2005; 237(1):123–131.
96. Fortner JG, Silva JS, Maj MC, Golbey RB, Cox EB, Maclean BA. Multivariate analysis of a personal series of 247 consecutive patients with liver metastases from colorectal cancer. Ann Surg 1984; 199:306–316.
97. Gibbs JF, Weber TK, Rodriguez-Bigas MA, Driscoll DL, Petrelli NJ. Intraoperative determinants of unresectability for patients with colorectal hepatic metastases. Cancer 1998; 82(7):1244–1249.
98. Castaing D, Emond J, Kunstlinger F, Bismuth H. Utility of operative ultrasound in the surgical management of liver tumors. Ann Surg 1986; 204:600–605.
99. Heiken JP, Weyman PJ, Lee JKT, et al. Detection of focal hepatic masses: prospective evaluation with CT, delayed CT, CT during arterial portography, and MR imaging. Radiology 1989; 171:47–51.
100. Soyer P. CT during arterial portography. European Radiol 1996; 6(3):349–357.
101. Soyer P, Levesque M, Elias D, Zeitoun G, Roche A. Detection of liver metastases from colorectal cancer: comparison of intraoperative US and CT during arterial portography. Radiology 1992; 183(2):541–544.
102. Nelson RC, Chezmar JL, Sugarbaker PH, Bernardino ME. Hepatic tumors: comparison of CT during arterial portography, delayed CT, and MR imaging for preoperative evaluation. Radiology 1989; 172(1):27–34.
103. Kim MJ, Kim JH, Chung JJ, Park MS, Lim JS, Oh YT. Focal hepatic lesions: detection and characterization with combination gadolinium- and superparamagnetic iron oxide-enhanced MR imaging. Radiology 2003; 228(3):719–726.
104. Dill-Macky MJ, Burns PN, Khalili K, Wilson SR. Focal hepatic masses: enhancement patterns with SH U 508A and pulse-inversion US. Radiology 2002; 222(1):95–102.
105. Imam K, Bluemke DA. MR imaging in the evaluation of hepatic metastases. Magn Reson Imaging Clin North Am 2000; 8(4):741–756.
106. Ward J, Guthrie JA, Wilson D, et al. Colorectal hepatic metastases: detection with SPIO-enhanced breath-hold MR imaging—comparison of optimized sequences. Radiology 2003; 228(3):709–718.
107. Seneterre E, Taourel P, Bouvier Y, et al. Detection of hepatic metastases: ferumoxides-enhanced MR imaging versus unenhanced MR imaging and CT during arterial portography. Radiology 1996; 200(3):785–792.
108. Ito K, Kato T, Tadokoro M, et al. Recurrent rectal cancer and scar: differentiation with PET and MR imaging. Radiology 1992; 182:549–552.

109. Strauss LG, Clorius JH, Schlag P, et al. Recurrence of colorectal tumors: PET evaluation. Radiology 1989; 170(2):329–332.
110. Beets G, Penninckx F, Schiepers C, et al. Clinical value of whole-body positron emission tomography with [18F]fluorodeoxyglucose in recurrent colorectal cancer. Br J Surg 1994; 81:1666–1670.
111. Fong Y, Saldinger PF, Akhurst T, et al. Utility of 18F-FDG positron emission tomography scanning on selection of patients for resection of hepatic colorectal metastases. Am J Surg 1999; 178(4):282–287.
112. Akhurst T, Fong Y. Positron emission tomography in surgical oncology. Adv Surg 2002; 36:309–331.
113. Ruers TJ, Langenhoff BS, Neeleman N, et al. Value of positron emission tomography with [F-18]fluorodeoxyglucose in patients with colorectal liver metastases: a prospective study. J Clin Oncol 2002; 20(2):388–395.
114. Delbeke D, Martin WH, Sandler MP, et al. Evaluation of benign vs malignant hepatic lesions with positron emission tomography. Arch Surg 1998; 133(5):510–515.
115. Zubeldia JM, Bednarczyk EM, Baker JG, Nabi HA. The economic impact of 18FDG positron emission tomography in the surgical management of colorectal cancer with hepatic metastases. Cancer Biother Radiopharm 2005; 20(4):450–456.
116. Beyer T, Townsend DW, Brun T, et al. A combined PET/CT scanner for clinical oncology. J Nucl Med 2000; 41(8):1369–1379.
117. Schussler-Fiorenza CM, Mahvi DM, Niederhuber J, Rikkers LF, Weber SM. Clinical risk score correlates with yield of PET scan in patients with colorectal hepatic metastases. J Gastrointest Surg 2004; 8(2):150–157.
118. Mala T, Edwin B, Gladhaug I, et al. A comparative study of the short-term outcome following open and laparoscopic liver resection of colorectal metastases. Surg Endosc 2002; 16(7):1059–1063.
119. Mala T, Edwin B, Rosseland AR, Gladhaug I, Fosse E, Mathisen O. Laparoscopic liver resection: experience of 53 procedures at a single center. J Hepatobiliary Pancreat Surg 2005; 12(4):298–303.
120. Mala T, Edwin B. Role and limitations of laparoscopic liver resection of colorectal metastases. Dig Dis 2005; 23(2):142–150.
121. Barbot DJ, Marks JH, Feld RI, Liu JB, Rosato FE. Improved staging of liver tumors using laparoscopic intraoperative ultrasound. J Surg Oncol 1997; 64:63–67.
122. Thaler K, Kanneganti S, Khajanchee Y, Wilson C, Swanstrom L, Hansen PD. The evolving role of staging laparoscopy in the treatment of colorectal hepatic metastasis. Arch Surg 2005; 140(8):727–734.
123. D'Angelica M, Fong Y, Weber S, et al. The role of staging laparoscopy in hepatobiliary malignancy: prospective analysis of 401 cases. Ann Surg Oncol 2003; 10(2):183–189.
124. Callery MP, Strasberg SM, Doherty GM, Soper NJ, Norton JA. Staging laparoscopy with laparoscopic ultrasonography: optimizing resectability in hepatobiliary and pancreatic malingnancy. J Am Coll Surg 1997; 185:33–39.
125. Jarnagin WR, Bodniewicz J, Dougherty E, Conlon K, Blumgart LH, Fong Y. A prospective analysis of staging laparoscopy in patients with primary and secondary hepatobiliary malignancies. J Gastrointest Surg 2000; 4(1):34–43.
126. Grobmyer SR, Fong Y, D'Angelica M, DeMatteo RP, Blumgart LH, Jarnagin WR. Diagnostic laparoscopy prior to planned hepatic resection for colorectal metastases. Arch Surg 2004; 139(12):1326–1330.
127. Fernandez-del Castillo CL, Warshaw AL. Pancreatic cancer. Laparoscopic staging and peritoneal cytology. Surg Oncol Clin North Am 1998; 7(1):135–142.
128. Parker GA, Lawrence W Jr, Horsley JS, III, et al. Intraoperative ultrasound of the liver affects operative decision making. Ann Surg 1989; 209:569–577.
129. Jarnagin WR, Bach AM, Winston CB, et al. What is the yield of intraoperative ultrasonography during partial hepatectomy for malignant disease? J Am Coll Surg 2001; 192(5):577–583.
130. Bismuth H, Castaing D, Garden OJ. The use of operative ultrasound in surgery of primary liver tumors. World J Surg 1987; 11(5):610–614.
131. Staren ED, Gambla M, Deziel DJ, et al. Intraoperative ultrasound in the management of liver neoplasms. Am Surg 1997; 63(7):591–596.
132. Makuuchi M, Hasegawa H, Yamazaki S, Takayasu K, Moriyama N. The use of operative ultrasound as an aid to liver resection in patients with hepatocellular carcinoma. World J Surg 1987; 11(5):615–621.
133. Torzilli G, Takayama T, Hui AM, Kubota K, Harihara Y, Makuuchi M. A new technical aspect of ultrasound-guided liver surgery. Am J Surg 1999; 178(4):341–343.
134. Weitz J, D'Angelica M, Jarnagin W, et al. Selective use of diagnostic laparoscopy prior to planned hepatectomy for patients with hepatocellular carcinoma. Surgery 2004; 135(3):273–281.

16 The Role of Ablative Therapy for the Treatment of Metastatic Tumors of the Liver

Kevin T. Watkins
Department of Surgery, State University of New York at Stony Brook, Stony Brook, New York, U.S.A.

Steven A. Curley
Department of Surgical Oncology, The University of Texas MD Anderson Cancer Center, Houston, Texas, U.S.A.

INTRODUCTION

The liver is the most common site of metastasis for most gastrointestinal malignancies. Liver metastases will occur in approximately 50% of patients diagnosed with primary colorectal cancer. In the past, development of liver metastases from colorectal cancer was associated with a very low probability of five-year survival. Liver resection as a therapy for metastatic colorectal cancer is now a well-accepted practice and has significantly improved survival in a selected group of patients (1–5). Although metastatic cancer is potentially a harbinger of systemic disease, local resection of liver metastases conveys a significant survival benefit. However, only 10% to 20% of patients who present with colorectal liver metastases are candidates for liver resection. The reasons for this include tumor location and number, presence of extrahepatic disease, and pre-existing comorbidities which preclude surgical resection. As liver resection complication rates have diminished, tumor number and the presence of limited or resectable extrahepatic disease have become more relative contraindications.

In the past when liver resection carried significant mortality and morbidity rates, local ablative techniques were developed to attempt local control of disease. The survival benefit following resection of liver metastases has led to a renewed emphasis to identify methods to treat patients with unresectable liver lesions. Chemoembolization, arterial infusion therapy, and local ablation techniques have all been employed. Of these techniques, local thermal ablative methods have produced the most interest in recent years.

There are generally two techniques employed to perform in situ hepatic tumor ablation; chemoablation and thermal ablation. Chemoablation requires direct instillation of sclerosing agents into tumors. Thermal ablation techniques use temperature as a direct or indirect method to cause cellular death in a specific region.

ABLATION TECHNIQUES

Ethanol Ablation

Direct intratumoral injection of ethanol has been used for local tumor ablation in the liver. The mechanism of tumor necrosis by ethanol is two-fold. The first is by direct diffusion of absolute ethanol into the cytoplasm that leads to cellular dehydration. Secondly, ethanol enters the circulation and causes endothelial cell damage that leads to platelet aggregation and thrombosis of small intratumoral vessels producing local tissue ischemia. As with other local tumor ablation techniques, the instillation of ethanol can be monitored with ultrasonography. The local tissue effects can be seen ultrasonographically but are ill-defined. The procedure has generally been performed with a percutaneous approach but has also been used at laparotomy. Ethanol ablation is employed for relatively small tumors (generally <3 cm diameter) due to the fact that the volume of ethanol required to ablate lesions is related to the tumor radius to the third power. For larger tumors, multiple sessions are employed to achieve tumor necrosis. Some of the problems associated with the use of ethanol ablation for metastatic lesions are the inconsistent diffusion of alcohol through metastatic lesions compared to primary hepatic malignancies (6).

Cryotherapy

Cryotherapy was one of the initial methods of thermal destruction of tumors reported in the literature. The technique involves the placement of cryoprobes into the tumor using ultrasound guidance. Utilizing liquid nitrogen to cool the probe, several freeze-and-thaw cycles are performed. The formation of an "ice ball" can be monitored with ultrasound to judge the extent of the zone of freezing. Larger lesions are produced by employing larger diameter or multiple probes. The thermal damage to the tissue is not direct. Tumor necrosis is achieved due to secondary mechanisms such as cell membrane rupture by ice crystals and electrolyte disturbances. As with other thermal ablative techniques, the heat sink effect of major vascular flow can cause difficulty with effective tumor necrosis near major vascular structures. This could leave potentially viable tumor at the vascular wall. The procedure can be performed during laparotomy, laparoscopy, or by a percutaneous approach.

Radiofrequency Ablation

Radiofrequency ablation (RFA) causes direct coagulative necrosis of tissues by frictional heating. A wide variety of probes for RFA are available at this time. Monopolar alternating electrical current is applied by a single or multiple array electrode positioned in the area of the tumor. Electrical current continuity is established through large surface area return electrodes (grounding pads) generally placed on the patients' thighs. Applied current causes ionic agitation in the region of the active electrode. This frictional energy leads to tissue heating. Cell death occurs with temperatures over 55°C to 60°C due to loss of cell membrane structural integrity and protein denaturation. Irreversible cellular damage is dependent on the final temperature reached and the duration of cell exposure to lethal temperatures.

There are a variety of methods by which electrodes achieve maximal diameter thermal injury. Variations in the intratumoral electrodes have been designed in attempts to increase the size of the zone of coagulative necrosis. Newer devices are becoming available which can employ bipolar energy and utilize two electrodes within the tumor and eliminate the need for a return electrode. This has the potential to eliminate the complication of return pad burns seen with the monopolar devices. The size of the thermal lesion is limited by the ability to continue propagation of the electrical energy into the tissues. Larger lesions are now able to be created by a variety of techniques including local infiltration of ionic or sclerosing agents (including ethanol) and by continuous monitoring of impedance and power adjustment to prevent tissue desiccation. As with cryotherapy, the procedure can be performed at laparotomy, laparoscopy, or as a percutaneous approach. Probe position is generally guided with ultrasound or CT scan. Lesion propagation can be followed with ultrasound although the borders of the lesion are generally ill-defined with ultrasound imaging. Final results are better identified with contrast-enhanced CT.

Laser Interstitial Thermotherapy

Laser interstitial thermotherapy (LIT) is similar to RFA in that it produces thermal necrosis. Heating by LIT is caused by a beam of coherent, monochromatic light. Light energy absorption by tissue adjacent to the laser fiber results in heating and vaporization. The ability to create an adequate size lesion is dependent on the tissue penetration by a given frequency of laser light. The most commonly used laser source is the Nd:YAG system. The use of low-power light allows lower absorption and higher scatter. This leads to more tissue penetration. Additionally, the thermal effect is propagated past the point of light absorption from convection and direct conduction of energy. The treatment times required for LIT are generally long, and single fiber systems cannot propagate large lesions. The procedure can be performed both during laparotomy and laparoscopy, as well as percutaneously.

Microwave Coagulation Therapy

Microwave coagulation therapy (MCT) uses dithermic heat energy to cause thermal coagulative necrosis. MCT utilizes a much higher frequency electromagnetic field. Polarization of water molecules in the alternating electromagnetic field leads to heating of intracellular water. The higher frequency energy allows for more localized energy but, as is the problem with other thermal techniques, causes reduction in tissue penetration. The therapy can be delivered during laparotomy, laparoscopy, or by a percutaneous approach.

PROCEDURAL MORBIDITY

In general, local tumor ablative therapies carry low complication rates. Cryotherapy is associated with the most significant complication rates. Many of these are related to the development of "cryoshock" which is due to a systemic inflammatory response to the breakdown products of cellular destruction. The overall morbidity rate of cryotherapy is 16% to 52% (7–9). The complications associated with cryotherapy include abscess, biloma, fistula, bile leak, renal insufficiency or failure and respiratory complications primarily due to pleural effusions. In a comparison of two consecutive prospective studies, cryoablation was shown to have a significantly higher complication rate versus RFA (10). Additionally, in this report, there was noted to be a significant increase in local tumor recurrence rate in those patients undergoing cryoablation. However, in another retrospective review of a prospectively maintained database, the local recurrence rate from RFA was 38% for lesions larger than 3 cm as opposed to a 17% recurrence for cryoablation of similar lesions, although this difference did not reach statistical significance (11). In the overall group, the local recurrence rate for RFA was 7% versus 15% for cryoablation. There was a comparable decrease in complications with RFA alone when compared to cryoablation.

Most therapies that apply heat to achieve thermal destruction are associated with similar morbidity and mortality rates. The mortality rates are less than 1% to 2% and the major morbidity rates have been reported to range from 3% to 40%. Some of the higher morbidity rates are associated with combination of thermal ablation and surgical resection. The major complications specifically associated with thermal ablation include biloma or abscess, biliary tract injury, jaundice, arrhythmias, and secondary thermal damage such as intestinal perforation or fistula.

OUTCOMES

Ethanol Injection

There is a paucity of long-term follow-up data on the use of ethanol injection for the treatment of hepatic metastases. Giovannini and Seitz (12) published a series of 40 patients with 55 lesions, 32 of colorectal origin who were treated with percutaneous ethanol injection. The total amount of alcohol delivered to a lesion was calculated using a standard volume formula with addition of a 10-mm margin. The injections were performed in weekly sessions with a maximum ethanol delivery per session of 10 mL. Tumor necrosis was followed by CT imaging and biopsy. Complete necrosis was obtained in 56% of the treated tumors. In the patients where a complete necrosis of tumor was obtained, there was an improvement in median survival from 21 to 38 months over the patients who did not obtain complete tumor necrosis.

Single-shot ethanol injection has been reported with higher complication rates (13). Livraghi et al. (14) reported this use in 30 patients with metastatic tumors. Likely due to the diffusion properties in larger metastatic tumors, the single-shot therapy was associated with few complete local responses. There was no definitive impact on survival in these patients.

Cryotherapy

There are several retrospective reviews recently with reasonable follow-up periods. Yan et al. (15) report on a retrospective review of 172 patients treated with cryotherapy. Additionally, these patients were treated with hepatic arterial infusion chemotherapy. Stage IV primary tumors were present in 43% of patients. Extrahepatic disease was present in 16% of the patients treated. Complete macroscopic tumor removal or destruction was obtained at the time of surgery in 85%. Preoperative carcinoembryonic antigen (CEA) measurements were obtained in 84% of patients and were only >100 ng/mL in 23%. The mean tumor size treated was 3.6 cm and the mean number of tumors was 4.2. Median follow-up time was 23 months. The median overall survival for the group was 28 months with a two- and five-year survival rate of 60% and

15%, respectively. In this series, local and systemic tumor recurrence information is not presented. Several prognostic factors were identified including age, tumor size and differentiation, low preoperative CEA levels, and complete eradication of metastatic disease although the definition of this is unclear.

For noncolorectal liver metastases, Rikkers et al. publish a retrospective review of 42 patients treated with cryoablation and/or resection (9). Out of 48 procedures performed in these 42 patients, 16 had cryoablation only and 7 had cryoablation in combination with resection. The majority of the cryoablations were performed in patients with neuroendocrine or ovarian primaries. The overall survival of patients was not dependent upon whether they received resection or cryotherapy. The median overall survival of patients in this series was 45 months.

In a prospective small series from Norway, 19 patients were treated with hepatic cryotherapy in 24 procedures (16). Unlike other studies that utilize intraoperative sonography, in this case the cryoablation lesions were followed with magnetic resonance imaging. Nine of the 19 patients also had simultaneous liver resection. For the cryoablated lesions there was a 44% local tumor recurrence rate.

In a retrospective review, Kerkar et al. (8) show results of cryoablation of 98 patients over a nine-year period. There was a wide range of tumors treated with 14% being primary hepatocellular carcinomas, 57% colorectal metastases, and 29% noncolorectal metastases. The median follow-up for the entire group was 54 months. Local recurrence at the lesion site occurred in 15% of patients with a lesion recurrence rate of 5%. The median recurrence free survival for the group was 20 months. Overall survival was not different between the noncolorectal and colorectal metastasis groups. The median survival of patients with colorectal metastases was 30 months. For the noncolorectal metastases group, the median survival was 24 months. The noncolorectal gastrointestinal metastases had a dismal survival with a median survival of nine months. The procedure-related mortality rate was 2% and there was a statistically significant difference in median survival of patients who had a major complication related to the procedure.

Radiofrequency Ablation

Of all ablative techniques, the largest volume of literature exists for RFA. However, to date there are no randomized trials that establish the true effectiveness of RFA. There are several prospective series of the use of RFA in the management of metastatic liver disease.

Gilliams and Lees (17) report on the outcome of 167 patients with colorectal metastases treated by percutaneous RFA. Within this group, 57% of patients presented with synchronous hepatic metastases. Additional liver treatments had been performed in these patients to include 26 liver resections and 22 LIT treatments that were performed prior to RFA. Chemotherapy was received by 80% of the patients with a 67% response rate. Roughly one-third of the patients had treated or stable extrahepatic disease or a perforated primary. The overall extent of extrahepatic disease in these patients cannot be elucidated from the data presented. Patients were enrolled if they had unresectable disease or declined surgery. It is unclear how many patients had surgically resectable disease but declined resection. Of those patients treated with RFA, 145 of the 167 had available follow-up CT scans. In these patients, there was a 16% local lesion recurrence rate. The median overall survival from time of RFA was 22 months with a five-year overall survival rate of 14%. Disease-free survival data is not presented in this series. There was no reported mortality and the overall complication rate appears to be less than 20%.

Solbiati et al. (18) published a series of 117 consecutive RFA treatments for colorectal metastases. All procedures were performed utilizing a percutaneous approach. In the 117 patients the authors reported, there were 179 tumors treated in 229 ablation sessions. All lesions treated were metachronous recurrences, however, two patients underwent liver resection for synchronous metastases at the time of their primary tumor resection. Prior resection of metastatic liver tumors had been performed in 21% of patients and 11% had extrahepatic disease. Not all patients had technically unresectable disease with 19% of the patients enrolled because of refusal to consent to surgery. Over 60% of patients were being treated for a single metastasis at the time of initial RFA. All but 11% of patients underwent some form of chemotherapy with all patients in this group having chemotherapy prior to RFA with 72% of patients continuing chemotherapy after RFA. The chemotherapy regimens utilized were not elucidated in the manuscript.

Median follow-up time in this study was just over two years. The estimated median survival was 36 months. The local tumor recurrence rate was 39% for all lesions treated. Of all patients treated, 55% experienced at least one local recurrence and 50 retreatments of lesions were performed after the initial RFA. The authors evaluated survival in patients with local recurrence who were retreated with RFA versus those who were not, but no comment was made as to how some patients were selected to undergo retreatment while others were not. There was no survival advantage noted in the patients who had retreatment. The complication rate was under 2% and no procedure-related mortalities were noted.

More recently, Berber et al. (19) looked at the predictors of survival after RFA in a prospective study. A total of 135 patients underwent RFA performed laparoscopically over a five-year time span. In this group, 80% had received some form of chemotherapy prior to RFA and 14% had undergone prior resection for liver metastases. Extrahepatic disease was present in 30% of patients and these patients were excluded from analysis for disease-free or progression-free survival. There was no statistically significant difference in survival for patients with extrahepatic disease versus those without. The median survival for patients from RFA was 29 months. Patients with a serum CEA value less than 200 ng/mL and smaller dominant tumor sizes had a statistically significant improvement in survival. These data are consistent with some of the data on prognostic factors of patients undergoing resection of colorectal liver metastases (5). Local tumor recurrence, morbidity and mortality rates are not listed.

There is little data on the efficacy of RFA as compared to standard therapies. A single prospective series looks at the results of resection, RFA, combined RFA and resection, or systemic chemotherapy (20). The study evaluated 358 consecutive patients surgically treated who had colorectal liver metastases. Patients who had resectable disease were treated with resection. Those who had technically unresectable disease were treated with either RFA alone or in combination with resection. Out of all patients, 70 (17%) underwent laparotomy but were not deemed candidates for local therapy and received chemotherapy alone. All patients had disease confined to the liver and no evidence of extrahepatic tumor. The overall survival was better with resection compared to RFA alone or RFA combined with resection. Tumor number was a significant prognostic factor for all groups. Most importantly the survival advantage for resection was seen even when resection was compared to RFA for a single lesion. Most importantly it should be noted that patients treated with RFA as some part of their therapy had a statistically significant improvement in survival over the group treated with chemotherapy alone. Local recurrence rates in the resection, resection with RFA, and RFA only groups were 2%, 5%, and 9%, respectively. There was no difference in the rate of distant metastases between these three groups. This study was prospective but not randomized. Patients were treated based on the number and location of their metastatic liver tumors.

Laser Interstitial Thermotherapy

Unlike RFA, there is limited data on the use of LIT for the treatment of liver metastases. In a series of 19 patients treated with LIT, there was no procedure-related mortality (21). All procedures were performed percutaneously with local anesthetic. In this series, all treatments were performed in patients with liver recurrence after prior resection of colorectal metastases. Chemotherapy was received by 79% of patients from the time of recurrence to LIT. One of the 19 patients experienced a tract site recurrence. Overall morbidity related to the procedure was 32%. The median survival after the procedure was 16 months.

More recently, Vogl et al. (22) published a prospective series of 603 patients treated with percutaneous LIT performed under local anesthetic. In this cohort, 14% were patients with potentially resectable disease who refused surgery. Patients with more than five lesions, a lesion larger than 5 cm, or extrahepatic disease were excluded. There was a 1.5% reported complication rate and a 0.3% mortality rate. Local lesional recurrence rate was 2.2%. Survival data is reported as time from initial diagnosis of metastatic lesions. For the entire cohort evaluated, the median survival was three-and-half years; no disease-free survival data was reported.

In a prospective series from Australia, 80 patients with 168 colorectal metastases were treated with LIT (23). All patients treated were deemed unresectable due to inability to achieve a complete resection and all had disease confined to the liver. Patients with tumors larger than 10 cm or more than five tumors were excluded. All patients were treated using a percutaneous technique with local anesthesia and sedation. The overall morbidity rate was 16% with one small bowel fistula that was treated without surgical intervention. The local recurrence rate six months after LIT was 33%. Repeat LIT was performed in 19 of these 26 patients, all with tumors less than 5 cm. The overall median survival rate was 35 months with a disease-free median survival of 25 months. Prognostic factors affecting patient outcomes included; prior history of hepatic resection, lack of treatment with chemotherapy before LIT, number and differentiation of tumors.

Microwave Coagulation Therapy

Microwave-induced coagulation of tissue is a new approach and there are limited series with long-term follow-up. In a series of 74 patients with hepatic metastases from various tumors, MCT was performed percutaneously with ultrasound guidance (24). The largest tumor treated was 6.8 cm. The two- and five-year survival rates were 60% and 29%, respectively. In multivariate analysis, liver recurrence, number of metastases, and tumor grade were all independent predictors of survival.

From Japan a prospective series of 52 patients with colorectal metastases were treated with MCT (25). Among these patients, only four treatments were performed percutaneously, and 25 patients had MCT combined with resection. The five-year survival rate in all the groups was 24%.

SUMMARY

The data on ablative techniques is difficult to interpret. The patient populations treated encompass a broad spectrum of metastatic disease (26–29). Several series report treatment of patients with almost one out of three patients having extrahepatic disease (Table 1). Even though liver resection is a local therapy for patients with isolated metastases, most physicians would agree that the patients have a systemic disease and the role for adjuvant therapies is continuing to change. There is no prospective ablation trial where the systemic therapy patients receive is controlled. More importantly, the treatment of metastatic colorectal cancer with systemic chemotherapy has been undergoing dramatic improvements. Median survival in patients treated with chemotherapy alone can approach 20 months (30). It is difficult to compare the more recent results from ablative techniques to historical controls of systemic chemotherapy alone. In one trial from M.D. Anderson, a control group of chemotherapy alone was available for comparison (20). There was a marginal improvement in patients treated with RFA in this study; however,

TABLE 1 Outcome Data—Hepatic Ablation Series

Study	Year	No. of patients	Type of therapy	Local recurrence rate (%)	Extrahepatic disease present (%)	Median survival (mo)	Median follow-up (mo)	References
Goering et al.	2002	42	Cryo/Op	NR	NR	45	48	(9)
Yan et al.	2003	172	Cryo/Op	NR	16.3	28	23	(15)
Kerkar et al.	2004	98	Cryo/Op	5	NR	33	54	(8)
Solbiati et al.	2001	117	RFA/Perc	39	NR	36	NR	(18)
Gilliams and Lees	2004	167	RFA/Perc	16	31	22	NR	(17)
Abdalla et al.	2004	158	RFA/Op	5–9	0	25–29	21	(20)
Elias et al.	2005	63	RFA/Op	7.1	27	36	27.6	(31)
Berber et al.	2005	135	RFA/Lap	46	30	29	NR	(19)
Vogl et al.	2003	603	LIT/Perc	2.1	0	35	NR	(22)
Christophi et al.	2004	80	LIT/Perc	33	NR	35	NR	(23)

Abbreviations: Cryo, cryoablation; Lap, laparoscopic; LIT, laser interstitial thermotherapy; NR, not reported; Op, laparotomy; Perc, percutaneous; RFA, radiofrequency ablation.

there is very significant bias with poor prognosis patients in the chemotherapy alone arm. With the available outcome data it seems that all forms of ablative techniques offer similar results.

In relation to procedure-related morbidity and mortality there are two series which show a higher procedure-related morbidity associated with cryotherapy over RFA (10,11). The majority of morbidity is related to the cryoshock phenomenon that is observed with cryotherapy. Other techniques such as RFA, LIT, and MCT, which use coagulative necrosis, do not have the same morbidity. The procedure-related morbidity also depends on the approach used to perform ablation in terms of laparotomy, laparoscopy, or percutaneous.

The question of which way to employ the ablative technique (surgical or percutaneous) also raises very interesting questions. Surgical application of the ablative techniques increases the risk due to general anesthesia with the added potential morbidity related to open surgical procedures. However, surgical application allows for more accurate staging of the hepatic disease as well as the presence of small volume extrahepatic disease. From the RFA data, it appears that percutaneous application is associated with a higher incidence of local tumor recurrence in comparison to RFA performed during laparotomy. This local recurrence rate does not appear to portend a worse prognosis with similar median survival (Table 1).

Although no randomized data exists to support the use of ablative techniques to treat liver metastases, there is also little drive to perform such trials. Caution needs to be advised when treating patients with resectable liver metastases from colorectal cancer. There is no data showing that ablation is equivalent to resection for colorectal liver metastases and data exists that for single isolated metastases it does not offer equivalent survival (10). In treating patients with unresectable metastatic disease, ablative techniques can be considered for therapy if patients have tumors amenable to ablative therapy. Further clinical data is necessary to make specific recommendations as to what patients may benefit from ablation of hepatic metastases.

REFERENCES

1. Jamison RL, Donohue JH, Nagorney DM, Rosen CB, Harmsen WS, Ilstrup DM. Hepatic resection for metastatic colorectal cancer results in cure for some patients. Arch Surg 1997; 132:505–510.
2. Scheele J, Stang R, Altendorf-Hoffman A, Paul M. Resection of colorectal liver metastases. World J Surg 1995; 19:59–71.
3. Choti MA, Sitzmann JV, Tiburi MF, et al. Trends in long-term survival following liver resection for hepatic colorectal metastases. Ann Surg 2002; 235:759–765.
4. Vauthey JN, Pawlik TM, Abdalla EK, et al. Is extended Hepatectomy for hepatobiliary malignancy justified? Ann Surg 2004; 239:722–730.
5. Fong Y, Fortner J, Sun RL, Brennan MF, Blumgart LH. Clinical score for predicting recurrence after hepatic resection for metastatic colorectal cancer: analysis of 1001 consecutive cases. Ann Surg 1999; 230:309–318.
6. Mazziotti A, Grazi GL, Gardini A, et al. An appraisal of percutaneous treatment of liver metastases. Liver Transpl Surg 1998; 4:271–275.
7. Yan DB, Clingan P, Morris DL. Hepatic cryotherapy and regional chemotherapy with or without resection for liver metastases from colorectal carcinoma, how many are too many? Cancer 2003; 98:320–330.
8. Kerkar S, Carlin AM, Sohn RL, et al. Long-term follow up and prognostic factors for cryotherapy of malignant liver tumors. Surgery 2004; 136:770–779.
9. Goering JD, Mahvi DM, Niederhuber JE, Chicks D, Rikkers LF. Cryoablation and liver resection for noncolorectal liver metastases. Am J Surg 2002; 183:384–389.
10. Pearson AS, Izzo F, Fleming RY, et al. Intraoperative radiofrequency ablation or cryoablation for hepatic malignancies. Am J Surg 1999; 178:592–599.
11. Bilchik AJ, Wood TF, Allegra D, et al. Cryosurgical ablation and radiofrequency ablation for unresectable hepatic malignant neoplasms. Arch Surg 2000; 135:657–664.
12. Giovannini M, Seitz JF. Ultrasound-guided percutaneous alcohol injection of small liver metastases. Results in 40 patients. Cancer 1994; 73:294–297.
13. Livraghi T, Lazzaroni S, Pellicano S, Ravasi S, Torzilli G, Vettori C. Percutaneous ethanol injection of hepatic tumors: single-session therapy with general anesthesia. Am J Roentgenol 1993; 161:1065–1069.
14. Livraghi T, Vettori C, Lazzaroni S. Liver metastases: results of percutaneous ethanol injection in 14 patients. Radiology 1991; 179:709–712.
15. Yan DB, Clingan P, Morris DL. Hepatic cryotherapy and regional chemotherapy with or without resection for liver metastases from colorectal carcinoma—how many are too many? Cancer 2003; 98:320–330.

16. Mala T, Edwin B, Mathisen O, et al. Cryoablation of colorectal liver metastases: minimally invasive tumour control. Scand J Gastroenterol 2004; 39:571–578.
17. Gilliams AR, Lees WR. Radio-frequency ablation of colorectal liver metastases in 167 patients. Eur Radiol 2004; 14:2261–2267.
18. Solbiati L, Livraghi T, Goldberg SN, et al. Percutaneous radio-frequency ablation of hepatic metastases from colorectal cancer: long-term results in 117 patients. Radiology 2001; 221:159–166.
19. Berber E, Pelley R, Siperstein AE. Predictors of survival after radiofrequency thermal ablation of colorectal cancer metastases to the liver: a prospective study. J Clin Oncol 2005; 23:1358–1364.
20. Abdalla EK, Vauthey JN, Ellis LM, et al. Recurrence and outcomes following hepatic resection, radiofrequency ablation, and combined resection/ablation for colorectal liver metastases. Ann Surg 2004; 239:818–825.
21. Shankar A, Lees WR, Gilliams AR, Lederman JA, Taylor I. Treatment of recurrent colorectal liver metastases by interstitial laser photocoagulation. Br J Surg 2000; 87:298–300.
22. Vogl TJ, Straub R, Eichler K, Sollner O, Mack MG. Colorectal carcinoma metastases in liver: laser-induced interstitial thermotherapy—local tumor control rate and survival data. Radiology 2004; 230:450–458.
23. Christophi C, Nikfarjam M, Malcontenti-Wilson C, Muralidharan V. Long-term survival of patients with unresectable colorectal liver metastases treated by percutaneous interstitial laser thermotherapy. World J Surg 2004; 28:987–994.
24. Liang P, Dong B, Yu X, et al. Prognostic factors for percutaneous microwave coagulation therapy of hepatic metastases. Am J Roentgenol 2003; 181:1319–1325.
25. Morita T, Shibata T, Okuyama M, et al. Microwave coagulation therapy for liver metastases from colorectal cancer. Gan To Kagaku Ryoho 2004; 31:695–699.
26. Mack MG, Straub R, Eichler K, Sollner O, Lehnert T, Vogl TJ. Breast cancer metastases in liver: laser-induced interstitial thermotherapy—local tumor control rate and survival data. Radiology 2004; 233:400–409.
27. Mateo R, Singh G, Jabbour N, Palmer S, Genzyk Y, Roman L. Optimal cytoreduction after combined resection and radiofrequency ablation of hepatic metastases from recurrent malignant ovarian tumors. Gynecol Oncol 2005; 97:266–270.
28. Vlastos G, Smith DL, Singletary SE, et al. Long-term survival after an aggressive surgical approach in patients with breast cancer hepatic metastases. Ann Surg Oncol 2004; 11:869–874.
29. Touzios JG, Kiely JM, Pitt SC, et al. Neuroendocrine hepatic metastases: does aggressive management improve survival? Ann Surg 2005; 241:776–785.
30. Kabbinavar F, Hurwitz HI, Fehrenbacher L, et al. Phase II, randomized trial comparing bevacizumab plus fluorouracil (FU)/leucovorin (LV) with FU/LV alone in patients with metastatic colorectal cancer. J Clin Oncol 2003; 21:60–65.
31. Elias D, Baton O, Sideris L, et al. Hepatectomy plus intraoperative radiofrequency ablation and chemotherapy to treat technically unresectable multiple colorectal liver metastases. J Surg Oncol 2005; 90:36–42.

17 The Role of Hepatic Arterial Infusion Chemotherapy in the Management of Patients with Hepatic Metastases from Colorectal Cancer

Archie N. Tse and Nancy E. Kemeny
Gastrointestinal Oncology Service, Solid Tumor Division, Department of Medicine, Memorial Sloan-Kettering Cancer Center, New York, New York, U.S.A.

PERSPECTIVE

Approximately one out of 17 people will develop colorectal cancer in their life time. In the United States, colorectal cancer accounts for an incidence of 149,000 cases and over 55,000 death in 2006 (1). About 50% to 60% of all patients with colorectal cancer develop distant disease with the liver as the first and most common site of metastasis. In a third of the cases, all metastases are confined to the liver.

The prognosis for patients with metastatic colorectal cancer is generally poor, with five-year survival rates of 5% or less. In carefully selected patients with metastatic colorectal cancer confined to the liver, complete surgical resection is the only curative option with a five-year survival rates of 25% to 37%, and 10-year rates of 20% to 22% (2–4).

It has been 40 years since Sullivan et al. first reported the administration of antimetabolite chemotherapy given by a prolonged hepatic arterial infusion (HAI) to patients with metastatic liver cancer (5). Multiple prospective trials evaluating HAI therapy have been performed in a number of clinical settings with merits demonstrated in multiple studies. Despite such a protracted period of investigation, the role of HAI therapy in the management of metastatic colorectal cancer has continued to evolve. The issue has become more complex due to the recent development of newer systemic regimens which incorporate more effective chemotherapeutic agents (irinotecan and oxaliplatin) (6–8) as well as targeted drugs (cetuximab and bevacizumab) (9–11) in the treatment of metastatic colorectal cancer. In this chapter, we will review the rationale of HAI therapy, the technical aspects of this approach, the unique complications associated with this form of treatment and their management, and the results of recent literature evaluating its efficacy, focusing on prospective randomized clinical trials. Finally, we will discuss the current role of HAI therapy in the management of colorectal hepatic metastases and the future challenges of this therapeutic modality.

RATIONALE FOR HEPATIC ARTERIAL INFUSION CHEMOTHERAPY

Until recently, the pyrimidine analog 5-fluorouracil (5-FU) had been the palliative standard for patients with metastatic colorectal cancer. It resulted in response rates of approximately 20% (12). The addition of leucovorin (LV) to 5-FU results in a higher response rate without significant improvement in survival (13). Changing the method of administration of 5-FU from bolus to continuous infusion can modestly improve response rates, without significant impact on survival (12). Thus, the poor response to 5-FU-based system chemotherapy provided the initial impetus for developing alternative approaches to the management of metastatic colorectal cancer. Regional chemotherapy by HAI is based on sound physiological and pharmacological grounds. First, liver metastases that grow beyond 2 to 3 mm are dependent on the hepatic artery for vascularization, whereas normal liver tissues are perfused by the portal vein (14,15). Second, HAI therapy allows delivery of increased local concentration of cytotoxic agents to hepatic metastases not achievable by systemic administration, especially for drugs with high systemic clearance (16). Third, first-pass hepatic extraction of certain drugs results in lower systemic concentrations and hence less systemic toxicities. Floxuridine (FUDR) is an example of such a drug with 94% to 99% extraction by the liver during the first pass, whereas only 19%

to 55% of 5-FU is extracted (17,18). This reduction in systemic exposure also allows higher or more frequent dosing of regional therapy.

TECHNICAL ASPECTS OF HEPATIC ARTERIAL INFUSION CHEMOTHERAPY

The Totally Implantable Pump

Early experience with regional chemotherapy involves the use of a percutaneously placed catheter attached to an external infusion device. Treatment required hospitalization and was often associated with a high incidence of complications such as catheter dislodgement, bleeding, thrombosis, and infection (19). Another approach is the implanted port which allows repeated access to the arterial system as well as attachment to an external portable pump for ambulatory treatment. However, these ports still had a high failure rate, particularly with regard to hepatic arterial thrombosis (20). The development of a totally implantable arterial-infusion pump in the late 1970s marked the modern era of HAI therapy (21). Slightly larger than a pacemaker, these pumps can provide a constant slow infusion of chemotherapy at infusion volumes of 30 to 50 mL. The constant flow of fluid is driven by the pressure generated from a self-charging system of fluorocarbon liquid present in the sealed chamber of the pump. Typically, the drug reservoir needs to be filled every two weeks with chemotherapy or heparinized saline. Most pumps also contain a side port that allows direct infusion into the catheter. The provision of a refillable drug chamber, freedom from an external infusion device, and a lower complication rate offer significant advantages over the other methods of delivery of HAI therapy. It has been shown that, when compared to surgically or percutaneously placed catheters attached to an external infusion device, the implantable pump can provide chemotherapy administration with less frequent treatment interruption (22,23). A recent, single-institution retrospective comparison of pumps versus ports found a lower therapy-relevant complication rate (30% vs. 47%) and higher complication-free survival (12.2 months vs. 7.3 months) in favor of pumps (24).

Preoperative Evaluation

Prior to pump placement, all patients should undergo a thorough radiographic evaluation to assess the extent of liver involvement, to confirm the absence of extra-hepatic disease, and to define the anatomy of the hepatic vasculature. A recent colonoscopy is also required for patients with metachronous disease. Patients with portal vein thrombosis are considered ineligible because of the risk of hepatic ischemia. Relative contraindications include hepatic replacement ≥40%, poor performance status, severe ascites, and hyperbilirubinemia (total bilirubin >2). Conventional arteriography was routinely performed in the past as part of the preoperative evaluation. However, more recently, this technique has been replaced by CT angiography which provides a non-invasive means for identifying any anomalous arterial anatomy. Patients with anatomical variants which would preclude perfusion of the entire liver should be excluded, although small vessels can often be ligated to allow for proper perfusion. In the majority of cases, complete and specific hepatic perfusion is obtainable. Additional tests such as PET scan can be helpful for further evaluation of equivocal findings identified on cross-sectional imaging studies.

Pump Placement

The primary goals of pump placement are to achieve complete perfusion of the liver and to prevent misperfusion of extra-hepatic tissues. The arterial supply of the liver is variable. Normal type I anatomy was seen 55% of the time when the gastroduodenal artery (GDA) arose from the common hepatic artery proximal to the takeoff of the left and right hepatic arteries (25). More common variants include trifurcation of the vessels with the GDA, right and left hepatic arteries arising from a common point (12%), replaced or accessory right gastric artery (15%) or left gastric artery (11%) (25).

Catheter positioning and ligation of the appropriate vessels will depend on the hepatic arterial anatomy. For normal type I anatomy, the catheter tip should be positioned in the GDA, and ligation of distal vessels supplying the stomach, duodenum, and pancreas should be carried out to avoid misperfusion of these organs. A prophylactic cholecystectomy is performed during pump placement to avoid the development of chemical-induced cholecystitis. Following pump placement, perfusion of the liver was checked intraoperatively by injection of either fluorescein or methylene blue through the pump. Postoperatively, liver flow scan using technician-labeled macroaggregated albumin should be performed to document adequate perfusion of both lobes and to rule out extra-hepatic perfusion. Any extra-hepatic perfusion should be confirmed with an arteriogram and the culprit vessel embolized, if possible (26).

HEPATIC ARTERIAL INFUSION CHEMOTHERAPY DOSING AND SCHEDULE

In a typical HAI regimen utilizing FUDR, a 14-day drug infusion is alternated with 14 days infusion of heparinized saline. There has been some confusion in the literature regarding FUDR dosing. The older publication often reported only the total instilled into the pump without correcting for the pump flow rate which is about 1 to 2 mL/day. A residual of 10 to 15 mL is typically retrieved during pump empty at the end of each 14-day cycle. Thus, the actual amount of FUDR delivered to the patient is less than that placed inside the pump. Recent literature reports FUDR dosing based on the amount of drug actually delivered (0.12–0.18 mg/kg/day). The calculated total FUDR dose (in mg) to be placed into drug chamber of the pump = [dose rate (mg/kg/day) × patient weight (kg) × pump volume (mL)] ÷ [pump flow rate (mL/day)]. For a 70-kg patient, receiving FUDR at 0.14 mg/mg/day via a 30-mL Cadman pump at a flow rate of 1.2 mL/day, this amounts to (0.14 mg/kg/day)(70 kg)(30 mL)/1.2 mL/day = 245 mg.

RESULTS OF RANDOMIZED TRIALS COMPARING HEPATIC ARTERIAL INFUSION WITH SYSTEMIC CHEMOTHERAPY IN PATIENTS WITH UNRESECTABLE COLORECTAL LIVER METASTASIS

Early phase II trials employing HAI FUDR given mainly by an external pump have reported encouraging response rates of 29% to 83% (27–31). This sets the stage for prospective, randomized phase III comparison between HAI therapy and systemic chemotherapy or best supportive care. Seven randomized studies were reported between 1987 and 1994 (Table 1) (32–38). One major conclusion that one can draw from these studies is that HAI therapy has resulted in higher tumor response rates than systemic chemotherapy. Since most individual trials are small and therefore not adequately powered to detect a small difference in overall survival (OS), two meta-analyses have been performed in order to determine whether HAI therapy confers a survival benefit over systemic chemotherapy (Table 1) (39,40).

The Meta-analysis Group in Cancer included individual patient data from six of seven randomized studies (39). The Northern California Oncology Group (NCOG) trial (34) (representing 143 patients) was excluded in survival analysis because individual patient data could not be retrieved. Five trials compared HAI FUDR with intravenous (i.v.) FUDR (three trials) or 5-FU (two trials). The remaining two studies compared HAI FUDR with an ad libitum control arm where patients could receive either systemic 5-FU or supportive care only. The overall response rate was 41% for patients assigned to HAI therapy and 14% for patients assigned to systemic chemotherapy [odds ratio = 0.25 (95% confidence interval (CI) = 0.16–0.40), $P < 10^{-10}$]. Whereas survival was longer in the HAI arm than in the control arm in six of seven studies, a statistically significant survival benefit was demonstrated in only two of the trials where an ad libitum control arm was used. Survival analyses from the meta-analysis showed a statistically significant relative-risk reduction of 27% for HAI therapy compared with control when all six trials were considered [HR = 0.73 (95% CI = 0.61–0.88), P = 0.0009]. However, when the trials that incorporated best supportive care in the control arms were excluded, the survival advantage of 19% was no longer statistically significant [overall survival: HAI 16 months vs. IV 12.2 months, HR 0.81 (95% CI = 0.62–1.05), P = 0.14] (39). A second meta-analysis by Harmantas et al. evaluated six trials, including the NCOG study, but excluded the trials with the ad libitum group as controls (40). Data were extracted from the individual articles, and found an improvement in one- and two-year survival (10% and 6%, respectively) although only the one-year survival was statistically significant (P = 0.041). A subgroup analyses of trials that did not allow crossover demonstrated one- and two-year survival of 19% and 9%, respectively, both of which were statistically significant (40).

There are several explanations as to why the improved response rates with HAI in the individual trials did not translate into greater survival benefit. First, a substantial number of

TABLE 1 Randomized Trials of HAI Chemotherapy for Unresectable Colorectal Liver Metastases

	Regimens		Number of patients		Received assigned treatment			Responses (CR + PR)		Median survival (mo)	
Trial	HAI	IV	HAI	IV	HAI	IV	Crossover	HAI	IV	HAI	IV
Kemeny et al. (MSKCC), 1987 (32)	FUDR	FUDR	48	51	94%	94%	Yes	50%	20%	17	12
Chang et al. (NCI), 1987 (33)	FUDR	FUDR	32	32	66%	92%	No	62%	17%	17[a]	12
Hohn et al. (NCOG), 1989 (34)	FUDR	FUDR	67	76	75%	86%	Yes	42%	10%	16.5	15.8
Wagman et al. (City of Hope), 1990 (35)	FUDR	FU	31	10	100%	100%	Yes	55%	20%	13.8	11.6
Martin et al. (NCCTG), 1990 (36)	FUDR	FU/LV	39	35	85%	100%	No	55%	20%	12.6	10.5
Rougier et al. (France), 1992 (37)	FUDR	FU/BSC	81	82	87%	50%	Yes	48%	21%	15[b]	11
Allen-Marsh et al. (UK), 1994 (38)	FUDR	FU/BSC	51	49	96%	20%	No	44%	9%	13.5[b]	7.5
Meta-analysis, 1996 (39)	FUDR	FUDR or FU or BSC	—	—	—	—	—	41%	14%	16.0 14.5[c]	12.2 10.1[c]
Harmantas et al. (Meta-analysis), 1996 (40)	FUDR	FUDR or FU	—	—	—	—	—	—	—	10%[b,d] 1-yr survival difference 6.4%[d] 2-yr survival difference	
Lorenz and Muller (German), 2000 (41)	FUDR 5-FU	FU/LV	54 57	57	69% 70%	91%	No	43% 45%	20%	12.7 18.7	17.6
Kerr et al. (MRC/EORTC), 2003 (42)	FU/LV	FU/LV	145	145	38%	75%	No	22%	19%	14.7	14.8
Kemeny et al. (CALGB), 2005 (43)	FUDR	FU/LV	68	67	87%	87%	No	48%	25%	24.4[b]	20

[a]Median survival calculated from Kaplan-Meir survival curve published in original citation (excluding patients with extrahepatic disease).
[b]Statistically different ($P < 0.05$) compared with control arm.
[c]Median survival comparing HAI with systemic chemotherapy were 16.0 versus 12.2; median survival comparing HAI with an ad libitum control arm were 14.5 versus 10.1.
[d]Percent survival difference after excluding Rougier et al. study; positive values favoring the HAI arm.
Abbreviations: BSC, best supportive care; CALGB, Cancer and Leukemia Group B; CR, complete response; EORTC, European Organization for Research and Treatment of Cancer; FUDR, floxuridine; 5-FU, 5-fluorouracil; HAI, hepatic arterial infusion; IV, intravenous; LV, leucovorin; MRC, Medical Research Council; MSKCC, Memorial Sloan-Kettering Cancer Center; NCI, National Cancer Institute; NCCTG, North Central Cancer Treatment Group; NCOG, Northern California Oncology Group; PR, partial response.

patients allocated to HAI treatment never received the assigned therapy because of technical problems with pump placement and unexpectedly high rates of extra-hepatic disease discovered at laparotomy (range 0–34%, Table 1). This may have led to an underestimation of benefit when using an intent-to-treat analysis. Second, the size of the individual trials was too small and therefore underpowered. To detect a 10% improvement in survival with a type I error of 5% and power of 80%, a trial would require more than 120 patients to each arm. No individual HAI therapy trial to date met this requirement. Third, three trials (MSKCC, NCOG, and City of Hope) allowed crossover of patients who progressed on systemic to HAI chemotherapy, which may have further diluted any survival benefit based on intent-to-treat. Finally, HAI therapy requires meticulous medical follow-up for toxicity management and dose modification, the lack of experience in certain centers in several trials may have led to increased toxicity and fewer cycles of therapy given, which may have offset any survival benefit.

Three further randomized studies have been reported since the publication of these two meta-analyses (41–43). Two of the trials were conduced in Europe. Unlike early randomized HAI chemotherapy trials which utilized FUDR, these two European studies evaluated HAI 5-FU (41,42). The German Coorperative Group conducted a three-arm comparison, where a total of 168 patients were randomized to: (*i*) HAI 5-FU/LV, (*ii*) HAI FUDR, or (*iii*) i.v. 5-FU/LV (41). Only 75% of patients randomized to the HAI arms received the assigned therapy. The median times to progression were 9.2 months for HAI 5-FU/LV, 5.9 months for HAI FUDR, and 6.6 months for i.v. 5-FU/LV (*P*-values of between-arm comparison did not reach significance after adjustment for three two-sided comparisons). Intra-hepatic response was significantly higher in patients treated with HAI therapy than those who received i.v. chemotherapy. Extra-hepatic progression was earlier in those patients treated with HAI FUDR than those who received either HAI or i.v. 5-FU/LV (Table 1) (41).

The Medical Research Council (MRC)/European Organization for Research and Treatment of Cancer (EORTC) groups compared between i.v. 5-FU/LV given by the de Gramont regimen and HAI 5-FU/LV (42). Crossover from the i.v. to the HAI arm was not allowed. This dose and schedule of HAI 5-FU/folinic acid were previously tested to produce the same level of systemic toxicity and "spill-over" steady-state venous 5-FU concentrations as that in the intravenous regimen. Thus, this trial should best be viewed as an HAI plus systemic versus systemic comparison. Based on an intent-to-treat analysis, median OS was 14.7 months for the HAI group and 14.8 months for the i.v. group [HR 1.04 (95% CI=0.80–1.33), P=0.79] (42). There was also no difference in progression-free survival between the two groups. The major criticism of this trial is the high attrition rate of patients randomized to the HAI arm. Thirty (22%) of those patients did not start their treatment because of problems with catheter insertion and another 39 (29%) of them had to stop therapy before receiving six cycles of treatment because of catheter failure. The HAI group received a median of only 2 cycles compared with 8.5 cycles for the systemic group (42). Of note, both of the above trials utilized subcutaneous ports rather than implantable pumps, which likely accounted for significant catheter-related problems (up to 36% of HAI patients in the MRC/EORTC trial).

A recently reported multi-institutional trial (Cancer and Leukemia Group B, CALGB) compared HAI FUDR, dexamethasone, LV to systemic 5-FU/LV in patients with unresectable hepatic metastasis from colorectal cancer (43). One hundred and thirty-five patients were randomized and no crossover was allowed between the two arms. This trial demonstrated that OS was significantly longer for HAI than systemic therapy (median survival 24.4 months vs. 20.0 months; P=0.0034) (43). Response rates (47% vs. 24%; P=0.012) and time to hepatic progression (9.8 months vs. 7.3 months, P=0.029) also favored HAI over systemic treatment (43). In addition to the usual clinical end-points, this trial also incorporates quality-of-life and cost-effectiveness analysis in its overall evaluation.

ADJUVANT HEPATIC ARTERIAL INFUSION THERAPY AFTER RESECTION OF COLORECTAL LIVER METASTASES

Although surgical resection represents the only curative option for colorectal cancer patients with hepatic metastasis, the five-year survival after liver resection in these patients is only about 30% (2,44). More than half of the patients who relapse have recurrent disease in the liver.

Adjuvant 5-FU-based systemic chemotherapy has not been shown to have a significant survival benefit (45–47). Taieb et al. evaluated the efficacy of sequential modern chemotherapy with intensified FOLFOX7 followed by FOLFIRI in 47 patients with resectable metastatic colorectal cancer (48). Thirty (64%) of the 47 patients developed recurrence during a median follow-up of 38 months (48). Nineteen (65%) of these recurrences involved the liver. Thus, the relapse rate after liver resection remains unacceptably high even with modern adjuvant systemic chemotherapy and alternative postoperative approaches are required. Based on the theoretical advantages of regional chemotherapy, investigators therefore embarked on studying HAI therapy in the adjuvant setting. Several small trials were undertaken to demonstrate both the feasibility and efficacy of this approach (35,49,50). Following these pilot studies, larger-scale prospective randomized studies have been conducted in an attempt to determine the impact of adjuvant HAI on survival following curative liver resection (Table 2).

In a multicenter German trial, patients who underwent liver resection were randomized to receive a six-month period of adjuvant HAI of continuous 5-FU plus a short infusion of folinic acid for five days every four weeks or observation only (51). In the first planned intent-to-treat interim analysis after inclusion of 226 patients and 91 deaths, the median survival was 34.5 months for patients who received adjuvant therapy versus 40.8 months for the control

TABLE 2 Randomized Trials of HAI Chemotherapy After Resection of Colorectal Liver Metastases

Trial	Regimens	Number of patients	Median time to hepatic progression (mo)	Median disease-free progression (mo)	Median OS (mo)
Lorenz et al. (German), 1998 (51)	HAI 5-FU + LV	108	21.6	14.2	34.5
	None	111	24	13.7	40.8
Kemeny et al. (MSKCC), 1999 (52)	HAI FUDR + IV FU/LV	74	Not reached	37.4[a]	72.2
	IV FU/LV	82	42.7	17.2	59.3 2-yr OS 72.2%[a] versus 59.3%
Lygidakis et al. (Greek), 2001 (55)	Half-dose HAI and half-dose IV mitomycin C + 5-FU + LV; HAI IL-2	62	79[a]	45.5[a]	79[a]
	IV chemotherapy, s.c. IL-2	60	44.5	19	66
Kemeny et al. (ECOG + SWOG), 2002 (54)	HAI FUDR + IV 5-FU	30	43.0%[a]	25.2%[a]	63.7 (47.5)[b]
	None	45	66.9% 4-yr liver recurrence rate in assessable patients	45.7% 4-yr recurrence rate in assessable patients	49.4 (34.2)[b]
Clancy et al. (Meta-analysis), 2005 (56)	FUDR or FU or immunochemotherapy	332	—	—	1.8[c] 1-yr survival difference
	None or FU/LV or oral UFT or oral FU or immunochemotherapy	354	—	—	9.6[c] 2-yr survival difference

[a]Statistically different ($P < 0.05$) compared with control arm.
[b]Median survival comparing HAI with systemic chemotherapy were 63.7 months versus 49.4 months and 47.5 months versus 34.2 months in assessable patients and for the whole group (intent-to-treat), respectively.
[c]Survival difference in months; positive values favoring the HAI arm.
Abbreviations: ECOG, Eastern Cooperative Oncology Group; FUDR, floxuridine; 5-FU, 5-fluorouracil; HAI, hepatic arterial infusion; IL-2, interleukin 2; IV, intravenous; LV, leucovorin; MSKCC, Memorial Sloan-Kettering Cancer Center; OS, overall survival; s.c., subcutaneous; SWOG, Southwest Oncology Group, UFT, uracil-tegafur.

group (51). Further accrual was stopped because the estimated reduction in the risk of death would be 15% at best but the increased risk of death was double at worst. No difference in time to progression, time to hepatic progression, and median OS was noted in an intention-to-treat analysis. When patients were analyzed "as treated," time to hepatic progression (45 months vs. 23 months) and time to progression or death (20 months vs. 12.6 months) were improved in the HAI arm (51). Several reasons may have contributed to the failure of the study. First, of the 108 patients randomized to adjuvant therapy, 24 did not receive the assigned treatment because of abnormal vascular anatomy, port-related complications, or unresectability. Of the 87 patients scheduled to receive adjuvant treatment, only 34 patients completed the protocol. Second, therapy was discontinued in 19 patients because of technical complications. Third, systemic toxicities (mainly stomatitis and nausea) are substantial because of incomplete extraction of 5-FU possibly exacerbated after liver resection.

A single-institution, randomized study performed at MSKCC compares adjuvant HAI FUDR/dexamethasone plus systemic 5-FU (with or without LV) with systemic therapy alone for six months following curative hepatic resection (52). Randomization was performed intraoperatively among 156 patients after complete resection of metastases, and patients were stratified based on number of metastases and prior treatment history. Ninety-two percent of patients received treatment as assigned. At the time of publication, there was significant improvement in a prespecified two-year actuarial survival rate in patients assigned to the regional plus systemic arm compared with the systemic alone arm (86% vs. 72%; $P=0.03$) (52). At two years, the hazard ratio for death was 2.34 among patients treated with systemic therapy alone, as compared with patients who received combined therapy (95% CI=1.10–4.98; $P=0.03$), after adjustment for important variables (52). The median survival was 72.2 months in the combined therapy group and 59.3 months in the monotherapy group. After two years, the rates of survival free of hepatic recurrence were 90% in the combined therapy group and 60% in the monotherapy group ($P < 0.001$), and the respective rates of progression-free survival were 57% and 42% ($P=0.07$) (52). Toxicity was higher (39%) in the combined therapy group requiring hospitalization for diarrhea, neutropenia, mucositis, or small bowel obstruction, compared with the monotherapy group (22%) ($P=0.02$). Biliary sclerosis requiring stents occurred in 6% of the combined group and 2% of the monotherapy group. There was no significant difference between the groups in therapy-related deaths (one combined, two monotherapy). The results of this trial have recently been updated after a median follow-up of 10.3 years (53). The difference in overall progression-free survival is now statistically significant, favoring the combined therapy arm (31.3 months vs. 17.2 months; $P=0.02$). Median OS is now 68.4 months in the group receiving combined therapy and 58.8 months in the monotherapy group ($P=0.10$). Ten-year survival rates are 41.1% and 27.2%, respectively (53). In patients with poor risk factors, the survival remained high at 10 years, 37% versus 16% for the combined group and systemic groups, respectively.

In an Intergroup Study [Eastern Cooperative Oncology Group (ECOG) later joined by Southwest Oncology Group (SWOG)], 109 patients were randomized preoperatively to receive either surgical resection of hepatic metastasis alone or surgery in combination with post-operative chemotherapy consisting of four 14-day cycles of HAI FUDR and twelve 14-day cycles of systemic continuous infusion of 5-FU (54). Because randomization was performed prior to surgery, a substantial proportion of patients were found in surgery to be ineligible for the study due to the presence of greater than three liver metastases, or extra-hepatic disease, or unresectable disease. Eleven patients from the control group and 22 from the chemotherapy group were removed from study, leaving only 45 and 30 patients in the control and treatment group, respectively, considered assessable. Despite these shortcomings, patients in the chemotherapy group had significant improvement in recurrence-free four-year survival compared to the control arm (25% vs. 46%; $P=0.04$) (54). Of note, this trial was not powered for OS. Of the 75 assessable patients, the median survival was 63.7 months for the chemotherapy arm and 49 months for the control arm ($P=0.06$) (54). Although cited as a criticism, these limitations also highlight the logistic difficulty in executing and completing randomized trials in an intergroup setting for such a technically demanding therapeutic approach.

One study conducted in Greece randomly assigned 112 patients after hepatic resection of colorectal metastases to receive locoregional chemoimmunotherapy plus systemic chemotherapy (Group A; $n=62$) or systemic immunochemotherapy alone (Group B; $n=60$) (55). This study differs from other HAI trials in that a lipiodol–urografin mixture was used as the carrier for both regional chemo- and immunotherapy. Patients received adjuvant immunochemotherapy up to six years. The median OS, survival free of hepatic recurrence, and overall disease-free survival were 79, 79, and 45.5 months, and 66, 44.5, and 19 months for Group A and Group B, respectively ($P=0.04$, 0.00003, and 0.00602, respectively) (55). Treatment-related toxicity was lower in patients of Group A with fewer hospitalizations necessary. The authors concluded that regional immunochemotherapy in combination with systemic chemotherapy resulted in an improved clinical outcome. One caveat is that eight patients in Group A (12.9%) had port-related complications and were excluded from the study because of treatment interruption.

Clancy et al. recently reported a meta-analysis of prospective trials evaluating adjuvant HAI after curative hepatic resection of metastasis (56). Seven studies were included in their analysis and six were randomized trials. Unlike the meta-analysis conducted for regional chemotherapy in unresectable disease, where HAI FUDR was employed for all the studies, the form of HAI therapy utilized in the adjuvant trials was quite heterogeneous, involving FUDR, 5-FU, immunochemotherapy, and two trials also utilized oral fluoropyrimidines. Further, the control arms were quite variable, including resection only (three trials), systemic treatment in the form of oral UFT (tagafur/uracil) or 5-FU, and i.v. chemotherapy with 5-FU/LV or chemoimmunocherapy. The OS difference (positive values favoring the HAI arm) was 1.8 months at 1 year (95% CI=–4.9 to 8.5; $P=0.59$) and 9.6 months at 2 years (95% CI=–2.2 to 21.4; $P=0.11$) postsurgery, respectively (56). Both the German (51) and ECOG (54) studies were considered to have a negative impact on survival in the HAI-treated group in the meta-analysis. This meta-analysis included all patients who entered, not the patients who were actually treated. In most studies, this does not make a difference, but in these two studies 36% and 32%, respectively, were not treated. However, it should be noted that the ECOG trial was powered to evaluate improvement in time to recurrence and hepatic disease-free survival, not OS. Despite meeting its primary end-point, this trial was regarded as a "negative" study because it was the actuarial one- and two-year survival of all 109 patients rather than those of the 75 assessable patients who were considered in the meta-analysis (54).

COST EFFECTIVENESS AND QUALITY-OF-LIFE ISSUES

HAI chemotherapy is often perceived as a complex and costly form of treatment. An important question is therefore whether the clinical benefits of HAI therapy worth the tradeoffs in its risks and whether it is cost-effective. The Meta-analysis Group in Cancer undertook an economic analysis on the additional cost of HAI therapy over that of conventional treatment using data from the meta-analysis performed by the group in 1996 (57). Health-care costs were computed for the entire duration of follow-up, and were based on actual costs (in 1995 U.S. dollars) at two trial centers, in Paris, France and Palo Alto, California, U.S.A. (57). The average cost per patient for HAI (which included the pump and its placement, initial hospitalization, administration of chemotherapy, and all related complications) was US $29,562 in Paris and US $25,208 in Palo Alto. The additional cost over control treatment (systemic chemotherapy in five trials, chemotherapy or best supportive care in two trials) was US $19,636 in Paris and US $19,280 in Palo Alto (57). Based on a mean gain of life expectancy of 3.2 months conferred by HAI therapy, the cost-effectiveness with respect to survival was US $73,635 per life-year in Paris and US $72,300 per life-year in Palo Alto. The authors concluded that the cost-effectiveness of HAI therapy was considered within the accepted range for therapies for serious medical conditions such as hemodialysis and organ transplantation. A more recent analysis was performed to compare costs and benefits of HAI therapy, systemic chemotherapy, and palliative care in two British randomized trials (58). In addition to the costs borne by the health-care system, societal costs (welfare costs and loss of earnings) were also computed for each type of management. HAI was more cost-effective than systemic chemotherapy (£31,892 vs. £41,527) with regard to the health care plus societal cost per life-year gained, and equally effective with regard to cost per normal quality of life gained (58). With the availability of multiple newer, more expensive agents for the treatment of metastatic colorectal cancer, economic analysis has become increasingly important in evaluating the cost-and-benefit ratios of regional versus systemic chemotherapy.

Four quality-of-life end-points (i.e., emotional well-being, physical functioning, social functioning, and the general health perceptions subscales) were assessed every three months during the 18-month follow-up period in the CALGB unresectable liver metastases study (43). Analyses of data at three and six months, while most of the patients were on active protocol treatment, demonstrated that the physical functioning of the HAI patients was better than that of those on systemic therapy at both three months ($P=0.038$) and six months ($P=0.024$) (43).

COMPLICATIONS OF HEPATIC ARTERIAL INFUSION THERAPY AND THEIR MANAGEMENT

Complications of HAI therapy can be divided into those related to the pump device and those secondary to chemotherapy. The development of a completely implantable HAI pump in the 1970s represents a significant stride in HAI research. Despite this technological advance, reports published as late as the 1990s continued to record pump complication rates of around 40%, although peri-operative mortality associated with pump placement was rare (<2%) (24,59–61). Pump-related complications include pump malfunction, pocket infection, catheter thrombosis or displacement, catheter erosion, arterial thrombosis or arterial dissection, extra-hepatic perfusion, and incomplete perfusion. In a recent retrospective analysis of the technical complications and durability of HAI pump in 544 patients, the incidence of pump complications was 22% (62). However, complications that occurred within 30 days after operation were more likely to be salvaged. These include extrahepatic perfusion, pump malfunction, pocket hematoma, and pump migration. Complications that occur late (>30 days from operation) are likely to be catheter occlusion or arterial thrombosis and are less likely to be salvaged (62). The long-term pump durability was excellent; failure rate was 9% at one year and 16% at two years (62). Only one out of 10 patients who underwent HAI therapy discontinued pump therapy in the course of therapy as a result of pump failure. These results are comparable to the pump-related complication rate of 16% recently reported from M.D. Anderson Cancer Center (63). Multivariate analysis identified single vessel cannulation of the GDA as an independent predictor of pump complications (64). The incidence of technical complications also varies considerably with surgeon's experience. In one study, the complication rate of pump placement was 37% for inexperienced surgeons and 7% for experienced surgeons (61).

Chemotherapy-associated complications include gastrointestinal toxicities (gastroduodenal inflammation or ulceration, and pancreatitis), chemical hepatitis, and sclerosing cholangitis. Gastroduodenal and pancreatic toxicities usually results from inadvertent perfusion and drug delivery to these organs. Persistent epigastric pain in patients on HAI therapy mandates prompt cessation of therapy and endoscopic evaluation. Methylene blue can be infused via the side port during upper endoscopy; if blue staining of the ulcer appears, an angiogram to identify and possibly embolize the aberrant vessel is warranted (26).

Chemical hepatitis with elevation of liver enzymes or bilirubin is a unique toxicity associated with HAI using FUDR, occurring in 42% of patients in early randomized trials (25). In some cases, progressive biliary sclerosis develops, which resembles idiopathic sclerosing cholangitis radiographically (65). Significant biliary sclerosis documented by endoscopic retrograde cholangiopancreatography (ERCP) occurred in 3% to 26% in earlier studies (25). A number of measures have been attempted to reduce the hepatic toxicities associated with HAI therapy. The addition of dexamethasone to FUDR has been shown to decrease hyperbilirubinemia, increase response rate, and perhaps even increase survival (66). The incidence of significant biliary sclerosis was reduced to only 5% to 6% in recent HAI trials where dexamethasone was given in conjunction with FUDR (43,67). Liver function should be monitored every two weeks while on therapy, and strict guidelines regarding dose reduction and/or cessation should be followed (Table 3). In most cases, appropriate dose reduction results in normalization of liver function tests. Patients with persistently elevated liver enzymes should undergo evaluation with ERCP or transhepatic cholangiography for the presence of biliary strictures which may be amendable for balloon dilatation and/or stenting. Other approaches in order to minimize

TABLE 3 Memorial Sloan-Kettering Cancer Center Guidelines for FUDR Dose Modification

	AST		FUDR dose
Reference value (ref)[a]	≤50 U/L	>50 U/L	
Current value[b]	0 to <3 × ref	0 to <2 × ref	100%
	3 to <4 × ref	2 to <3 × ref	80%
	4 to <5 × ref	3 to <4 × ref	50%
	≥5 × ref	≥4 × ref	Hold
If held, restart when	<4 × ref	<3 × ref	50% of last dose given
	Alkaline phosphatase		
Reference value (ref)	≤90 U/L	>90 U/L	
Current value	0 to <1.5 × ref	0 to <1.2 × ref	100%
	1.5 to >2 × ref	1.2 to 1.5 × ref	50%
	≥2 × ref	≥1.5 × ref	Hold
If held, restart when	<1.5 × ref	<1.2 × ref	25% of last dose given
	Total bilirubin		
Reference value (ref)	≤1.2 mg/dL	>1.2 mg/dL	
Current value	0 to <1.5 × ref	0 to <1.2 × ref	100%
	1.5 to <2 × ref	1.2 to <1.5 × ref	50%
	≥2 × ref	≥1.5 × ref	Hold
If held, restart when	<1.5 × ref	<1.2 × ref	25% of last dose given

[a]Reference value is the value obtained on the day patient received last FUDR dose.
[b]Current value is the value obtained at pump emptying or on the day of planned treatment (whichever is higher).
Abbreviations: AST, aspartate aminotransferase; FUDR, floxuridine.

hepatic toxicity include circadian modifications of HAI and alternating between FUDR and 5-FU (68,69).

THE ROLE OF REGIONAL CHEMOTHERAPY IN THE ERA OF MODERN SYSTEMIC TREATMENT

Despite a 40-year long investigation, the precise role of HAI therapy in the management of patients with hepatic metastasis from colorectal cancer has not been clearly defined. Apart from the technically demanding nature of this approach, one major difficulty faced in HAI research is that the appropriate systemic treatment with which regional therapy is being compared has always been a "moving target." Early HAI therapy trials were carried out in a time period where fluoropyrimidines were considered the standard systemic treatment. With the advent of more effective cytotoxic as well as biologic agents, a more relevant issue is, therefore, to determine how HAI therapy can be incorporated into the armamentarium of colorectal patient care. In the remaining portion of this chapter, we will focus our discussion on the recent advances of HAI therapy in the context of contemporary systemic treatment.

Three general approaches were undertaken to improving the efficacy of HAI in the setting of newer agents:

1. Combining HAI therapy with modern systemic treatment.
2. Studying newer agents for HAI chemotherapy.
3. Identifying clinical settings where HAI therapy can be effectively applied.

COMBINING HEPATIC ARTERIAL INFUSION THERAPY WITH CONTEMPORARY SYSTEMIC CHEMOTHERAPY

Irinotecan is a topoisomerase I poison with proven efficacy in first- and second-line treatment of metastatic colorectal cancer (6,7,70). Systemic treatment with oxaliplatin, a third-generation platinum, in combination with 5-FU and LV (FOLFOX) has now been approved by the Food and Drug Administration for the adjuvant treatment of resected Stage III colorectal cancer as well as for the first- and second-line treatment of metastatic disease (8,71,72). With the availability of 5-FU and these two new drugs, the median survival of patients with metastatic colorectal cancer is about 20 months, an outcome approaches or exceeds that was achievable using HAI as the primary therapy in highly selected patients. Combining HAI therapy with these newer systemic chemotherapeutic agents should in theory improve hepatic response and also delay extra-hepatic progression. Several studies have been undertaken to evaluate the feasibility of this approach. Thirty-eight patients with unresectable hepatic metastases were treated in a phase I trial of concurrent systemic irinotecan and HAI FUDR at MSKCC (Table 4). The maximum tolerated dose (MTD) was 100 mg/m^2 of irinotecan weekly for three weeks every four weeks with concurrent HAI FUDR (0.16 mg/kg/day × pump volume/flow rate) plus dexamethasone for 14 days of a 28-day cycle. Diarrhea and myelosuppression were dose-limiting. The response rate was 74%, median time to progression 8.1 months, and median survival 17.2 months. Thirteen of the 16 (81%) patients who received prior irinotecan showed a partial response (PR) to treatment (73).

The combination of HAI FUDR with systemic oxaliplatin has also been evaluated in a phase I study where patients were assigned to receive two different oxaliplatin-containing systemic regimens (Table 4) (74). In Group A, patients receive HAI FUDR in combination with escalating doses of systemic oxaliplatin and irinotecan. In group B, patients receive HAI FUDR plus systemic oxaliplatin at 100 mg/m^2, LV at 400 mg/m^2, and escalating doses of continuous infusion of 5-FU. Systemic treatment was given every two weeks. Sixty-nine percent of the 36 patients were previously treated with irinotecan. An impressive 90% (Group A) and 89% (Group B) response rates were obtained (74). In Group A, seven of 21 patients were able to undergo liver resection, and two patients had no remaining tumor. The MTD for Group A was oxaliplatin 100 mg/m^2 and irinotecan 150 mg/m^2, not dissimilar to the recommended dose of oxaliplatin 85 mg/m^2 and irinotecan 200 mg/m^2 when given without HAI therapy. The MTD of 5-FU in Group B was 1400 mg/m^2, somewhat lower than what is usually given in systemic regimens (2000–2400 mg/m^2 over 48 hours) (Table 4) (74). Taken together, these results indicate that modern systemic chemotherapy can be successfully incorporated into regional therapy with

TABLE 4 Summary of Trials Combining HAI Therapy with Newer Systemic Agents for Unresectable Colorectal Liver Metastases

Trial	Number of patients	HAI	MTD of systemic agent	RR (%)	Med THP (mo)	Med TEP (mo)	Med TTP (mo)	Med survival (mo)	Prior systemic chemotherapy
Kemeny et al. (43)	68	FUDR + LV + Dex	None	47	9.8	7.7	5.3	24.4[a]	First line
Kemeny et al. (90)	38	FUDR + Dex	100 mg/m^2 3 out of 4 wk irinotecan	74	8.5	9.0	8.1	17.2[a]	All received prior chemotherapy (42% received prior irinotecan)
Kemeny et al. (74)	21	FUDR + Dex	100 mg/m^2 oxaliplatin + 150 mg/m^2 irinotecan every 2 wk	90	16.4	16.9		28[a] 37[b]	89% received prior chemotherapy (69% received prior irinotecan)
Kemeny et al. (74)	15	FUDR + Dex	100 mg/m^2 oxaliplatin + 400 mg/m^2 LV + 1400 mg/m^2 5-FU (CIV over 24 hr)	87	9.4	10.8		22[a] 35[b]	

[a]Calculated from time to pump placement.
[b]Calculated from time from initial diagnosis of liver metastasis.
Abbreviations: CIV, continuous infusion; Dex, dexamethasone; FUDR, floxuridine; 5-FU, 5-fluorouracil; HAI, hepatic arterial infusion; LV, leucovorin; Med, median; MSKCC, Memorial Sloan-Kettering Cancer Center; MTD, maximum tolerated dose; RR, response rate; TEP, time-to-extra-hepatic progression; THP, time-to-hepatic progression; TTP, time-to-progression.

promising activity and manageable toxicities. Further, neoadjuvant HAI therapy after tumor progression on first-line treatment can occasionally render patients resectable; as a result, transforming a palliative therapy into a potentially curative treatment.

The National Surgical Adjuvant Breast and Bowel Project has completed a feasibility trial using HAI FUDR in combination with systemic oxaliplatin and capecitabine, an oral fluoropyrimidine, in patients with resected or ablated liver metastases from colorectal cancer. A randomized phase III study (C-09) comparing oxaliplatin and capecitabine with or without HAI therapy is underway.

It has been shown that combining monoclonal antibodies targeting the epidermal growth factor receptor (cetuximab) or the vascular endothelial growth factor (bevacizumab) with cytotoxic agents can lead to an improved tumor response (9,11,75). In principle, this concept should also apply to HAI therapy. To date, trials of HAI chemotherapy in combination with antiangiogenesis agents or epidermal growth factor receptor inhibitors have not been reported in either the metastatic or adjuvant setting. One important concern is whether bevacizumab can be safely given to patients who have undergone hepatic resection given the possibility that an antiangiogenesis agent may affect liver regeneration. This question is currently being addressed in an ongoing phase II trial at MSKCC where patients were randomized to adjuvant HAI FUDR plus systemic chemotherapy with or without bevacizumab following hepatic resection.

EVALUATION OF NEWER CYTOTOXIC AGENTS FOR HEPATIC ARTERIAL INFUSION THERAPY

Based on the established activity of IV irinotecan and oxaliplatin in advanced colorectal cancer, these newer agents have also been evaluated for HAI therapy. van Riel et al. conducted a phase II trial in pretreated colorectal cancer patients where HAI irinotecan was given as a five-day continuous infusion at 20 mg/m^2/day every three weeks (76). Of the 22 evaluable patients, only 3 patients (14%) had a PR. Major toxicities were vomiting and diarrhea. Fiorentini et al. reported the results of a phase II study, where HAI irinotecan was given as a 30-minute short infusion at 200 mg/m^2 every 3 weeks (77). A higher response rate was observed (4 PR in 12 patients). Grade 2 diarrhea and myelosuppression were found in 41% and 50% of the patients, respectively. Based on its pharmacokinetic properties, one would have predicted that irinotecan may not be the ideal candidate drug for HAI therapy. Thus, in a prior phase I and pharmacokinetic study, van Riel et al. have shown that HAI irinotecan resulted in a higher conversion of irinotecan to its active metabolite SN-38 compared with IV irinotecan given at the same dose rate, presumably due to the high carboxyl esterase content of the liver (78). However, the steady-state plasma level of SN-38 was equal or higher after HAI than after IV infusion. Therefore, despite a first-pass hepatic clearance of the parent drug after HAI, systemic exposure to SN-38 was not reduced. This is in sharp contrast to using FUDR for HAI therapy where an almost complete first-pass hepatic extraction of drug can be achieved, resulting in minimal systemic toxicity (17). In accord with this concept, side effects were remarkably similar between HAI and i.v. administration of irinotecan. Regional advantage of HAI irinotecan therefore lies only in the achievement of high local concentration of the drug.

Single-agent activity of HAI oxaliplatin has been demonstrated in two clinical trials. Mancuso et al. evaluated HAI oxaliplatin given at 20 mg/m^2/day for five days every three weeks (79). A 46% response rate was noted in 15 patients. In a phase I/II study of single-agent HAI oxaliplatin given as a 30-minute infusion every three weeks, Fiorentini et al. reported an MTD of 150 mg/m^2. A PR rate of 33% was noted in four out of 12 patients (33%) (80). These response rates are impressive given the low single-agent activity of IV oxaliplatin in advanced colorectal cancer (71). The overall toxicities of HAI oxaliplatin were very similar to those observed following systemic administration of the drug with the exception of abdominal pain. Severe right upper quadrant/epigastric pain (in the absence of chemical hepatitis or sclerosing cholangitis) was noted by Mancuso et al. to be dose-limiting in 41% of the patients (80). Interestingly, the abdominal pain was unrelieved by nonsteriodal anti-inflammatory drugs and opioids but could be prevented by tricyclic antidepressants, raising the possibility of an acute sensory neuropathy to the hepatobiliary system induced by HAI oxaliplatin.

Several trials have studied HAI oxaliplatin in combination with intravenous chemotherapy. In a phase I and pharmacokinetic study of HAI oxaliplatin given in combination with intravenous folinic acid and 5-FU, Kern et al. reported a recommended phase II dose of 125 mg/m^2 (81). Ten of 18 evaluable patients achieved a complete or partial response (59%). Ducreux et al. studied a similar regimen in a phase II trial and found an objective response rate of 79% (82). Three out of 14 patients were able to undergo a complete resection of their liver metastasis. In a combined HAI oxaliplatin, folinic acid, 5-FU, and mitomycin C study, pharmacokinetic analysis revealed an estimated liver extraction ratio of 0.47 for oxaliplatin (83).

The antimetabolite gemcitabine has the pharmacological properties of being a good candidate drug for regional chemotherapy. Gemcitabine demonstrates rapid systemic clearance with a plasma half-life of approximately 17 minutes. In an ongoing phase I study at our center, we evaluate escalating doses as well as escalating infusion duration of HAI gemcitabine in patients who have progressed on FUDR-based HAI therapy. Our preliminary data have indicated that gemcitabine is extracted up to 85% by the liver and no biliary toxicities were seen in all 19 patients thus far (84).

IDENTIFICATION OF CLINICAL SETTINGS APPROPRIATE FOR REGIONAL CHEMOTHERAPY

Hepatic Arterial Infusion Chemotherapy as Second-Line Treatment

Leonard et al. have recently reviewed the response rates and survival data from trials evaluating second-line chemotherapy after irinotecan or oxaliplatin failure. The response rates were generally less than 20% and median survival is around 10 months (85). For example, Tournigand et al. reported response rates of 15% with FOLFOX6 and 4% with FOLFIRI, respectively (86). As described above, HAI therapy when combined with newer cytotoxic agents has demonstrated encouraging second-line activity (up to 90%) even in patients who had progressed on modern chemotherapy (Table 4). Dose-finding trials combining HAI with newer chemotherapeutic drugs have now been completed, and randomized trials of HAI plus systemic chemotherapy versus the most active systemic chemotherapy alone should allow determination of the best second-line approach.

Although HAI treatment provides an excellent control of liver metastasis, development of extra-hepatic disease remains a major issue. In addition to developing treatment strategy that combines both HAI with systemic agents, the ability to identify patients whose tumors are likely to stay confined to the liver will undoubtedly increase the success rate of regional therapy. To this end, using HAI therapy in the second-line setting should, in theory, select for those patients who are less likely to develop rapid extra-hepatic progression. Alternatively, biomarker discovery using gene expression profiling technique may help to distinguish subgroups of colorectal cancers with low likelihood for extra-hepatic spread—a potential area of research that is currently wide open.

Neoadjuvant Use of Hepatic Arterial Infusion Therapy

As mentioned above, hepatic resection offers a chance for long-term survival in a small but finite percentage of patients with liver metastasis. With the advent of more effective systemic chemotherapy, liver resection should routinely be reconsidered in those patients who were previously considered unresectable but had showed objective response to treatment. In a recent review by Leonard et al. of the current data on neoadjuvant chemotherapy followed by hepatic resection treatment using modern systemic chemotherapy containing oxaliplatin and/or irinotecan has demonstrated a secondary complete resection rate of 3.3% to 41% (85). Most of the trials included in the review involve chemotherapy-naïve patients. The report by Adam et al. represents one of the largest series of this nature (87). In that study, 701 patients with unresectable colorectal cancer were treated with neoadjuvant chemotherapy using chronomodulated 5-FU, LV, and oxaliplatin. Ninety-five patients (13.5%) were found to be resectable on reevaluation and underwent a potentially curative resection. The actuarial five-year survival for the post neoadjuvant resection group was 34% (87).

Several studies evaluated the utility of HAI therapy in the neoadjuvant setting. Most of the studies have used HAI FUDR or 5-FU with or without systemic chemotherapy. Complete hepatic metastasis resection rate following neoadjuvant HAI therapy varies among different studies, ranges between 3.4% and 47% (85). As mentioned above, 7 out of 21 patients with initially unresectable liver metastases who received second-line treatment with HAI and systemic oxaliplatin-based chemotherapy were able to undergo liver resection without complications.

An outstanding question is whether those patients who were rendered resectable after tumor "downstaging" using HAI therapy enjoy the same disease-free survival as those who undergo de novo resection. A cautionary note has been raised by Meric et al. indicating that of the 18 patients who underwent secondary complete surgical resection and/or local ablation after tumor downstaging with neoadjuvant HAI, the one-year disease-free survival rate was only 6% despite a one-year OS of 83% (88). The authors suggested that the fact that most of their patients had progressed during systemic chemotherapy might signify more aggressive tumors at presentation. In accord with this concept, a recent report by Adam et al. has shown that tumor progression during neoadjuvant treatment represents a poor prognosis factor for long-term survival even after potentially curative hepatectomy (89). At this juncture, it is impossible to compare the merits between systemic and HAI chemotherapy in the neoadjuvant setting, and randomized studies will be required to determine the optimal approach.

CONCLUSIONS

A large body of knowledge has been accumulated over the past 40 years with regard to the use of HAI chemotherapy. Parallel progress in systemic cytotoxic and targeted therapies have made the management of patients with liver-only metastatic colorectal cancer increasingly, albeit excitingly, complex. Improvement in surgical techniques, the development of implantable pumps, and adherence to strict dose modification guidelines in HAI treatment have increased the feasibility of this therapeutic approach. Early randomized trials in patients with unresectable liver metastases have demonstrated a higher response rate with HAI than systemic chemotherapy although evaluation of survival benefit of HAI was plagued by technical complications, preventable toxicities, and methodological flaws. The more recently reported CALGB trial has shown a survival advantage with HAI FUDR when compared with the then standard systemic chemotherapy. Dose-finding studies combining HAI with newer agents have been completed and have yielded impressive response rates in the second-line and neoadjuvant settings. Encouraging results have also been seen in trials using newer chemotherapeutic agents such as oxaliplatin delivered by HAI. For patients who have undergone complete resection of hepatic colorectal metastases, the adjuvant use of HAI FUDR has resulted in delay in hepatic relapse and improved OS in two years. The development of extra-hepatic relapse remains a problem and therefore well-conducted randomized studies comparing HAI in combination with newer systemic agents versus newer systemic agents alone are ongoing. We have identified potential areas where HAI therapy can be optimized so that this approach can be added to the therapeutic armamentarium for colorectal cancer (Table 5).

TABLE 5 Optimization of HAI Therapy in Liver-Only Metastatic Colorectal Cancer

Issue	Remedy
Control of intrahepatic disease	Incorporate modern systemic chemotherapy and targeted treatment into HAI therapy Develop newer agent for HAI therapy
Control of extrahepatic disease	Incorporate modern systemic chemotherapy and targeted treatment into HAI therapy Select for patients with liver-confined disease by either clinical history or molecular markers
HAI toxicities	Combine dexamethasone with FUDR Careful monitoring of liver function with dose modification in case of hepatic toxicity Develop newer agents for HAI therapy with nonoverlapping toxicities
Pump complications	Preoperative evaluation Hepatic flow scan to rule out extrahepatic perfusion Placement of pump by experienced surgeons at high-volume centers

Abbreviations: FUDR, floxuridine; HAI, hepatic arterial infusion.

REFERENCES

1. Jemal A, Siegel R, Ward E, et al. Cancer Statistics 2006. CA Cancer J Clin 2006; 56(2):106–130.
2. Nordlinger B, Guigiet M, Vaillant JC, et al. Surgical resection of colorectal carcinoma metastases to the liver. Cancer 1996; 77:1254–1262.
3. Jamison R, Donohur J, Nagorney D, et al. Hepatic resection for metastatic colorectal cancer results in cure for some patients. Arch Surg 1997; 132:505–511.
4. Fong Y, Fortner J, Sun RL, Brennan MF, Blumgart LH. Clinical score for predicting recurrence after hepatic resection for metastatic colorectal cancer: analysis of 1001 consecutive cases. Ann Surg 1999; 230(3):309–318; discussion 318–321.
5. Sullivan RD, Norcross JW, Watkins E Jr. Chemotherapy of metastatic liver cancer by prolonged hepatic-artery infusion. N Engl J Med 1964; 270:321–327.
6. Saltz LB, Cox JV, Blanke C, et al. Irinotecan plus fluorouracil and leucovorin for metastatic colorectal cancer. Irinotecan Study Group. N Engl J Med 2000; 343(13):905–914.
7. Douillard JY, Cunningham D, Roth AD, et al. Irinotecan combined with fluorouracil compared with fluorouracil alone as first-line treatment for metastatic colorectal cancer: a multicentre randomised trial. Lancet 2000; 355(9209):1041–1047.
8. Goldberg RM, Sargent DJ, Morton RF, et al. A randomized controlled trial of flurouracil plus leucovorin, irinotecan, and oxaliplatin combinations in patients with previously untreated metastatic colorectal cancer. J Clin Oncol 2004; 1(22):23–30.
9. Saltz LB, Meropol NJ, Loehrer PJ Sr, Needle MN, Kopit J, Mayer RJ. Phase II trial of cetuximab in patients with refractory colorectal cancer that expresses the epidermal growth factor receptor. J Clin Oncol 2004; 22(7):1201–1208.
10. Cunningham D, Humblet Y, Siena S, et al. Cetuximab monotherapy and cetuximab plus irinotecan in irinotecan-refractory metastatic colorectal cancer. N Engl J Med 2004; 351:337–345.
11. Hurwitz H, Fehrenbacher L, Novotny W, et al. Bevacizumab plus irinotecan, fluorouracil, leucovorin for metastatic colorectal cancer. N Engl J Med 2004; 350:2335–2342.
12. Efficacy of intravenous continuous infusion of fluorouracil compared with bolus administration in advanced colorectal cancer. Meta-analysis group in cancer. J Clin Oncol 1998; 16(1):301–308.
13. Advanced Colorectal Cancer Meta-analysis Project. Modulation of fluorouracil by leucovorin in patients with advanced colorectal cancer: evidence in terms of response rate. J Clin Oncol 1992; 10(6):896–903.
14. Breedis C, Young C. The blood supply of neoplasms in the liver. Am J Pathol 1954; 30:969.
15. Ackerman NB. The blood supply of experimental liver metastases. IV. Changes in vascularity with increasing tumor growth. Surgery 1974; 75(4):589–596.
16. Collins JM. Pharmacologic rationale for regional drug delivery. J Clin Oncol 1984; 2:498–504.
17. Ensminger WD, Rosowsky A, Raso V. A clinical pharmacological evaluation of hepatic arterial infusions of 5-fluoro-2-deoxyuridine and 5-fluorouracil. Cancer Res 1978; 38:3789–3792.
18. Ensminger WD, Gyves JW. Clinical pharmacology of hepatic arterial chemotherapy. Semin Oncol 1983; 10:176–183.
19. Barone RM, Byfield JE, Goldfarb PB, Frankel S, Ginn C, Greer S. Intra-arterial chemotherapy using an implantable infusion pump and liver irradiation for the treatment of hepatic metastases. Cancer 1982; 50(5):850–862.
20. Wickremeskera J, Cannan R, Stubs R. Hepatic artery access ports: recognizing and avoiding the problems. Aust NZ J Surg 2000; 70(7):496–502.
21. Blackshear PJ, Dorman FD, Blackshear PL Jr, Varco RL, Buchwald H. The design and initial testing of an implantable infusion pump. Surg Gynecol Obstet 1972; 134(1):51–56.
22. Yasuda S, Noto T, Ikeda M, et al. Hepatic arterial infusion chemotherapy using implantable reservoir in colorectal liver metastasis. GanTo Kagaku Ryoho 1990; 8:1815–1819.
23. Fordy C, Burke D, Earlam S, Twort P, Allen-Mersh TG. Treatment interruptions and complications with two continuous hepatic artery floxuridine infusion systems in colorectal liver metastases. Br J Cancer 1995; 72(4):1023–1025.
24. Heinrich S, Petrowsky H, Schwinnen I, et al. Technical complications of continuous intra-arterial chemotherapy with 5-fluorodeoxyuridine and 5-fluorouracil for colorectal liver metastases. Surgery 2003; 133(1):40–48.
25. Skitzki JJ, Chang AE. Hepatic artery chemotherapy for colorectal liver metastases: technical considerations and review of clinical trials. Surg Oncol 2002; 11(3):123–135.
26. Bloom AI, Gordon RL, Ahl KH, et al. Transcatheter embolization for the treatment of misperfusion after hepatic artery chemoinfusion pump implantation. Ann Surg Oncol 1999; 6(4):350–358.
27. Oberfield RA, McCaffrey JA, Polio J, Clouse ME, Hamilton T. Prolonged and continuous percutaneous intra-arterial hepatic infusion chemotherapy in advanced metastatic liver adenocarcinoma from colorectal primary. Cancer 1979; 44(2):414–423.
28. Weiss G, Garnick M, Osteen R, et al. Long-term arterial infusion of 5-fluorouracil for liver metastases using an implantable infusion pump. J Clin Oncol 1983; 1:337–344.
29. Balch CM, Urist MM, Soong SJ, McGregor M. A prospective phase II clinical trial of continuous FUDR regional chemotherapy for colorectal metastases to the liver using a totally implantable drug infusion pump. Ann Surg 1983; 198(5):567–573.

30. Kemeny N, Conti JA, Cohen A, et al. Phase II study of hepatic arterial floxuridine, leucovorin, and dexamethasone for unresected liver metastases from colorectal carcinoma. J Clin Oncol 1994; 12: 2288–2295.
31. Arai Y, Inaba Y, Takeuchi Y, Ariyoshi Y. Intermittent hepatic arterial infusion of high-dose 5FU on a weekly schedule for liver metastases from colorectal cancer. Cancer Chemother Pharmacol 1997; 40(6):526–530.
32. Kemeny N, Daly J, Reichman B, Geller N, Botet J, Oderman P. Randomized study of intrahepatic versus systemic infusion of fluorodeoxyuridine in patients with liver metastases from colorectal carcinoma. Ann Intern Med 1987; 107:459–465.
33. Chang AE, Schneider PD, Sugarbaker PH. A prospective randomized trial of regional versus systemic continuous 5-fluorodeoxyuridine chemotherapy in the treatment of colorectal liver metastases. Ann Surg 1987; 206:685–693.
34. Hohn D, Stagg R, Friedman M, et al. A randomized trial of continuous intravenous versus hepatic intra-arterial floxuridine in patients with colorectal cancer metastatic to the liver: The Northern California Oncology Group Trial. J Clin Oncol 1989; 7:1646–1654.
35. Wagman L, Kemeny M, Leong L, et al. A prospective randomized evaluation of the treatment of colorectal cancer metastatic to the liver. J Clin Oncol 1990; 8:1885–1893.
36. Martin JKJ, O'Connell MG, Wieland HS, et al. Intra-arterial floxuridine vs systemic fluorouracil for hepatic metastases from colorectal cancer. A randomized trial. Arch Surg 1990; 125:1022–1027.
37. Rougier P, Laplanche A, Huguier M, et al. Hepatic arterial infusion of floxuridine in patients with liver metastases from colorectal carcinoma: long-term results of a prospective randomized trial. J Clin Oncol 1992; 10:1112–1118.
38. Allen-Mersh T, Earlam S, Fordy C, Abrams K, Houghton J. Quality of life and survival with continuous hepatic artery floxuridine infusion for colorectal liver metastases. Lancet 1994; 344:1255–1260.
39. Reappraisal of HAI in the treatment of nonresectable liver metastases from colorectal carcinoma. Meta-analysis group in cancer. J Natl Cancer Inst 1996; 88(5):252–258.
40. Harmantas A, Rotstein LE, Langer B. Regional versus systemic chemotherapy in the treatment of colorectal carcinoma metastatic to the liver. Is there a survival difference? Meta-analysis of the published literature. Cancer 1996; 78(8):1639–1645.
41. Lorenz M, Muller HH. Randomized, multicenter trial of fluorouracil plus leucovorin administered either via hepatic arterial or intravenous infusion versus fluorodeoxyuridine administered via hepatic arterial infusion in patients with nonresectable liver metastases from colorectal carcinoma. J Clin Oncol 2000; 18(2):243–254.
42. Kerr DJ, McArdle CS, Ledermann J, et al. Intrahepatic arterial versus intravenous fluorouracil and folinic acid for colorectal cancer liver metastases: a multicentre randomised trial. Lancet 2003; 361(9355):368–373.
43. Kemeny N, Niedzwiecki DHD, Hollis DR, et al. Hepatic arterial infusion versus systemic therapy for hepatic metastases from colorectal cancer a randomized trial of efficacy, quality of life, and molecular markers. (CALGB 9481) J Clin Oncol 2006; 24(9):1395-1403.
44. Fong Y, Salo J. Surgical therapy of hepatic colorectal metastasis. Semin Oncol 1999; 26(5):514–523.
45. O'Connell MJ, Adson MA, Schutt AJ, Rubin J, Moertel CG, Ilstrup DM. Clinical trial of adjuvant chemotherapy after surgical resection of colorectal cancer metastatic to the liver. Mayo Clin Proc 1985; 60:517–520.
46. Portier G, Elias D, Bouche O, et al. Multicenter randomized trial of adjuvant fluorouracil and folinic acid compared with surgery alone after resection of colorectal liver metastases: FFCD ACHBTH AURC 9002 trial. J Clin Oncol 2006; 24(31):4952–4953.
47. Langer B, Blieberg H, Labianca, et al. Fluorouracil (FU) plus l-leucovorin (i-LV) versus observation after potentially curative resection of liver or lung metastases from colorectal cancer (CRC): results of the ENG (EORTC/NCIC CTG/GIVO) randomized trial. Proc Am Soc Clin Oncol 2002; 21:149a.
48. Taieb J, Artru P, Paye F, et al. Intensive systemic chemotherapy combined with surgery for metastatic colorectal cancer: results of a phase II study. J Clin Oncol 2005; 23(3):502–509.
49. Moriya Y, Sugihara K, Hojo K, Makuuchi M. Adjuvant hepatic intra-arterial chemotherapy after potentially curative hepatectomy for liver metastases from colorectal cancer: a pilot study. Eur J Surg Oncol 1991; 17(5):519–525.
50. Curley SA, Roh MS, Chase JL, Hohn DC. Adjuvant hepatic arterial infusion chemotherapy after curative resection of colorectal liver metastases. Am J Surg 1993; 166(6):743–746; discussion 746–748.
51. Lorenz M, Muller HH, Schramm H, et al. Randomized trial of surgery versus surgery followed by adjuvant hepatic arterial infusion with 5-fluorouracil and folinic acid for liver metastases of colorectal cancer. German Cooperative on Liver Metastases (Arbeitsgruppe Lebermetastasen). Ann Surg 1998; 228(6):756–762.
52. Kemeny N, Huang Y, Cohen AM, et al. Hepatic arterial infusion of chemotherapy after resection of hepatic metastases from colorectal cancer. N Engl J Med 1999; 341(27):2039–2048.
53. Kemeny NE, Gonen M. Hepatic arterial infusion after liver resection. N Engl J Med 2005; 352(7): 734–735.

54. Kemeny MM, Adak S, Gray B, et al. Combined-modality treatment for resectable metastatic colorectal carcinoma to the liver: surgical resection of hepatic metastases in combination with continuous infusion of chemotherapy—an intergroup study. J Clin Oncol 2002; 20(6):1499–1505.
55. Lygidakis NJ, Sgourakis G, Vlachos L, et al. Metastatic liver disease of colorectal origin: the value of locoregional immunochemotherapy combined with systemic chemotherapy following liver resection. Results of a prospective randomized study. Hepatogastroenterology 2001; 48(42):1685–1691.
56. Clancy TE, Dixon E, Perlis R, Sutherland FR, Zinner MJ. Hepatic arterial infusion after curative resection of colorectal cancer metastases: a meta-analysis of prospective clinical trials. J Gastrointest Surg 2005; 9(2):198–206.
57. Durand-Zaleski I, Roche B, Buyse M, et al. Economic implications of hepatic arterial infusion chemotherapy in treatment of nonresectable colorectal liver metastases. Meta-analysis Group in Cancer. J Natl Cancer Inst 1997; 89(11):790–795.
58. Durand-Zaleski I, Earlam S, Fordy C, Davies M, Allen-Mersh TG. Cost-effectiveness of systemic and regional chemotherapy for the treatment of patients with unresectable colorectal liver metastases. Cancer 1998; 83(5):882–888.
59. Hohn DC, Rayner AA, Economou JS, Ignoffo RJ, Lewis BJ, Stagg RJ. Toxicities and complications of implanted pump hepatic arterial and intravenous floxuridine infusion. Cancer 1986; 57(3): 465–470.
60. Curley SA, Chase JL, Roh MS, Hohn DC. Technical considerations and complications associated with the placement of 180 implantable hepatic arterial infusion devices. Surgery 1993; 114(5):928–935.
61. Campbell KA, Burns RC, Sitzmann JV, Lipsett PA, Grochow LB, Niederhuber JE. Regional chemotherapy devices: effect of experience and anatomy on complications. J Clin Oncol 1993; 11(5):822–826.
62. Allen PJ, Nissan A, Picon AI, et al. Technical complications and durability of hepatic artery infusion pumps for unresectable colorectal liver metastases: an institutional experience of 544 consecutive cases. J Am Coll Surg 2005; 201(1):57–65.
63. Scaife CL, Curley SA, Izzo F, et al. Feasibility of adjuvant hepatic arterial infusion of chemotherapy after radiofrequency ablation with or without resection in patients with hepatic metastases from colorectal cancer. Ann Surg Oncol 2003; 10(4):348–354.
64. Allen PJ, Nissan AI, Picon A, et al. Technical complications and durability of hepatic artery infusion pumps for unresectable colorectal liver metastases: an institutional experience of 544 consecutive cases. J Am Coll Surg 2005;201(1):57–65.
65. Kemeny M, Battifora H, Flayney D, et al. Sclerosing cholangitis after continuous hepatic artery infusion of FUDR. Ann Surg 1985; 202:176–181.
66. Kemeny N, Steiter K, Niedzweiecki D, et al. A randomized trial of intrahepatic infusion of fluorouridine (FUDR) with dexamethasone versus FUDR alone in the treatment of metastatic colorectal cancer. Cancer 1992; 69:327–334.
67. Kemeny N. Randomized study of hepatic arterial infusion (HAI) and systemic chemotherapy (SYS) versus SYS alone as adjuvant therapy after resection of hepatic metastases from colorectal cancer. ASCO 1999; 18:2.
68. Hrushesky WJ, von Roemeling R, Lanning RM, Rabatin JT. Circadian-shaped infusions of floxuridine for progressive metastatic renal cell carcinoma. J Clin Oncol 1990; 8(9):1504–1513.
69. Stagg R, Venook A, Chase J, et al. Alternating hepatic intra-arterial floxuridine and fluorouracil: a less toxic regimen for treatment of liver metastases from colorectal cancer. J Natl Cancer Inst 1991; 83:423–428.
70. Rothenberg M, Cox JV, DeVore RF, et al. A multicentre phase II trial of weekly irinotecan (CPT-11) in patients with previously treated colorectal carcinoma. Cancer 1999; 85:786–795.
71. Rothenberg ML, Oza AM, Bigelow RH, et al. Superiority of oxaliplatin and fluorouracil–leucovorin compared with either therapy alone in patients with progressive colorectal cancer after irinotecan and fluorouracil–leucovorin: interim results of a phase III trial. J Clin Oncol 2003; 21:2059–2069.
72. Andre T, Boni C, Mounedji-Boudiaf L, et al. Oxaliplatin, fluorouracil, and leucovorin as adjuvant treatment for colon cancer. N Engl J Med 2004; 350(23):2343–2351.
73. Kemeny N, Gonen M, Sullivan D, et al. Phase I study of hepatic arterial infusion of floxuridine and dexamethasone with systemic irinotecan for unresectable hepatic metastases from colorectal cancer. J Clin Oncol 2001; 19(10):2687–2695.
74. Kemeny N, Fong Y, Jarnagin W, et al. A phase I trial of systemic oxaliplatin combinations with hepatic arterial infusion in patients with unresectable liver metastases from colorectal cancer. J Clin Oncol 2005;23(22):4888–4896.
75. Cunningham D, Humblet Y, Siena S, et al. Cetuximab monotherapy and cetuximab plus irinotecan in irinotecan-refractory metastatic colorectal cancer. N Engl J Med 2004; 351(4):337–345.
76. van Riel JM, van Groeningen CJ, de Greve J, Gruia G, Pinedo HM, Giaccone G. Continuous infusion of hepatic arterial irinotecan in pretreated patients with colorectal cancer metastatic to the liver. Ann Oncol 2004; 15(1):59–63.
77. Fiorentini G, Lucci SR, Giovanis P, Cantore M, Guadagni S, Papiani G. Irinotecan hepatic arterial infusion chemotherapy for hepatic metastases from colorectal cancer: results of a phase I clinical study. Tumori 2001; 87:388–390.

78. van Riel JM, van Groeningen CJ, Kedde MA, et al. Continuous administration of irinotecan by hepatic arterial infusion: a phase I and pharmacokinetic study. Clin Cancer Res 2002; 8(2):405–412.
79. Mancuso A, Giuliani R, Accettura C, et al. Hepatic arterial continuous infusion (HACI) of oxaliplatin in patients with unresectable liver metastases from colorectal cancer. Anticancer Res 2003; 23(2C):1917–1922.
80. Fiorentini G, Rossi S, Dentico P, et al. Oxaliplatin hepatic arterial infusion chemotherapy for hepatic metastases from colorectal cancer: a phase I–II clinical study. Anticancer Res 2004; 24(3b):2093–2096.
81. Kern W, Beckert B, Lang N, et al. Phase I and pharmacokinetic study of hepatic arterial infusion with oxaliplatin in combination with folinic acid and 5-fluorouracil in patients with hepatic metastases from colorectal cancer. Ann Oncol 2001; 12(5):599–603.
82. Ducreux M, Ychou M, Laplanche A, et al. Intra-arterial hepatic chemotherapy (IAHC) with oxaliplatin (O) combined with intravenous treatment with 5FU+folinic acid (FA) in hepatic metastases of colorectal cancer (HMCC). Proc Am Soc Clin Oncol 2003; 22:278.
83. Guthoff I, Lotspeich E, Fester C, et al. Hepatic artery infusion using oxaliplatin in combination with 5-fluorouracil, folinic acid and mitomycin C: oxaliplatin pharmacokinetics and feasibility. Anticancer Res 2003; 23(6D):5203–5208.
84. Tse A, Kemeny N, Raggio G, Morse M. A phase I clinical and pharmacokinetic study of escalating doses of fixed rate and escalating infusion duration of gemcitabine given via an intrahepatic pump for patients with hepatic metastases. 2006 ASCO Annual Meeting Proceedings, Part I. 2006; 24(S18):14035.
85. Leonard GD, Brenner B, Kemeny NE. Neoadjuvant chemotherapy before liver resection for patients with unresectable liver metastases from colorectal carcinoma. J Clin Oncol 2005; 23(9):2038–2048.
86. Tournigand C, Andre T, Achille E, et al. FOLFIRI followed by FOLFOX6 or the reverse sequence in advanced colorectal cancer: a randomized GERCOR study. J Clin Oncol 2004; 22(2):229–237.
87. Adam R, Avisar E, Ariche A, et al. Five-year survival following hepatic resection after neoadjuvant therapy for nonresectable colorectal. Ann Surg Oncol 2001; 8(4):347–353.
88. Meric F, Patt YZ, Curley SA, et al. Surgery after downstaging of unresectable hepatic tumors with intra-arterial chemotherapy. Ann Surg Oncol 2000; 7(7):490–495.
89. Adam R, Pascal G, Castaing D, et al. Tumor progression while on chemotherapy: a contraindication to liver resection for multiple colorectal metastases? Ann Surg 2004; 240(6):1052–1061; discussion 1061–1064.
90. Kemeny N, Gonen M, Sullivan D, et al. Phase I study of hepatic arterial infusion of floxuridine and dexamethasone with systemic irinotecan for unresectable hepatic metastases from colorectal cancer. J Clin Oncol 2001; 19(10):2687–2695.

18 The Role of Combined Modality Therapy for Anal Cancer

Kyriakos Papadopoulos
South Texas Accelerated Research Therapeutics, South Texas Oncology and Hematology, San Antonio, Texas, U.S.A.

Charles R. Thomas
Department of Radiation Medicine, Oregon Health and Sciences University, Portland, Oregon, U.S.A.

SQUAMOUS-CELL CANCER OF THE ANAL CANAL

Squamous-cell cancer (SCC) of the anal canal is an uncommon malignancy, with an annual incidence in the heterosexual population of one to two per 100,000. It occurs more frequently in women, with an increasing incidence in human immunodeficiency virus (HIV)-infected individuals. The majority of patients present with locoregional disease, of these 20% to 30% will develop distant metastases. What constitutes the most appropriate therapy for anal cancer has undergone significant evolution over the past three decades.

Risk Factors and Pathogenesis

A number of epidemiologic studies have linked sexual practices and genital viral infections to the development of anal cancer. A case control study in women and heterosexual men demonstrated that the relative risk of anal cancer is highest in those with 10 or more sexual partners or a history of anal warts and sexually transmitted infections (1). Receptive anal sex is a risk factor in both men and women. Smoking increases the risk of anal cancer up to fivefold in premenopausal women (2). Human papillomavirus type 16 has been implicated in the pathogenesis of anal intraepithelial neoplasia and invasive anal cancer (3). Whether HIV infection is directly involved in the pathogenesis of anal cancer remains unclear, but HIV infection predisposes to anal papillomavirus infection and an associated increased risk of anal cancer (4,5).

The Nonsurgical Treatment of Anal Cancer

Radiation Therapy

The intent of therapy for anal cancer is cure with the least morbidity. Traditionally, the primary treatment for SCC of the anal canal was abdominoperineal resection (APR). Depending on tumor stage, five-year survival after APR was 48% to 71% (6–10). Locoregional recurrence was common and ranged from 18% to 27%.

Contemporary studies for patients receiving radiotherapy alone reported similar five-year survival of 42% to 94%, but with typical sphincter preservation and colostomy-free survival of between 56% and 74% (11–16). Proponents of brachytherapy (BRT), with or without external-beam radiation therapy (EBRT), reported five-year survival rates of 60% to 65% and locoregional control rates of 75% to 79% (17–19). Retrospective studies show excellent local control and survival of >85% at five years obtained by radiotherapy alone for early stage T1-2 anal cancer (20,21). For in situ (Tis) and T1 tumors <1 m, treated with sphincter preserving resection and radiation (EBRT +/− BRT), Ortholan et al. report five-year overall and disease-free survival of 94% and 89%, respectively (22). Toxicity was acceptable, with only grade 1–2 late toxicity occurred in 27% of patients, less in those receiving <60 Gy (14%) than ≥60 Gy (37%). As with surgery, patients with larger tumors (>5 cm) or nodal involvement had poorer outcome with five-year survival of <60% (20,23,24). The optimal dose, intensity, and duration of radiotherapy either alone, or for that matter in combination with chemotherapy, as discussed later, remain to be defined. Radiation therapy, was thus considered an acceptable alternative to surgery, particularly for patients who might otherwise not be suitable surgical candidates. There is no randomized trial comparing these two modalities of treatment.

Chemoradiotherapy

The classic report in 1974 by Nigro et al., of complete pathologic response found at the time of APR in three patients with anal cancer treated with preoperative low-dose radiation (30–35 Gy) and concomitant 5-fluorouracil (5-FU) [1000 mg/m^2 continuous infusion (CI) days 1–4] and mitomycin (MMC) (10–15 mg/m^2 day 1), was a landmark both in the treatment of anal cancer and for proponents of combined-modality therapy (25). The concept emerged that anal cancer was curable without the need for radical surgery. Subsequent confirmation of the efficacy of concomitant chemoradiation therapy, with five-year survival rates and complete tumor regression rates of 60% to 90%, established this nonsurgical approach to SCC of the anal canal as the treatment of choice (12,15,26,27). The obvious benefit to nonsurgical therapy is the potential for sphincter preservation in 60% to 70% of patients, without apparent compromise in overall survival. Salvage surgical resection was generally performed only if residual tumor was present after initial chemoradiotherapy. No randomized trial comparing primary surgery to concomitant chemoradiation therapy for anal cancer has been nor is likely to be performed.

Radiation Therapy Vs. Chemoradiotherapy

The questions addressed in recent prospective trials of anal cancer therapy have focused on the role and efficacy of concomitant chemotherapy in locoregional control and sphincter preservation, and in determining the optimal chemotherapy regimen in terms of efficacy and toxicity for concomitant use with radiation.

The benefit of chemoradiotherapy compared to radiotherapy alone in improving local control of tumor was suggested in retrospective studies (12,17). Two prospective randomized phase III trials confirmed the utility of concomitant chemotherapy and radiation therapy in improving local control and reducing the need for colostomy in patients with anal cancer (Table 1). The United Kingdom Coordinating Committee on Cancer Research (UKCCCR) anal cancer trial (ACT I) randomized 585 patients with anal cancer to radiotherapy alone (45 Gy in 20–25 fractions, followed after six weeks by a booster of 15 Gy) or the same radiotherapy with chemotherapy (MMC-C 12 mg/m^2 day 1, 5-FU 1000mg/m^2 days 1–4 and days 29–32). In total, six deaths (2%) were attributed to chemoradiation among the 283 patients thus treated. At three years, local control was better in patients treated with chemoradiotherapy compared to radiation alone (61% vs. 39%). Disease-specific mortality at three years was higher in the radiotherapy patients (28% vs. 39%). Of note was the significant advantage to chemoradiotherapy in avoiding local recurrence even in T1 and T2 stage patients (28). In the second trial, the European Organization for Research and Treatment of Cancer (EORTC) randomized 110 patients to locally advanced anal cancer to radiotherapy alone (45 Gy in 25 fractions, followed six weeks later by a booster of 15–20 Gy) or with chemotherapy (MMC-C 15 mg/m^2 on day 1, 5-FU 750mg/m^2 on days 1–5 and days 29–33). There was one treatment death in the chemoradiotherapy group. Chemoradiation resulted in a higher complete response (CR) rate (80% vs. 54%). At five years, the chemoradiotherapy group had significantly better colostomy-free interval (70% vs. 40%) and local control (68% vs. 50%). No difference in overall survival was demonstrated in either study, likely reflecting the effectiveness of APR as salvage therapy for persistent or locally recurrent disease.

Efficacy of Chemotherapy Regimens

In a series of prospectively designed, sequential nonrando mized studies, Cunningham et al. showed the combination of MMC and 5-FU given concomitantly with radiation therapy to be more effective than 5-FU and radiation alone with respect to five-year, disease-specific survival rates (76% vs. 64%), local control (86% vs. 60%), and the likelihood of conservation of anorectal function (29). The prospectively randomized phase III Eastern Cooperative Oncology Group (ECOG)/Radiation Therapy Oncology Group (RTOG) 87-04 of 310 patients addressed the role of MMC in chemoradiotherapy (30). Patients with T1-4 tumors were randomized to receive radiotherapy (45–50.4 Gy in 25–28 fractions) and 5-FU (1000 mg/m^2 days 1–4 and days 29–32) or the same therapy with MMC (10 mg/m^2 day 1 and 29) (Table 1). Re-evaluation by biopsy at six weeks after therapy was performed. Patients with less than a CR received salvage chemoradiation with 5-FU and cisplatin. Abdominoperineal resection was performed if CR was not achieved at follow up after a further six weeks. An improved four-year disease-free (73% vs. 51%) and colostomy-free survival (71% vs. 59%) was conferred by the addition of MMC, particularly to patients with larger (T3/T4) tumors. Although associated with increased acute toxicity, this trial confirmed the favorable contribution of MMC to the regimen for chemoradiotherapy.

A sizable number of patients with locally advanced anal tumors receiving chemoradiotherapy will still ultimately require salvage APR. In an attempt to improve outcome and reduce toxicity, several investigators have examined the role of cisplatin, a potentially more effective chemotherapy agent and radiosensitizer, as a substitute for MMC. In a retrospective analysis, Hung et al. reported their experience with 92 patients treated with protracted daily infusion of cisplatin (4 mg/m^2/day) and 5-FU (250 mg/m^2/day) during radiation therapy (55 Gy in six weeks without a planned break) (31). The five-year survival rate was 85%, and colostomy-free survival was 82% with no patient requiring colostomy for symptom control. Local control was achieved in 83% of patients (T1/T2 90% and T3/T4 72%). The regimen was well-tolerated with <5% grade 4 acute toxicity. In another retrospective series, 95 patients were treated with cisplatin (25-mg/m^2/day bolus) and 5-FU (1000 mg/m^2/day) on days 1–4 of high-dose EBRT, followed at eight weeks by a boost with 192 Iridium implant. Five-year overall survival was 84%, and the cancer-specific survival was 90%. Locoregional control was 80% and the colostomy-free survival was 71% (32).

Two prospective phase II trials investigated the efficacy of cisplatin and 5-FU with radiotherapy (33,34) (Table 2). In an Italian study, 35 patients with anal cancer were treated with two cycles (or three cycles in eight patients) of chemotherapy (5-FU 750 mg/m^2 CI days 1–4 and cisplatin 100 mg/m^2 on day 1) starting on days 1 and 21 of radiation (33). Concurrent radiotherapy was given at a daily dose of 1.8 Gy up to a total dose of 36–38 Gy in four weeks with a boost dose of 18–24 Gy in 10 fractions. Complete response occurred in 33 patients (94%) and 86% were colostomy-free. The authors note that the response rate and toxicity of cisplatin and 5-FU compared favorably with their experience with 5-FU and MMC (35), but with a lower recurrence rate (6% vs. 24%). The ECOG phase II (E4292) trial of radiation therapy, 5-FU, and cisplatin for patients with T1-4 anal cancer treated 19 patients with radiation therapy (59.4 Gy in 33 fractions with a two-week treatment gap at 36 Gy). Concomitant chemotherapy consisted of 5-FU (1000 mg/m^2 days 1–4) and cisplatin (75 mg/m^2 day 1) with a second cycle when the radiation therapy was resumed. CR rate was 68%, with 79% of patients experiencing significant grade ≥3 toxicity and one treatment-related death. As all these studies used higher doses of radiation, comparison with MMC–based chemoradiotherapy regimens is made with caution.

The chemosensitivity of anal cancer to cisplatin-based regimens has suggested a potential role for neoadjuvant chemotherapy, particularly in patients with large tumors (Table 3). A phase II study of the Cancer and Leukemia Group B (CALGB) treated 45 patients with T3-4 tumors with two cycles of neoadjuvant cisplatin (100 mg/m^2 day 1) and 5-FU (1000 mg/m^2/day days 1–5) every four weeks, followed by radiation with 5-FU and MMC as per the RTOG 87-04 study. Induction chemotherapy led to a response rate of 65% (CR 18%) and 91% (CR 82%) after completion of therapy. At four years of follow up, overall patient survival was 68% , of which 61% were disease free and 50% colostomy free (36). This regimen constitutes the experimental arm of the current phase III RTOG 98-11 study. Peiffert et al. reported a phase II trial of two cycles each of neoadjuvant and concomitant cisplatin (80 mg/m^2 day 1) and 5-FU (800 mg/m^2 CI days 1–4) with split-course radiotherapy in 80 patients (37). Response rate after neoadjuvant therapy was 61% (CR 10%), and 98% (CR 93%) after completion of treatment. Three-year overall, relapse-free, and colostomy-free survival were 86%, 70%, and 73%, respectively. This regimen is in phase III testing in the Fondation Francaise de Cancerologie Digestive (FFCD) 98-04/ACCORD-3 trial.

Combined Modality Therapy as Salvage Treatment

Approximately 10% to 20% of patients will have residual disease after primary chemoradiotherapy. Anal cancer may continue to regress for weeks or months following therapy (29). Outside a clinical trial, as practiced in many instances, if residual disease is present at six-week post-treatment evaluation, patients are followed for a further six weeks. If there is no further response or progression, then salvage therapy is performed; otherwise, observation is continued, if the lesion is regressing.

Following the initial report by Flam et al. (38), the role of cisplatin-based chemotherapy as salvage for persistent disease after primary MMC-based chemoradiotherapy was further examined in the ECOG/RTOG 87-04 trial (30). Therapy consisted of radiotherapy (9 Gy to the primary site) with 5-FU (1000 mg/m^2 days 1–4) and cisplatin (100 mg/m^2 day 2). Of 22 assessable patients receiving salvage chemoradiotherapy, 50% were rendered disease free as assessed 12 weeks after initial therapy. There is some uncertainty whether this response rate is confounded by the tendency of anal cancer to continue to regress following initial therapy. Notwithstanding, the outcome of salvage CMT with cisplatin approximates that achieved with salvage APR. There is no clinical study comparing salvage chemoradiation to APR.

Sequelae and Limitations of Chemoradiotherapy for Squamous-Cell Anal Cancer

Chemoradiotherapy has replaced surgical resection as the treatment of choice for anal cancer, based on local disease control rates of 60% to 90% with sphincter preservation. The untested assumption is that the impact of sphincter preservation on quality-of-life (QOL) outweighs any acute and late morbidity relating to combination chemoradiotherapy. In practice, many patients are unable to tolerate or require dose modification of one or both components of the chemoradiotherapy. Furthermore, although sphincter preservation can be attained with chemoradiation, the issue of late toxicities, particularly sphincter dysfunction, has been less well addressed.

Acute grade 3–4 toxicities of chemoradiotherapy occur in 23% to 50% of patients (30,39,40). These toxicities include those predominantly caused by radiotherapy, such as skin reactions and diarrhea and those caused by chemotherapy, namely nausea, vomiting, mucositis, neutropenia, and infection. Most acute toxicities are acceptable to patients primarily because they tend to be self limiting, and supportive care measures to manage these toxicities continue to improve. Radiotherapy contributes substantially to acute toxicity. Attempts to attenuate these effects have included planned breaks in therapy and limiting dose and normal tissue exposure. Whether these maneuvers, while reducing toxicity, might affect efficacy, is unclear. Radiation dose may be an important determinant of response for larger tumors, with patients receiving ≥54-Gy EBRT achieving better local control (77–90% vs. 50–61%) than those receiving a lesser dose (41,42). Two phase II trials designed to administer higher doses of radiation (59.4–59.6 Gy), including a two-week break after 36 Gy, did not show any benefit over conventional radiotherapy (34,43). There is nonrandomized evidence suggesting a reduction in local control following intentional or unintentional breaks in radiotherapy (42,44), but no randomized trial has addressed the issues of duration and dose of radiotherapy. Toxic deaths in randomized chemoradiotherapy trials approximate 2% (30,39,40). By comparison, operative mortality for patients undergoing primary APR has been reported between 2% and 5%.

Late complications associated with radiation and chemotherapy can adversely affect the QOL of patients. Grade 3–4 complications occur in 10% to 19% of patients (17,20,27,29,45,46). Frequent late effects of chemoradiotherapy include chronic diarrhea, dysuria due to proctitis, chronic pelvic pain, fractures and sexual dysfunction (27,45,47). Complications of the anal canal occur in 15% to 30% of patients and include anal necrosis, stenosis, fistulae or ulceration, and anal incontinence (particularly if there was sphincter involvement by tumor). The incidence of radionecrosis in patients treated with BRT is 2% to 9% (48–50). In general, treatment-related anorectal complications require APR or colostomy in 3% to 6% of patients (39,40,44). In a retrospective study of 144 patients treated with radiation and chemotherapy, factors contributing to late toxicity included anatomical tumor extent and delivered dose of radiation. Patients receiving <39.6 Gy had a 7% complication rate, while those treated with ≥39.6 Gy had a 23% complication rate (45). Daily radiation-fraction dose is associated with rate and severity of late complications in some but not all studies (20,29).

The ECOG/RTOG 87-04 study confirmed that MMC significantly increases acute hematologic toxicity (18% vs. 3%) when combined with 5-FU and radiation therapy (30). Whether addition of 5-FU and MMC chemotherapy potentiates the side effects associated with radiotherapy was evaluated in the randomized phase III EORTC and UKCCCR trials. In the EORTC trial, acute side effects, such as diarrhea and skin reactions, were not different between the two treatment arms. Notably, reduction in the second cycle of chemotherapy was needed in 37% of patients, predominantly for myelosuppression. Except for more anal-canal ulcers in patients receiving chemoradiotherapy (18% vs. 4%), late toxicities were similar to those receiving only radiation. The increased incidence of ulcers may be explained by improved responses in the chemoradiotherapy patients. The UKCCCR ACT I trial reported more acute hematologic and nonhematologic toxicity in the chemoradiotherapy group compared to the radiotherapy alone group, while late morbidity was similar. Ten patients (3%) in each group required surgery for functional problems or radionecrosis. These cumulative data would suggest that addition of chemotherapy does not substantially increase late toxicity in patients with anal cancer treated with chemoradiotherapy.

An impetus to replacing MMC with cisplatin in chemoradiation regimens was the goal of reduced acute and late toxicity. Comparison of toxicities associated with 5-FU and MMC or cisplatin-based chemoradiation is difficult due to the lack of standard toxicity grading and absence of randomized trials. In a retrospective study of protracted cisplatin and 5-FU infusion and 55-Gy radiation, Hung et al. report acute toxicity in 75% of 92 patients, including diarrhea, skin desquamation, and nausea (31). However, only 5% of patients experienced grade 4 acute toxicity, and, unlike MMC-containing regimens, no patients experienced severe hematologic toxicity. Only two patients had anal complications and none required colostomy for incontinence or pain. A similar low rate of grade ≥3 acute and late toxicity is reported for a 5-FU and cisplatin regimen administered on days 1–4 every three weeks during radiation (33). In contrast, the high-dose radiation, 5-FU and cisplatin regimen utilized in the ECOG E4292 study, resulted in 63% grade ≥3 hematologic toxicity and 37% grade ≥4 toxicity (34).

Very few studies formally assess QOL in anal cancer patients who have had successful sphincter-preserving chemoradiotherapy. A Canadian study of 50 patients reported significant decreases in global and disease-specific aspects of QOL (51). By contrast, a Swiss study of 41 patients showed that, except for increased diarrhea and possibly decreased sexual role function, QOL was similar to the population-based sample (52). Similarly, Vordermark reported that long-term QOL was acceptable in most colostomy-free survivors of anal cancer, with normal anal function or complete continence ranging from 56% to 100% (53). All these studies are fraught with methodologic weaknesses; current and future randomized trials will hopefully provide an opportunity for reliable prospective assessment of QOL.

Patients at Potentially Increased Risk for Treatment-Related Adverse Events—Elderly and Human Immunodeficiency Virus-Infected Patients

Elderly patients, particularly those with poor performance status, may find it difficult to tolerate full-dose radiation and chemotherapy. Of the three randomized phase III studies in anal cancer, the EORTC trial was restricted to patients aged <76 years, while both the UKCCCR ACT I and ECOG/RTOG 87-04 trials had no age restriction. Neither of these latter studies specifically reports tolerance or outcome for the subset of elderly patients. In the UKCCCR study, frail elderly patients were excluded and the dose of MMC was reduced from 12 to 10 mg/m^2 in patients older than 70 years. Following fatal toxicity owing to sepsis in two elderly patients, a further protocol amendment lowered the MMC dose to 8 mg/m^2 in patients >80 years with the addition of co-trimoxazole prophylaxis. A study reported by Allal et al. suggests that with modified chemotherapy doses (5-FU 600 mg/m^2), tolerance and outcome are comparable with younger patients (54). Charnley et al. treated 16 elderly patients with 30 Gy and concurrent chemotherapy (5-FU 600 mg/m^2 CI days 1–4 of radiotherapy) (55). At a median follow up of 16 months, local control was 73% (13/16) and disease-specific survival 86%. The treatment was well tolerated with only one patient experiencing any grade 3 toxicity. These results of modified chemoradiation in elderly and poor performance patients are encouraging. Further exploration of oral regimens incorporating capecitabine rather than 5-FU for this population is ongoing.

In HIV-positive patients, the availability of highly active antiretroviral therapy (HAART) has not impacted anal cancer in terms of incidence and overall survival (56). Optimal therapy for advanced HIV patients with anal cancer is not well defined. Advanced HIV-infected patients tend to have poorer tolerance to chemoradiotherapy and shorter time to cancer-related death (57,58). Clinical data are limited, but attenuated radiation alone or surgical excision can be considered as alternatives in patients with small lesions. Patients with CD4 counts <200/µl or those with a history of opportunistic infections may experience increased morbidity with standard chemoradiotherapy and require close monitoring and timely treatment adjustment. In patients with adequate CD4 counts, standard chemoradiotherapy appears tolerable with equivalent efficacy (59–61).

Current Studies

The prognosis of anal cancer remains poor, particularly for patients with T3-4 tumors. Current randomized phase III trials are addressing the questions of alternative schedules and doses of chemotherapy and radiation therapy to try and improve outcome of untreated patients with anal cancer. The randomized ACT II trial has a 2 x 2 design, with patients receiving radiation and concurrent 5-FU (1000 mg/m^2 days 1–4 and 29–32) and either MMC (12 mg/m^2 day 1) or cisplatin (60 mg/m^2 days 1 and 29). Radiation therapy (50.4 Gy in 28 fractions) is given without a planned break. The second randomization compares two further cycles of 5-FU and cisplatin with observation after completion of CMT. This trial should answer the question of whether cisplatin is more effective and tolerable than MMC and the utility of cisplatin-based adjuvant therapy. Preliminary results on toxicity and outcome suggest that chemoradiation and adjuvant chemotherapy can be given without interruption and with acceptable toxicity.

Neoadjuvant 5-FU and cisplatin is tested in both the RTOG-9811 and FFCD 98-04/ACCORD-3 trials. The RTOG-9811 trial compares radiation and concurrent 5-FU/MMC with the experimental regimen of two cycles of neoadjuvant 5-FU and cisplatin followed by radiation with concurrent 5-FU/cisplatin. Radiation to 59.6 Gy is administered to patients with residual disease and all T3-4 and node-positive patients. If the cisplatin regimen proves more effective, the study design precludes determination of whether this is due to the neoadjuvant therapy or substitution of MMC for cisplatin during radiation. In the FFCD trial, patients are randomized between neoadjuvant 5-FU/cisplatin and no neoadjuvant therapy. All patients receive 5-FU/cisplatin and concurrent radiation (45 Gy in 25 fractions) followed by randomization to low-dose (15 Gy in eight fractions) or high-dose (20–25 Gy in 11–14 fractions) boost.

Treatment Recommendations

Newly diagnosed patients with anal cancer should undergo accurate staging, utilizing appropriate clinical and imaging techniques (62). Tumor size is the most important prognostic indicator in the SCC of the anal canal (19,63). Tumors <2 cm are cured in 90% of cases, and those >5 cm in less than 50% of cases (19). The EORTC randomized trial identified positive nodes, male gender, and skin ulceration as negative prognostic factors (40).

If a clinical trial is available, eligible patients should be encouraged to participate. For patients treated outside a trial setting, stage and performance status should guide treatment selection.

Patients with T1–T2 N0 disease should be offered chemoradiotherapy as standard therapy, supported by data from the ACT I randomized trial (39). In the United States, the most commonly used chemoradiotherapy regimen is radiation, 5-FU, and MCC as given in the RTOG 87-04 study (30). The RTOG 87-04 trial showed that the addition of MMC to 5-FU and radiation did not significantly impact colostomy rate reduction in T1-2 tumors. In immunocompromised or poor performance patients with small tumors, reduction of MMC dose can be considered. Radiotherapy as a single modality remains a viable consideration for patients with small tumors (<2 cm) unwilling or unable to tolerate combined modality therapy (19,29,50). For these patients, BRT with or without EBRT can yield similar local control and survival rates as chemoradiotherapy and can be offered in centers with the appropriate expertise, but is associated with increased incidence of radionecrosis even in experienced hands. Patients with small tumors (<1 cm), not involving the anal sphincter, can be offered excision with radiation therapy (50–60 Gy) (22).

Treatment of locally advanced anal cancer (T1-2 N1-3, T3-4 any N) with concomitant radiation and chemotherapy is a standard of care on the bases of large randomized trials (30,39,40). Patients with bulky disease can be considered candidates for cisplatin-based

(*Text continuous on page 208*)

TABLE 1 Randomized Phase III Trials of Chemoradiotherapy in Patients with Squamous-Cell Cancer of the Anal Canal

Trial	Patients (TNM stage)	Therapy	Boost/salvage therapy	CR %	LC % (yrs)	CFS % (yrs)	OS % (yrs)	Severe early toxicity %	% late toxicity	Surgery for complications %
UKCCCR[a]-ACT I	279	45-Gy EBRT	15-Gy EBRT or 25-Gy BRT[b]	—	39 (3)	—	58 (3)	16	38	3.6
		or			($P < 0.0001$)		ns	($p = 0.03$)	ns	
	283 (T1-4)	45-Gy EBRT + 5-FU 1 g/m^2 days 1–4 and 29–32 MMC 12 mg/m^2 day 1	15-Gy EBRT or 25-Gy BRT[b]	—	61 (3)	—	65 (3)	34	42	3.5
EORTC	51	45-Gy EBRT	15- to 20-Gy EBRT or BRT[c]	54	50 (5)	40 (5)	52 (5)	58	29 (4% anal ulcers)	3.8
		or			($P = 0.02$)	($P = 0.002$)	ns	ns		5.9
	52 (T3-4 T1-2 N1-3)	45-Gy EBRT + 5-FU 750 mg/m^2 days 1–5 and 29–33 MMC 15 mg/m^2 day 1	15- to 20-Gy EBRT or BRT[c]	80	68 (5)	72 (5)	57 (5)	78	43 (18% anal ulcers)	
RTOG/ ECOG	145	45 Gy + 5.4 Gy +[d] 5-FU 1 g/m^2 days 1–4 and 29–32	9 Gy + 5-FU and cisplatin 100 mg/m^2	86	—	59 (4)	67 (4)	7	1	—
		or				($p = 0.014$)	ns	($p < 0.001$)	ns	
	146 (T1-4)	45 Gy + 5.4 Gy +[d] 5-FU 1 g/m^2 days 1–4 and 29–32 MMC 10 mg/m^2 days 1 and 29	9 Gy + 5-FU and cisplatin 100 mg/ m^2	92	—	71 (4)	76 (4)	20	5	—

[a]Study included 23% of patients with anal margin cancers.
[b]Boost given after six weeks if ≥50% response, and if the response was ≤50%, the patient underwent resection.
[c]Boost given after six weeks—15 Gy if complete response, 20 Gy if partial response. If < partial response after initial therapy, patient underwent resection.
[d]Boost given for positive nodes or palpable residual disease after 45 Gy. If biopsy was positive six weeks after initial treatment, planned salvage therapy with 5-FU, cisplatin and radiation was administered.
Abbreviations: BRT, brachytherapy; CFS, colostomy-free survival; CR, complete response; EBRT, external-beam radiation therapy; ECOG, Eastern Cooperative Oncology Group; EORTC, European Organization for Research and Treatment of Cancer; LC, local control; MMC, mitomycin C; OS, overall survival; RTOG, Radiation Therapy Oncology Group; TNM, tumor node metastases; UKCCCR, United Kingdom Coordinating Committee on Cancer Research; 5-FU, fluorouracil; ns, not significant.

TABLE 2 Prospective Phase II Trials of Chemoradiotherapy Incorporating Cisplatin in Patients with Squamous-Cell Cancer of the Anal Canal

Trial	Patients (TNM stage)	Chemoradiotherapy	Boost	Median follow-up	CR %	LC %	CFS %	OS % (yrs)	Severe early toxicity %	Surgery for complications %
Doci	35 (T1-3)	36 to 38-Gy EBRT + 5-FU 750 mg/m^2 days 1–4 and 22–25 Cisplatin 100 mg/m^2 days 1 and 22	18 to 24-Gy EBRT[a]	37 mo	94	94	86	94 (3)	11	3
Martenson ECOG E4292	19 (T1-4)	36 Gy + 9-Gy EBRT (starting on day 43 after two weeks' break) + 5-FU 1 g/m^2 days 1–4 and 43–46 Cisplatin 75 mg/m^2 days 1 and 43	14.4-Gy EBRT[b]	33 mo	68	79			79	

[a]Median dose of 57 Gy delivered over six weeks.
[b]Total dose of 59.4 Gy in 33 fractions over 60 days.
Abbreviations: CFS, colostomy-free survival; CR, complete response; EBRT, external-beam radiation therapy; ECOG, Eastern Cooperative Oncology Group; LC, local control; OS, overall survival; TNM, tumor node metastases; 5-FU, fluorouracil.

TABLE 3 Prospective Phase II Trials of Neoadjuvant Cisplatin-Based Combined Modality Therapy in Patients with Squamous-Cell Cancer of the Anal Canal

Trial	Patients (stage)	Phase of treatment	Chemoradiotherapy	CR %	CFS % (yrs)	OS % (yrs)	Grade 3/4 early toxicity	NV/D	Neutropenia	Mucositis	Cutaneous %
Peiffert	80 (T1-4)	Neoadjuvant	5-FU 1 g/m^2 days 1–4, wks 1 and 5 Cisplatin 80 mg/m^2 day 1, wks 1 and 5	10	73 (3)	86 (3)	Cycle 1 Cycle 2	11/0 13/0	3 4	1 0	0 0
		+ Concomitant	45 Gy + 5-FU 1 g/m^2 days 57–60 and 85–88 Cisplatin 80 mg/m^2 days 57 and 85	67			Cycle 3 Cycle 4	10/8 7/7	4 3	2 0	16 15
		+ Boost	20-Gy EBRT or 15-Gy BRT[b]	94[a]							
Meropol	45	Neoadjuvant	5-FU 1 g/m^2 days 1–5, wks 1 and 5 Cisplatin 100 mg/m^2 day 1 wks 1 and 5	18	50 (4)	68 (4)		22/6	44	39	—
CALGB	(T3-4)	+ Concomitant	45 Gy wks 9–16[c] + 5-FU 1 g/m^2 days 1–4, wks 9 and 15 MMC 10 mg/m^2 day 1 wks 9 and 15								
		+ Salvage	9 Gy wk 19 + 5-FU 800 mg/m^2 days 1–5 cisplatin 100 mg/m^2 day 1 wk 19	82				8/10	43	3	—

[a]Includes four abdominoperitoneal resection patients.
[b]Boost given four to eight weeks after completion of chemoradiation.
[c]Planned break of two weeks after 30.6 Gy.
Abbreviations: BRT, brachytherapy; CALGB, cancer and leukemia group B; CFS, colostomy-free survival; CR, complete response; EBRT, external–beam radiation therapy; LC, local control; MMC, mitomycin C; NV/D, Nausea Vomiting/Diarrhea; OS, overall survival; 5-FU, fluorouracil.

neoadjuvant chemotherapy on the basis of two well-executed phase II trials (36,64). Patients who have residual disease following MMC-based chemoradiotherapy may benefit from salvage therapy with reradiation, cisplatin, and 5-FU (30,65). Abdominoperineal resection remains standard therapy for locoregional relapse. In patients unwilling to undergo surgery, cisplatin, 5-FU and reradiation can be considered.

Despite salvage therapy for locoregional relapse, overall five-year survival is 50%, with 10–33% of patients dying with systemic disease, predominantly involving the liver and lungs. Chemotherapy options are limited for patients with recurrence who have failed salvage cisplatin-based chemotherapy and surgery. Patients in these circumstances should be encouraged to enter clinical trials. The survival benefit of systemic therapy for patients with metastatic cancer is unclear. Cisplatin and 5-FU in the treatment of metastatic anal cancer shows encouraging responses, and is well tolerated (66).

CONCLUSION

Despite the absence of randomized trials to support current practice, chemoradiotherapy has supplanted surgical resection as the standard of care for SCC of the anal canal, on the strength of retrospective and prospective trials showing similar survival, but with the advantage of sphincter preservation in the majority of patients. Chemoradiotherapy is however not without significant acute and late morbidity that can adversely affect the patient's QOL.

Current ongoing trials will hopefully answer some of the important questions regarding the role of radiation and neoadjuvant, concomitant, and adjuvant chemotherapy and define the most appropriate and least-toxic therapy for patients with anal cancer. Establishing the best standard of care will provide a platform to investigate newer cytotoxic and targeted therapies and emerging radiation technology.

REFERENCES

1. Friis S, Kjaer SK, Frisch M, Mellemkjaer L, Olsen JH. Cervical intraepithelial neoplasia, anogenital cancer, and other cancer types in women after hospitalization for condylomata acuminata. J Infect Dis 1997; 175(4):743–748.
2. Frisch M, Fenger C, van den Brule AJ, et al. Variants of squamous cell carcinoma of the anal canal and perianal skin and their relation to human papillomaviruses. Cancer Res 1999; 59(3):753–757.
3. Frisch M, Glimelius B, van den Brule AI, et al. [Sexually transmitted infection as a cause of anal cancer]. Ugeskr Laeger 1998; 160(49):7109–7117.
4. Palefsky JM. Human papillomavirus infection and anogenital neoplasia in human immunodeficiency virus-positive men and women. J Natl Cancer Inst Monogr 1998; 23:15–20.
5. Critchlow CW, Surawicz CM, Holmes KK, et al. Prospective study of high grade anal squamous intraepithelial neoplasia in a cohort of homosexual men: influence of HIV infection, immunosuppression and human papillomavirus infection. Aids 1995; 9(11):1255–1262.
6. Beahrs OH, Wilson SM. Carcinoma of the anus. Ann Surg 1976; 184(4):422–428.
7. Boman BM, Moertel CG, O'Connell MJ, et al. Carcinoma of the anal canal. A clinical and pathologic study of 188 cases. Cancer 1984; 54(1):114–125.
8. Greenall MJ, Quan SH, Stearns MW, Urmacher C, DeCosse JJ. Epidermoid cancer of the anal margin. Pathologic features, treatment, and clinical results. Am J Surg 1985; 149(1):95–101.
9. Hardcastle JD, Bussey HJ. Results of surgical treatment of squamous cell carcinoma of the anal canal and anal margin seen at St. Mark's Hospital 1928–66. Proc R Soc Med 1968; 61(6):629–630.
10. Pintor MP, Northover JM, Nicholls RJ. Squamous cell carcinoma of the anus at one hospital from 1948 to 1984. Br J Surg 1989; 76(8):806–810.
11. Cantril ST, Green JP, Schall GL, Schaupp WC. Primary radiation therapy in the treatment of anal carcinoma. Int J Radiat Oncol Biol Phys 1983; 9(9):1271–1278.
12. Cummings B, Keane T, Thomas G, Harwood A, Rider W. Results and toxicity of the treatment of anal canal carcinoma by radiation therapy or radiation therapy and chemotherapy. Cancer 1984; 54(10):2062–2068.
13. Newman G, Calverley DC, Acker BD, Manji M, Hay J, Flores AD. The management of carcinoma of the anal canal by external beam radiotherapy, experience in Vancouver 1971–1988. Radiother Oncol 1992; 25(3):196–202.
14. Martenson JA, Jr., Gunderson LL. External radiation therapy without chemotherapy in the management of anal cancer. Cancer 1993; 71(5):1736–1740.
15. Allal A, Kurtz JM, Pipard G, et al. Chemoradiotherapy versus radiotherapy alone for anal cancer: a retrospective comparison. Int J Radiat Oncol Biol Phys 1993; 27(1):59–66.

16. Doggett SW, Green JP, Cantril ST. Efficacy of radiation therapy alone for limited squamous cell carcinoma of the anal canal. Int J Radiat Oncol Biol Phys 1988; 15(5):1069–1072.
17. Papillon J, Montbarbon JF. Epidermoid carcinoma of the anal canal. A series of 276 cases. Dis Colon Rectum 1987; 30(5):324–333.
18. Ng Ying Kin NY, Pigneux J, Auvray H, Brunet R, Thomas L, Denepoux R. Our experience of conservative treatment of anal canal carcinoma combining external irradiation and interstitial implant: 32 cases treated between 1973 and 1982. Int J Radiat Oncol Biol Phys 1988; 14(2):253–259.
19. Peiffert D, Bey P, Pernot M, et al. Conservative treatment by irradiation of epidermoid cancers of the anal canal: prognostic factors of tumoral control and complications. Int J Radiat Oncol Biol Phys 1997; 37(2):313–324.
20. Touboul E, Schlienger M, Buffat L, et al. Epidermoid carcinoma of the anal canal. Results of curative-intent radiation therapy in a series of 270 patients. Cancer 1994; 73(6):1569–1579.
21. Myerson RJ, Kong F, Birnbaum EH, et al. Radiation therapy for epidermoid carcinoma of the anal canal, clinical and treatment factors associated with outcome. Radiother Oncol 2001; 61(1):15–22.
22. Ortholan C, Ramaioli A, Peiffert D, et al. Anal canal carcinoma: early-stage tumors </=10 mm (T1 or Tis): therapeutic options and original pattern of local failure after radiotherapy. Int J Radiat Oncol Biol Phys 2005; 62(2):479–485.
23. Eschwege F, Lasser P, Chavy A, et al. Squamous cell carcinoma of the anal canal: treatment by external beam irradiation. Radiother Oncol 1985; 3(2):145–150.
24. James RD, Pointon RS, Martin S. Local radiotherapy in the management of squamous carcinoma of the anus. Br J Surg 1985; 72(4):282–285.
25. Nigro ND, Vaitkevicius VK, Considine B, Jr. Combined therapy for cancer of the anal canal: a preliminary report. Dis Colon Rectum 1974; 17(3):354–356.
26. Nigro ND. An evaluation of combined therapy for squamous cell cancer of the anal canal. Dis Colon Rectum 1984; 27(12):763–766.
27. Tanum G, Tveit K, Karlsen KO, Hauer-Jensen M. Chemotherapy and radiation therapy for anal carcinoma. Survival and late morbidity. Cancer 1991; 67(10):2462–2466.
28. Northover J, Meadows H, Ryan C, Gray R. Combined radiotherapy and chemotherapy for anal cancer. Lancet 1997; 349:205–206.
29. Cummings BJ, Keane TJ, O'Sullivan B, Wong CS, Catton CN. Epidermoid anal cancer: treatment by radiation alone or by radiation and 5-fluorouracil with and without mitomycin C. Int J Radiat Oncol Biol Phys 1991; 21(5):1115–1125.
30. Flam M, John M, Pajak TF, et al. Role of mitomycin in combination with fluorouracil and radiotherapy, and of salvage chemoradiation in the definitive nonsurgical treatment of epidermoid carcinoma of the anal canal: results of a phase III randomized intergroup study. J Clin Oncol 1996; 14(9):2527–2539.
31. Hung A, Crane C, Delclos M, et al. Cisplatin-based combined modality therapy for anal carcinoma: a wider therapeutic index. Cancer 2003; 97(5):1195–1202.
32. Gerard JP, Ayzac L, Hun D, et al. Treatment of anal canal carcinoma with high dose radiation therapy and concomitant fluorouracil-cisplatinum. Long-term results in 95 patients. Radiother Oncol 1998; 46(3):249–256.
33. Doci R, Zucali R, La Monica G, et al. Primary chemoradiation therapy with fluorouracil and cisplatin for cancer of the anus: results in 35 consecutive patients. J Clin Oncol 1996; 14(12):3121–3125.
34. Martenson JA, Lipsitz SR, Wagner H, Jr., et al. Initial results of a phase II trial of high dose radiation therapy, 5-fluorouracil, and cisplatin for patients with anal cancer (E4292): an Eastern Cooperative Oncology Group study. Int J Radiat Oncol Biol Phys 1996; 35(4):745–749.
35. Doci R, Zucali R, Bombelli L, Montalto F, Lamonica G. Combined chemoradiation therapy for anal cancer. A report of 56 cases. Ann Surg 1992; 215(2):150–156.
36. Meropol NJ, Niedzwiecki D, Shank B, et al. Combined-modality therapy of poor prognosis anal canal carcinoma: a phase II study of the Cancer and Leukemia Group B (CALGB). 2005 Gastrointestinal Cancers Symposium 2005:Abstr 238.
37. Peiffert D, Giovannini M, Ducreux M, et al. High-dose radiation therapy and neoadjuvant plus concomitant chemotherapy with 5-fluorouracil and cisplatin in patients with locally advanced squamous-cell anal canal cancer: final results of a phase II study. Ann Oncol 2001; 12(3):397–404.
38. Flam MS, John MJ, Mowry PA, Lovalvo LJ, Ramalho LD, Wade J. Definitive combined modality therapy of carcinoma of the anus. A report of 30 cases including results of salvage therapy in patients with residual disease. Dis Colon Rectum 1987; 30(7):495–502.
39. Epidermoid anal cancer: results from the UKCCCR randomised trial of radiotherapy alone versus radiotherapy, 5-fluorouracil, and mitomycin. UKCCCR Anal Cancer Trial Working Party. UK Co-ordinating Committee on Cancer Research. Lancet 1996; 348(9034):1049–1054.
40. Bartelink H, Roelofsen F, Eschwege F, et al. Concomitant radiotherapy and chemotherapy is superior to radiotherapy alone in the treatment of locally advanced anal cancer: results of a phase III randomized trial of the European Organization for Research and Treatment of Cancer Radiotherapy and Gastrointestinal Cooperative Groups. J Clin Oncol 1997; 15(5):2040–2049.
41. Hughes LL, Rich TA, Delclos L, Ajani JA, Martin RG. Radiotherapy for anal cancer: experience from 1979–1987. Int J Radiat Oncol Biol Phys 1989; 17(6):1153–1160.

42. Constantinou EC, Daly W, Fung CY, Willett CG, Kaufman DS, DeLaney TF. Time-dose considerations in the treatment of anal cancer. Int J Radiat Oncol Biol Phys 1997; 39(3):651–657.
43. John M, Pajak T, Flam M, et al. Dose escalation in chemoradiation for anal cancer: preliminary results of RTOG 92-08. Cancer J Sci Am 1996; 2(4):205–211.
44. Allal AS, Mermillod B, Roth AD, Marti MC, Kurtz JM. The impact of treatment factors on local control in T2-T3 anal carcinomas treated by radiotherapy with or without chemotherapy. Cancer 1997; 79(12):2329–2335.
45. Allal AS, Mermillod B, Roth AD, Marti MC, Kurtz JM. Impact of clinical and therapeutic factors on major late complications after radiotherapy with or without concomitant chemotherapy for anal carcinoma. Int J Radiat Oncol Biol Phys 1997; 39(5):1099–1105.
46. Wagner JP, Mahe MA, Romestaing P, et al. Radiation therapy in the conservative treatment of carcinoma of the anal canal. Int J Radiat Oncol Biol Phys 1994; 29(1):17–23.
47. John M, Flam M, Palma N. Ten-year results of chemoradiation for anal cancer: focus on late morbidity. Int J Radiat Oncol Biol Phys 1996; 34(1):65–69.
48. Papillon J, Mayer M, Montbarbon JF, Gerard JP, Chassard JL, Bailly C. A new approach to the management of epidermoid carcinoma of the anal canal. Cancer 1983; 51(10):1830–1837.
49. Papillon J, Montbarbon JF, Gerard JP, Chassard JL, Ardiet JM. Interstitial curietherapy in the conservative treatment of anal and rectal cancers. Int J Radiat Oncol Biol Phys 1989; 17(6):1161–1169.
50. Sandhu AP, Symonds RP, Robertson AG, Reed NS, McNee SG, Paul J. Interstitial iridium-192 implantation combined with external radiotherapy in anal cancer: ten years experience. Int J Radiat Oncol Biol Phys 1998; 40(3):575–581.
51. Jephcott CR, Paltiel C, Hay J. Quality of life after non-surgical treatment of anal carcinoma: a case control study of long-term survivors. Clin Oncol (R Coll Radiol) 2004; 16(8):530–535.
52. Allal AS, Sprangers MA, Laurencet F, Reymond MA, Kurtz JM. Assessment of long-term quality of life in patients with anal carcinomas treated by radiotherapy with or without chemotherapy. Br J Cancer 1999; 80(10):1588–1594.
53. Vordermark D, Sailer M, Flentje M, Thiede A, Kolbl O. Curative-intent radiation therapy in anal carcinoma: quality of life and sphincter function. Radiother Oncol 1999; 52(3):239–243.
54. Allal AS, Obradovic M, Laurencet F, et al. Treatment of anal carcinoma in the elderly: feasibility and outcome of radical radiotherapy with or without concomitant chemotherapy. Cancer 1999; 85(1):26–31.
55. Charnley N, Choudhury A, Chesser P, Cooper RA, Sebag-Montefiore D. Effective treatment of anal cancer in the elderly with low-dose chemoradiotherapy. Br J Cancer 2005; 92(7):1221–1225.
56. Bower M, Powles T, Newsom-Davis T, et al. HIV-associated anal cancer: has highly active antiretroviral therapy reduced the incidence or improved the outcome? J Acquir Immune Defic Syndr 2004; 37(5):1563–1565.
57. Holland JM, Swift PS. Tolerance of patients with human immunodeficiency virus and anal carcinoma to treatment with combined chemotherapy and radiation therapy. Radiology 1994; 193(1):251–254.
58. Kim JH, Sarani B, Orkin BA, Young HA, White J, Tannebaum I, et al. HIV-positive patients with anal carcinoma have poorer treatment tolerance and outcome than HIV-negative patients. Dis Colon Rectum 2001; 44(10):1496–1502.
59. Cleator S, Fife K, Nelson M, Gazzard B, Phillips R, Bower M. Treatment of HIV-associated invasive anal cancer with combined chemoradiation. Eur J Cancer 2000; 36(6):754–758.
60. Hoffman R, Welton ML, Klencke B, Weinberg V, Krieg R. The significance of pretreatment CD4 count on the outcome and treatment tolerance of HIV-positive patients with anal cancer. Int J Radiat Oncol Biol Phys 1999; 44(1):127–131.
61. Peddada AV, Smith DE, Rao AR, Frost DB, Kagan AR. Chemotherapy and low-dose radiotherapy in the treatment of HIV-infected patients with carcinoma of the anal canal. Int J Radiat Oncol Biol Phys 1997; 37(5):1101–1105.
62. Khatri VP, Chopra S. Clinical presentation, imaging, and staging of anal cancer. Surg Oncol Clin N Am 2004; 13(2):295–308.
63. Schlienger M, Krzisch C, Pene F, et al. Epidermoid carcinoma of the anal canal treatment results and prognostic variables in a series of 242 cases. Int J Radiat Oncol Biol Phys 1989; 17(6):1141–1151.
64. Peiffert D, Seitz JF, Rougier P, et al. Preliminary results of a phase II study of high-dose radiation therapy and neoadjuvant plus concomitant 5-fluorouracil with CDDP chemotherapy for patients with anal canal cancer: a French cooperative study. Ann Oncol 1997; 8(6):575–581.
65. Flam MS, John M, Lovalvo LJ, et al. Definitive nonsurgical therapy of epithelial malignancies of the anal canal. A report of 12 cases. Cancer 1983; 51(8):1378–1387.
66. Ajani JA, Carrasco CH, Jackson DE, Wallace S. Combination of cisplatin plus fluoropyrimidine chemotherapy effective against liver metastases from carcinoma of the anal canal. Am J Med 1989; 87(2):221–224.

19 The Role of Surgery for Squamous-Cell Cancer of the Anal Canal

Dimitra G. Barabouti
James H. Quillen VA Medical Center, Mountain Home, Tennessee, U.S.A.

W. Douglas Wong
Department of Surgery, Memorial Sloan-Kettering Cancer Center and Cornell University Medical College, New York, New York, U.S.A.

The current mainstay of treatment for squamous-cell carcinoma (SCCa) of the anal canal is combined chemotherapy and radiation (CRT). In the 1970s, Nigro and his coworkers demonstrated that CRT produced local control rates similar to those of surgery, while offering the additional advantage of sphincter preservation (1–4). Several subsequent studies (including large, prospective randomized trials) have confirmed the superiority of combined CRT, compared to RT alone, in achieving local control and improving survival (5). A randomized prospective trial by the Radiation Therapy Oncology Group/Eastern Cooperative Oncology Group suggested that in large tumors (equal to or greater than 5 cm), the addition of mitomycin C improves local control (83% complete response rate), colostomy-free survival, and disease-free survival, although it is associated with greater hematologic toxicity (6).

The complete response rates of initial CRT for anal SCCa range from 75% to 95%, leaving 5% to 25% with persistent disease (7,8). Another 10% to 30% of patients can be expected to recur at a later date. Local failure is frequently isolated, without distant metastases, and is therefore potentially amenable to salvage surgery. Currently, surgery is considered for those patients who fail initial CRT (having either residual or recurrent disease) or those who develop toxic side effects and must therefore discontinue treatment. Additionally, patients with persistent or recurrent inguinal lymphadenopathy after groin RT may benefit from lymphadenectomy.

This review discusses the indications for surgical treatment of anal SCCa, the results of relevant studies, and the practice followed at Memorial Sloan-Kettering Cancer Center (MSKCC).

SURGERY FOR RESIDUAL AND RECURRENT ANAL SQUAMOUS-CELL CARCINOMA

Previous studies on the outcomes of salvage surgery after initial CRT for anal SCCa are retrospective, and the majority of these are small. Residual disease has been determined by positive biopsy less than six months following the end of treatment. Recurrence is usually determined by positive biopsy more than six months after cessation of treatment.

Some information on salvage surgery after CRT can be gleaned from studies reporting the overall experience of single institutions in treating anal SCCa. In 1994, Tanum reported on the outcomes of a study of 94 patients with anal SCCa treated with CRT at the Norwegian Radium Hospital in Oslo between 1983 and 1989 (9). There were 11 cases of local recurrence, of which nine cases were treated with salvage abdominoperineal resection (APR). Of this small group, six patients were alive and free of disease after three years of follow-up.

Longo et al. retrospectively studied outcomes for 164 patients treated for anal SCCa in 159 Veterans Affairs hospitals from 1987 to 1991 (10). Recurrent disease was identified in 29% of the patients, and multivariate analysis identified initial stage and method of treatment as predictors for recurrence. Fifty-three percent of patients who underwent salvage APR ($n=17$) were alive at the conclusion of follow-up, compared to only 19% of those treated with salvage chemotherapy with or without RT ($n=15$).

In 1998, Grabenbauer et al. published their experience with treatment of anal SCCa (11). A total of 62 patients received CRT over a period of 11 years. At five years, actuarial cancer-related survival, disease-free survival, and colostomy-free survival rates were 81%, 76%, and 86%, respectively. The authors identified higher tumor stage and nodal disease as predictors of poor outcome. Seven patients had local failure and were treated with salvage APR, with long-term control in four.

Faynsod et al. performed a retrospective analysis of 81 patients treated for anal SCCa at Harbor-UCLA Medical Center over a period of 36 years. They reported 100% disease-free survival, at three years, for five patients who had local recurrence after CRT and were treated with salvage APR (12).

Deniaud-Alexandre et al. reported on outcomes for 305 patients with anal SCCa treated with RT over a 25-year period at Tenon Hospital, Paris (13). Their overall results were good, showing better response rates for early stage tumors (complete response was 96% for T1 lesions, 87% for T2 lesions, 79% for T3 lesions, and 44% for T4 lesions). The authors treated approximately half of those patients who had residual disease (27 out of 61) or recurrent disease (20 out of 37) with salvage APR, reporting an overall local control rate (with or without salvage therapy) of 84%.

Nguyen et al. studied 51 anal SCCa patients treated with CRT at the Oschsner Clinic, in order to identify those at higher risk for residual or recurrent disease and subsequent need for a stoma (14). Their analysis indicated that initial tumor size, but not RT dose, was significantly associated with the need for a stoma. Nodal disease was the only independent predictor of mortality. The authors suggested that patients with large tumors on presentation are more likely to require a stoma eventually for persistent or recurrent disease.

The studies focusing on salvage surgery for anal SCCa after CRT are mostly small, and report on oncologic outcome and morbidity of surgery as well as potential prognostic factors. Two of these studies show disappointingly high rates of surgical failure. In a study by Zelnick et al., nine patients with anal SCCa were treated with salvage APR after failing CRT (15). Eight patients had residual disease, and one patient had local recurrence. The outcome was poor, with 89% (eight of nine) dying of disease progression. Smith et al. also reported dismal results with salvage APR in their study of 22 patients, with 18 (82%) patients dying of recurrent disease in a mean time of 19 months (16). Of note, 10 of these 18 patients had residual disease left at the time of surgery. In contrast, two women with T4 disease extending into the vagina achieved long-term survival following salvage APR and posterior vaginectomy.

The remainder of the dedicated salvage surgery studies report more favorable local control and survival rates, as well as similar morbidity rates. Van der Waal et al. retrospectively studied 17 patients treated with salvage APR after CRT failure (17). Twelve patients had persistent disease, and five had recurrent disease. Prolonged survival was achieved in about half of these patients, with five-year actuarial survival of 47%. Tumor size greater than 5.0 cm and age over 55 years were predictive of poor outcome. There was a significant incidence of perineal wound complications; this was higher in patients with omental flap reconstruction, compared to those with muscle flap reconstruction of the perineal defect.

Ghouti et al. recently published a retrospective study of 36 anal SCCa patients treated with salvage APR after initial CRT (18). Twenty-three patients (64%) developed recurrent disease following surgery, in a mean interval of 30 months. Overall five-year survival was 69%. There was no significant difference in five-year survival between patients with persistent disease ($n=15$) and patients with local recurrence ($n=21$). Perineal morbidity was significant, with a 70% incidence of wound breakdown.

An interesting and somewhat controversial issue is the difference in oncologic outcome, seen in several studies, between patients with residual disease and patients with recurrent disease. Pocard et al. studied 21 patients with residual (11) or recurrent (10) anal SCCa who underwent APR following initial RT (19). The overall survival rate at three years after surgery was 58%. The group with residual disease fared significantly better than the group with recurrent disease, with an overall survival rate of 72% at three years (vs. 29%) and 60% at five years (vs. zero).

Other studies, however, contradict Pocard's observations. Bai et al. retrospectively reviewed 16 anal SCCa patients treated with salvage surgery, after failure of initial RT, over a period of 16 years at the Cancer Hospital of Chinese Academy of Medical Sciences (20). Of 16 patients, 14 patients underwent APR and 2 patients had transanal excision. Long-term (10-year) survival was achieved in 38% of these patients ($n = 6$). For patients who succumbed to disease, the mean survival time following surgery was 16 months. In this study, five patients with recurrent disease had better 10-year survival overall than 11 patients with persistent disease. The outcome of salvage surgery appeared to correlate with initial stage, as the majority of survivors had a smaller tumor, without nodal disease, on presentation. Complications related to the perineal wound occurred in eight patients.

Similar results were obtained by Nilsson et al., in a study of 35 patients with local failure after CRT who were treated with salvage APR at the Stockholm Health Care Region (21). Five-year survival in this group was 52%. Patients with local recurrence did significantly better than patients with persistent disease, with a five-year survival rate of 82% versus 33%. There was significant morbidity related to the perineal wound, including wound infections and delayed healing (66%).

Allal et al. reported comparable findings in their study of 42 anal SCCa patients with local failure after CRT at the Geneva University Hospital, Switzerland (22). In this group, APR was considered the salvage treatment of choice in cases of potentially curable disease. Local excision was performed only in patients considered unfit for APR, or those with very limited failures. Overall, 26 of the 42 patients (62%) underwent potentially curative salvage surgery; specifically, 23 had APR and 3 underwent local excision. All those who were not candidates for potential surgical salvage died of disease progression in a mean interval of 11 months. Initial early tumor stage appeared to correlate with better outcome; 41% of patients without nodal disease at presentation were salvaged successfully, as opposed to only 17% of patients with lymph node involvement. Moreover, salvage proved unfeasible in all patients with initial T4 tumors. The 26 patients treated with salvage surgery had an overall five-year survival of 45%, with five-year local and locoregional control rates of 53% and 43%, respectively. Patients with local recurrence after initial complete response to CRT had a better outcome, with 10 of 22 (45%) achieving long-term survival. In contrast, patients with residual disease after CRT did poorly, with only one patient alive after salvage APR at the conclusion of follow-up.

Overall, patients with recurrent disease after CRT appear to have a better outcome when compared to those with residual disease. This difference may be related to the advanced initial tumor stage of many patients with persistent disease following CRT. Alternatively, it may be related to the more aggressive biologic phenotypes of tumors that are resistant to chemoradiotherapy.

The experience at MSKCC with salvage surgery for anal SCCa after failure of CRT was initially reported by Ellenhorn et al. in 1994, in a study of 38 patients: 24 with residual disease and 14 with local recurrence (23). Actuarial five-year survival was 44%. Twenty-three patients developed recurrent disease after salvage APR. Inguinal lymphadenopathy at initial presentation, fixation of tumor to the pelvic sidewall, and pathologic involvement of the perirectal at were identified as predictors of poor outcome.

In 2004, Akbari et al. updated the MSKCC data in a retrospective analysis of 62 anal SCCa patients treated with salvage surgery (24). Five patients underwent inguinal lymphadenectomy only for regional disease, and were analyzed separately. Overall 5-year survival was 33% (median, 34 months). Patients undergoing potentially curative resections ($n = 47$) had a five-year survival of 40% (median, 49 months). Patients with local recurrence after CRT had a five-year survival of 51%, higher than that of patients with persistent disease (31%). After potentially curative resections, most recurrences (74%) were locoregional and were seen within two years (79%). Five-year recurrence-free survival was 46%.

On univariate analysis, the study identified tumor size >5 cm, or adjacent organ involvement, lymph node involvement, and positive margins as predictors of decreased survival. However, tumor size or adjacent organ involvement at salvage lacked statistical significance in predicting survival on multivariate analysis. Independent predictors of decreased survival were the presence of lymph node disease, and positive margins at salvage. It is likely that tumor size and nodal status are correlated, with nodal status being the more dominant prognostic factor. In the potentially curative subgroup, independent predictors of poor outcome (survival and recurrence) included nodal disease at salvage and persistence of disease after CRT.

Some have proposed salvage CRT instead of surgery. In 1996, Flam et al. reported the results of additional pelvic RT (9 Gy), 5-fluorouracil (5-FU), and cisplatin for persistent local disease, documented by biopsies four to six weeks after initial CRT for anal SCCa (6). Of 22 patients receiving this salvage regimen, 11 (50%) were alive without disease at four years, but only four patients avoided APR. The significance of these results is uncertain, since the effect of RT continues for some time following completion of CRT, making it a possibility that some patients who have positive biopsies a few weeks after treatment may, on longer follow-up, be seen to achieve complete disease remission. Furthermore, although chemotherapy with low-dose RT may be feasible for patients initially treated with moderate RT doses (range, 45–50 Gy), its safety and efficacy in those who have previously received high RT doses (≥60 Gy) are questionable.

In summary, salvage APR carries significant morbidity, mostly related to the perineal wound. This is not unexpected, since delayed healing of perineal wounds is common following RT therapy. RT dose does not appear to influence the incidence of delayed perineal healing (20). Salvage APR provides ultimate disease control and long-term survival for approximately 50% of patients with operable local failure after initial CRT. Potentially favorable prognostic factors include recurrence (vs. persistence) after CRT, absence of nodal disease at salvage, and negative margins. Early detection of persistent or recurrent disease after CRT is essential (Fig. 1). Our surveillance protocol at MSKCC includes endorectal ultrasound examination and CT scanning of the abdomen and pelvis, at frequent intervals, for a total follow-up period of six years.

SURGERY AS AN ALTERNATIVE TO COMBINED CHEMOTHERAPY AND RADIATION

Surgery for anal SCCa is an alternative for patients who are unable to complete CRT due to significant side effects, or for patients who are not candidates for CRT (such as those with previous history of pelvic RT). Special consideration has been given to patients with HIV/AIDS, especially if they have a history of fecal incontinence, chronic diarrhea, or poor performance status. Early reports suggested that these patients might suffer increased toxicity if treated with CRT for anal SCCa (25,26). However, in today's era of highly active anti-retroviral therapy (HAART), recent reports suggest low toxicity, better tolerance, and a trend toward better survival for HIV patients treated with CRT for anal SCCa, if they are receiving concomitant HAART (27,28).

The literature on surgery for anal SCCa in HIV patients is extremely limited. Tarantino and Bernstein reported briefly on their experience with such cases in a study evaluating endoanal ultrasound in the staging of patients with anal SCCa (29). Of 12 patients with anal SCCa staged by endoanal ultrasound (EAUS), 5 selected APR and the remaining 7 underwent CRT. Four of the patients who chose surgery were HIV positive, with a history of fecal incontinence, chronic diarrhea, or poor performance status. The fifth patient had received pelvic RT for another primary malignancy, and was not a candidate for additional RT treatment.

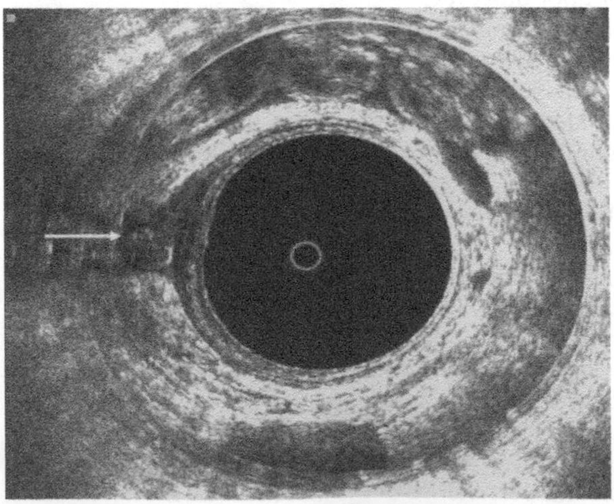

FIGURE 1 This endorectal ultrasound image demonstrates an extraluminal perirectal recurrence of a squamous-cell carcinoma of the anus, initially treated with the Nigro protocol.

In all five patients, surgical staging correlated with ultrasound staging. There were no cases of residual disease in the seven patients treated with CRT. However, this study did not include long-term follow-up and survival outcome.

SURGERY FOR INGUINAL LYMPH NODE DISEASE

Inguinal lymph nodes are usually included in the RT field when anal SCCa patients are treated with CRT. Lee et al. reported on the University of Florida experience with elective inguinal lymph node RT in 164 patients with pelvic malignancies at risk for inguinal nodal metastases (30). Primary sites included the anal canal, distal rectum, and the distal genitourinary (GU) tract. In 148 patients, both groins were clinically negative; 16 patients had unilateral clinical lymphadenopathy. The authors reported a 96% inguinal lymph node control rate and minimal complications, with a follow-up of at least two years. They concluded that elective inguinal RT is effective and safe in patients with pelvic malignancies who are at risk for inguinal nodal disease.

Conversely, Gerard et al. advocated a selective approach in the management of inguinal nodal disease, based on their retrospective analysis of 270 patients with anal SCCa treated with RT in Lyon over a 16-year period (31). No routine groin RT was performed. Patients with metastatic inguinal lymph nodes were treated with inguinal dissection and postoperative RT. Synchronous inguinal metastases were observed in 10% of patients ($n=27$; the rate was 16% for patients with T3–T4 lesions); the five-year overall survival rate in this subgroup was 54%. Metachronous inguinal metastases were seen in 19 patients (8%), and the five-year overall survival rate of these patients was 41%. The authors noted that, when the primary tumor was clearly located on a single lateral side of the anal canal, the nodal metastases always involved the ipsilateral groin (36 of 36 synchronous or metachronous tumors).

From the same group, Bobin et al. recently published a series on 35 patients with clinically N0 cancers of the anal canal who underwent sentinel inguinal lymph node (SILN) biopsy (32). Of this group, 33 had SCCa and 2 had anal melanomas. The SILN was positive in seven cases with SCCa, and in both melanomas. After 18 months of follow-up, the SILN negative cases showed no evidence of inguinal nodal disease. The authors suggested that SILN biopsy can be used to stage anal canal cancers, in order to avoid unnecessary prophylactic inguinal lymph node RT.

MSKCC patients with anal SCCa treated with CRT routinely receive bilateral groin RT. For persistent or recurrent isolated inguinal lymph node disease, we perform selective lymphadenectomy (Fig. 2). The literature on this approach is scarce. An older report by Greenall et al. on 67 patients with recurrent SCCa tumors of the anal canal suggested that patients with

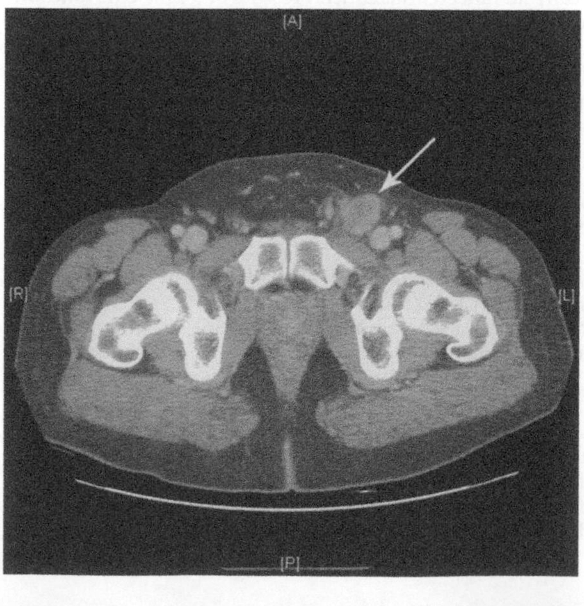

FIGURE 2 This CT image demonstrates a large recurrent metastatic left inguinal lymph node in an HIV-positive patient with squamous-cell carcinoma of the anus, initially treated with radiation therapy. *Abbreviation*: CT, computed tomography.

recurrence in the inguinal lymph nodes have relatively good prognosis (55% five-year survival after lymphadenectomy), and recommended treatment with groin dissection (33). In our institution's study by Akbari et al., five patients had isolated inguinal nodal recurrence and underwent inguinal lymph node dissection, with good results (24). Three patients remained free of disease, one died of distant recurrence, and another had local nodal recurrence.

SUMMARY

Salvage APR is potentially curative in select patients with anal SCCa after failure of initial CRT. Patients with local recurrence following initial complete response to CRT, negative nodal disease at salvage, and/or negative margins at salvage have a more favorable prognosis. Appropriate preoperative selection is crucial, in order to exclude patients with distant metastases or locally unresectable disease. The morbidity of surgery is significant, mainly involving the perineal wound. Salvage inguinal lymphadenectomy after CRT failure can also control disease. Areas worthy of future investigation may include the potential benefit of additional treatment after salvage APR. Additionally, the role of salvage CRT merits further investigation, especially for those patients presenting with poor prognostic factors for salvage surgery.

REFERENCES

1. Nigro ND, Vaitkevicius VK, Considine B. Combined therapy for cancer of the anal canal: a preliminary report. Dis Colon Rectum 1974; 17:354–356.
2. Buroker TR, Nigro ND, Bradley G, et al. Combined therapy for cancer of the anal canal: follow-up report. Dis Colon Rectum 1977; 20:677–678.
3. Nigro ND. An evaluation of combined therapy for Squamous-cell carcinoma of the anal canal. Dis Colon Rectum 1984; 27:763–766.
4. Sawyers JL. Current management of carcinoma of the anus and perianus. Am Surg 1977; 43(7):424–429.
5. UKCCCR Anal Cancer Trial Working Party. UK Co-ordinating Committee on Cancer Research. Epidermoid anal cancer: results from the UKCCCR randomised trial of radiotherapy alone versus radiotherapy, 5-fluorouracil, and mitomycin. Lancet 1996; 348:1049–1054.
6. Flam M, John M, Pajak TF, et al. Role of mitomycin in combination with fluorouracil and radiotherapy, and of salvage chemoradiation in the definitive nonsurgical treatment of epidermoid carcinoma of the anal canal: results of a phase III randomized intergroup study. J Clin Oncol 1996; 14: 2527–2539.
7. Nilsson PJ, Svensson C, Goldman S, Ljungqvist O, Glimelius B. Epidermoid anal cancer: a review of a population-based series of 308 consecutive patients treated according to prospective protocols. Int J Radiat Oncol Biol Phys 2005; 61(1):92–102.
8. Bartelink H, Roelofsen F, Eschwege F, et al. Concomitant radiotherapy and chemotherapy is superior to radiotherapy alone in the treatment of locally advanced anal cancer: results of a phase III randomized trial of the European Organization for Research and Treatment of Cancer Radiotherapy and Gastrointestinal Cooperative Groups. J Clin Oncol 1997; 15(5):2040–2049.
9. Tanum G. Treatment of relapsing anal carcinoma. Acta Oncol 1993; 32(1):33–35.
10. Longo WE, Vernava AM 3rd, Wade TP, Coplin MA, Virgo KS, Johnson FE. Recurrent Squamous-cell carcinoma of the anal canal. Predictors of initial treatment failure and results of salvage therapy. Ann Surg 1994; 220:40–49.
11. Grabenbauer GG, Matzel KE, Schneider IH, et al. Sphincter preservation with chemoradiation in anal canal carcinoma: abdominoperineal resection in selected cases? Dis Colon Rectum 1998; 41(4):441–450.
12. Faynsod M, Vargas HI, Tolmos J, et al. Patterns of recurrence in anal canal carcinoma. Arch Surg 2000; 135:1090–1093.
13. Deniaud-Alexandre E, Touboul E, Tiret E, et al. Results of definitive irradiation in a series of 305 epidermoid carcinomas of the anal canal. Int J Radiat Oncol Biol Phys 2003; 56(5):1259–1273.
14. Nguyen WD, Mitchell KM, Beck DE. Risk factors associated with requiring a stoma for the management of anal cancer. Dis Colon Rectum 2004; 47(6):843–846.
15. Zelnick RS, Haas PA, Ajlouni M, Szilagyi E, Fox TA Jr. Results of abdominoperineal resections for failures after combination chemotherapy and radiation therapy for anal canal cancers. Dis Colon Rectum 1992; 35:574–577.
16. Smith AJ, Whelan P, Cummings BJ, Stern HS. Management of persistent or locally recurrent epidermoid cancer of the anal canal with abdominoperineal resection. Acta Oncol 2001; 40(1):34–36.
17. Van der Wal BC, Cleffken BI, Gulec B, Kaufman HS, Choti MA. Results of salvage abdominoperineal resection for recurrent anal carcinoma following combined chemoradiation therapy. J Gastrointest Surg 2001; 5(4):383–387.

18. Ghouti L, Houvenaeghel G, Moutardier V, et al. Salvage abdominoperineal resection after failure of conservative treatment in anal epidermoid cancer. Dis Colon Rectum 2005; 48(1):16–22.
19. Pocard M, Tiret E, Nugent K, Dehni N, Parc R. Results of salvage abdominoperineal resection for anal cancer after radiotherapy. Dis Colon Rectum 1998; 41(12):1488–1493.
20. Bai YK, Cao WL, Cao JD, Liang J, Shao YF. Surgical salvage therapy of anal canal cancer. World J Gastroenterol 2004; 10(3):424–426.
21. Nilsson PJ, Svensson C, Goldman S, Glimelius B. Salvage abdominoperineal resection in anal epidermoid cancer. Br J Surg 2002; 89:1425–1429.
22. Allal AS, Laurencet FM, Reymond MA, Kurtz JM, Marti MC. Effectiveness of surgical salvage therapy for patients with locally uncontrolled anal carcinoma after sphincter-conserving treatment. Cancer 1999; 86(3):405–409.
23. Ellenhorn JD, Enker WE, Quan SH. Salvage abdominoperineal resection following combined chemotherapy and radiotherapy for epidermoid carcinoma of the anus. Ann Surg Oncol 1994; 1(2):105–110.
24. Akbari RP, Paty PB, Guillem JG, et al. Oncologic outcomes of salvage surgery for epidermoid carcinoma of the anus initially managed with combined modality therapy. Dis Colon Rectum 2004; 47(7):1136–1144.
25. Chadha M, Rosenblatt EA, Malamud S, Pisch J, Berson A. Squamous-cell carcinoma of the anus in HIV-positive patients. Dis Colon Rectum 1994; 37:861–865.
26. Holland JM, Swift PS. Tolerance of patients with human immunodeficiency virus and anal carcinoma to treatment with combined chemotherapy and radiation therapy. Radiology 1994; 193:251–254.
27. Stadler RF, Gregorcyk SG, Euhus DM, Huber PJ, Simmang CL. Outcome of HIV-infected patients with invasive squamous-cell carcinoma of the anal canal in the era of highly active antiretroviral therapy. Dis Colon Rectum 2004; 47(8):1305–1309.
28. Blazy A, Hennequin C, Gornet JM, et al. Anal carcinomas in HIV-positive patients: high-dose chemoradiotherapy is feasible in the era of highly active antiretroviral therapy. Dis Colon Rectum 2005; 48(6):1176–1181.
29. Tarantino D, Bernstein MA. Endoanal ultrasound in the staging and management of squamous-cell carcinoma of the anal canal: potential implications of a new ultrasound staging system. Dis Colon Rectum 2002; 45(1):16–22.
30. Lee WR, McColough WM, Mendenhall WM, Marcus RB, Parsons JT, Million RR. Elective inguinal lymph node irradiation for pelvic carcinomas. The University of Florida experience. Cancer 1993; 72(6):2058–2065.
31. Gerard JP, Chapet O, Samiei F, et al. Management of inguinal lymph node metastases in patients with carcinoma of the anal canal: experience in a series of 270 patients treated in Lyon and review of the literature. Cancer 2001; 92:77–84.
32. Bobin JY, Gerard JP, Chapet O, Romestaing P, Isaac S. Lymphatic mapping and inguinal sentinel lymph node biopsy in anal canal cancers to avoid prophylactic inguinal irradiation. Cancer Radiother 2003; 7(suppl 1):85s–90s.
33. Greenall MJ, Magill GB, Quan SH, DeCosse JJ. Recurrent epidermoid cancer of the anus. Cancer 1986; 57(7):1437–1441.

20 Pancreatic Adenocarcinoma: A Rationale for the Surgical Approach

Cletus A. Arciero and John P. Hoffman
Fox Chase Cancer Center, Philadelphia, Pennsylvania, U.S.A.

Pancreatic adenocarcinoma remains a therapeutic challenge for clinicians. It is estimated that in 2005 there will be 32,180 new cases of adenocarcinoma of the pancreas and 31,800 deaths (1). Worldwide, the incidence of pancreatic adenocarcinoma is 236,306, with annual death rates over 227,000 (2). Recently there has been an improved survival in patients diagnosed with pancreatic adenocarcinoma, but this increased survival is only from 3% (1983–1985) to 4% (1998–2002) (1). Most patients diagnosed with pancreatic adenocarcinoma are likely to die from their disease.

The surgical treatment of pancreatic adenocarcinoma continues to evolve since the first procedure done 93 years ago. Walter Kausch described the first successful two-stage pancreaticoduodenectomy for a periampullary tumor in 1912 (3). Whipple and colleagues popularized the pancreaticoduodenectomy in the 1930s and 1940s through their publications (4–6). The procedure was first utilized for periampullary tumors exclusively, but later was applied to adenocarcinoma of the head of the pancreas. Pancreaticoduodenectomy for pancreatic head adenocarcinoma, distal pancreatectomy for body/tail adenocarcinoma, and total pancreatectomy for diffuse, resectable tumors have become the surgical modalities to treat pancreatic adenocarcinoma. Due to the late presentation and the decreased incidence of pancreatic adenocarcinoma of the body and tail, distal and total pancreatectomies make up only a small proportion of curative resections performed. Today, most consider the surgical management of resectable pancreatic adenocarcinoma as standard of care.

There has been much debate as to the success of these procedures and the rationale for such "radical" approaches to this deadly disease process. As advances are made in the realm of radiation therapy, chemotherapy, and now biologic/targeted therapies, the role of surgical intervention in adenocarcinoma of the pancreas perhaps needs redefining. The role surgery should play in the treatment of pancreatic adenocarcinoma perhaps is best answered by examining the surgical approaches and their effect on the patient and the disease process. Close examination of the morbidity and mortality surrounding the procedures themselves, particularly pancreaticoduodenectomy is crucial. Ultimately, the true role for surgical intervention is defined by survival and whether a survival advantage is gained through surgical resection. Quality-of-life is also an important variable, for both potentially curative and palliative surgical procedures.

MORBIDITY AND MORTALITY

Early arguments against surgical resection for pancreatic adenocarcinoma centered on the high rate of morbidity and mortality. In the late 1960s and early 1970s, 30-day operative mortality rates ranged from 10.3% to 41% (7–11). Even more patients suffered from postoperative morbidity. There were many who felt that the mortality rate from pancreatic resection was greater than the survival rate offered by the surgery, and therefore surgical resection was not warranted (11,12). But that argument is no longer valid. There have been several changes over the past 20 years that have dramatically decreased the mortality associated with pancreatic resections.

One important factor has been the establishment of specialty centers (13–15). Recent studies have indicated that the 30-day mortality associated with pancreatic surgery is less than 5% in high-volume centers (performing greater than 13 pancreatic resections per year) (16).

This rate is even lower (3.1%) in the hands of the most experienced surgeons (defined as a surgeon who performs more than four pancreatic resections per year). Another factor has been the improvement of perioperative care, from the operating room to the intensive care unit to the surgical ward. Advances in anesthesia and critical care have combined to decrease mortality rates for most major surgeries. Most published reports today have a much lower mortality rate than 30 years ago. Morbidity rates of ~30% predominate, and 30-day operative mortality rates are consistently ~3%. Morbidity and mortality associated with the pancreatic resection is no longer the survival-limiting factor in patients with resectable pancreatic adenocarcinoma.

SURGICAL APPROACH

There has also been much debate on the utility/futility of surgical resection for adenocarcinoma of the pancreas (17–22). In an attempt to improve survival rates, many have investigated more aggressive surgical approaches. These aggressive approaches include extended lymphadenectomies and *en bloc* resections, including celiac axis, hepatic artery, superior mesenteric, and portal veins when involved. Modifications of the pancreaticoduodenectomy have also been introduced in an attempt to decrease the morbidity while maintaining an equal survival rate. These various approaches have helped to define the optimal surgical intervention in patients with pancreatic adenocarcinoma.

Extended Lymphadenectomy

Fortner first presented extended lymphadenectomy for pancreatic adenocarcinoma as a technique in 1973 (23). The "regional pancreatectomy" included a radical pancreaticoduodenectomy including the transpancreatic portion of the portal vein. The celiac axis, superior mesenteric artery, and the middle colic artery occasionally were included with the specimen and reconstructed. Extended lymphadenectomy has differed in many of the studies. Additional lymph nodes in regions not usually part of a pancreaticoduodenectomy specimen have included para-aortic nodes from the diaphragmatic hiatus to the inferior mesenteric artery laterally to the renal hila, hepatic hilum, and celiac and superior mesenteric arterial nodal regions (23–25). The goal is to remove all disease, including any lymph node metastases. This was supported by several Japanese studies that claimed a survival advantage for those patients undergoing a more aggressive surgical resection (26–30). The conclusion drawn from these retrospective studies was that an *en bloc* excision of all possible disease regions improves survival. It should be pointed out that the patients in these series were treated without the addition of radiation therapy or chemotherapy. Furthermore, no phase III trials have been done.

After these reports, multiple prospective, randomized trials were constructed to examine the extent of lymphadenectomy and its effect on morbidity, mortality, and survival. Pedrazzoli and colleagues examined 81 patients, 40 undergoing standard pancreaticoduodenectomy and 41 undergoing pancreaticoduodenectomy with extended (360°) lymphadenectomy (31). The extended procedure involved total SMA clearance as well as aortocaval lymphadenectomy. Analysis revealed little difference between the two groups with the exception of a longer operative time in patients undergoing extended lymphadenectomy. There was a trend toward a survival advantage in the extended lymphadenectomy grouping those with N1 nodes, but it was not significant. Capussito et al. also showed a trend toward better survival in patients undergoing an extended lymph node dissection (32). Two larger studies by Yeo et al. without the extensive SMA dissection, failed to show any significant difference in survival. The more recent study examined 294 patients, and found the only significant differences between the groups to be an increased hospital stay, increased number of lymph nodes removed, and increased morbidity in the extended group. Operative mortality and overall survival was not significantly different between the groups. Quality-of-life studies on the same group of patients also failed to show any difference between the two groups (33).

There may be minor trends toward improved survival in patients undergoing extended lymphadenectomy, but there appears to be no long-term benefit to undertaking this more aggressive approach. There are few randomized trials examining this approach, and they contain relatively low numbers of patients. Logic would dictate resection of all possible disease, to include diseased lymph nodes. In selected patients, this aggressive approach may be warranted. But studies to date have failed to present a convincing argument for routine extended lymphadenectomy in patients with pancreatic adenocarcinoma.

Venous Resection

In a similar approach, and often combined with extended lymphadenectomy, venous resections as part of an *en bloc* resection have also been studied. The approach is designed to allow for an R0 resection in a patient that would otherwise either be unresectable or undergo a R1/2 resection with its known low survival (21,34–36). Since patients with documented vessel invasion preoperatively are often deemed unresectable, the majority of the studies examining portal or superior mesenteric vein resections are retrospective in nature. But, there are some small, prospective studies that have attempted to address the utility of this approach.

Fuhrman et al. examined their prospectively gathered database and compared patients who underwent SMV/PV resection and those who did not (37). There was significant increase in blood loss, transfusion requirement, and operative time, but morbidity was equivalent. Unfortunately, survival data were not provided. Bachellier et al. examined 52 patients undergoing SMV/PV resection versus 185 patients undergoing a standard resection (38). Again, there was an increase in blood loss and operative time for the venous resection group. However, there was no difference noted in survival between the two groups. Their results did confirm that the most important factor influencing survival was actually the presence of negative margins. Van Geenen et al. echoed those results, stating that in fact the positive margin is often in the body of the pancreas rather than at the SMV/PV margins (39). Several more recent studies have also noted similar rates of morbidity, mortality, and survival between patients undergoing SMV/PV resections and those who undergo standard resections (32,40–42). Undergoing a margin negative resection is the most important factor for survival, not the operative approach to attaining that negative margin. Resection of the SMV/PV confluence allows for an R0 resection in patients that might otherwise be unresectable and therefore is advisable in selected cases.

Other aggressive approaches, such as total pancreatectomy, have little additional support in the literature mainly due to relatively low numbers of patients undergoing these procedures. Total pancreatectomy is performed relatively infrequently, and therefore it is hard to draw definitive conclusions. Karpoff et al. presented their experience with 28 patients with pancreatic adenocarcinoma who underwent total pancreatectomy (43). The overall morbidity and mortality for the procedure was consistent with other pancreatic resections, but the median survival was a modest 7.9 months. Lim et al. in their examination of all patients undergoing pancreatic resection found similar results in terms of morbidity, mortality, and survival (44). Total pancreatectomy can provide an R0 resection with acceptable operative morbidity and mortality. But, survival in this group of patients is lower than those undergoing pancreaticoduodenectomy and the postoperative diabetes can often be severe or even lethal. Total pancreatectomy can be utilized in a select group of patients, that is, those with diffuse pancreatic cancer, although its long-term survival benefit is questionable.

Pylorus Preserving Pancreaticoduodenectomy

In contrast to the more aggressive resections mentioned, there were also movements toward a more tolerable pancreatic resection. In an attempt to decrease the morbidity surrounding pancreaticoduodenectomy (PD), Watson introduced a pylorus-preserving technique in 1944 (45). This technique applied a less aggressive approach to pancreatic head adenocarcinoma, preserving the stomach, the pylorus, and a portion of the duodenum. By maintaining more anatomy of the gastrointestinal tract, it was hoped that the morbidity associated with PD might be decreased. There were concerns that the pylorus-preserving pancreaticoduodenectomy (PPPD) would lead to a decreased overall survival owing to its less radical scope. But, there were numerous retrospective examinations that found no difference in survival when comparing PPPD with the standard PD, although the numbers for these studies were small (46–48). In fact, many felt that the morbidity and mortality surrounding PPPD was actually less than that of PD. Prospective studies were undertaken to examine this technique and its effect on morbidity, mortality, and survival. A small study by Lin et al. found equivalent morbidity and mortality rates and no significant difference in survival (49). Seiler et al. performed a larger study that revealed a trend toward lower morbidity with the pylorus-preserving technique, but overall no difference in mortality or survival (50). A recent analysis of the long-term results of this study again revealed no differences between the two surgical approaches (51). Tran et al. examined 170 patients randomized to receive either PD or PPPD (52). Their results revealed little difference in morbidity such as leak, hemorrhage, abscess formation or rates of re-operation. There were also equivalent rates of mortality and survival between groups. These results were echoed by a more recent examination of PD versus PPPD by Yeo et al. The standard and the pylorus-preserving pancreaticoduodenectomies were equivalent procedures, with minimal difference in morbidity, mortality, or survival (53). Most authors advocate the PPPD in all cases except those where the operative margin may be in jeopardy due to involvement of or near the first portion of the duodenum, or the blood supply of the pylorus appears tenuous.

Surgical Palliation

Curative resection is the goal in the majority of surgical oncology endeavors. But, with aggressive neoplasms such as pancreatic adenocarcinoma, palliation is often the only option. Palliation for pancreatic adenocarcinoma can take many forms, and some researchers believe that a "curative" pancreatic resection is truly just a more extensive palliative procedure. But, most agree that operative palliation for pancreatic cancer refers to biliary and/or gastroduodenal bypass. Biliary bypass is often performed by endoscopy, and success rates have steadily increased, thereby decreasing the need for surgical intervention (54–56). But, bypassing duodenal obstructions is still a difficult issue for endoscopic management and thus remains largely a surgical issue. In studies comparing nonsurgical versus surgical treatment of duodenal obstruction, the nonsurgical group had late obstruction in 9% to 14% of patients versus 0% to 4% in the surgical group (57–59).

The early experience with pancreatic resections was wrought with high morbidity and mortality as previously noted. Many researchers at the time undertook examining whether bypass procedures would actually be equivalent to the more extensive and more dangerous approach of resection. Mongé examined a small series of patients with resectable pancreatic adenocarcinoma who underwent palliative bypass procedure (biliary and/or gastrojejunal) (60). He found that survival for this group averaged 12 months, which was greater than the survival of patients with unresectable disease who underwent bypass and less than those undergoing curative resection. Despite the high operative mortality of the time, Mongé concluded that resection provided better palliation of symptoms than bypass procedures, even if the patient did not enjoy a prolonged survival. But, Shapiro's similar study several years later failed to show any significant difference between the resected group and the bypass group in terms of palliation or survival (12). A large series by Sarr and Cameron also showed that patients undergoing palliative bypass had improved survival and quality of life compared with those who only underwent exploration without bypass (61). Several years later, Wade et al. found that although biliary/gastric bypass did not improve survival compared to those who did not undergo bypass, they did have better palliation of their symptoms (62).

To better define palliation in terms of surgical intervention, Bakkevold and Kambestad undertook a prospective examination of palliation comparing curative resection, bypass, and no surgical intervention (63). Their research confirmed the findings of Mongé, with patients undergoing resection enjoying the best palliation of symptoms. However, those patients that were bypassed did have palliation of symptoms and were able to engage in more daily living activities than those who received no surgical therapy. These results were confirmed in a later study performed by Kyiomonis et al. (19).

Over the last 15 years, the increasing utilization of minimally invasive approaches to palliation have gained favor and the exact role that palliative surgery should play in pancreatic adenocarcinoma has again been addressed in the recent literature. Espat et al. examined all patients with locally advanced or metastatic disease identified on staging laparoscopy (64). This group was examined in terms of future operative procedures required due to obstruction. They found that 98% of patients in fact did not need an open operative procedure for obstruction, either biliary or gastroduodenal. They concluded that bypasses were indicated for patients who were symptomatic and could not be palliated via minimally invasive/endoscopic techniques. But, their median follow-up for patients was 5.9 months, and the median survival for those with locally advanced disease was 7.8 months. Also, follow-up was usually by phone interview only. Therefore, there could be a number of patients with the development of symptoms that were not discovered during this study.

In contrast, Sohn et al. presented their data concerning operative palliative bypass (biliary, duodenal, or both) and found that their patients had excellent (>96%) palliation of their symptoms (65). They agreed that minimally invasive techniques are effective at palliating obstructive symptoms, but noted that there is a relatively high rate of stenosis/re-obstruction requiring intervention that is not seen in those patients that are operatively bypassed. Nieveen van Dijkum et al. compared patients undergoing endoscopic biliary stent placement versus those undergoing an operative double-bypass procedure (66). They found that overall morbidity and mortality were equivalent between the two groups. Although the numbers studied were small, they found no benefit to patients being treated "less invasively" with endoscopic stenting.

Multiple studies have found that a proportion of patients will develop gastric outlet obstruction during the course of their disease (17–21%) (61,67–69). Up to 50% of patients with pancreatic adenocarcinoma will have nausea and vomiting at presentation, with only a portion exhibiting radiographic evidence of obstruction (70). Lillemoe et al. randomized 87 patients discovered at exploration to have unresectable disease to surgical bypass or no bypass. Despite no preoperative indications of a pending obstruction, 19% of the nonbypass patients developed obstruction while 0% of the bypass patients developed obstruction (71). They also found, consistent with previous studies, that patients undergoing a gastrojejunal bypass during exploration for possible resection have little increase in morbidity and mortality (61,67–69,71,72). But, patients undergoing a second procedure due to the development of obstruction can exhibit mortality rates approaching 25%. Thus, they advocate prophylactic gastrojejunostomy in patients undergoing exploration for possible curative resection who are found to have locally advanced or metastatic disease.

Another surgical approach for palliation is the palliative pancreaticoduodenectomy. Lillemoe et al. performed a retrospective examination of patients with pancreatic adenocarcinoma. They compared 64 patients that underwent R1/R2 PDs with a group of 62 patients who underwent exploration, 87% of whom underwent palliative bypass and the other 13% had explorations only. Analysis of these two groups showed equivalent morbidity and mortality rates, although there was a longer hospital stay for those who underwent resection. But, there was a significant survival advantage to those patients who underwent a palliative pancreaticoduodenectomy. The conclusion was that palliative resections could be undertaken at high-volume centers that did not have high operative-mortality rates with improved palliation and modestly improved survival. The criticisms of this body of research revolve around the retrospective nature of the work and that the patients who had R1/R2 resections had been approached with a planned R0 resection that was either discovered late in the dissection to be impossible or discovered on permanent sectioning to be impossible. However, palliative pancreaticoduodenectomy may provide a role in the management of pancreatic adenocarcinoma, especially with the advent of directed chemotherapeutic and biologic therapies.

Despite institutional biases, palliative surgical interventions do have a role in the management of pancreatic adenocarcinoma. In patients with locally advanced or metastatic disease, surgical palliation can provide a durable solution to obstruction, either gastroduodenal or biliary. Endoscopic or percutaneous biliary drainage should be performed when feasible, but surgical biliary drainage is very effective at treating obstructive jaundice. Gastrojejunostomy can provide palliation in a patient population where a significant percentage will develop signs/symptoms of gastric outlet obstruction if they are not already symptomatic. In centers that are adept at minimally invasive surgery, accomplishing these bypasses laparoscopically is ideal. But, open-bypass procedures still allow for excellent palliation with low morbidity and mortality.

OVERALL SURVIVAL

There has always been debate surrounding the survival statistics in patients with pancreatic adenocarcinoma. Even today, there is a wide variation in survival statistics between different treatment centers. The majority of the debate in the literature began in 1978 with Gudjonnson's article in Cancer (73). The argument he presented tried to explain many of the discrepancies in the literature that had been noted to date. Examining 100 patients (1960–1971) diagnosed with adenocarcinoma of the pancreas, he noted that only 61 patients had histologic confirmation. This led to a review of the literature encompassing over 60 studies and 15,000 patients with pancreatic adenocarcinoma. Overall, only about half of all patients diagnosed with adenocarcinoma of the pancreas had pathologic confirmation of the diagnosis. When examining all patients, operative mortality ranged from 0% to 100% (average 22%) and five year actual survival ranged from 0% to 28.5%. When examining all patients diagnosed with pancreatic adenocarcinoma, only 0.4% survived five years. The wide discrepancies in survival were explained by a lack of consistent pathologic diagnoses and the exclusion of 30-day mortalities in overall survival. He concluded that most survival statistics were inflated and that some of the five-year survivors were actually patients who had never undergone any resection. He questioned the utility of surgical intervention in patients with pancreatic adenocarcinoma due to the high morbidity/mortality rates and the lack of convincing survival benefit. Gudjonsson followed up this report with a more expanded critique in 1987 (74). He examined his own experience and then reviewed over 37,000 patients cited in the literature. He noted that most patients do not survive five years, and that the lone five-year survivor in his cohort did not even undergo pancreatic resection. He felt that surgical resection was futile and that surgery should truly be reserved for diagnosis and palliative procedures that is, bypass.

However, the resection of pancreatic adenocarcinoma was still viewed by most clinicians as holding the only possibility for cure in these patients. Promising reports began to surface in the literature in the early 1990s. Trede et al. published their experience with 118 patients, all with pathologically confirmed adenocarcinoma (34). They reported no operative mortalities with a five-year actuarial survival of 24%. There were no survivors past 24 months that had pathologically positive margins at resection while the R0 group enjoyed a five-year actuarial survival of 36%. Cameron et al. followed with a report showing a median survival of 11.9 months and a five-year actuarial survival of 19% (75). They also noted that factors contributing to shortened survival times included tumors greater than 2 cm, tumors showing vascular invasion, and the presence of lymph node metastasis. Geer and Brennan examined 799 patients diagnosed with pancreatic adenocarcinoma, 18% of whom underwent curative resection (76). The five-year actuarial survival was 24% (median survival 18 months) in those undergoing resection and 0% in those who did not. When examining all patients with pancreatic adenocarcinoma, the five-year survival was only 1.25%. These studies showed increased survival in patients undergoing curative pancreatic resection, and a survival benefit when compared to patients not undergoing resection.

But, Gudjonsson was undeterred. He published another critical assessment of surgical resections of pancreatic adenocarcinoma (77). Examining 340 papers, he estimated the total number of patients with pancreatic adenocarcinoma based on previous data stating that ~80% of all patients with pancreatic adenocarcinoma undergo exploration. Based on these estimations, he determined an overall five-year survival for patients diagnosed with pancreatic adenocarcinoma of only 0.4%. He stated that higher survival rates noted by other authors were based upon (*i*) multiple reports of overlapping data allowing for survivors to be over-represented (*ii*) the exclusion of 30-day mortalities from survival statistics, and (*iii*) the reporting of actuarial survival versus actual survival.

Gudjonsson noted 22 long-term survivors (>5 years) that had not undergone a pancreatic resection. He also stated that since most reports of survival are based on pancreaticoduodenectomies performed, nonresected survivors are vastly undercounted. His viewpoint was that if there were long-term survivors without surgical resection, why undertake such a morbid procedure? He felt that millions of dollars were wasted each year on pancreatic resections with minimal survival benefit gained. But, examination of the data reveals that these 22 unresected patients comprised less than 10% of survivors in his study. The other 90% underwent surgical resection. Therefore, if surgical resection were abandoned, there would be over 278 long-term survivors lost by not performing curative resections. Further critiques of his assessment were quick to point out that Gudjonsson had derived many of his numbers from the 1970s and 1980s, prior to the clinical application of multimodality therapy. He therefore drew incorrect conclusions as to the true role of curative resections in pancreatic adenocarcinoma (13,17,20). They also pointed out that Gudjonsson's claim of 10% five-year survival in the un-resected group was likely due to misdiagnoses (ampullary cancer or benign lesions), which Gudjonsson himself stated was often a failing in many studies examining pancreatic adenocarcinoma.

Studies began to grow in patient numbers. The combination of improvements in diagnostic workups and pathologic methods led to more accurate analyses. Most modern studies ensured histological confirmation of the diagnosis of pancreatic adenocarcinoma prior to patient inclusion in any study, and found that resection improved survival and showed a clear benefit to nonresectional interventions. Bramhall et al. examined 13,560 patients with pathology proven pancreatic adenocarcinoma (78). The five-year survival for patients undergoing resection was 9.7%, in stark contrast to the five-year survival rates of those undergoing bypass, exploration only, or only supportive care. (0.8%, 0.4%, and 0%, respectively). They also noted an increase in five-year survival rates when comparing 1957 to 1976 (2.6%) and 1977 to 1986 (9.7%) (78). Yeo et al. at John's Hopkins noted an increased survival as well, with a five-year actuarial survival of 26% with a median survival of 18 months (79). In examining their experience over the preceding decades, they found that median survival was 7.5 months in the 1970s, 14 months in the 1980s, and 17.5 months in the 1990s. They also noted that patients with R0 resections fare much better than patients with even microscopically positive margins. Conlon et al. noted similar results with 684 patients (1983–1989) (80). Overall five-year survival was 1.8% with a median survival of six months, but those undergoing curative resection had median survival of 14.3 months. In terms of patients not treated with resection, studies examining those patients with locally advanced pancreatic adenocarcinoma and treated only with chemotherapy and/or radiotherapy, survival was less than 7 to 11 months (81–86). In particular, Imamura et al. performed the only randomized trial comparing curative resection versus radiochemotherapy alone for resectable pancreatic adenocarcinoma (86). They noted that the resection group survived longer (>17 months vs. 11 months) and had greater one-year survival (62% vs. 32%). Only four patients survived at least 24 months, and all were in the resection group. Overall, multiple studies have shown the survival benefit for patients of undergoing curative resection (34,79,87–89).

The last several years have shown stabilization in the survival statistics for patients undergoing pancreatic resection. The five-year survival rate is now consistently ~20%, with certain factors showing survival advantages such as node negativity and small tumor size (44,88,90–93). Those patients with cancers discovered early and undergoing R0 resections have the better survival rates. The survival rates now appear consistent over the last 10 years, with little increase in survival noted. The overall goal of curative surgical resections is to remove all disease from the patient. Despite the approach, whether it is a "radical" or a pylorus preserving, a R0 resection is the desired result. The benefit of an R0 resection makes intuitive sense, and has been proven to be a significant prognostic factor in many studies (34,79,87–89). Many investigators have found that a negative margin is the only true independent prognostic factor (87–89). Regardless of the type of resection undertaken, a curative resection is the goal and a significant factor in survival (38,39,41,94). Research thus far has shown that more extensive resections can be undertaken with minimal change in morbidity or mortality to achieve a margin-negative pancreatic resection.

Ever since the late 1970s, there has been an intense interest in discovering adjuvant therapies. Bakkevold et al. examined the use of adjuvant chemotherapy alone. They noted an early increase in median survival, but failed to show a long-term survival benefit (95). A larger study actually exhibited evidence of a decrease in survival in patients treated with adjuvant chemotherapy versus those receiving no adjuvant therapy (96).

Adjuvant chemotherapy combined with radiation therapy has shown more promise. Studies by GITSG and EORTC showed a survival advantage for patients that received adjuvant chemoradiation therapy (97,98). But, both studies were criticized due to inadequate radiation doses and suboptimal chemotherapy dosings. A more recent study examining chemoradiation was the European Study Group for Pancreatic Cancer-1 trial (ESPAC-1) (99). This study showed a survival advantage for patients receiving adjuvant chemotherapy, but interestingly, those receiving radiation therapy actually exhibited a survival disadvantage. This study has been heavily criticized due to missing follow-up data, failure of patients to receive the prescribed protocol therapy, and failures of radiation therapy quality assurance. Although there are indications that adjuvant chemotherapy could provide a survival advantage, results regarding radiation therapy are inconclusive.

The adjuvant or neoadjuvant role of targeted therapies in pancreatic adenocarcinoma remains unknown. Potential targets such as matrix metalloproteinases showed early promise, but had overall disappointing results (100–102). Epidermal growth factor receptor agents continue to be examined, with promising early results in patients exhibiting a tumor response to treatment (103). Vascular epidermal growth factor (VEGF) has also been examined and been found to be elevated in pancreatic adenocarcinoma. An anti-VEGF (bevacizumab) therapy combined with Gemcitabine in unresectable patients was found to show tumor responses in some patients in early Phase I/II studies (104). Although targeted therapy as a part of the multimodality treatment of pancreatic adenocarcinoma is promising, its role is yet to be truly defined.

CONCLUSIONS

Pancreatic adenocarcinoma remains a fatal disease. There are few long-term survivors from pancreatic adenocarcinoma. A small proportion of patients with this disease are able to undergo curative pancreatic resection. For this subgroup of patients, a significant survival advantage is gained, as well as excellent palliation from their disease process. Despite increasing five-year survival rates in patients undergoing successful pancreatic resections, the majority of these patients will eventually succumb to the disease. Surgical resection is currently the only chance for cure in patients afflicted with this disease. More patients could have this if the cancers were discovered at an earlier stage. It is clear that the most important factor is the ability to resect all disease. Palliative intervention has shown to benefit patients and allows for a better quality of life. But, the reality is that despite a "curative" resection, most patients with adenocarcinoma of the pancreas will have disease recurrence. Surgical resection is not the sole therapy for pancreatic adenocarcinoma. The multimodality approach appears to hold promise in the treatment of pancreatic adenocarcinoma. With the plateau of survival benefit from surgery alone reached, it will be important to expand the realm of clinical trials to identify active agents against pancreatic cancer.

A curative resection combined with newer chemotherapeutic agents may lead to a prolonged survival. As advances in targeted therapies arise, the 'palliative' resections may truly become "curative." For now, complete resection of disease combined with a clinical trial of neoadjuvant/adjuvant therapy is the best hope for patients stricken with this deadly disease.

REFERENCES

1. ACS. Estimated New Cancer Cases and Deaths by Sex for All Sites, US; 2005.
2. Parkin DM, Bray F, Ferlay J, Pisani P. Global cancer statistics, 2002. CA Cancer J Clin 2005; 55(2):74–108.
3. Kausch W. Das carcinom der papilla duodeni und seine radikale entfernung. Beitr Kiln Chir 1912; 78:439–451.
4. Whipple A, Parsons N, Mullins C. Treatment of carcinoma of the ampulla of Vater. Ann Surg 1935; 102:763–779.
5. Whipple A. Present-day surgery of the pancreas. N Engl J Med 1942; 226:515–518.
6. Whipple A. Observations on radical surgery for lesions of the pancreas. Surg Gynecol Obstet 1946; 82:62.
7. Gilsdorf R, Spanos, P. Factors influencing morbidity and mortality in pancreaticoduodenectomy. Ann Surg 1973; 177:332–337.
8. Gray L, Crook JN, Cohn I. Carcinoma of the pancreas. Proc Natl Cancer Conf 1973; 7:503–510.
9. Aston SJ, Longmire WP Jr. Pancreaticoduodenal resection. Twenty years' experience. Arch Surg 1973; 106(6):813–817.
10. Bowden L, McNeer G, Pack GT. Carcinoma of the head of the pancreas; five year survival in four patients. Am J Surg 1965; 109:578–582.
11. Crile G Jr. The advantages of bypass operations over radical pancreatoduodenectomy in the treatment of pancreatic carcinoma. Surg Gynecol Obstet 1970; 130(6):1049–1053.
12. Shapiro TM. Adenocarcinoma of the pancreas: a statistical analysis of biliary bypass vs Whipple resection in good risk patients. Ann Surg 1975; 182(6):715–721.
13. Gordon TA, Cameron JL. Management of patients with carcinoma of the pancreas. J Am Coll Surg 1995; 181(6):558–560.

14. Parks RW, Bettschart V, Frame S, Stockton DL, Brewster DH, Garden OJ. Benefits of specialisation in the management of pancreatic cancer: results of a Scottish population-based study. Br J Cancer 2004; 91(3):459–465.
15. Lieberman MD, Kilburn H, Lindsey M, Brennan MF. Relation of perioperative deaths to hospital volume among patients undergoing pancreatic resection for malignancy. Ann Surg 1995; 222(5):638–645.
16. Birkmeyer JD, Stukel TA, Siewers AE, Goodney PP, Wennberg DE, Lucas FL. Surgeon volume and operative mortality in the United States. N Engl J Med 2003; 349(22):2117–2127.
17. Bruckner HW, Farber LA, Fier CM. Definitive surgery for duct cell carcinomas of the pancreas. J Am Coll Surg 1996; 183(3):292–294.
18. Gudjonsson B. Management of patients with carcinoma of the pancreas. J Am Coll Surg 1996; 183(3):290–291.
19. Kymionis GD, Konstadoulakis MM, Leandros E, et al. Effect of curative versus palliative surgical treatment for stage III pancreatic cancer patients. J R Coll Surg Edinb 1999; 44(4):231–235.
20. Douglass HO Jr, Smith JL. Carcinoma of the pancreas: critical analysis of costs, results of resections, and the need for standardized reporting. J Am Coll Surg 1996; 183(3):291–294.
21. Nitecki SS, Sarr MG, Colby TV, van Heerden JA. Long-term survival after resection for ductal adenocarcinoma of the pancreas. Is it really improving? Ann Surg 1995; 221(1):59–66.
22. Bradley EL III. Pancreatoduodenectomy for pancreatic adenocarcinoma: triumph, triumphalism, or transition? Arch Surg 2002; 137(7):771–773.
23. Fortner JG. Regional resection of cancer of the pancreas: a new surgical approach. Surgery 1973; 73(2):307–320.
24. Fortner JG, Kim DK, Cubilla A, Turnbull A, Pahnke LD, Shils ME. Regional pancreatectomy: en bloc pancreatic, portal vein and lymph node resection. Ann Surg 1977; 186(1):42–50.
25. Fortner JG, Klimstra DS, Senie RT, Maclean BJ. Tumor size is the primary prognosticator for pancreatic cancer after regional pancreatectomy. Ann Surg 1996; 223(2):147–153.
26. Nagakawa T, Konishi I, Ueno K, Ohta T, Kayahara M, Miyazaki I. Extended radical pancreatectomy for carcinoma of the head of the pancreas. Hepatogastroenterology 1998; 45(21):849–854.
27. Nagakawa T, Nagamori M, Futakami F, et al. Results of extensive surgery for pancreatic carcinoma. Cancer 1996; 77(4):640–645.
28. Kayahara M, Nagakawa T, Ueno K, Ohta T, Takeda T, Miyazaki I. An evaluation of radical resection for pancreatic cancer based on the mode of recurrence as determined by autopsy and diagnostic imaging. Cancer 1993; 72(7):2118–2123.
29. Satake K, Nishiwaki H, Yokomatsu H, et al. Surgical curability and prognosis for standard versus extended resection for T1 carcinoma of the pancreas. Surg Gynecol Obstet 1992; 175(3):259–265.
30. Imaizumi T, Hanyu F, Harada N, Hatori T, Fukuda A. Extended radical Whipple resection for cancer of the pancreatic head: operative procedure and results. Dig Surg 1998; 15(4):299–307.
31. Pedrazzoli S, DiCarlo V, Dionigi R, et al. Standard versus extended lymphadenectomy associated with pancreatoduodenectomy in the surgical treatment of adenocarcinoma of the head of the pancreas: a multicenter, prospective, randomized study. Lymphadenectomy Study Group. Ann Surg 1998; 228(4):508–517.
32. Capussotti L, Massucco P, Ribero D, Vigano L, Muratore A, Calgaro M. Extended lymphadenectomy and vein resection for pancreatic head cancer: outcomes and implications for therapy. Arch Surg 2003; 138(12):1316–1322.
33. Nguyen TC, Sohn TA, Cameron JL, et al. Standard vs. radical pancreaticoduodenectomy for periampullary adenocarcinoma: a prospective, randomized trial evaluating quality of life in pancreaticoduodenectomy survivors. J Gastrointest Surg 2003; 7(1):1–9; discussion 9–11.
34. Trede M, Schwall G, Saeger HD. Survival after pancreatoduodenectomy. 118 consecutive resections without an operative mortality. Ann Surg 1990; 211(4):447–458.
35. Willett CG, Lewandrowski K, Warshaw AL, Efird J, Compton CC. Resection margins in carcinoma of the head of the pancreas. Implications for radiation therapy. Ann Surg 1993; 217(2):144–148.
36. Willett CG, Warshaw AL, Convery K, Compton CC. Patterns of failure after pancreaticoduodenectomy for ampullary carcinoma. Surg Gynecol Obstet 1993; 176(1):33–38.
37. Fuhrman GM, Leach SD, Staley CA, et al. Rationale for en bloc vein resection in the treatment of pancreatic adenocarcinoma adherent to the superior mesenteric–portal vein confluence. Pancreatic Tumor Study Group. Ann Surg 1996; 223(2):154–162.
38. Bachellier P, Nakano H, Oussoultzoglou PD, et al. Is pancreaticoduodenectomy with mesentericoportal venous resection safe and worthwhile? Am J Surg 2001; 182(2):120–129.
39. van Geenen RC, ten Kate FJ, de Wit LT, van Gulik TM, Obertop H, Gouma DJ. Segmental resection and wedge excision of the portal or superior mesenteric vein during pancreatoduodenectomy. Surgery 2001; 129(2):158–163.
40. Shibata C, Kobari M, Tsuchiya T, et al. Pancreatectomy combined with superior mesenteric–portal vein resection for adenocarcinoma in pancreas. World J Surg 2001; 25(8):1002–1005.
41. Nakagohri T, Kinoshita T, Konishi M, Inoue K, Takahashi S. Survival benefits of portal vein resection for pancreatic cancer. Am J Surg 2003; 186(2):149–153.

42. Poon RT, Fan ST, Lo CM, et al. Pancreaticoduodenectomy with en bloc portal vein resection for pancreatic carcinoma with suspected portal vein involvement. World J Surg 2004; 28(6):602–608.
43. Karpoff HM, Klimstra DS, Brennan MF, Conlon KC. Results of total pancreatectomy for adenocarcinoma of the pancreas. Arch Surg 2001; 136(1):44–47; discussion 48.
44. Lim JE, Chien MW, Earle CC. Prognostic factors following curative resection for pancreatic adenocarcinoma: a population-based, linked database analysis of 396 patients. Ann Surg 2003; 237(1):74–85.
45. Watson K. Carcinoma of the ampulla of Vater. Successful radical resection. Br J Surg 1944; 31:368–373.
46. Tsao JI, Rossi RL, Lowell JA. Pylorus-preserving pancreatoduodenectomy. Is it an adequate cancer operation. Arch Surg 1994; 129(4):405–412.
47. Braasch JW, Deziel DJ, Rossi RL, Watkins E Jr, Winter PF. Pyloric and gastric preserving pancreatic resection. Experience with 87 patients. Ann Surg 1986; 204(4):411–418.
48. Takao S, Aikou T, Shinchi H, et al. Comparison of relapse and long-term survival between pylorus-preserving and Whipple pancreaticoduodenectomy in periampullary cancer. Am J Surg 1998; 176(5):467–470.
49. Lin PW, Lin YJ. Prospective randomized comparison between pylorus-preserving and standard pancreaticoduodenectomy. Br J Surg 1999; 86(5):603–607.
50. Seiler CA, Wagner M, Sadowski C, Kulli C, Buchler MW. Randomized prospective trial of pylorus-preserving vs. classic duodenopancreatectomy (Whippl'e procedure): initial clinical results. J Gastrointest Surg 2000; 4(5):443–452.
51. Seiler CA, Wagner M, Bachmann T, et al. Randomized clinical trial of pylorus-preserving duodenopancreatectomy versus classical Whipple resection-long term results. Br J Surg 2005; 92(5):547–566.
52. Tran KT, Smeenk HG, van Eijck CH, et al. Pylorus preserving pancreaticoduodenectomy versus standard Whipple procedure: a prospective, randomized, multicenter analysis of 170 patients with pancreatic and periampullary tumors. Ann Surg 2004; 240(5):738–745.
53. Yeo CJ, Cameron JL, Lillemoe KD, et al. Pancreaticoduodenectomy with or without distal gastrectomy and extended retroperitoneal lymphadenectomy for periampullary adenocarcinoma, part 2: randomized controlled trial evaluating survival, morbidity, and mortality. Ann Surg 2002; 236(3):355–366; discussion 366–368.
54. Arguedas MR, Heudebert GH, Stinnett AA, Wilcox CM. Biliary stents in malignant obstructive jaundice due to pancreatic carcinoma: a cost-effectiveness analysis. Am J Gastroenterol 2002; 97(4):898–904.
55. Lichtenstein DR, Carr-Locke DL. Endoscopic palliation for unresectable pancreatic carcinoma. Surg Clin North Am 1995; 75(5):969–988.
56. Indar AA, Lobo DN, Gilliam AD, et al. Percutaneous biliary metal wall stenting in malignant obstructive jaundice. Eur J Gastroenterol Hepatol 2003; 15(8):915–919.
57. Bornman PC, Harries-Jones EP, Tobias R, Van Stiegmann G, Terblanche J. Prospective controlled trial of transhepatic biliary endoprosthesis versus bypass surgery for incurable carcinoma of head of pancreas. Lancet 1986; 1(8472):69–71.
58. Shepherd HA, Royle G, Ross AP, Diba A, Arthur M, Colin-Jones D. Endoscopic biliary endoprosthesis in the palliation of malignant obstruction of the distal common bile duct: a randomized trial. Br J Surg 1988; 75(12):1166–1168.
59. Smith AC, Dowsett JF, Russell RC, Hatfield AR, Cotton RB. Randomised trial of endoscopic stenting versus surgical bypass in malignant low-bileduct obstruction. Lancet 1994; 334(8938):1655–1660.
60. Monge JJ. Survival of patients with small carcinomas of the head of the pancreas. Biliary-intestinal bypass vs. pancreatoduodenectomy. Ann Surg 1967; 166(6):908–912.
61. Sarr MG, Cameron JL. Surgical management of unresectable carcinoma of the pancreas. Surgery 1982; 91(2):123–133.
62. Wade TP, Neuberger TJ, Swope TJ, Virgo KS, Johnson FE. Pancreatic cancer palliation: using tumor stage to select appropriate operation. Am J Surg 1994; 167(1):208–212; discussion 212–213.
63. Bakkevold KE, Kambestad B. Palliation of pancreatic cancer. A prospective multicentre study. Eur J Surg Oncol 1995; 21(2):176–182.
64. Espat NJ, Brennan MF, Conlon KC. Patients with laparoscopically staged unresectable pancreatic adenocarcinoma do not require subsequent surgical biliary or gastric bypass. J Am Coll Surg 1999; 188(6):649–655; discussion 655–657.
65. Sohn TA, Lillemoe KD, Cameron JL, Huang JJ, Pitt HA, Yeo CJ. Surgical palliation of unresectable periampullary adenocarcinoma in the 1990s. J Am Coll Surg 1999; 188(6):658–666; discussion 666–669.
66. Nieveen van Dijkum EJ, Romijn MG, Terwee CB, et al. Laparoscopic staging and subsequent palliation in patients with peripancreatic carcinoma. Ann Surg 2003; 237(1):66–73.
67. Sohn TA, Yeo CJ, Cameron JL, et al. Resected adenocarcinoma of the pancreas—616 patients: results, outcomes, and prognostic indicators. J Gastrointest Surg 2000; 4(6):567–579.
68. Watanapa P, Williamson RC. Surgical palliation for pancreatic cancer: developments during the past two decades. Br J Surg 1992; 79(1):8–20.
69. Singh SM, Longmire WP Jr, Reber HA. Surgical palliation for pancreatic cancer. The UCLA experience. Ann Surg 1990; 212(2):132–139.

70. Lillemoe KD, Sauter PK, Pitt HA, Yeo CJ, Cameron JL. Current status of surgical palliation of periampullary carcinoma. Surg Gynecol Obstet 1993; 176(1):1–10.
71. Lillemoe KD, Cameron JL, Hardacre JM, et al. Is prophylactic gastrojejunostomy indicated for unresectable periampullary cancer? A prospective randomized trial. Ann Surg 1999; 230(3):322–328; discussion 328–330.
72. Lillemoe KD. Palliative therapy for pancreatic cancer. Surg Oncol Clin North Am 1998; 7(1):199–216.
73. Gudjonsson B, Livstone EM, Spiro HM. Cancer of the pancreas: diagnostic accuracy and survival statistics. Cancer 1978; 42(5):2494–2506.
74. Gudjonsson B. Cancer of the pancreas. 50 years of surgery. Cancer 1987; 60(9):2284–2303.
75. Cameron JL, Crist DW, Sitzmann JV, et al. Factors influencing survival after pancreaticoduodenectomy for pancreatic cancer. Am J Surg 1991; 161(1):120–124; discussion 124–125.
76. Geer RJ, Brennan MF. Prognostic indicators for survival after resection of pancreatic adenocarcinoma. Am J Surg 1993; 165(1):68–72; discussion 72–73.
77. Gudjonsson B. Carcinoma of the pancreas: critical analysis of costs, results of resections, and the need for standardized reporting. J Am Coll Surg 1995; 181(6):483–503.
78. Bramhall SR, Allum WH, Jones AG, Allwood A, Cummins C, Neoptolemos JP. Treatment and survival in 13,560 patients with pancreatic cancer, and incidence of the disease, in the West Midlands: an epidemiological study. Br J Surg 1995; 82(1):111–115.
79. Yeo CJ, Cameron JL, Lillemoe KD, et al. Pancreaticoduodenectomy for cancer of the head of the pancreas. 201 patients. Ann Surg 1995; 221(6):721–731; discussion 731–733.
80. Conlon KC, Klimstra DS, Brennan MF. Long-term survival after curative resection for pancreatic ductal adenocarcinoma. Clinicopathologic analysis of 5-year survivors. Ann Surg 1996; 223(3): 273–279.
81. Whitehead RP, Benedetti JK, Abbruzzese JL, et al. A phase II study of high-dose 24 hour continuous infusion 5-FU and leucovorin and low-dose PALA for patients with advanced pancreatic adenocarcinoma: a Southwest Oncology Group Study. Invest New Drugs 2004; 22(3):335–341.
82. Furuse J, Kinoshita T, Kawashima M, et al. Intraoperative and conformal external-beam radiation therapy with protracted 5-fluorouracil infusion in patients with locally advanced pancreatic carcinoma. Cancer 2003; 97(5):1346–1352.
83. Feliu J, Mel R, Borrega P, et al. Phase II study of a fixed dose-rate infusion of gemcitabine associated with uracil/tegafur in advanced carcinoma of the pancreas. Ann Oncol 2002; 13(11):1756–1762.
84. Azria D, Ychou M, Jacot W, et al. Treatment of unresectable, locally advanced pancreatic adenocarcinoma with combined radiochemotherapy with 5-fluorouracil and cisplatin. Pancreas 2002; 25(4): 360–365.
85. Blackstock AW, Tepper JE, Niedwiecki D, Hollis DR, Mayer RJ, Tempero MA. Cancer and leukemia group B (CALGB) 89805: phase II chemoradiation trial using gemcitabine in patients with locoregional adenocarcinoma of the pancreas. Int J Gastrointest Cancer 2003; 34(2–3):107–116.
86. Imamura M, Doi R, Imaizumi T, et al. A randomized multicenter trial comparing resection and radiochemotherapy for resectable locally invasive pancreatic cancer. Surgery 2004; 136(5):1003–1011.
87. Wagner M, Redaelli C, Lietz M, Seiler CA, Friess H, Buchler MW. Curative resection is the single most important factor determining outcome in patients with pancreatic adenocarcinoma. Br J Surg 2004; 91(5):586–594.
88. Richter A, Niedergethmann M, Sturm JW, Lorenz D, Post S, Trede M. Long-term results of partial pancreaticoduodenectomy for ductal adenocarcinoma of the pancreatic head: 25-year experience. World J Surg 2003; 27(3):324–329.
89. Millikan KW, Deziel DJ, Silverstein JC, et al. Prognostic factors associated with resectable adenocarcinoma of the head of the pancreas. Am Surg 1999; 65(7):618–623; discussion 623–624.
90. Ahmad NA, Lewis JD, Ginsberg GG, et al. Long term survival after pancreatic resection for pancreatic adenocarcinoma. Am J Gastroenterol 2001; 96(9):2609–2615.
91. Sasson AR, Hoffman JP, Ross EA, Kagan SA, Pingpank JF, Eisenberg BL. En bloc resection for locally advanced cancer of the pancreas: is it worthwhile? J Gastrointest Surg 2002; 6(2):147–157; discussion 157–158.
92. Kuhlmann KF, de Castro SM, Wesseling JG, et al. Surgical treatment of pancreatic adenocarcinoma; actual survival and prognostic factors in 343 patients. Eur J Cancer 2004; 40(4):549–558.
93. Cleary SP, Gryfe R, Guindi M, et al. Prognostic factors in resected pancreatic adenocarcinoma: analysis of actual 5-year survivors. J Am Coll Surg 2004; 198(5):722–731.
94. Hartel M, Wente MN, Di Sebastiano P, Friess H, Buchler MW. The role of extended resection in pancreatic adenocarcinoma: is there good evidence-based justification? Pancreatology 2004; 4(6): 561–566.
95. Bakkevold KE, Arnesjo B, Dahl O, Kambestad B. Adjuvant combination chemotherapy (AMF) following radical resection of carcinoma of the pancreas and papilla of Vater—results of a controlled, prospective, randomized multicentre study. Eur J Cancer 1993; 29A(5):698–703.
96. Takada T, Amano H, Yasuda H, et al. Is postoperative adjuvant chemotherapy useful for gallbladder carcinoma? A phase III multicenter prospective randomized controlled trial in patients with resected pancreaticobiliary carcinoma. Cancer 2002; 95(8):1685–1695.

97. Kalser MH, Ellenberg SS. Pancreatic cancer. Adjuvant combined radiation and chemotherapy following curative resection. Arch Surg 1985; 120(8):899–903.
98. Klinkenbijl JH, Jeekel J, Sahmoud T, et al. Adjuvant radiotherapy and 5-fluorouracil after curative resection of cancer of the pancreas and periampullary region: phase III trial of the EORTC gastrointestinal tract cancer cooperative group. Ann Surg 1999; 230(6):776–782; discussion 782–784.
99. Neoptolemos JP, Stocken DD, Friess H, et al. A randomized trial of chemoradiotherapy and chemotherapy after resection of pancreatic cancer. N Engl J Med 2004; 350(12):1200–1210.
100. Bramhall SR, Rosemurgy A, Brown PD, Bowry C, Buckels JA. Marimastat as first-line therapy for patients with unresectable pancreatic cancer: a randomized trial. J Clin Oncol 2001; 19(15): 3447–3455.
101. Bramhall SR, Schulz J, Nemunaitis J, Brown PD, Baillet M, Buckels JA. A double-blind placebo-controlled, randomized study comparing gemcitabine and marimastat with gemcitabine and placebo as first line therapy in patients with advanced pancreatic cancer. Br J Cancer 2002; 87(2):161–167.
102. Moore MJ, Hamm J, Dancey J, et al. Comparison of gemcitabine versus the matrix metalloproteinase inhibitor BAY 12-9566 in patients with advanced or metastatic adenocarcinoma of the pancreas: a phase III trial of the National Cancer Institute of Canada Clinical Trials Group. J Clin Oncol 2003; 21(17):3296–3302.
103. Xiong HQ, Abbruzzese JL. Epidermal growth factor receptor-targeted therapy for pancreatic cancer. Semin Oncol 2002; 29(5 suppl 14):31–37.
104. Kindler HL, Stadler WM. Bevacizumab plus gemcitabine is an active combination in patients with advanced pancreatic cancer: interim results of an ongoing Phase II trial from the University of Chicago Phase II Consortium. Proceedings from the Gastrointestinal Cancers Symposium (ASCO, SSO, ASTRO, AGA), 2004 [Abstract #86].

21 The Role of Radiation Therapy for the Treatment of Pancreatic Adenocarcinoma

Johanna Bendell
Division of Oncology and Transplantation, Duke University Medical Center, Durham, North Carolina, U.S.A.

Christopher Willett
Department of Radiation Oncology, Duke University Medical Center, Durham, North Carolina, U.S.A.

INTRODUCTION

Pancreatic cancer remains one of the greatest challenges in oncology. In the year 2005, there will be an estimated 32,180 new cases of pancreatic cancer in the United States and 31,900 estimated deaths from the disease, making pancreatic cancer the fourth leading cause of cancer death in the United States (1). At present, surgery is the only means of cure. Unfortunately, only 5% to 25% of patients present with tumors amenable to resection. Historically, patients who do undergo resection for localized pancreatic carcinoma have a long-term survival of approximately 20% and a median survival of 13 to 20 months (2). Recent data suggest that the survival of patients who undergo resection of their pancreatic cancer may be improving, with new three-year survival rates around 30% (3). Patients who present with unresectable, locally advanced pancreatic cancer have a median survival of approximately 9 to 13 months, with rare long-term survival. The highest percentage (40–45%) of patients present with metastatic disease, which carries a shorter median survival of only three to six months (4). The high mortality rate of pancreatic cancer is due to the high incidence of metastatic disease at the time of diagnosis, a fulminant clinical course, and the lack of adequate systemic therapies.

For patients with nonmetastatic disease, radiation therapy can be combined with chemotherapy in an effort to offer patients a better chance of longer survival. However, the optimal treatment for these patients remains controversial. New research is being done to evaluate improving treatment for these patients with better radiation techniques, different chemotherapeutic agents, and the incorporation of novel "molecularly targeted" agents into therapy. This chapter will review the data that exist on the role of radiation therapy in the treatment of localized pancreatic adenocarcinoma, as well as comment on current and future areas of research.

ADJUVANT THERAPY

After surgical resection of pancreatic cancer, recurrence rates range from 50% to 90% for local recurrence and 40% to 90% for distant recurrence, most commonly in the liver and/or peritoneum (5–8). For this reason, adjuvant radiation therapy, chemotherapy, and combined radiation- and chemotherapy have been studied in this setting in an attempt to improve patient outcomes (Table 1). However, despite multiple trials, a definitive role for adjuvant therapy for resected pancreatic cancer has not been established.

Prospective Trials

The Gastrointestinal Tumor Study Group (GITSG) in conducted the first prospective trial of adjuvant chemoradiotherapy for patients with resected pancreatic cancer and negative surgical margins. These patients were randomized to external beam radiation therapy (EBRT) of 40 Gy delivered in split-course fashion with concurrent 5-fluorouracil (5-FU; 500 mg/m^2) given as an intravenous bolus on the first three and last three days of radiation, followed by maintenance

TABLE 1 Prospective, Randomized Trials for Adjuvant Therapy for Pancreatic Cancer

Series	No. of patients	Median survival (mo)	Two-year survival (%)	Five-year survival (%)
GITSG (9)				
Treatment	21	21.0	43	19
Observation	22	10.9	18	5
Treatment (expanded cohort) (10)	30	18.0	46	NA
EORTC (11)				
Treatment	60	17.1	37	20
Observation	54	12.6	23	10
ESPAC-1 (12,13)				
Pooled data				
Chemotherapy	244	19.7	NA	NA
No chemotherapy	237	14.0	NA	NA
Chemoradiation	178	15.5	NA	NA
No chemoradiation	180	16.1	NA	NA
2 × 2 Factorial				
Chemotherapy	147	20.1	40	21
No chemotherapy	142	15.5	30	8
Chemoradiation	145	15.9	29	10
No chemoradiation	144	17.9	41	20

Abbreviations: EORTC, European Organization for Research and Treatment of Cancer; ESPAC-1, European Study Group for Pancreatic Cancer 1; GITSG, Gastrointestinal Tumor Study Group.

5-FU for two years or until disease progression, or to observation only (9). This trial was stopped early secondary to slow accrual (43 patients over eight years), and a positive interim analysis found that patients treated on the chemoradiotherapy arm had a positive survival benefit. Patients who received chemoradiotherapy had a longer median survival (21 months vs. 11 months) and a higher two-year survival (43% vs. 19%). Additional 30 patients were then enrolled to receive adjuvant chemoradiation. These additional patients confirmed the survival outcomes seen in the original trial, with median survival of 18 months and a two-year survival of 46% (10). The GITSG trial was criticized for many reasons: only 9% of patients received the two-year maintenance chemotherapy, the radiation dose was low, the number of patients was small, slow accrual, an unusually poor survival for the surgical control group, 25% of patients did not begin adjuvant therapy until over 10 weeks after resection, and 32% of the original treatment arm had violations of the scheduled radiation therapy. Nevertheless, this trial resulted in chemoradiation therapy being accepted as appropriate adjuvant therapy in the United States.

A second study sponsored by the European Organization for Research and Treatment of Cancer (EORTC) sought to confirm the findings of the original GITSG study. In this trial, 218 patients with resected pancreas or periampullary cancers were randomly assigned to receive 40 Gy of EBRT in a split-dose fashion with concurrent continuous infusional 5-FU (25 mg/kg/day) or observation alone (11). This study showed no significant improvement ($P = 0.208$) in median survival (24 months vs. 19 months) or two-year survival (51% vs. 41%). Interestingly, only 114 of the patients enrolled in trial had pancreatic cancer, the remaining patients had ampullary tumors. Subset analysis of the patients with primary pancreatic tumors showed a two-year survival of 34% for treated patients versus 26% for the control group ($P = 0.099$). Criticisms of this trial include: there was no maintenance chemotherapy given in the treatment arm, patients with positive surgical margins were allowed in trial with no prospective assessment, the radiation dose was low, low numbers of patients, and 20% of patients assigned to treatment never received treatment.

The European Study Group for Pancreatic Cancer (ESPAC) then conducted the largest trial evaluating adjuvant therapy for pancreatic cancer, ESPAC-1. Treating physicians were allowed to enroll their patients in any one of the three parallel randomized studies: (*i*) chemoradiation versus no chemoradiation ($n = 69$), chemoradiation was 20 Gy over two weeks with 5-FU (500 mg/m^2) on days 1 to 3, then repeated after a two-week break; (*ii*) chemotherapy versus no chemotherapy ($n = 192$), chemotherapy was bolus 5-FU (425 mg/m^2) and leucovorin (20 mg/m^2) given for five days every 28 days for six months; and (*iii*) a 2 × 2 factorial design of

289 patients enrolled in chemoradiotherapy ($n = 73$), chemotherapy ($n = 75$), chemoradiotherapy with maintenance chemotherapy ($n = 72$), or observation ($n = 69$) (12,13). The data from the treatment groups from all three parallel trials were then pooled for analysis. There was no survival difference between the 175 patients who received adjuvant chemoradiation and the 178 patients who did not receive therapy (median survival 15.5 months vs. 16.1 months, $P=0.24$). There was, however, a survival benefit found for the patients who received adjuvant chemotherapy ($n=238$) compared to those who did not ($n=235$) (median survival 19.7 months vs. 14 months, $P=0.0005$). On further follow-up, the five-year survival rate for the patients who received chemotherapy was 21% versus 8% for those who did not.

Like its predecessors, the ESPAC-1 trial had many criticisms: (*i*) Physicians and patients were allowed to choose which of the three parallel trials to enroll in, creating potential bias. (*ii*) Patients could receive "background" chemoradiation or chemotherapy if decided by their physician. Approximately, one-third of the patients enrolled in the chemotherapy versus no chemotherapy trial received "background" chemoradiation therapy or chemotherapy. (*iii*) The radiation was given in a split-dose fashion, with the treating physician judging the final treatment dose (40 Gy vs. 60 Gy). (*iv*) In the chemoradiation versus no chemoradiation trial, no maintenance adjuvant chemotherapy was given, similar to the EORTC trial. The conclusion of the ESPAC-1 trial was that, although no benefit is seen from adjuvant chemoradiation therapy, there was a benefit to adjuvant chemotherapy.

Single-Institution Experiences

Reports of single-institution experiences with adjuvant therapy for pancreatic cancer have served to provide some additional evidence to the benefit of adjuvant therapy. The largest of these series is from the Johns Hopkins Medical Institutions, where investigators reported the results of a retrospective analysis of 174 patients who had chosen either: (*i*) EBRT (40–45 Gy) with two three-day courses of 5-FU at the beginning and end of radiation, followed by weekly bolus 5-FU (500 mg/m^2) for four months ($n=99$), (*ii*) EBRT (50.4–57.6 Gy) to the pancreatic bed plus prophylactic hepatic irradiation (23.4–27 Gy) given with infusional 5-FU (200 mg/m^2/day) plus leucovorin (5 mg/m^2/day) for 5 out of 7 days of the week for four months ($n=21$), or no therapy ($n=53$) (14). Patients who received adjuvant chemoradiation had a median survival of 20 months compared to 14 months for patients who were not treated. Two-year survival was 44% and 30%, respectively. There was no survival advantage to the more intensive adjuvant therapy. A follow-up report from this group of 616 patients with resected pancreatic cancer found adjuvant chemoradiation treatment as a strong predictor of outcome, with a hazard ratio of 0.5 (15).

In addition to the Johns Hopkins series, small series from the Mayo Clinic and the University of Pennsylvania have also reported survival benefit to adjuvant chemoradiation therapy. In these series, the EBRT dosed in a range of 45 to 54 Gy in combination with 5-FU-based therapy yielded a superior five-year survival compared to no therapy (17% vs. 4% and 43% vs. 35%, respectively) (16,17). A series of Medicare patients from the surveillance epidemiology and end results (SEER) database have found an improved median and three-year survival for patients who received adjuvant chemoradiation therapy than those who did not (29 months vs. 12.5 months, 45% vs. 30%, respectively) (3). However, it must be noted that in all of these retrospective analyses, there is a possible bias toward the treatment of better-risk patients.

Data with the highest observed survival after adjuvant therapy for pancreatic cancer come from a phase II trial done at Virginia Mason University. Results from 43 of 53 enrolled patients in this study were reported in 2003. These patients were treated with EBRT to 50 Gy with concurrent chemotherapy with 5-FU (200 mg/m^2/day) continuous infusion, cisplatin 30 mg/m^2 weekly, and IFN-α 3 million units subcutaneously every other day. After completion of chemoradiation, patients received 5-FU (200 mg/m^2/day) continuous infusion in weeks 10 through 15 and 18 through 23 (18). The median survival, two-year overall survival, and five-year overall survival were 44 months, 58%, and 45%, respectively. With these encouraging data came significant toxicity, with 70% of patients experiencing grade 3 common terminology criteria (CTC) toxicities, and 42% of patients requiring hospitalization. The American College of Surgeons Oncology Group has opened a larger, multicenter, phase II trial of 100 patients to further investigate this regimen.

Newer Chemotherapy Agents

The results of the numerous clinical trials of adjuvant therapy for pancreatic cancer leave many questions unanswered with no definitive answer as to the optimal treatment for these patients. In addition, newer chemotherapy agents such as gemcitabine and molecularly targeted agents have emerged, and the possible benefit of their addition to adjuvant therapy has yet to be reported in larger trials. Based on the results of a prospective randomized trial, gemcitabine has become the standard first line agent in patients with advanced pancreatic cancer. Burris and colleagues randomized 160 previously untreated patients with advanced and metastatic pancreatic cancer to receive either gemcitabine or 5-FU. Patients who received gemcitabine had a statistically improved median survival, one-year survival rate, and clinical benefit compared to patients who received 5-FU (19). In radiobiologic models, gemcitabine has also been observed to be a potent radiosensitizer. Although the mechanism of action is not yet defined, a key event appears to be inhibition of ribonucleotide reductase, producing depletion of d-adenosine triphosphate pools, followed by cell-cycle redistribution into S phase. These events lower the threshold for radiation-induced apoptosis (20). Gemcitabine, a potent radiosensitizer, has been studied in phase I and II studies in combination with radiation. A recent phase II trial of twice-weekly gemcitabine at 40 mg/m2 given with concurrent EBRT to 50.4 Gy has reported results for 38 patients with a median survival of 14.5 months (21). A phase I study of full-dose gemcitabine at 1000 mg/m2 found a maximum tolerated dose (MTD) of concurrent EBRT to be 39 Gy to the pancreatic bed. Median survival for the 32 patients in this study was 16.5 months (22). A recently reported randomized phase III trial from Europe evaluated 368 patients with resected pancreatic cancer. They were either treated with weekly gemcitabine (1000 mg/m2 weekly on days 1, 8, and 15 for six four-week cycles) or observation (23). Patients who received gemcitabine had a significantly longer disease-free survival than those in the observation-only arm (14.2 months vs. 7.5 months).

Current Trials

There are several ongoing large clinical trials that are attempting to further clarify the role of adjuvant therapy for pancreatic cancer. The first is Radiation Therapy Oncology Group (RTOG) and GI Intergroup Trial 9704. This is a phase III study of 519 patients with resected pancreatic cancer randomized to either: three weeks of continuous infusional 5-FU at 250 $mg/m^2/day$, followed by chemoradiation (50.4 Gy in 1.8 Gy daily fractions with continuous infusional 5-FU at 250 $mg/m^2/day$), then two four-week courses of continuous infusional 5-FU at 250 $mg/m^2/day$ with two weeks rest between courses to begin three to five weeks after completion of chemoradiation, or three weekly doses of gemcitabine at 1000 $mg/m^2/wk$ followed by the same 5-FU-based chemoradiation as in the first arm, followed by three months of gemcitabine 1000 mg/m^2 given weekly 3 out of every four weeks. Accrual to this trial has been completed. In Europe and Australia, ESPAC-3 has enrolled over 500 patients of a planned 990. Originally, this study randomized patients with resected pancreatic cancer into one of three arms: 5-FU (425 mg/m^2) and leucovorin (20 mg/m^2) given days for five days every 28 days for six months, gemcitabine (1000 mg/m^2) given weekly over 30 minutes for three out of four weeks for six months, or observation. However, with the release of the matured ESPAC-1 data confirming a survival benefit to chemotherapy over observation, the observation arm has now been dropped from this trial. Notably, radiation therapy has been excluded from this trial.

NEOADJUVANT THERAPY

Even after undergoing curative resection for pancreatic cancer, 80% to 85% of patients will recur. In addition, positive margins or nodal disease increases this rate of recurrence to 90% (24,25). The use of neoadjuvant chemoradiation offers another possible way to improve upon these figures for several reasons: (*i*) approximately 25% of patients do not receive adjuvant therapy in a timely manner after surgery or do not receive it at all (15,26); (*ii*) given the high recurrence rates after surgical resection, pancreatic cancer is likely a systemic disease at the time of diagnosis in 80% to 85% of patients who appear to have resectable disease (27,28), and with neoadjuvant therapy, 20% to 40% of patients will be spared the morbidity of resection because their metastatic disease becomes clinically apparent (29); (*iii*) preoperative therapy could theoretically be less toxic and more effective as the chemotherapy and radiation would be given without the postsurgical issues of small bowel in the radiation field and decreased oxygenation and decreased drug delivery to the remaining tumor bed (30); and (*iv*) patients with local and unresectable lesions may be able to be downstaged to allow for surgical resection.

5-Fluorouracil-Based Regimens

Small initial studies of neoadjuvant radiation with and without continuous infusion 5-FU established the tolerability of this regimen, but showed no improvement in survival or resectability for these patients (31–35). For this reason, further studies were done increasing the radiation dose, with different chemotherapy regimens, and with intraoperative radiation therapy (IORT) at the time of surgery.

The Eastern Cooperative Oncology Group (ECOG) treated 53 patients with potentially resectable pancreatic cancer with 5-FU (1000 mg/m^2/day) continuous infusion on days 2 to 5 and 29 to 32 of radiation, mitomycin (10 mg/m^2) on day 2, and EBRT to 50.4 Gy (36). Nine (17%) of the treated patients developed either local progression of disease or distant metastases and were not surgical candidates, 11 patients (21%) had metastatic disease at surgery, and complete resection was possible in 24 of the 41 patients taken to surgery. For the patients who underwent resection, the median survival was 16 months, and 10 months for the entire group. The poor survival for the patients who did undergo resection was likely due to three of the patients having positive peritoneal cytology, four having lymph node metastases, 13 having close surgical margins, and four needing resection of the superior mesenteric vein (SMV). In addition, over 50% of the treated patients required hospitalization due to treatment toxicity.

At M.D. Anderson Cancer Center, multiple trials of neoadjuvant 5-FU-based chemoradiation have been performed. The first trial treated 28 patients with 5-FU (300 mg/m^2/day) continuous infusion with concurrent EBRT of 50.4 Gy over 5.5 weeks (35). Patients who underwent surgical resection also received IORT. Twenty-five percent of patients had evidence of metastatic disease on preoperative restaging. Fifteen percent had metastatic disease that was found on laparoscopy. For the patients who underwent surgery median survival was 18 months, and 41% had a pathologic partial response to therapy. However, 33% of patients treated in this study required hospitalization for gastrointestinal toxicity from therapy. For this reason, the next trials from this group focused on rapid fractionation EBRT. A prospective trial of 35 patients treated with EBRT to 30 Gy (3 Gy per fraction for 10 fractions) with concurrent 5-FU (300 mg/m^2/day) continuous infusion found grade 3 nausea and vomiting in only 9% of patients with no grade 4 toxicities (37). Twenty-seven patients were taken to surgery and 20 patients underwent resection and IORT to 10 to 15 Gy. Locoregional recurrence occurred in only two for the 20 resected patients. Median survival for patients who underwent surgery was 25 months with a three-year survival of 23%.

Gemcitabine-Based Regimens

Several phase I studies have attempted to use the radiosensitization effects and the improved efficacy in advanced pancreatic cancer of gemcitabine in the neoadjuvant setting. A phase I study of twice-weekly gemcitabine in combination with EBRT of 50.4 Gy in 28 fractions for patients with localized pancreatic cancer found a MTD of 50 mg/m^2 twice a week (38). Another phase I study of full dose gemcitabine in combination with EBRT (39) dosed gemcitabine at 1000 mg/m^2 over 30 minutes on days 1, 8, and 15 of a 28 day cycle, with radiation theraphy directed at the primary tumor alone starting at a radiation dose of 24 Gy in 1.6 Gy fractions. The MTD of the radiation was 36 Gy in 2.4 Gy fractions. The dose-limiting toxicities were vomiting and gastroduodenal ulceration. The phase II trial of this regimen enrolled 41 patients with resectable or locally advanced pancreatic cancer. Eight of the 32 evaluable patients for toxicity showed grade 3 GI toxicity, grade 3 fatigue, and one unexplained death (40). Survival data are not yet available. Another trial of weekly gemcitabine at a dose of 400 mg/m^2 for seven doses plus concurrent ERBT to 30 Gy in 10 fractions over two weeks, beginning three days after first gemcitabine dose has preliminary results reported (41). Of the 86 patients treated, all received the total dose of radiation, but only 45% received the full dose of gemcitabine.

Forty-three percent of patients were hospitalized prior to surgery. However, 86% of patients went to laparotomy with 73% undergoing a successful tumor resection, and 59% of tumor specimens had >50% tumor necrosis. The median survival was 37 months.

Gemcitabine has also been studied in combination with other chemotherapy agents and EBRT in the neoadjuvant setting. A phase I study of 19 patients with pancreatic cancer evaluated the MTD of cisplatin when given with gemcitabine at 1000 mg/m^2 weekly with EBRT to 36 Gy given in 2.4 Gy fractions (42). Cisplatin was given on days 1 and 15 following gemcitabine. The MTD of cisplatin was 40 mg/m^2. Another trial by the M.D. Anderson Cancer Center group evaluated a treatment schedule of gemcitabine (750 mg/m^2) and cisplatin (30 mg/m^2) given every 14 days for four treatments, followed by four weekly doses of gemcitabine at 400 mg/m^2 concurrent with 30 Gy of EBRT given as 3 Gy fractions over two weeks, beginning two days after the first dose of gemcitabine (43). Preliminary results from 37 patients showed that 67% underwent resection, with 70% of the pathologic specimens showing necrosis of >50% of the tumor. This regimen, however, had significant toxicity, with 62% of patients requiring hospitalization, most due to biliary stent occlusion.

Taxane-Based Regimens

In radiobiologic models, paclitaxel may result in enhanced radiosensitization through (*i*) synchronization of tumor cells at G2/M, a relatively radiosensitive phase of cell cycle and (*ii*) tumor reoxygenation after apoptotic clearance of paclitaxel-damaged cells. Pisters and colleagues from M.D. Anderson Cancer Center have examined the use of paclitaxel as a radiation sensitizer in the neoadjuvant setting for pancreatic cancer (44). In this trial, 35 patients received paclitaxel 60 mg/m^2 weekly with concurrent EBRT to 30 Gy. Eighty percent underwent resection with 21% percent of pathology specimens showing >50% tumor necrosis. The three-year survival for the patients who underwent preoperative therapy and resection was 28%. Hospitalization was required in 11% of patients for toxicity, primarily nausea and vomiting. These preliminary data show an increased toxicity without a significant improvement compared to histologic response rate or overall survival for this paclitaxel-based regimen.

Targeted Therapies/Future Directions

Future directions for neoadjuvant therapy include the incorporation of novel, targeted agents with ERBT alone or with chemoradiation, and newer radiation therapy techniques. The use of targeted therapies is based on impressive phase II data combining targeted agents with chemotherapy in the metastatic pancreatic cancer setting. A phase II trial of the vascular endothelial growth factor (VEGF) inhibitor, bevacizumab, in combination with gemcitabine for patients with advanced pancreatic cancer (45) has shown response rate of 27% compared to 5.6% historically for gemcitabine alone (46), and a one-year survival of 53% compared to <20%, respectively. A phase II trial of an epidermal growth factor receptor (EGFR) inhibitor, cetuximab, in combination with gemcitabine for patients with advanced pancreatic cancer has shown a one-year survival of 33% (47). In addition, a randomized controlled phase III trial of gemcitabine plus or minus erlotinib, another EGFR inhibitor, has shown a 23.5% increase in overall survival with the addition of erlotinib compared to gemcitabine alone (48). No trials of these agents in the neoadjuvant setting have yet been reported, but preliminary results are available in the locally advanced setting. The use of IORT technique and three-dimensional conformal radiation therapy is further discussed in the locally advanced section.

LOCALLY ADVANCED THERAPY

Patients with locally advanced carcinoma of the pancreas compose a group of patients with an intermediate prognosis between resectable and metastatic patients. These patients have pancreatic tumors which are defined as surgically unresectable, but have no evidence of distant metastases. A tumor is considered to be unresectable if it has one of the following features: (*i*) extensive peripancreatic lymph node involvement and/or distant metastases (typically to the liver or peritoneum), (*ii*) encasement or occlusion of the SMV or SMV/portal vein confluence, or (*iii*) direct involvement of the superior mesenteric artery (SMA), inferior vena cava, aorta, or celiac axis. However, recent advances in surgical techniques may allow for resection of selected patients with tumors involving the SMV (49). Combined treatment with radiation and chemotherapy increases median survival for patients with locally advanced cancers to approximately 9 to 13 months, but rarely results in long-term survival. The therapeutic options of patients with locally advanced pancreatic cancer include EBRT with 5-FU chemotherapy, IORT, and more recently EBRT with novel chemotherapeutic and target agents. In evaluating the results of these various therapies, it is useful to remember that a median survival of three to six months has been reported for this subset of patients undergoing palliative gastric or biliary bypass only (50).

Prospective Trials

With the exception of one trial, conventional EBRT for locally advanced pancreatic cancer has been shown to improve survival when combined with 5-FU compared to EBRT alone or chemotherapy alone (Table 2). The Mayo Clinic undertook an early randomized trial in the 1960s in which 64 patients with locally unresectable, nonmetastatic pancreatic adenocarcinoma received 35 to 40 Gy of EBRT with concurrent 5-FU versus the same EBRT schedule plus placebo. A significant survival advantage was seen for patients receiving EBRT with 5-FU versus EBRT only (10.4 months vs. 6.3 months) (51).

GITSG followed with a similar study comparing EBRT alone to EBRT with concurrent and maintenance 5-FU. One hundred and ninety-four eligible patients with surgically confirmed unresectable and nonmetastatic pancreatic adenocarcinoma were randomized to receive 60 Gy of split-course EBRT alone, 40 Gy of split-course EBRT with two to three cycles of concurrent bolus 5-FU chemotherapy, or 60 Gy of split-course EBRT using a similar chemotherapy regimen. Patients in the latter groups received maintenance 5-FU after EBRT completion. The EBRT alone arm was closed early as a result of an inferior survival rate. The median one-year survival rate in the two combined modality therapy arms was 38% and 36%, respectively, versus 11% in the EBRT alone arm (52).

The second GITSG trial of this series randomized 157 eligible patients with unresectable disease to 60 Gy split-course EBRT with concurrent and maintenance 5-FU from the previous trial or 40 Gy continuous course radiation with weekly concurrent doxorubicin chemotherapy, followed by maintenance doxorubicin and 5-FU. A significant increase in treatment-related toxicity was seen in the doxorubicin arm. However, no survival difference was observed between the two groups (median survival 37 weeks vs. 33 weeks) (53). No clinical benefit was seen in substituting adriamycin for 5-FU.

TABLE 2 Prospective Randomized Trials for Locally Advanced, Unresectable Pancreatic Cancer

Series	No. of patients	Median survival (mo)	Local failure (%)	One-year survival (%)	Eighteenth-month survival (%)
Mayo Clinic (51)					
EBRT (35–40 Gy/3–4 wk) only	32	6.3	NS	6	6
EBRT (35–40 Gy/3–4 wk) + 5-FU	32	10.4	NS	22	13
GITSG (52,77)					
EBRT (60 Gy/10 wk) only	25	5.3	24	10	5
EBRT (40 Gy/6 wk) + 5-FU	83	8.4	26	35	20
EBRT (60 Gy/10 wk) + 5-FU	86	11.4	27	46	20
GITSG (53)					
EBRT (60 Gy/10 wk) + 5-FU	73	8.5	58 (first site)	33	15
EBRT (40 Gy/4 wk) + doxorubicin	70	7.6	51 (first site)	27	17
GITSG (54,78)					
EBRT (54 Gy/6 wk) + 5-FU and SMF	22	9.7	45 (first site)	41	18
SMF only	21	7.4	48 (first site)	19	0
ECOG (55)					
EBRT (40 Gy/4 wk) + 5-FU	47	8.3	32	26	11
5-Flurouracil only	44	8.2	32	32	21

Abbreviations: EBRT, external beam radiation therapy; ECOG, Eastern Cooperative Oncology Group; 5-FU, 5-fluorouracil; GITSG, Gastrointestinal Tumor Study Group; SMF, streptozocin, mitomycin-C, and 5-FU.

A follow-up GITSG trial compared chemotherapy alone to chemoradiation, again in surgically confirmed unresectable tumors. Forty-three patients were randomized to receive combination streptozocin, mitomycin-C, and 5-FU (SMF) chemotherapy or 54 Gy of EBRT with two cycles of concurrent bolus 5-FU chemotherapy, followed by adjuvant SMF chemotherapy. The chemoradiation arm demonstrated a significant survival advantage over the chemotherapy alone arm (one year survival of 41% vs. 19%) (54).

In contrast to the results of the prior studies, the ECOG reported no benefit to chemoradiation versus chemotherapy only. In this study, patients with unresectable, nonmetastatic pancreatic or gastric adenocarcinoma were randomized to receive either 5-FU chemotherapy alone or 40 Gy EBRT with concurrent bolus 5-FU week one. Patients with locally recurrent disease as well as patients undergoing surgery with residual disease were eligible for this trial. In the 91 analyzable pancreatic patients, no survival difference was observed between the two groups (median survival 8.2 months vs. 8.3 months) (55).

Continuous Infusional 5-Fluorouracil

The idea that continuous infusion 5-FU allows for increased cumulative drug dose to be given without a significant increase in toxicity and for a more protracted radiosensitization effect relative to bolus 5-FU has prompted its study in locally advanced pancreatic cancer. Other trials of other gastrointestinal sites have shown an increased survival using continuous infusion 5-FU (56). Phase I and phase II trials have been done in pancreatic cancer, showing that the use of infusional 5-FU is without excessive treatment-related toxicity and is effective (57–59). These phase I trials from ECOG found the MTD of continuous infusion 5-FU to be 250 mg/m^2, the dose-limiting toxicity being gastrointestinal. The progression-free survival at one year was 40% with a median survival of 11.9 months. The two-year survival rate for this trial was 18%. No randomized trials have been published, but combined radiation therapy with infusional 5-FU is now commonly used, and combinations of chemotherapy with infusional 5-FU and radiation therapy for locally advanced pancreatic cancer are under investigation. In addition, capecitabine, an oral 5-FU analog, in combination with radiation therapy for the treatment of pancreatic cancer has been reported (60). Dosing of capecitabine has been extrapolated from combined modality trials in rectal cancer to be about 1600 mg/m^2 divided BID during radiation treatment (61). No randomized trials have been reported with this combination.

In summary, with the exception of one study, conventional EBRT combined with 5-FU chemotherapy has been shown to offer a modest survival benefit for patients with locally advanced unresectable pancreatic cancer compared to radiation alone or chemotherapy alone. The most favorable median survival duration and two-year survival rate for EBRT plus 5-FU are approximately 10 months and 12%, respectively. Because of these results, EBRT with 5-FU-based chemotherapy has become a frequently employed therapy for these patients.

Increased External Beam Radiation Therapy Dosing

Because of the limited tolerance of normal tissue in the upper abdomen (liver, kidney, spinal cord, and bowel) to EBRT, total doses of only 45 to 54 Gy in 25 to 30 Gy fractions, have usually been given. For an unresectable tumor, this dose of radiation is inadequate, as demonstrated by the high rates of tumor progression and poor survival seen in both prospective and retrospective studies. For example, local progression occurred as first site of failure in 58% of patients treated to 60 Gy with concurrent 5-FU in the second GITSG trial (53). Similarly, the Mayo Clinic reported a local failure rate of 72% for 122 patients with unresectable pancreatic cancer treated with an EBRT dose of 40 to 60 Gy (62). An attempt has been made to evaluate whether an increased dose of radiation may improve outcomes. In a report from Thomas Jefferson University Hospital, 46 evaluable patients with unresectable disease by laparotomy were treated with 63 to 70 Gy EBRT with or without chemotherapy. Despite high-dose EBRT, the local failure rate was 78% (63).

Conversion of Locally Advanced Disease to Resectable

Because surgical resection of the primary tumor remains the only potentially curative treatment for pancreatic cancer, preoperative radiation has been studied to assess its ability to convert locally unresectable pancreatic cancer to resectable disease. In a study from New England Deaconess Hospital, 16 patients with locally advanced unresectable pancreatic cancer were treated neoadjuvantly with 5-FU chemotherapy and 45 Gy of EBRT and infusional 5-FU. Of these 16 patients, only two (13%) were able to undergo resection (34). Similarly, investigators from Duke University reported that only 2 (8%) of 25 patients with locally advanced pancreatic cancer treated with 45 Gy of EBRT and 5-FU (with or without cisplatin or mitomycin C) subsequently underwent complete resection with negative margins (64). A prospective study of 87 patients with locally advanced pancreatic cancer from Memorial Sloan-Kettering Cancer Center treated with combined modality therapy found that 3 patients achieved a complete response. These patients were taken for resection, and two were found to still have locally advanced disease and one was resected with negative margins only to recur and die 18 months later (65). These and other studies indicate that it is unlikely that currently utilized neoadjuvant chemoradiation can convert unresectable lesions to resectable ones and thereby increase the number of patients potentially cured with combined modality therapy. It is important to remember that broadening the definition of a locally advanced pancreatic cancer will give the appearance of more optimistic results. If, however, one maintains a stringent CT-based definition of locally advanced pancreatic cancer that includes only arterial involvement (SMA or celiac axis invasion) or superior mesenteric or portal vein encasement or occlusion, successful downstaging to allow complete surgical resection will be an uncommon event with contemporary chemoradiation approaches.

Intraoperative Radiation Therapy

Because of the poor local control and results achieved with conventional EBRT and chemotherapy, specialized radiation therapy techniques that increase the radiation dose to the tumor volume have been used to improve local tumor control without increasing normal tissue morbidity. These include iodine-125 implants or IORT as a dose escalation technique in combination with external beam irradiation and chemotherapy. A lower incidence of local failure in most series and improved median survival in some have been reported with these techniques when compared with conventional external beam irradiation, but it is uncertain whether this is due to superior treatment or case selection (62).

A recent study from investigators of the Massachusetts General Hospital reported the results of 150 patients treated with IORT and external beam irradiation and chemotherapy (64). Although the study spanned nearly 25 years, it is relevant because it shows for the first time that long-term survival is possible for patients with unresectable pancreatic cancer. Even though the three- and five-year survival rates (7%, 4%) are modest, they are not markedly different than the results reported in contemporary trials of resected pancreatic cancer patients (20%, 10%) or patients undergoing palliative pancreaticoduodenectomy (6.3%, 1.6%), especially when taking into account those patients with smaller tumors as measured by the size of the IORT treatment applicator. For 25 patients treated with a small diameter applicator (5 or 6 cm), the two- and three-year actuarial survival rates were 27% and 17%, respectively. Furthermore, this study shows that postoperative and late treatment related toxicity rates were acceptable. These study results support further study of selected patients with small, unresectable tumors into innovative protocols employing IORT.

Newer Chemotherapeutic Agents

Because of the high incidence of hepatic and peritoneal metastases and poor results with standard chemoradiotherapy, current and future research efforts include evaluation of EBRT with newer systemic agents (gemcitabine and paclitaxel). Interest in these agents is based on both their systemic cytotoxic effects and their radiosensitizing properties. At present, numerous investigators are pursuing phase I and II studies combining EBRT with gemcitabine. Investigators from Wake Forest University and the University of North Carolina have recently reported the results of a phase I trial of twice-weekly gemcitabine and 50.4 Gy of concurrent upper abdominal EBRT in 19 patients with unresectable/inoperable pancreatic adenocarcinoma. In this study, the MTD of gemcitabine was 40 mg/m^2. At this dose level, gemcitabine was well tolerated. Of eight patients with a minimum follow-up of 12 months, three remain alive, and one of the three has no evidence of disease progression (66). Following this trial, the Cancer and Leukemia Group B (CALGB) began a phase II study of this regimen for locally advanced pancreatic cancer. Data from this trial show a median overall survival of 8.2 months for 38 patients enrolled (67). Using an alternate dosing scheme, McGinn et al. (39) investigated weekly full-dose gemcitabine combined with radiation therapy at escalating doses in a phase I trial of 37 patients with locally advanced or incompletely resected pancreatic cancer. These patients received two cycles of gemcitabine at 1000 mg/m^2 on days 1, 8, and 15 of a 28-day cycle with concurrent EBRT during the first three weeks. An optimal dose of 36 Gy in 2.4 Gy fractions was determined and recommended for a phase II trial which has completed accrual (40).

Gemcitabine has also been studied in combination with 5-FU and radiation. ECOG performed a phase I trial of continuous infusion 5-FU at 200 mg/m^2, weekly gemcitabine at 50 to 100 mg/m^2, and 59.4 Gy of EBRT (68). The patients in this trial showed a significant amount of toxicity, the five out of seven patients experiencing dose-limiting toxicities of gastric or duodenal ulcers, thrombocytopenia, or Stevens–Johnson syndrome. Because of these toxicities, the authors concluded that the combination of gemcitabine, 5-FU, and EBRT was not appropriate. However, the Massachusetts General Hospital, Dana Farber Cancer Center, and Brigham and Women's Hospital conducted a phase I/II study of continuous infusion 5-FU with weekly gemcitabine and concurrent 50.4 Gy of EBRT for locally advanced pancreatic cancer. In this study, the MTD of weekly gemcitabine was 200 mg/m^2 when given with continuous infusion 5-FU at 200 mg/m^2 and concurrent EBRT. In this study, 32 patients were treated (13 at the MTD), and the severe toxicities were limited to one patient experiencing a grade 3 gastrointestinal bleed. The reason behind this is thought to be the lower dose of EBRT given, smaller treatment fields, and the continuous infusion 5-FU was given five days out of the week instead of seven (C. Fuchs, preliminary data). This dosage is now being used for investigation in a phase II, multicenter trial through CALGB.

In a phase I trial at Brown University evaluating paclitaxel and 50 Gy of EBRT for patients with unresectable pancreatic and gastric cancers, the MTD of weekly paclitaxel with conventional irradiation was 50 mg/m^2 (69). The response rate was 31% among 13 evaluable pancreatic cancer patients. In the Brown University phase II study employing 50 Gy of EBRT with 50 mg/m^2/wk of paclitaxel, 6 (33%) of 18 evaluable pancreatic cancer patients have had a partial response; stable disease has been observed in 7 patients (39%); only 1 patient (6%) has had local tumor progression after completion of treatment; and 4 patients (22%) have developed distant metastases. These data have led to an RTOG phase II study evaluating paclitaxel with EBRT for patients with unresectable pancreatic cancer (70). The median survival of 109 patients in this study was 11.2 months (95% CI: 10.1, 12.3) with estimated one- and two-year survivals of 43% and 13%, respectively. External irradiation plus concurrent weekly paclitaxel was well tolerated when given with large-field radiotherapy. The median survival is better than historical results achieved with irradiation and fluoropyrimidines. These data provided the basis for a RTOG trial using paclitaxel and irradiation combined with a second radiation sensitizer, gemcitabine, and a farnesyl transferase inhibitor.

Chemoradiation Effects on Quality-of-Life

Despite the potential survival benefits for patients with locally advanced pancreatic cancer receiving radiation therapy and chemotherapy, these gains are modest. With rare exception, all patients will ultimately succumb to their disease. In spite of this, significant palliative benefit can be achieved by chemoradiation. Pain, anorexia, fatigue, and clinical wasting are relatively common symptoms, which significantly impact on the patient's quality of life. Although poorly documented in many studies, using the aforementioned techniques (including IORT), reports from larger series indicate that complete pain relief can be obtained in as much as 50% to 80% of patients (71). Using EBRT alone with or without chemotherapy, approximately 35% to 65% of patients will experience pain resolution as well as some improvement in wasting and obstructive symptoms (53,72,73). Definite but less dramatic improvements in performance status and anorexic symptoms may be observed as well (72,73). Because of the high rate of mortality associated with this disease, quality of life should be one of the important endpoints in study design for these patients.

Newer Radiation Techniques

Three-dimensional conformal radiation therapy is being integrated into the treatment of a variety of malignancies, including intra-abdominal tumors. This CT-based treatment allows implementation of "unconventional" beam orientations, permitting coverage of the target volume with reductions in irradiation of nontarget tissues compared to conventional techniques. For example, an important technical consideration in the radiation treatment of pancreatic cancer is minimizing kidney irradiation, given the marked radiosensitivity of this organ. By optimizing beam orientation and weighting, significant reductions in renal irradiation have been achieved relative to standard techniques without significantly increasing the dose to other surrounding organs (74).

Further refinement of this approach is now being obtained by the use of intensity-modulated radiation therapy. With this new technology, inverse treatment planning can be performed, permitting computer-based treatment optimization versus a standard "trial and error" planning approach. Secondly, a computer-controlled, nonuniform radiation treatment can be delivered to the target permitting an even more precise and conformal dose pattern with further reductions in normal tissue irradiation. Evolution of these techniques will likely result in improved treatment tolerance and reduction of late morbidity. This is especially critical in this era of intensive chemoradiation protocols with their potential toxicity.

Chemotherapy Alone

Although local control rates have been improved by innovations in radiation therapy, systemic failure remains a major obstacle in improving the long-term survivorship. Because of the high rates of distant metastases and poor overall survival results, some investigators have questioned the value of radiation therapy in the treatment of this subset of patients. A phase III trial led by the ECOG is randomizing locally advanced pancreatic cancer patients to gemcitabine chemotherapy only or EBRT and gemcitabine.

Targeted Therapies/Future Directions

As the biological basis of cancer is better understood, the use of cancer-specific targeted therapies are being increasingly investigated. There is preclinical evidence for either additive or synergistic effects for several of these approaches (such as antibodies against and VEGF and EGFR) with both chemotherapy and radiation therapy, making these approaches especially promising. The RTOG is currently undertaking a phase II study combining bevacizumab, an anti-VEGF antibody with EBRT and capecitabine in the treatment of this group of patients. Erlotinib is an oral EGFR inhibitor recently shown to improve survival in patients with metastatic pancreatic cancer when used in combination with gemcitabine versus gemcitabine alone (48). A phase I study of erlotinib, gemcitabine, and radiation therapy for patients with locally advanced pancreatic cancer has found an MTD of erlotinib 100 mg daily, gemcitabine 40 mg/m^2 biweekly, and EBRT of 50.4 Gy (75). Of eight patients treated, seven have stable disease, and one patient was taken for R1 resection. Another phase I study has established an MTD for the combination of erlotinib, gemcitabine, paclitaxel, and radiation therapy for patients with locally advanced pancreatic cancer (76).

Pancreatic cancer remains one of the most formidable challenges in oncology. Newer imaging modalities have improved staging, thus facilitating treatment decisions. In the past 30 years, modest improvements in median survival have been attained for patients with locally advanced tumors treated by chemoradiation protocols. However, no significant impact on long-term survival has been accomplished. Local tumor control has been improved by the use of specialized radiation techniques permitting safe dose escalation. Even with these techniques, it is not clear that a survival benefit is achieved given the proclivity of metastases in this malignancy. Trials are underway testing newer systemic agents that also act as potent radiosensitizers.

Despite the recognized limitations of current therapy, palliation can be achieved for a high percentage of patients by combined modality treatment. Quality of life should be considered a paramount endpoint in the care and protocol design of these patients. In patients with marginal or poor performance status, gemcitabine administration alone represents a reasonable alternative to combined modality therapy. Significant improvements in long-term survival will likely be achieved through exploitation of the basic biologic anomalies of this malignancy.

REFERENCES

1. Jemal A, Murray T, Ward E, et al. Cancer statistics, 2005. CA Cancer J Clin 2005; 55(1):10–30.
2. Geer RJ, Brennan MF. Prognostic indicators for survival after resection of pancreatic adenocarcinoma. Am J Surg 1993; 165(1):68–72; discussion 73.
3. Lim JE, Chien MW, Earle CC. Prognostic factors following curative resection for pancreatic adenocarcinoma: a population-based, linked database analysis of 396 patients. Ann Surg 2003; 237(1):74–85.
4. Evans D, Abbruzzese J, Willett C. Cancer of the Pancreas. 6th ed. Philadelphia: Lippincott, Williams, and Wilkins, 2001.
5. Tepper J, Nardi G, Sutt H. Carcinoma of the pancreas: review of MGH experience from 1963 to 1973. Analysis of surgical failure and implications for radiation therapy. Cancer 1976; 37(3):1519–1524.
6. Griffin JF, Smalley SR, Jewell W, et al. Patterns of failure after curative resection of pancreatic carcinoma. Cancer 1990; 66(1):56–61.
7. Ozaki H. Improvement of pancreatic cancer treatment from the Japanese experience in the 1980s. Int J Pancreatol 1992; 12(1):5–9.
8. Westerdahl J, Andren-Sandberg A, Ihse I. Recurrence of exocrine pancreatic cancer—local or hepatic? Hepatogastroenterology 1993; 40(4):384–387.
9. Kalser MH, Ellenberg SS. Pancreatic cancer. Adjuvant combined radiation and chemotherapy following curative resection. Arch Surg 1985; 120(8):899–903.
10. Gastrointestinal Tumor Study Group. Further evidence of effective adjuvant combined radiation and chemotherapy following curative resection of pancreatic cancer. Cancer 1987; 59(12):2006–2010.
11. Klinkenbijl JH, Jeekel J, Sahmoud T, et al. Adjuvant radiotherapy and 5-fluorouracil after curative resection of cancer of the pancreas and periampullary region: phase III trial of the EORTC gastrointestinal tract cancer cooperative group. Ann Surg 1999; 230(6):776–782; discussion 782–784.
12. Neoptolemos JP, Dunn JA, Stocken DD, et al. Adjuvant chemoradiotherapy and chemotherapy in resectable pancreatic cancer: a randomised controlled trial. Lancet 2001; 358(9293):1576–1585.
13. Neoptolemos JP, Stocken DD, Friess H, et al. A randomized trial of chemoradiotherapy and chemotherapy after resection of pancreatic cancer. N Engl J Med 2004; 350(12):1200–1210.
14. Yeo CJ, Abrams RA, Grochow LB, et al. Pancreaticoduodenectomy for pancreatic adenocarcinoma: postoperative adjuvant chemoradiation improves survival. A prospective, single-institution experience. Ann Surg 1997; 225(5):621–633; discussion 633–636.
15. Sohn TA, Yeo CJ, Cameron JL, et al. Resected adenocarcinoma of the pancreas-616 patients: results, outcomes, and prognostic indicators. J Gastrointest Surg 2000; 4(6):567–579.
16. Foo ML, Gunderson LL, Nagorney DM, et al. Patterns of failure in grossly resected pancreatic ductal adenocarcinoma treated with adjuvant irradiation +/− 5 fluorouracil. Int J Radiat Oncol Biol Phys 1993; 26(3):483–489.
17. Whittington R, Bryer MP, Haller DG, Solin LJ, Rosato EF. Adjuvant therapy of resected adenocarcinoma of the pancreas. Int J Radiat Oncol Biol Phys 1991; 21(5):1137–1143.
18. Picozzi VJ, Kozarek RA, Traverso LW. Interferon-based adjuvant chemoradiation therapy after pancreaticoduodenectomy for pancreatic adenocarcinoma. Am J Surg 2003; 185(5):476–480.
19. Burris HA 3rd, Moore MJ, Andersen J, et al. Improvements in survival and clinical benefit with gemcitabine as first-line therapy for patients with advanced pancreas cancer: a randomized trial. J Clin Oncol 1997; 15(6):2403–2413.
20. Lawrence TS, Eisbruch A, Shewach DS. Gemcitabine-mediated radiosensitization. Semin Oncol 1997; 24(2 suppl 7):S7-24–S7-28.
21. Blackstock A, Mornex F, Partensky C, et al. Phase II trial of adjuvant gemcitabine and external beam radiation in the treatment of completely resected adenocarcinoma of the pancreas. In: GI ASCO, 2004.
22. Allen AM, Zalupski MM, Robertson JM, et al. Adjuvant therapy in pancreatic cancer: phase I trial of radiation dose escalation with concurrent full-dose gemcitabine. Int J Radiat Oncol Biol Phys 2004; 59(5):1461–1467.
23. Neuhaus P, Oettle H, Post S, et al. A randomised, prospective, multicenter, phase III trial of adjuvant chemotherapy with gemcitabine vs. observation in patients with resected pancreatic cancer. In: Proc Am Soc Clin Oncol, 2005.
24. Willett CG, Lewandrowski K, Warshaw AL, Efird J, Compton CC. Resection margins in carcinoma of the head of the pancreas. Implications for radiation therapy. Ann Surg 1993; 217(2):144–148.
25. Cameron JL, Crist DW, Sitzmann JV, et al. Factors influencing survival after pancreaticoduodenectomy for pancreatic cancer. Am J Surg 1991; 161(1):120–124; discussion 124–125.

26. Spitz FR, Abbruzzese JL, Lee JE, et al. Preoperative and postoperative chemoradiation strategies in patients treated with pancreaticoduodenectomy for adenocarcinoma of the pancreas. J Clin Oncol 1997; 15(3):928–937.
27. Evans DB, Pisters PW, Lee JE, et al. Preoperative chemoradiation strategies for localized adenocarcinoma of the pancreas. J Hepatobiliary Pancreat Surg 1998; 5(3):242–250.
28. Wayne JD, Abdalla EK, Wolff RA, Crane CH, Pisters PW, Evans DB. Localized adenocarcinoma of the pancreas: the rationale for preoperative chemoradiation. Oncologist 2002; 7(1):34–45.
29. Raut CP, Evans DB, Crane CH, Pisters PW, Wolff RA. Neoadjuvant therapy for resectable pancreatic cancer. Surg Oncol Clin North Am 2004; 13(4):639–661, ix.
30. White RR, Tyler DS. Neoadjuvant therapy for pancreatic cancer: the Duke experience. Surg Oncol Clin North Am 2004; 13(4):675–684, ix–x.
31. Pilepich MV, Miller HH. Preoperative irradiation in carcinoma of the pancreas. Cancer 1980; 46(9):1945–1949.
32. Kopelson G. Curative surgery for adenocarcinoma of the pancreas/ampulla of Vater: the role of adjuvant pre or postoperative radiation therapy. Int J Radiat Oncol Biol Phys 1983; 9(6):911–915.
33. Ishikawa O, Ohhigashi H, Teshima T, et al. Clinical and histopathological appraisal of preoperative irradiation for adenocarcinoma of the pancreatoduodenal region. J Surg Oncol 1989; 40(3):143–151.
34. Jessup JM, Steele G Jr, Mayer RJ, et al. Neoadjuvant therapy for unresectable pancreatic adenocarcinoma. Arch Surg 1993; 128(5):559–564.
35. Evans DB, Rich TA, Byrd DR, et al. Preoperative chemoradiation and pancreaticoduodenectomy for adenocarcinoma of the pancreas. Arch Surg 1992; 127(11):1335–1339.
36. Hoffman JP, Lipsitz S, Pisansky T, Weese JL, Solin L, Benson AB 3rd. Phase II trial of preoperative radiation therapy and chemotherapy for patients with localized, resectable adenocarcinoma of the pancreas: an Eastern Cooperative Oncology Group Study. J Clin Oncol 1998; 16(1):317–323.
37. Pisters PW, Abbruzzese JL, Janjan NA, et al. Rapid-fractionation preoperative chemoradiation, pancreaticoduodenectomy, and intraoperative radiation therapy for resectable pancreatic adenocarcinoma. J Clin Oncol 1998; 16(12):3843–3850.
38. Pipas JM, Mitchell SE, Barth RJ Jr, et al. Phase I study of twice-weekly gemcitabine and concomitant external-beam radiotherapy in patients with adenocarcinoma of the pancreas. Int J Radiat Oncol Biol Phys 2001; 50(5):1317–1322.
39. McGinn CJ, Zalupski MM, Shureiqi I, et al. Phase I trial of radiation dose escalation with concurrent weekly full-dose gemcitabine in patients with advanced pancreatic cancer. J Clin Oncol 2001; 19(22):4202–4208.
40. McGinn CJ, Talamonti MS, Small W, et al. A phase II trial of full-dose gemcitabine with concurrent radiation therapy in patients with resectable or unresectable non-metastatic pancreatic cancer. In: GI ASCO, 2004.
41. Wolff RA, Evans DB, Crane CH, et al. Initial results of preoperative gemcitabine (GEM)-based chemoradiation for resectable pancreatic adenocarcinoma. In: Proc Am Soc Clin Oncol, 2002.
42. Muler JH, McGinn CJ, Normolle D, et al. Phase I trial using a time-to-event continual reassessment strategy for dose escalation of cisplatin combined with gemcitabine and radiation therapy in pancreatic cancer. J Clin Oncol 2004; 22(2):238–243.
43. Wolff RA, Crane CH, Xiong HQ, et al. Preliminary analysis of preoperative systemic gemcitabine (GEM) and cisplatin (CIS) followed by GEM-based chemoradiation for resectable pancreatic adenocarcinoma. In: Proc Am Soc Clin Oncol, 2004.
44. Pisters PW, Wolff RA, Janjan NA, et al. Preoperative paclitaxel and concurrent rapid-fractionation radiation for resectable pancreatic adenocarcinoma: toxicities, histologic response rates, and event-free outcome. J Clin Oncol 2002; 20(10):2537–2544.
45. Kindler H, Friberg G, Stadler W, et al. Bevacizumab plus gemcitabine is an active combination in patients with advanced pancreatic cancer: interim results of an ongoing phase II trial from the University of Chicago Phase II Consortium. In: ASCO Gastrointestinal Cancers Symposium, 2004.
46. Berlin JD, Catalano P, Thomas JP, Kugler JW, Haller DG, Benson AB 3rd. Phase III study of gemcitabine in combination with fluorouracil versus gemcitabine alone in patients with advanced pancreatic carcinoma: Eastern Cooperative Oncology Group Trial E2297. J Clin Oncol 2002; 20(15):3270–3275.
47. Xiong HQ, Abbruzzese JL. Epidermal growth factor receptor-targeted therapy for pancreatic cancer. Semin Oncol 2002; 29(5 suppl 14):31–37.
48. Moore M, Goldstein D, Hamm J, et al. Erlotinib improves survival when added to gemcitabine in patients with advanced pancreatic cancer. A phase III trial of the National Cancer Institute of Canada Clinical Trials Group [NCIC-CTG]. In: ASCO Gastrointestinal Cancers Symposium, 2005.
49. Leach SD, Lee JE, Charnsangavej C, et al. Survival following pancreaticoduodenectomy with resection of the superior mesenteric-portal vein confluence for adenocarcinoma of the pancreatic head. Br J Surg 1998; 85(5):611–617.
50. Gunderson LL, Haddock MG, Burch P, Nagorney D, Foo ML, Todoroki T. Future role of radiotherapy as a component of treatment in biliopancreatic cancers. Ann Oncol 1999; 10(suppl 4):291–295.

51. Moertel CG, Childs DS Jr, Reitemeier RJ, Colby MY Jr, Holbrook MA. Combined 5-fluorouracil and supervoltage radiation therapy of locally unresectable gastrointestinal cancer. Lancet 1969; 2(7626):865–867.
52. Moertel CG, Frytak S, Hahn RG, et al. Therapy of locally unresectable pancreatic carcinoma: a randomized comparison of high dose (6000 rads) radiation alone, moderate dose radiation (4000 rads + 5-fluorouracil), and high dose radiation + 5-fluorouracil: The Gastrointestinal Tumor Study Group. Cancer 1981; 48(8):1705–1710.
53. Gastrointestinal Tumor Study Group. Radiation therapy combined with Adriamycin or 5-fluorouracil for the treatment of locally unresectable pancreatic carcinoma. Cancer 1985; 56(11):2563–2568.
54. Gastrointestinal Tumor Study Group. Treatment of locally unresectable carcinoma of the pancreas: comparison of combined-modality therapy (chemotherapy plus radiotherapy) to chemotherapy alone. J Natl Cancer Inst 1988; 80(10):751–755.
55. Klaassen DJ, MacIntyre JM, Catton GE, Engstrom PF, Moertel CG. Treatment of locally unresectable cancer of the stomach and pancreas: a randomized comparison of 5-fluorouracil alone with radiation plus concurrent and maintenance 5-fluorouracil—an Eastern Cooperative Oncology Group study. J Clin Oncol 1985; 3(3):373–378.
56. O'Connell MJ, Martenson JA, Wieand HS, et al. Improving adjuvant therapy for rectal cancer by combining protracted-infusion fluorouracil with radiation therapy after curative surgery. N Engl J Med 1994; 331(8):502–507.
57. Whittington R, Neuberg D, Tester WJ, Benson AB 3rd, Haller DG. Protracted intravenous fluorouracil infusion with radiation therapy in the management of localized pancreaticobiliary carcinoma: a phase I Eastern Cooperative Oncology Group Trial. J Clin Oncol 1995; 13(1):227–232.
58. Boz G, De Paoli A, Innocente R, et al. Radiotherapy and continuous infusion 5-fluorouracil in patients with nonresectable pancreatic carcinoma. Int J Radiat Oncol Biol Phys 2001; 51(3):736–740.
59. Osti MF, Costa AM, Bianciardi F, et al. Concomitant radiotherapy with protracted 5-fluorouracil infusion in locally advanced carcinoma of the pancreas: a phase II study. Tumori 2001; 87(6):398–401.
60. Ben-Josef E, Shields AF, Vaishampayan U, et al. Intensity-modulated radiotherapy (IMRT) and concurrent capecitabine for pancreatic cancer. Int J Radiat Oncol Biol Phys 2004; 59(2):454–459.
61. Vaishampayan UN, Ben-Josef E, Philip PA, et al. A single-institution experience with concurrent capecitabine and radiation therapy in gastrointestinal malignancies. Int J Radiat Oncol Biol Phys 2002; 53(3):675–679.
62. Roldan GE, Gunderson LL, Nagorney DM, et al. External beam versus intraoperative and external beam irradiation for locally advanced pancreatic cancer. Cancer 1988; 61(6):1110–1116.
63. Whittington R, Solin L, Mohiuddin M, et al. Multimodality therapy of localized unresectable pancreatic adenocarcinoma. Cancer 1984; 54(9):1991–1998.
64. Willett CG, Del Castillo CF, Shih HA, et al. Long-term results of intraoperative electron beam irradiation (IOERT) for patients with unresectable pancreatic cancer. Ann Surg 2005; 241(2):295–299.
65. Kim HJ, Czischke K, Brennan MF, Conlon KC. Does neoadjuvant chemoradiation downstage locally advanced pancreatic cancer? J Gastrointest Surg 2002; 6(5):763–769.
66. Blackstock AW, Bernard SA, Richards F, et al. Phase I trial of twice-weekly gemcitabine and concurrent radiation in patients with advanced pancreatic cancer. J Clin Oncol 1999; 17(7):2208–2212.
67. Blackstock AW, Tepper JE, Niedwiecki D, Hollis DR, Mayer RJ, Tempero MA. Cancer and leukemia group B (CALGB) 89805: phase II chemoradiation trial using gemcitabine in patients with locoregional adenocarcinoma of the pancreas. Int J Gastrointest Cancer 2003; 34(2–3):107–116.
68. Talamonti MS, Catalano PJ, Vaughn DJ, et al. Eastern Cooperative Oncology Group Phase I trial of protracted venous infusion fluorouracil plus weekly gemcitabine with concurrent radiation therapy in patients with locally advanced pancreas cancer: a regimen with unexpected early toxicity. J Clin Oncol 2000; 18(19):3384–3389.
69. Safran H, Akerman P, Cioffi W, et al. Paclitaxel and concurrent radiation therapy for locally advanced adenocarcinomas of the pancreas, stomach, and gastroesophageal junction. Semin Radiat Oncol 1999; 9(2 suppl 1):53–57.
70. Rich T, Harris J, Abrams R, et al. Phase II study of external irradiation and weekly paclitaxel for nonmetastatic, unresectable pancreatic cancer: RTOG-98-12. Am J Clin Oncol 2004; 27(1):51–56.
71. Termuhlen PM, Evans DB, Willett CG. IORT in Pancreatic Cancer. Totowa, NJ: Humana Press, 1999.
72. Haslam JB, Cavanaugh PJ, Stroup SL. Radiation therapy in the treatment of irresectable adenocarcinoma of the pancreas. Cancer 1973; 32(6):1341–1345.
73. Dobelbower RR Jr, Borgelt BB, Strubler KA, Kutcher GJ, Suntharalingam N. Precision radiotherapy for cancer of the pancreas: technique and results. Int J Radiat Oncol Biol Phys 1980; 6(9):1127–1133.
74. Steadham AM, Liu HH, Crane CH, Janjan NA, Rosen, II. Optimization of beam orientations and weights for coplanar conformal beams in treating pancreatic cancer. Med Dosim 1999; 24(4):265–271.
75. Kortmansky J, O'Reilly E, Minsky B, et al. A phase I trial of erlotinib, gemcitabine, and radiation for patients with locally-advanced, unresectable pancreatic cancer. In: ASCO Gastrointectinal Cancers Symposium, 2005.

76. Iannitti D, Dipetrillo T, Barnett J, et al. Erlotinib and chemoradiation followed by maintenance erlotinib for locally advanced pancreatic cancer: a phase I study. In: ASCO Gastrointestinal Cancers Symposium, 2005.
77. The Gastrointestinal Tumor Study Group. A multi-institutional comparative trial of radiation therapy alone and in combination with 5-fluorouracil for locally unresectable pancreatic carcinoma. Ann Surg 1979; 189(2):205–208.
78. The Gastrointestinal Tumor Study Group. Phase II studies of drug combinations in advanced pancreatic carcinoma: fluorouracil plus doxorubicin plus mitomycin C and two regimens of streptozotocin plus mitomycin C plus fluorouracil. J Clin Oncol 1986; 4(12):1794–1798.

22 Does Adjuvant Chemotherapy Improve Outcomes in Pancreatic Adenocarcinoma?

Andrew H. Ko and Margaret A. Tempero
Comprehensive Cancer Center, University of California, San Francisco, San Francisco, California, U.S.A.

INTRODUCTION

Pancreatic cancer currently represents the fourth leading cause of cancer-related mortality in the United States, with most recent cancer statistics indicating that an estimated 31,800 individuals will die of this disease in 2005 (1). Five-year survival rate for all stages combined is approximately 3% to 4%—the lowest of any cancer site (1). Approximately 15% of all patients have operable disease at the time of diagnosis. However, despite improvements in staging evaluation, surgical techniques, and immediate postoperative care, with accumulating evidence that perioperative mortality can be reduced if pancreatic cancer operations are performed at high-volume centers, the five-year survival rate in patients undergoing a potentially "curative" resection remains only 15% to 20% (1,2). These modest outcomes are a direct reflection of the high rates of both local and distant recurrence that occur in these patients, with the vast majority of relapses occurring within 24 months of the time of surgery (3). This chapter will address the mounting evidence to support the role for adjuvant therapy, in particular, chemotherapy, in decreasing the likelihood of recurrence and improving survival rates.

EVIDENCE FROM RANDOMIZED PHASE III STUDIES

Randomized multicenter phase III studies conducted by three separate groups have been pivotal in shaping our understanding of the role and benefit of adjuvant therapy for resected pancreatic cancer over the past several decades. Each of these studies, however, arrived at different conclusions regarding the utility of adjuvant chemotherapy and/or radiation in this disease setting. Additionally, as will be pointed out, each must additionally be interpreted in light of significant methodologic flaws that limit how much we should glean from their findings.

Gastrointestinal Tumor Study Group

The first randomized clinical trial to investigate the role of adjuvant therapy in pancreatic cancer was conducted by the Gastrointestinal Tumor Study Group (GITSG) (4). From 1974 to 1982, resected patients were randomized to receive either no further treatment or combined chemoradiation followed by chemotherapy. Chemoradiation consisted of 4000 cGy of external beam radiation, split into two two-week courses separated by two weeks, with bolus 5-fluorouracil (5-FU) given at 500 mg/m^2 daily for three consecutive days at the start of each 2000-cGy course. The same dose of bolus 5-FU was then administered on a weekly basis for two years after completion of radiation or until development of recurrent disease. This trial demonstrated a statistically significant improvement for the treatment arm in terms of both median survival (20 vs. 11 months, adjusted $p=0.03$) and actuarial two-year survival rates (43% vs. 18%) (Table 1). However, the study has been criticized for its low accrual rate (43 evaluable patients over eight-plus years, resulting in study termination before reaching its original accrual goal), and for the fact that nearly one-quarter of patients (24%) randomized to the treatment arm never received the adjuvant therapy owing to poor or prolonged postoperative recovery. Nevertheless, this trial has been the basis on which 5-FU-based radiation has been adopted as the de facto standard of care for postoperative pancreatic cancer patients at many institutions. A confirmatory study subsequently performed by the GITSG registered an additional cohort of 30 patients to the adjuvant treatment arm (5). This study validated the findings of the original trial, with an actuarial two-year survival in treated patients of 46%.

Following the GITSG trial, a number of centers published their experience using similar strategies of 5-FU-based chemoradiation, with minor modifications of dosing and schedule. Foo et al. performed a retrospective analysis of 29 patients treated at the Mayo clinic with chemoradiation (either split-course or continuous-course radiation, median total dose of 54 Gy) (6). Ninety-three percent of patients received concomitant 5-FU with radiation, typically involving two three-day courses of bolus treatment. Median two- and five-year survival rates were 48% and 12%, respectively, results not markedly dissimilar to those in the GITSG trial. Obviously, a selection bias needs to be considered, given the retrospective and nonrandomized nature of this small study.

The Johns Hopkins group, meanwhile, has the largest single-institutional series of postoperative treatment for pancreatic cancer, with Yeo et al. initially publishing results of a prospective study of 174 patients who had undergone resection for pancreatic cancer at their hospital between 1991 and 1995 (7). Patients during this time period were offered, in nonrandomized fashion, three options for postoperative treatment: (*i*) standard therapy with external beam radiation to the pancreatic bed to 4000–4500 cGy (split course was encouraged but not required), given with two three-day courses of 5-FU (500 $mg/m^2/day$) during weeks 1 and 5, and followed by bolus 5-FU (500 $mg/m^2/day$) weekly for four months; (*ii*) intensive therapy with higher doses of external beam radiation to the pancreatic bed (5040–5760 cGy) plus prophylactic hepatic irradiation (2340–2700 cGy), given concurrently with and followed for four months by continuous infusion of 5-FU (200 $mg/m^2/day$) and leucovorin five of seven days a week; and (*iii*) no further chemotherapy or radiation. While no difference was detected between the standard and intensive therapy groups, both groups did demonstrate a prolonged median survival compared to the no-treatment group (19.5 vs. 13.5 months, $P=0.003$). More recently, the Hopkins group performed a retrospective analysis of 616 patients who underwent surgical resection at their institution between 1984 and 1999 (2). By univariate analysis, median survival for patients receiving adjuvant chemoradiation (primarily 5-FU based) was 19 months, compared to 11 months for those receiving no further treatment ($p < 0.0001$). Differences in five-year survival were also seen (20% vs. 9%). Again, the retrospective, nonrandomized nature of this analysis needs to be appreciated, as selection bias—more robust patients who recovered rapidly postoperatively may have been more likely to receive adjuvant therapy, although they may have had better outcomes regardless—may certainly have played an important role in the differences reported.

European Organization for Research and Treatment of Cancer

A larger study performed by the European Organization for Research and Treatment of Cancer (EORTC) randomized 218 patients who had undergone curative resection of a cancer of the pancreatic head or periampullary region (including distal common bile duct, papilla of Vater, or duodenum) to receive either adjuvant chemoradiation or no further treatment (8). The treatment regimen differed somewhat from that used in the GITSG study. Radiation was again given in a split-course design. However, in this European study, 5-FU concurrently with radiotherapy was administered as a continuous infusion (25 mg/kg/day) for zero to five days at the start of each course of radiation, and no additional chemotherapy was given afterward. Survival data for the 114 patients with pancreatic head cancer showed a trend toward improved median survival in the treatment arm (17.1 vs. 12.6 months), although this difference did not achieve statistical significance ($P=0.099$). Both two- and five-year actuarial survival rates were better in patients receiving chemoradiation; again, these differences were not statistically significant (37% vs. 23% at two years, and 20% vs. 10% at five years, respectively) (Table 1). On these bases, the EORTC study investigators concluded that adjuvant 5-FU-based chemoradiation as an adjuvant treatment for this group of patients should not be given routinely.

However, several important caveats need to be highlighted in interpreting this study. First, similar to the GITSG trial, a substantial proportion of patients (approximately 20%) randomized to the treatment arm never ended up receiving therapy. Second, the trial included a number of early-stage patients with very small tumors; almost 16% of those with pancreatic head tumors were a pathologic stage T1. Both of these factors could conceivably have contributed to the lack of a statistically significant survival difference seen in this study. Third, because the study

TABLE 1 Comparison of Gastrointestinal Tumor Study Group and European Organization for Research and Treatment of Cancer Randomized Phase III Trials

	Treatment		*n*	Median survival (mo)	Log-rank *P* value	Estimated two-year survival (%)
GITSG (4)	Control arm	Observation	22	11	0.03	15
	Treatment arm	5-FU/XRT → 5-FU x 2 yr[a]	21	20		42
EORTC (8)	Control arm	Observation	54	12.6	0.099	23
	Treatment arm	5-FU/XRT[b]	60	17.1		37

[a]Two courses of 2000 rad, each over 10 days, separated by two weeks, plus concurrent bolus 5-FU 500 mg/m^2 x three days at the beginning of each course, followed by weekly 5-FU 500 mg/m^2 x two years.
[b]Two courses of 2000 rad each over 10 days, separated by two weeks, plus concurrent infusional 5-FU 25 mg/kg x 0–5 days with each course of radiation.
Abbreviations: EORTC, European Organization for Research and Treatment of Cancer; 5-FU, 5-fluorouracil; GITSG, Gastrointestinal Tumor Study Group; XRT, radiation therapy.

included cancers of both the pancreatic head and the periampullary region, it was underpowered to detect a true difference in each separate group. Fourth, patients with positive resection margins were included in the study without appropriate stratification. Finally, and perhaps most critically, this study did not include in its design any period of chemotherapy alone for patients on the treatment arm. The potential benefit lost by not maintaining patients on 5-FU, or some other form of systemic therapy, after completion of chemoradiation is unknown (8).

European Study Group for Pancreatic Cancer

A great deal of attention has recently been focused on results reported by the European Study Group for Pancreatic Cancer (ESPAC). This group undertook a large multicenter trial (referred to as ESPAC-1) with the intention of examining the roles of both chemoradiation and chemotherapy in the adjuvant setting for patients with pancreatic cancer (9,10). The study used a two-by-two factorial design whereby patients were randomly assigned after surgery to one of four options: (*i*) chemotherapy alone (5-FU 425 mg/m^2 plus leucovorin 20 mg/m^2, both administered for five consecutive days every 28 days' time in six cycles); (*ii*) chemoradiation alone (given as a split course, consisting of a 20-Gy dose given in 10 daily fractions, with bolus 5-FU 500 mg/m^2 during the first three days of treatment, then repeated again after a two-week break); (*iii*) both treatments (chemoradiation followed by chemotherapy); or (*iv*) neither treatment. A total of 289 patients were enrolled, with the goal of yielding combined data of approximately 140 patients for each of the two main comparisons: chemotherapy versus no chemotherapy (groups 1 and 3 vs. groups 2 and 4), and chemoradiation versus no chemoradiation (groups 2 and 3 vs. groups 1 and 4). The trial was powered to detect a difference in mortality at two years of more than 20%. The median tumor size in each treatment group was 3 cm, and approximately half of the patients had node-positive disease. Resection margins were positive in 16% to 19% of tumor specimens.

With a median follow up of 47 months, patients who received chemotherapy had a median survival of 20.1 months compared with 15.5 months for those who did not receive chemotherapy (hazard ratio 0.71; P=0.009), with a two-year survival estimate of 40% versus 30%, respectively (Table 2). By contrast, patients who received chemoradiation appeared to fare more poorly than those who did not receive chemoradiation—median survival for the two groups was 15.9 months versus 17.9 months (hazard ratio 1.28; P=0.05), with a two-year survival estimate of 29% versus 41%. Rates of local recurrence were not improved in patients who received chemoradiation. Quality-of-life surveys did not reveal any significant difference among any of the treatment groups within 12 months after resection.

These provocative data led the study investigators to conclude that the standard of care for patients following resection of pancreatic cancer should consist of adjuvant chemotherapy, and not chemoradiation. Given that the deleterious effect of chemoradiation does not begin to occur until 14 months after randomization (discounting the possibility of treatment-associated morbidity and mortality contributing to the worse outcomes), the authors speculate

TABLE 2 Results of European Study Group for Pancreatic Cancer-1

Results from each separate treatment group in 2-by-2 factorial design

	n	Regimen	Median survival (mo)
Observation	69	N/A	16.9
Chemotherapy alone	75	Bolus 5-FU 425 mg/m 2 x 5 days q 28 days x 6 mo	21.6
Chemoradiation alone	73	20-Gy XRT in 10 fractions in split course x 2; concurrent bolus 5-FU 500 mg/m^2 on first 3 days of each course	13.9
Chemoradiation → chemotherapy	72	Same regimens as (2) and (3)	19.9

Analysis of combined groups

	n	Median survival (mo)	*P* value	Estimated two-year survival (%)	Estimated five-year survival (%)
Groups receiving chemotherapy (2+4)	147	20.1	0.009	40	21
Groups not receiving chemotherapy (1+3)	142	15.5		30	9
Groups receiving chemoradiation (3+4)	145	15.9	0.05	29	10
Groups not receiving chemoradiation (1+2)	144	17.9		41	20

Abbreviations: 5-FU, 5-fluorouracil; XRT, radiation therapy.
Source: From Ref. 10.

that chemoradiation delays the administration of potentially effective systemic treatment, the latter of which may in fact represent the most critical factor in improving survival.

Before immediately discarding radiation as a useful modality in the adjuvant setting, however, one should recognize the limitations of the ESPAC-1 study. There is the real possibility that chemoradiation in this trial was administered in a suboptimal fashion. Standard radiation treatment today typically consists of 45 Gy with an additional 5.4-Gy boost to the tumor, without any intervening treatment break. Furthermore, radiosensitizing doses of a fluoropyrimidine are more commonly administered as a continuous infusion throughout the course of radiation. Although these approaches have never been formally compared to the strategy chosen by the ESPAC investigators, it is reasonable to speculate whether they may have produced better outcomes than those seen in ESPAC-1. As an additional note, it is worth pointing out that this trial did not include a quality assurance plan for the radiation treatment, an important variable that may have further skewed the results seen in patients receiving radiation.

As this study was analyzed on an intent-to-treat basis, it is also important to consider the percentage of patients in each group who did not receive their intended treatment. Of note, 70% of those assigned to chemoradiotherapy received the total planned dose, and only 9% did not receive any radiation. Conversely, a third of all patients assigned to chemotherapy ended up receiving fewer than six full cycles, and an additional 17% did not get any chemotherapy at all. Thus, while the possibility exists that fuller doses of chemoradiation may have altered the study findings somewhat, the greater likelihood is that this trial, if anything, *underestimated* the potential benefit of systemic therapy. As will be discussed, these findings provide adequate justification for the exploration of other, potentially more active agents than bolus 5-FU in the adjuvant setting.

STRATEGIES BEYOND BOLUS 5-FLUOROURACIL

Other Fluoropyrimidine-Based Approaches

The question of whether bolus 5-FU represents the optimal chemotherapeutic agent to use in the adjuvant setting, both for radiosensitization and for systemic control of disease, is an important one which needs to be addressed. Certainly in other gastrointestinal malignancies, such as advanced colorectal cancer, administration of 5-FU as a continuous infusion rather than in bolus fashion confers distinct advantages in terms of response rate and survival outcomes (11,12). The infusional administration of 5-FU has furthermore become an appropriate standard of care for radiosensitization and is commonly used in adjuvant chemoradiation for esophagogastric and rectal cancers. Relatively recent data to support the use of oral capecitabine as a potentially more potent radiosensitizer (13) offers an additional agent worth exploring in this disease setting, an argument further buttressed by the antitumor activity seen using this drug in advanced pancreatic cancer (14).

Evidence already exists to support the potential efficacy of infusional 5-FU in the postoperative setting. Whittington et al. out of the University of Pennsylvania reported the outcomes of 72 resected patients seen at their institution between 1981 and 1989 (15). These patients were treated in three distinct patterns representative of the chronologic change in hospital policy during that time period. The earliest group of patients received no adjuvant treatment; the second group received adjuvant radiation therapy (4500–6300 cGy depending on the presence of positive surgical margins) either alone or with bolus 5-FU (500 mg/m^2/day × three days during weeks 1 and 5); and the third group received radiation concurrently with a modified chemotherapy regimen consisting of continuous infusion of 5-FU (1000 mg/m^2/day × four days during weeks one and five) plus one dose of mitomycin-C (10 mg/m^2) on the first day of treatment. In addition to a lower rate of local recurrence in the third group, both two- and three-year survival rates were higher (47% vs. 22% vs. 11% three-year survival in groups 3, 1, and 2, respectively). It is uncertain whether these results reflect a time-dependent bias given the nonrandomized nature of this study; nevertheless, they do lend credence to the idea that refinement of the chemotherapy regimen may have a significant impact on survival in postoperative patients.

Based on the aforementioned study, the Eastern Cooperative Oncology Group (ECOG) subsequently performed a phase I trial in patients with unresectable or recurrent pancreatic and bile duct carcinomas to evaluate the maximal tolerated dose (MTD) of continuous infusion of 5-FU that could be given concurrently throughout radiation therapy (59.4 Gy in 33 fractions) (16). The MTD of infusional 5-FU was found to be 250 mg/m^2/day, with oral mucositis representing the dose-limiting toxicity in this study.

Results from other institutions confirm that administration of 5-FU as a continuous infusion is comparable or superior to bolus dosing when used in the adjuvant setting together with radiation. Spitz et al. reported a three-year survival rate of 39% for 19 postoperative patients treated at M.D. Anderson with a combination of radiation (50.4 Gy in 28 fractions) and infusional 5-FU (300 mg/m^2/day, five days per week) (17). Mehta et al. treated 52 patients at Stanford University with radiation (45 Gy in 1.8-Gy fractions, plus a boost to the tumor bed in patients who had a positive resection margin to a total of 54 Gy) and concomitant infusional 5-FU (200–250 mg/m^2/day, seven days/week), and reported a median survival of 32 months with a three-year survival rate of 39% (18).

More intensified regimens combining 5-FU with other agents have also been explored in the adjuvant setting. The Virginia Mason group (19,20) published their results using a novel interferon-based chemoradiation protocol in the postoperative setting. Forty-three patients with resected pancreatic cancer received external beam radiation to a total of 4500–5400 cGy over 25 fractions, together with concurrent continuous infusion of 5-FU (200 mg/m^2 daily from days 1–35), weekly cisplatin at 30 mg/m^2, and interferon-α subcutaneously at a dose of 3 million units every other day throughout the course of radiation. Following completion of chemoradiation, two more five-week courses of infusional 5-FU (200 mg/m^2) were administered, spaced apart by three weeks. At the time of publication in 2003, median survival had not yet been reached with a mean follow-up time of 31.9 months, and actuarial survival at one, two, and five years was 95%, 64%, and 55%, respectively. These remarkable results were achieved in spite of a high percentage of subjects having node-positive disease (84%) and extracapsular extension of disease (70%). However, the tradeoff for this potentially efficacious regimen was a high incidence of moderate to severe toxicities, which developed in 70% of patients. Forty-two percent of patients required hospitalization due to treatment-associated toxicities, most commonly nausea, vomiting, diarrhea, and dehydration. Nevertheless, based on these encouraging survival results, the American College of Surgeons Oncology Group (ACOSOG) has opened a larger multicenter phase II trial (Z05031) to confirm the findings reported in this study.

Chakravarthy et al. (21) reported their experience using a novel regimen for resected pancreatic and periampullary cancers, in which patients received bolus administration of 5-FU ($400\ mg/m^2$) and leucovorin ($20\ mg/m^2$ on days 1–3) every four weeks, dipyridamole (75-mg orally, four times per day on days 0–3 every eight weeks), and mitomycin C ($10\ mg/m^2$ on day 1), concurrently with external beam radiation. Radiation treatment in this study consisted of split-course 5000 cGy given over 20 fractions with a two-week rest after the first 10 fractions. This was followed by four months of the same chemotherapy beginning one month following completion of chemoradiation. In general, the regimen was well tolerated, with 42% to 47% of patients experiencing grade 3 or 4 hematologic toxicities during chemotherapy or chemoradiation. For the 29 patients with pancreatic cancer treated on this protocol, median survival was 16 months.

Gemcitabine in Adjuvant Setting

Gemcitabine (Gemzar®, Eli Lilly), a deoxycytidine analog, is currently the only chemotherapeutic agent approved for the treatment of advanced pancreatic cancer. Approval of this drug was based on a randomized, phase III clinical study in which 126 previously untreated patients with advanced pancreatic cancer received either weekly infusions of gemcitabine or bolus 5-FU (22). The primary study end point was clinical benefit response, a parameter consisting of the composite of decreased pain intensity or analgesic consumption, improved performance status, or increased weight. This study showed that gemcitabine was significantly superior to 5-FU with regard to clinical benefit response (24% vs. 5% of patients, respectively, $P=0.0022$) and median survival (5.7 vs. 4.4 months, $P=0.0025$), in addition to one-year survival rate (18% for gemcitabine compared with 2% for 5-FU). It now represents the standard of care for patients with advanced disease. Multiple studies have since evaluated gemcitabine in combination with other cytotoxic or biologic agents, including a number of recently reported randomized phase III trials (23–26). Several regimens, such as gemcitabine in combination with a platinum agent (oxaliplatin or cisplatin), were demonstrated to produce improvements in response rate and time to tumor progression compared with gemcitabine monotherapy; although statistically significant differences in overall survival were not achieved, this may have been a reflection of the studies being underpowered (24,26). Most recently, investigators from the National Cancer Institute of Canada reported the first randomized phase III trial to demonstrate a statistically significant improvement in survival for patients receiving a gemcitabine-containing combination, that of gemcitabine plus erlotinib, an oral epidermal growth factor receptor inhibitor. Survival patients receiving combination treatment was superior to that of patients receiving single-agent gemcitabine (hazard ratio 0.81, $P=0.025$), although the actual difference in median survival was only two weeks (6.37 vs. 5.91 months) (27).

It has logically followed that gemcitabine has been, or is being actively, studied as a component of adjuvant treatment. As a sequel to their ESPAC-1 trial, ESPAC study investigators have developed a follow-up study (ESPAC-3 trial) in which patients with resected pancreatic cancer are randomized to one of three arms: bolus 5-FU/leucovorin (daily times five days, every 28 days for six cycles), standard-infusion gemcitabine (weekly times three weeks out of four for six cycles), or observation alone. Based on the conclusions drawn from ESPAC-1, suggesting a possible deleterious effect of chemoradiation in the adjuvant setting, no radiation has been included in the study design. The study was subsequently modified to eliminate the observation-alone arm, given the positive effects seen with chemotherapy in ESPAC-1. This trial, with a targeted accrual goal of 660 patients, is still enrolling at the time of this writing.

Neuhaus et al. recently reported preliminary results from a multicenter, phase III trial (CONKO-001) in which 368 resected patients were randomized to receive either no further treatment postoperatively or six months of chemotherapy alone with gemcitabine (28). Eighty-six percent of patients had T3 or T4 tumors, and 72% had node-positive disease. Median disease-free survival for gemcitabine-treated patients by Kaplan–Meier analysis was 13.4 months, compared to 6.9 months in the observation arm, a highly statistically significant finding (log-rank $p < 0.01$). This improvement in disease-free survival translated into a trend toward improved overall survival in favor of gemcitabine (median 22.1 vs. 20.2 months), although this difference did not reach statistical significance (log-rank $p < 0.06$). The relatively modest difference in median survival may be attributed in part to the fact that most patients in the control group received gemcitabine at the time of relapse.

Another phase III clinical trial, this one sponsored by the Radiation Therapy Oncology Group (RTOG) (97-04), compared gemcitabine to 5-FU for postoperative adjuvant treatment of resected pancreatic cancer. Unlike the ESPAC-3 study, this trial also incorporated chemoradiation into its study design for both treatment arms, with all patients receiving 5040 cGy of radiation concurrently with continuous infusion of 5-FU administered (250 $mg/m^2/day$). Patients who were randomized to the gemcitabine arm received one cycle of gemcitabine (1000 mg/m^2 weekly x three weeks) prechemoradiation and an additional three cycles postchemoradiation (each cycle consisting of weekly treatment times three out of four). Those randomized to the 5-FU arm received 5-FU as a continuous infusion for three weeks (250 $mg/m^2/day$) prechemoradiation and two cycles of 5-FU postchemoradiation (one cycle=four weeks of continuous infusion at 250 $mg/m^2/day$, followed by two weeks of rest). Patients were stratified according to nodal status, the presence of positive surgical margins, and tumor size ($\geq$ or $\leq$3 cm). This trial enrolled 538 patients, 442 of whom were eligible for analysis when the data were first presented in 2006 (29). Treatment arms were balanced except for T stage, of which more T3/T4 tumors were enrolled on the gemcitabine-containing arm than the 5-FU-containing arm (81% vs. 70%, $p = 0.0062$). One-third of all patients had positive surgical margins, and two-thirds had involved lymph nodes. When analyzing patients with pancreatic head tumors only ($n = 381$), the study investigators found statistically significant improvements in median and 3-year survival in patients receiving gemcitabine-based adjuvant treatment (20.6 months and 32%, compared to 16.9 months and 21% for patients receiving 5-FU-based adjuvant therapy; $p = 0.033$). These statistically significant differences did not hold when all patients, those with pancreatic tumors involving the body and tail as well as the head, were included.

Furthermore, in vitro studies have demonstrated the radiosensitizing properties of gemcitabine (30), and hence this agent has also been evaluated as a component in combined-modality therapy. In a phase I trial for patients with locally advanced pancreatic cancer, Blackstock et al. demonstrated that twice-weekly gemcitabine at 40 mg/m^2 was the MTD that could be delivered with concurrent full-dose radiation (50.4 Gy) (31). Conversely, given that maximizing systemic therapy during the course of radiation may be the most critical aspect in improving patients' long-term clinical outcomes, Allen et al. performed a phase I trial in patients with resectable pancreatic cancer to determine the MTD of radiation that could be delivered to the primary tumor bed in combination with full-dose gemcitabine (1000 mg/m^2 weekly times three) following surgery (32). These investigators found that 39 Gy, administered over 15 fractions, was the MTD, and that this dose provided an adequate degree of locoregional control.

In another phase II study, van Laethem et al. also demonstrated the feasibility of combining gemcitabine with radiation in the postoperative setting, in their case treating 22 resected patients with a combination regimen consisting of gemcitabine (1000 $mg/m^2/dose$, days 1 and 8 of a 21 day cycle) times three cycles, followed by split-course radiation (20 Gy in 2-Gy fraction times two courses, separated by a two-week rest) given with concurrent gemcitabine (300-mg/m^2 weekly) (33). Twenty-two percent of patients experienced grade 3 or 4 nausea/vomiting. With a median follow-up time of 15 months, they reported a median overall survival of 15 months. Following up on this study, the EORTC is currently conducting a phase II/III trial with two main goals: first, to further define the role of gemcitabine in the adjuvant treatment of pancreatic cancer; and second, to determine by direct head-to-head comparison whether the addition of chemoradiation confers any additional benefit to chemotherapy alone in this setting. For this study design, patients are randomized to receive either gemcitabine-based chemotherapy (three out of four weeks, times two cycles) followed by gemcitabine-based chemoradiation for six weeks; or gemcitabine-based chemotherapy alone (three out of four weeks, times four cycles).

Other Approaches to Adjuvant Therapy

Instead of standard cytotoxic therapy and/or radiation, investigators have also sought other alternative, potentially less toxic approaches to potentially improve patients' long-term prospects following pancreatic cancer surgery. Jaffee et al. from Johns Hopkins performed a phase I trial testing an allogeneic tumor vaccine in 14 patients with resected pancreatic cancer (34). These investigators created a cancer vaccine using two pancreatic cancer cell lines established from primary pancreatic tumor specimens that were stably transfected to express granulocyte-macrophage colony-stimulating factor (GM-CSF). At high doses of vaccine ($\geq 10 \times 10^7$ cells), three patients developed increased delayed-type hypersensitivity (DTH) responses to autologous tumor cells, providing the provocative suggestion of antitumor immunity. Subsequent studies demonstrated induction of CD8-positive T-cell responses in these patients to mesothelin, an antigen consistently upregulated in most pancreatic cancers (35). Although it would be premature to draw any conclusions, patients with increased DTH also had impressive disease-free survival times of greater than 25 months. These same investigators subsequently reported their phase II experience in 60 patients with resected pancreatic cancer (88% node-positive, 30% with positive margins) who received a total of 5 vaccinations before and after 5-FU-based chemoradiation. With a median follow-up of 3 years, the median survival for these patients was 26.8 months, with impressive 1- and 2-year survival rates of 88% and 76%, respectively (36). Further studies will be required to determine whether this vaccine, or other immunotherapy-based approaches, has a role either in place of or in addition to standard chemotherapy in the postoperative adjuvant setting.

IS THERE A ROLE FOR NEOADJUVANT TREATMENT?

As noted previously, up to one-quarter of patients are unable to receive planned adjuvant treatment following pancreatic cancer resection because of a prolonged or complicated postoperative course, a problem which could potentially be obviated by administering the treatment before surgery. Another theoretical advantage for neoadjuvant therapy is the possibility that the disease might "declare" itself during a preoperative period of receiving some form of therapy, either causing too much debilitation to permit the rigors of an aggressive operation, or producing overt metastatic disease within a short time frame that had not initially been detectable on imaging studies. In either scenario, the patient would be spared a morbid and perhaps unnecessary surgical procedure. Finally, the possibility exists that up-front treatment allows radiation to be delivered to well-oxygenated tumor cells prior to surgical devascularization, and increases the likelihood of the surgeon obtaining negative margins, an important prognostic factor in postoperative survival.

A number of single-institution studies have been reported which address this issue of timing of chemoradiation relative to surgery. Evans et al. first reported the feasibility of administering chemoradiation preoperatively in 28 patients with localized pancreatic cancer (37). The regimen consisted of 5040 cGy of external-beam radiation with concurrent continuous infusion of 5-FU (300 mg/m^2/day), with restaging performed four to five weeks after completion of treatment. Five of the 28 patients (17.9%) were found to have metastatic disease at the time of restaging. Of the 23 patients who went on laparatomy, three had metastatic disease detected intraoperatively; an additional three had a locally unadvanced unresectable primary pancreatic tumor; and 17 were able to undergo successful completion of pancreaticoduodenectomy.

These same investigators subsequently evaluated recurrence and survival rates in 39 patients treated with this same regimen plus 10 Gy of electron-beam intraoperative radiation (38). In this study, 82% of patients were able to undergo resection with negative margins. However, 29 patients subsequently developed recurrent disease, most commonly involving the liver (53%), with 11% developing an isolated local or peritoneal recurrence. Median survival of this entire cohort of patients was 19 months, with a five-year actuarial survival rate of 19%. Because of a high rate of gastrointestinal toxicity seen in patients treated with this preoperative regimen, Evans et al. modified the radiation component to a rapid-fractionation method (30 Gy delivered in 3-Gy daily fractions over two weeks, instead of the standard 50.4 Gy in 1.8 fractions over 5.5 weeks), with the same dosing of 5-FU as given previously (39). The toxicity profile using this rapid-fractionation chemoradiation was much more favorable, with a comparable median survival (20 months) for those patients who received all components of planned treatment (57% of the cohort). In total, evaluation of all 132 patients from 1990 to 1999 who received preoperative chemoradiation followed by pancreaticoduodenectomy at M.D. Anderson, showed an overall median survival from the time of tissue diagnosis of 21 months (40).

Despite the theoretical advantages of administering preoperative therapy for resectable pancreatic cancer, it remains difficult to establish whether such an approach results in improved patient outcomes when compared to postoperative treatment. Certainly, it can be argued that by delaying surgery, patients may be losing their window of opportunity to undergo a potentially curative operation, and therefore such a strategy is risky. Additionally, whereas most experienced surgeons do not require a preoperative pancreatic biopsy for patients with potentially resectable pancreatic cancer (41), one might argue that tissue confirmation is required prior to the delivery of systemic and/or radiation treatment, an extra invasive step that would subject patients to further risk (42). Finally, for patients presenting with obstructive jaundice, a delay in surgery might necessitate endobiliary decompression. Several reports have suggested increased morbidity and mortality after Whipple resection in patients who undergo preoperative biliary drainage (43,44), although this finding is not conclusive (45–47).

Spitz et al. reported their five-year institutional experience (again, from M.D. Anderson) in 142 patients with resectable pancreatic head cancer, of which 41 underwent preoperative therapy per protocol and 19 received postoperative 5-FU-based chemoradiation (17). No significant differences were observed between the two groups in terms of either toxicity or survival between the two groups (median survival of 19.2 vs. 22 months, respectively), although obviously, these data have to be interpreted in light of the nonrandomized retrospective nature of this analysis. The fact that the combined number of 60 in this analysis was far less than the total original number of patients studied reflects the large fraction of patients in both arms who failed to receive all components of their planned therapy for various reasons. For example, 43% of patients treated preoperatively did not undergo pancreaticoduodenectomy, most commonly because of disease extent detected pre- or intraoperatively. Conversely, 24% of patients who underwent resection of their localized pancreatic cancer and were subsequently supposed to receive postoperative chemoradiation never received the chemoradiation owing to delayed postoperative recovery, results consistent with the original GITSG study described earlier.

A pilot study conducted at Fox Chase Cancer Center demonstrated the feasibility and efficacy of preoperative chemoradiation using a slightly modified regimen consisting of 5-FU, mitomycin, and concurrent external-beam radiation (48). An impressive median survival of 45 months from the time of tissue diagnosis was reported for patients undergoing curative resection. Based on these encouraging results, the ECOG conducted a multi-institutional phase II trial using a similar preoperative regimen (49). Treatment included six consecutive weeks of radiation therapy to a total of 5040 cGy; continuous infusion of 5-FU (1000 mg/m^2/day) from days 2–5 and 29–32 of radiation; and mitomycin 10 mg/m^2 on day 2. Of 53 patients able to be analyzed, 12 did not proceed onto surgery because of progressive disease, treatment-related toxicity, intercurrent illness or death; an additional 17 who underwent laparotomy did not have a resection owing to intraoperative findings of local or extrapancreatic spread. This left 24 patients who received all planned components of treatment (chemoradiation plus resection). Median survival in this group of patients was 15.7 months compared with 9.7 months for the entire group. These suboptimal results were felt likely the result of unfavorable prognostic features among the resected group of patients, including 13 who had tumor within 2 mm of the surgical margins, three with positive peritoneal cytology, and four who required superior mesenteric vein resection.

To date, the issue of timing of combined-modality therapy for resectable disease remains unsettled. The theoretical advantages of neoadjuvant treatment need to be counterbalanced by the concern of delaying or even preventing potentially curative surgery. Use of neoadjuvant therapy for pancreatic cancer that appears to be operable, therefore, while an attractive concept, should be limited to the clinical trial setting at the present time.

ONGOING CONTROVERSIES AND FUTURE DIRECTIONS

Despite three decades of ongoing study, no consensus has been arrived at in terms of the appropriate treatment for patients who have undergone resection of their pancreatic cancer. The ESPAC-1 study has brought to the forefront the question of the role radiation therapy should play in the design of future studies of adjuvant treatment of pancreatic cancer. Certainly, the limitations of that study have to be taken into account, especially with regard to what may in fact represent an outdated approach to the administration of both the radiation treatment and the concurrent chemotherapy. Radiation is typically thought to reduce the risk of locoregional disease recurrence; however, if it delays or prevents the administration of optimal doses of systemic treatment, then whether, and at what point, it should be incorporated into a postoperative treatment plan needs to be considered carefully.

Another important research area is to identify whether other agents besides gemcitabine and fluoropyrimidines will prove to be useful in the adjuvant setting. Combining gemcitabine with other cytotoxic agents, such as platinum compounds, may be of some benefit, if one extrapolates from the advanced disease setting. Several cooperative group trials are also investigating newer biologic agents for patients with locally advanced and metastatic disease, most commonly evaluating whether the addition of these agents to gemcitabine improves survival compared with gemcitabine alone. Included among these "targeted" therapies are the recombinant humanized antibody against the vascular endothelial growth factor, bevacizumab (Avastin®, Genentech, South San Francisco), and the antibody directed against the epidermal growth factor receptor, cetuximab (Erbitux®, Bristol-Myers Squibb, Princeton, NJ, U.S.A.) (50,51). As noted previously, a recently completed randomized phase III study demonstrated a very modest survival advantage with the addition of the oral tyrosine kinase inhibitor erlotinib (Tarceva®, Genentech, South San Francisco) to gemcitabine in patients with advanced disease (27). Thus, one or more of these agents may prove to be useful in the adjuvant setting as well, although this certainly requires further rigorous testing before being put into clinical practice.

Finally, it remains unclear whether adjuvant therapy should be offered to all patients; for example, does the subgroup of patients with very early stage (T1), node-negative tumors benefit from postoperative treatment, or should such treatment be reserved for individuals with larger tumors, node-positive disease, and/or close or positive resection margins? Furthermore, aside from these clinical characteristics, are there other defining molecular features—that is, specific genes that mediate chemosensitivity or radiosensitivity—that will help guide therapeutic decision making, including which patients may benefit more from adjuvant therapy and the choice of which agents to use? As we move forward into an era of molecular diagnostics for the treatment of cancer, such a time may come when we are able to offer an individualized "patient-tailored" approach to arrive at these important decisions for this patient population.

REFERENCES

1. Jemal A, Murray T, Ward E, et al. Cancer statistics, 2005. CA Cancer J Clin 2005; 55:10–30.
2. Sohn TA, Yeo CJ, Cameron JL, et al. Resected adenocarcinoma of the pancreas-616 patients: results, outcomes, and prognostic indicators. J Gastrointest Surg 2000; 4:567–579.
3. Sperti C, Pasquali C, Piccoli A, Pedrazzoli S. Recurrence after resection for ductal adenocarcinoma of the pancreas. World J Surg 1997; 21:195–200.
4. Kalser MH, Ellenberg SS. Pancreatic cancer. Adjuvant combined radiation and chemotherapy following curative resection. Arch Surg 1985; 120:899–903.
5. Further evidence of effective adjuvant combined radiation and chemotherapy following curative resection of pancreatic cancer. Gastrointestinal Tumor Study Group. Cancer 1987; 59:2006–2010.
6. Foo ML, Gunderson LL, Nagorney DM, et al. Patterns of failure in grossly resected pancreatic ductal adenocarcinoma treated with adjuvant irradiation +/- 5 fluorouracil. Int J Radiat Oncol Biol Phys 1993; 26:483–489.
7. Yeo CJ, Abrams RA, Grochow LB, et al. Pancreaticoduodenectomy for pancreatic adenocarcinoma: postoperative adjuvant chemoradiation improves survival. A prospective, single-institution experience. Ann Surg 1997; 225:621–33; discussion 633–636.
8. Klinkenbijl JH, Jeekel J, Sahmoud T, et al. Adjuvant radiotherapy and 5-fluorouracil after curative resection of cancer of the pancreas and periampullary region: phase III trial of the EORTC gastrointestinal tract cancer cooperative group. Ann Surg 1999; 230:776–782; discussion 782–784.
9. Neoptolemos JP, Dunn JA, Stocken DD, et al. Adjuvant chemoradiotherapy and chemotherapy in resectable pancreatic cancer: a randomised controlled trial. Lancet 2001; 358:1576–1585.
10. Neoptolemos JP, Stocken DD, Friess H, et al. A randomized trial of chemoradiotherapy and chemotherapy after resection of pancreatic cancer. N Engl J Med 2004; 350:1200–1210.
11. de Gramont A, Bosset JF, Milan C, et al. Randomized trial comparing monthly low-dose leucovorin and fluorouracil bolus with bimonthly high-dose leucovorin and fluorouracil bolus plus continuous infusion for advanced colorectal cancer: a French intergroup study. J Clin Oncol 1997; 15:808–815.

12. Efficacy of intravenous continuous infusion of fluorouracil compared with bolus administration in advanced colorectal cancer. Meta-analysis Group In Cancer. J Clin Oncol 1998; 16:301–308.
13. Sawada N, Ishikawa T, Sekiguchi F, Tanaka Y, Ishitsuka H. X-ray irradiation induces thymidine phosphorylase and enhances the efficacy of capecitabine (Xeloda) in human cancer xenografts. Clin Cancer Res 1999; 5:2948–2953.
14. Cartwright TH, Cohn A, Varkey JA, et al. Phase II study of oral capecitabine in patients with advanced or metastatic pancreatic cancer. J Clin Oncol 2002; 20:160–164.
15. Whittington R, Bryer MP, Haller DG, Solin LJ, Rosato EF. Adjuvant therapy of resected adenocarcinoma of the pancreas. Int J Radiat Oncol Biol Phys 1991; 21:1137–1143.
16. Whittington R, Neuberg D, Tester WJ, Benson AB, III, Haller DG. Protracted intravenous fluorouracil infusion with radiation therapy in the management of localized pancreaticobiliary carcinoma: a phase I Eastern Cooperative Oncology Group Trial. J Clin Oncol 1995; 13:227–232.
17. Spitz FR, Abbruzzese JL, Lee JE, et al. Preoperative and postoperative chemoradiation strategies in patients treated with pancreaticoduodenectomy for adenocarcinoma of the pancreas. J Clin Oncol 1997; 15:928–937.
18. Mehta VK, Fisher GA, Ford JM, et al. Adjuvant radiotherapy and concomitant 5-fluorouracil by protracted venous infusion for resected pancreatic cancer. Int J Radiat Oncol Biol Phys 2000; 48:1483–1487.
19. Nukui Y, Picozzi VJ, Traverso LW. Interferon-based adjuvant chemoradiation therapy improves survival after pancreaticoduodenectomy for pancreatic adenocarcinoma. Am J Surg 2000; 179: 367–371.
20. Picozzi VJ, Kozarek RA, Traverso LW. Interferon-based adjuvant chemoradiation therapy after pancreaticoduodenectomy for pancreatic adenocarcinoma. Am J Surg 2003; 185:476–480.
21. Chakravarthy A, Abrams RA, Yeo CJ, et al. Intensified adjuvant combined modality therapy for resected periampullary adenocarcinoma: acceptable toxicity and suggestion of improved 1-year disease-free survival. Int J Radiat Oncol Biol Phys 2000; 48:1089–1096.
22. Burris HA, III, Moore MJ, Andersen J, et al. Improvements in survival and clinical benefit with gemcitabine as first-line therapy for patients with advanced pancreas cancer: a randomized trial. J Clin Oncol 1997; 15:2403–2413.
23. Richards DA, Kindler HL, Oettle H, Ramanathan R. A randomized phase III study comparing gemcitabine + pemetrexed versus gemcitabine in patients with locally advanced and metastatic pancreas cancer, Proceedings of the American Society of Clinical Oncology, New Orleans, Vol. 23, 2004.
24. Louvet C, Labianca L, Hammel P, Lledo G, DeBraud F. GemOx (gemcitabine + oxaliplatin) versus Gem (gemcitabine) in non resectable pancreatic adenocarcinoma: final results of the GERCOR / GISCAD Intergroup Phase III. Proceedings of the American Society of Clinical Oncology, New Orleans, Vol. 23, 2004:314.
25. Van Cutsem E, van de Velde H, Karasek P, et al. Phase III trial of gemcitabine plus tipifarnib compared with gemcitabine plus placebo in advanced pancreatic cancer. J Clin Oncol 2004; 22:1430–1438.
26. Heinemann V, Quietzsch D, Gieseler F, et al. A phase III trial comparing gemcitabine plus cisplatin vs. gemcitabine alone in advanced pancreatic carcinoma. Proceedings of the American Society of Clinical Oncology, Chicago, IL, Vol. 22, 2003:250.
27. Moore MJ, Goldstein D, Hamm J, et al. Erlotinib improves survival when added to gemcitabine in patients with advanced pancreatic cancer. A phase III trial of the National Cancer Institute of Canada Clinical Trials Group, 2005 Gastrointestinal Cancers Symposium, Hollywood, FL, 2005:121.
28. Oettle H, Post S, Heuhaus P, et al. Adjuvant chemotherapy with gemcitabine vs. observation in patients undergoing curative-intent resection of pancreatic cancer. JAMA 2007; 297:267–277.
29. Regine W, Winter K, Abrams R, et al. RTOG 9704 a phase III study of adjuvant pre and post chemoradiation 5-FU vs gemcitabine for resected pancreatic adenocarcinoma. Proceedings of the American Society of Clinical Oncology; Atlanta, 2006; 24:180S.
30. Lawrence TS, Eisbruch A, McGinn CJ, Fields MT, Shewach DS. Radiosensitization by gemcitabine. Oncology (Huntingt) 1999; 13:55–60.
31. Blackstock AW, Bernard SA, Richards F, et al. Phase I trial of twice-weekly gemcitabine and concurrent radiation in patients with advanced pancreatic cancer. J Clin Oncol 1999; 17:2208–2212.
32. Allen AM, Zalupski MM, Robertson JM, et al. Adjuvant therapy in pancreatic cancer: phase I trial of radiation dose escalation with concurrent full-dose gemcitabine. Int J Radiat Oncol Biol Phys 2004; 59:1461–1467.
33. Van Laethem JL, Demols A, Gay F, et al. Postoperative adjuvant gemcitabine and concurrent radiation after curative resection of pancreatic head carcinoma: a phase II study. Int J Radiat Oncol Biol Phys 2003; 56:974–980.
34. Jaffee EM, Hruban RH, Biedrzycki B, et al. Novel allogeneic granulocyte-macrophage colony-stimulating factor-secreting tumor vaccine for pancreatic cancer: a phase I trial of safety and immune activation. J Clin Oncol 2001; 19:145–156.
35. Thomas AM, Santarsiero LM, Lutz ER, et al. Mesothelin-specific CD8(+) T cell responses provide evidence of in vivo cross-priming by antigen-presenting cells in vaccinated pancreatic cancer patients. J Exp Med 2004; 200:297–306.

36. Laheru D, Yeo C, Biedrzycki B, et al. A safety and efficacy trial of lethally irradiated allogeneic pancreatic tumor cells transfected with the GM-CSF gene in combination with adjuvant chemoradiotherapy for the treatment of adenocarcinoma of the pancreas. Gastrointestinal Cancers Symposium; Orlando, 2007. Abstract 106.
37. Evans DB, Rich TA, Byrd DR, et al. Preoperative chemoradiation and pancreaticoduodenectomy for adenocarcinoma of the pancreas. Arch Surg 1992; 127:1335–1339.
38. Staley CA, Lee JE, Cleary KR, et al. Preoperative chemoradiation, pancreaticoduodenectomy, and intraoperative radiation therapy for adenocarcinoma of the pancreatic head. Am J Surg 1996; 171: 118–124; discussion 124–125.
39. Pisters PW, Abbruzzese JL, Janjan NA, et al. Rapid-fractionation preoperative chemoradiation, pancreaticoduodenectomy, and intraoperative radiation therapy for resectable pancreatic adenocarcinoma. J Clin Oncol 1998; 16:3843–3850.
40. Breslin TM, Hess KR, Harbison DB, et al. Neoadjuvant chemoradiotherapy for adenocarcinoma of the pancreas: treatment variables and survival duration. Ann Surg Oncol 2001; 8:123–132.
41. Temudom T, Sarr MG, Douglas MG, Farnell MB. An argument against routine percutaneous biopsy, ERCP, or biliary stent placement in patients with clinically resectable periampullary masses: a surgical perspective. Pancreas 1995; 11:283–288.
42. Wayne JD, Abdalla EK, Wolff RA, Crane CH, Pisters PW, Evans DB. Localized adenocarcinoma of the pancreas: the rationale for preoperative chemoradiation. Oncologist 2002; 7:34–45.
43. Sohn TA, Yeo CJ, Cameron JL, Pitt HA, Lillemoe KD. Do preoperative biliary stents increase postpancreaticoduodenectomy complications? J Gastrointest Surg 2000; 4:258–267; discussion 267–268.
44. Heslin MJ, Brooks AD, Hochwald SN, Harrison LE, Blumgart LH, Brennan MF. A preoperative biliary stent is associated with increased complications after pancreatoduodenectomy. Arch Surg 1998; 133:149–154.
45. Pisters PW, Hudec WA, Lee JE, et al. Preoperative chemoradiation for patients with pancreatic cancer: toxicity of endobiliary stents. J Clin Oncol 2000; 18:860–867.
46. Martignoni ME, Wagner M, Krahenbuhl L, Redaelli CA, Friess H, Buchler MW. Effect of preoperative biliary drainage on surgical outcome after pancreatoduodenectomy. Am J Surg 2001; 181:52–59; discussion 87.
47. Pisters PW, Hudec WA, Hess KR, et al. Effect of preoperative biliary decompression on pancreaticoduodenectomy-associated morbidity in 300 consecutive patients. Ann Surg 2001; 234:47–55.
48. Hoffman JP, Weese JL, Solin LJ, et al. A pilot study of preoperative chemoradiation for patients with localized adenocarcinoma of the pancreas. Am J Surg 1995; 169:71–77; discussion 77–78.
49. Hoffman JP, Lipsitz S, Pisansky T, Weese JL, Solin L, Benson AB, III. Phase II trial of preoperative radiation therapy and chemotherapy for patients with localized, resectable adenocarcinoma of the pancreas: an Eastern Cooperative Oncology Group Study. J Clin Oncol 1998; 16:317–323.
50. Kindler HL, Friberg G, Singh DA, et al. Phase II trial of bevacizumab plus gemcitabine in patients with advanced pancreatic cancer. J Clin Oncol 2005; 23:8033–8040.
51. Xiong HQ, Rosenberg A, LoBuglio A, et al. Cetuximab, a monoclonal antibody targeting the epidermal growth factor receptor, in combination with gemcitabine for advanced pancreatic cancer: a multicenter phase II Trial. J Clin Oncol 2004; 22:2610–2616.

23 Carcinoma of the Gallbladder and Bile Ducts

James S. Tomlinson and William Jarnagin
Division of Surgical Oncology, Department of Surgery, University of California, Los Angeles, Los Angeles, California, U.S.A.

INTRODUCTION

Cancers arising from the gallbladder or biliary epithelium account for approximately 15% of hepatobiliary neoplasms. This amounts to approximately 7500 new diagnoses per year in the United States. Gallbladder cancer is the most common site, accounting for 60% of the biliary tract cancer. The remaining 40% are referred to as cholangiocarcinomas and are distributed throughout the extrahepatic and intrahepatic biliary tree (1). Coupling the uncommon incidence of these tumors with their commonly advanced stage at presentation greatly hampers efforts to conduct meaningful randomized clinical trials. Complete resection is associated with the best survival and is the most effective therapy but is usually only possible in a minority of patients. Palliating the effects of biliary obstruction is thus often the primary therapeutic goal. Chemotherapy and radiation therapy have not been proven to reduce the incidence of recurrence after resection nor to improve survival. In addition, only a few chemotherapeutic agents have demonstrated marginal activity in patients with unresectable disease. It must be emphasized that meaningful controlled data comparing different treatment modalities are largely nonexistent. This chapter focuses on primary malignancies of the biliary tree, with an emphasis on current treatment paradigms for the most common of these tumors: hilar cholangiocarcinoma and gallbladder carcinoma.

CHOLANGIOCARCINOMA

General Considerations

Epidemiology

The incidence of bile duct tumors in large autopsy series varies from 0.01% to 0.2% and may constitute about 2% of all reported cancers (2). It is an uncommon cancer with an incidence of 1–2 per 100,000 in the United States (3). The majority of patients are more than 65 years, and the peak incidence occurs in the eighth decade of life (3). Cholangiocarcinomas are generally classified according to their site of origin within the biliary tree (Fig. 1), with those involving the biliary confluence, or hilar cholangiocarcinoma, the most common and accounting for approximately 60% of all cases (4–7). Twenty to thirty percent of cholangiocarcinomas originate in the lower bile duct, while approximately 10% arise within the intrahepatic biliary tree and will present as an intrahepatic mass (8–10). Less than 10% of patients will present with multifocal or diffuse involvement of the biliary tree (11). Recent reports have documented rising incidence and mortality rates associated with intrahepatic cholangiocarcinoma (IHC), which may be related to chronic hepatitis C infection.

Natural History

The vast majority of patients with unresectable bile duct cancer die within six months to a year of diagnosis, usually from liver failure or infectious complications secondary to biliary obstruction (2,4,12,13). The prognosis has been considered worse for lesions affecting the confluence of the bile ducts and better for lesions of the distal bile duct close to the papilla, which probably reflects the greater complexity and difficulty in effectively managing proximal lesions more so than differences in biologic behavior. Indeed, it has been shown that location within the biliary tree (proximal vs. distal) has no impact on survival provided that complete resection is achieved (5). On the other hand, anatomic site-related differences in biological

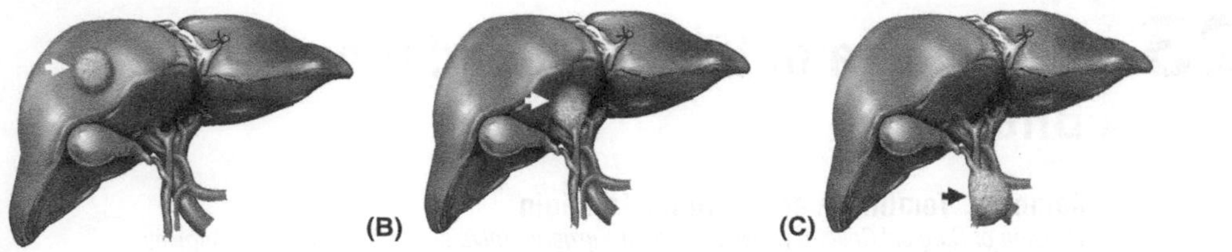

FIGURE 1 Schematic representation of sites of origin of cholangiocarcinoma. Intrahepatic (**A**), hilar (**B**), distal (**C**).

behavior may well exist but are not well-defined, and their clinical relevance remains unclear. IHC, unlike tumors of the extrahepatic bile ducts, rarely cause jaundice or biliary tract-related sepsis. Patients often present with advanced lesions due to the absence of symptoms with small intrahepatic tumors. Multifocal hepatic disease, likely the result of intrahepatic vascular spread, is not uncommon. Patients with disease not amenable to resection usually die of hepatic failure within 12 months, secondary to diffuse liver involvement, or inanition related to advanced malignant disease.

Etiology

In the West, most cases of cholangiocarcinoma are sporadic and have no obvious risk factors. However, certain pathologic conditions are associated with an increased incidence, the most common of which is primary sclerosing cholangitis (PSC). PSC is an autoimmune disease characterized by inflammation of the periductal tissues, ultimately resulting in multifocal strictures of the intrahepatic and extrahepatic bile ducts (14,15). Seventy to eighty percent of patients with PSC have associated ulcerative colitis; by contrast only a minority of those with ulcerative colitis develop PSC (14). The natural history of PSC is variable, and the true incidence of cholangiocarcinoma is unknown. In a Swedish series of 305 patients followed for over several years, 8% of patients eventually developed cancer. On the other hand, occult cholangiocarcinoma has been reported in up to 40% of autopsy specimens and up to 36% of liver explants from patients with PSC (14,16). Patients with cholangiocarcinoma associated with PSC are often not candidates for resection because of multifocal disease or severe underlying hepatic dysfunction. It is important to recognize that medical or surgical treatment of coexisting ulcerative colitis does not alter the subsequent risk of developing cholangiocarcinoma (14–17).

Congenital biliary cystic disease (i.e., choledochal cysts) is also associated with a well-described, increased risk for the development of biliary tract cancer (18,19), primarily when not recognized and treated early in life (19,20). The reason for this strong association is unclear but appears to be related to an abnormal choledochopancreatic duct junction, which predisposes to reflux of pancreatic secretions into the biliary tree, chronic inflammation and bacterial contamination (19–22). A similar mechanism may also explain the increased incidence of cholangiocarcinoma reported in patients subjected to transduodenal sphincteroplasty. In a series of 119 patients subjected to this procedure for benign conditions, Hakamada et al. (23) found a 7.4% incidence of cholangiocarcinoma over a period of 18 years.

In Japan and parts of Southeast Asia, hepatolithiasis is a well-known risk factor for cholangiocarcinoma, arising in 10% of those affected. This condition arises from chronic portal bacteremia and portal phlebitis, leading to intrahepatic pigment stone formation, obstruction of intrahepatic ducts, recurrent episodes of cholangitis, and stricture formation (24,25). Biliary parasites (*Clonorchis sinensis*, *Opisthorchis viverrini*) are also prevalent in parts of Asia and are similarly associated with an increased risk of cholangiocarcinoma (16). In Thailand, where approximately 7 million people are infested with *Opisthorchis*, the annual incidence of cholangiocarcinoma is 87 per 100,000 (26).

Histopathology

In considering extrahepatic cholangiocarcinoma, the overwhelming majority are adenocarcinomas and often well-differentiated. The majority are firm, sclerotic tumors with often a paucity of cellular components within a dense fibrotic, desmoplastic background. As a consequence, a nondiagnostic preoperative biopsy is often encountered (3,27,28). Papillary tumors represent a less common morphologic variant, accounting for approximately 10% of tumors arising from the extrahepatic biliary tree (27). Papillary tumors are soft and friable, may be associated with little transmural invasion and are characterized by a mass that expands rather than contracts the duct. Although papillary tumors may grow to significant size, they often arise from a well-defined stalk, with the bulk of the tumor mobile within the ductal lumen. Recognition of this variant is important since they are more often resectable and have a more favorable prognosis than the other types (16,29).

Hilar cholangiocarcinoma is typically highly invasive within the hepatoduodenal ligament. Direct invasion of the liver or perihepatic structures, such as the portal vein or hepatic artery, is a common feature and has important clinical implications regarding resectability (27). The liver is also a common site of metastatic disease, as are the regional lymph node basins, but spread to distant extra-abdominal sites is uncommon at initial presentation (4,30). These tumors also have a propensity for longitudinal spread along the duct wall and periductal tissues, which is an important pathologic feature of cholangiocarcinomas as it pertains to the margin of resection (27). There may be substantial extension of tumor beneath an intact epithelial lining, as much as 2 cm proximally and 1 cm distally (31). The full tumor extent may thus be underestimated by radiographic studies and may not be appreciated on palpation. This predilection for submucosal extension underscores the importance of frozen section analysis of the duct margins during operation to ensure a complete resection.

In considering IHC, gross examination usually reveals a gray scirrhous mass, which is usually infiltrative with a poorly defined tumor edge. Histopathologically, these tumors are adenocarcinomas and the diagnosis of intrahepatic or peripheral cholangiocarcinoma should be considered in all patients presenting with a presumptive diagnosis of metastatic adenocarcinoma in whom a primary lesion is not documented, particularly if they have a single, solitary hepatic mass. A small number of IHCs show different patterns with focal areas of papillary carcinoma with mucus production, signet ring cells, squamous cell, mucoepidermoid and spindle cell variants (32). Usually positive immunohistochemical staining includes carcinoembryonic antigen (CEA), tumor markers CA50 and CA19-9. K-ras mutations have also been detected in 70% of IHCs (33,34). Thirty percent of patients with peripheral cholangiocarcinoma will have peritoneal or hepatic metastases at presentation and many of these will not be detected until staging laparotomy or laparoscopy is undertaken. Over three quarters of patients dying of cholangiocarcinoma have metastases in regional lymph nodes, hepatic parenchyma, or the peritoneal cavity, and 10% will have either pulmonary or bone metastases (32).

Cholangiocarcinoma Involving the Proximal Bile Ducts (Hilar Cholangiocarcinoma)

Clinical Presentation

The early symptoms of hilar cholangiocarcinoma are nonspecific, with abdominal pain, discomfort, anorexia, weight loss, and/or pruritus seen in about one-third of patients (7,16,35,36). Most patients come to attention because of jaundice or abnormal liver function tests. Although most patients eventually become jaundiced, this may not be present in cases of incomplete biliary obstruction (i.e., right or left hepatic duct), which may go unrecognized for months. These patients are often further evaluated and diagnosed because of an elevated alkaline phosphatase or gamma glutamyltransferase. Pruritus may precede jaundice by some weeks, and this symptom should prompt an evaluation, especially if associated with abnormal liver function tests. Patients with papillary tumors of the hilus may give a history of intermittent jaundice. Small fragments of tumor may detach from a friable papillary tumor of the right or left hepatic duct and pass into the common hepatic duct. Physical exam findings are often nonspecific but may provide some useful information. Jaundice will usually be obvious. Patients with pruritus often have multiple excoriations of the skin. The liver may be enlarged and firm as a result of biliary tract obstruction. The gallbladder is usually decompressed and nonpalpable with hilar obstruction. Thus, a palpable gallbladder suggests a more distal obstruction or an alternative diagnosis. Rarely, patients with long-standing biliary obstruction and/or portal vein involvement may have findings consistent with portal hypertension.

In patients with cholangiocarcinoma and no previous biliary intervention, cholangitis is rare at initial presentation, despite a 30% incidence of bacterial contamination (37,38). Endoscopic or percutaneous instrumentation will significantly increase the incidence of bacterial contamination and the risk of infection. In fact, the incidence of bacterbilia is nearly 100% after endoscopic biliary intubation, and cholangitis is more common (38). Bacterial contamination of the biliary tract in partial obstruction is not always clinically apparent. The presence of overt or subclinical infection at the time of surgery is a major source of postoperative morbidity and mortality. *Escherichia coli*, *Klebsiella*, and *Enterococcal* species are the most common pathogens identified. However, this spectrum of organisms may change after endoscopic or percutaneous intubation, both of which are associated with greater morbidity and mortality following surgical resection or palliative bypass for hilar cholangiocarcinoma. In an analysis of 71 patients who underwent either resection or palliative biliary bypass for proximal cholangiocarcinoma, all patients stented endoscopically and 62% of those stented percutaneously had bacterbilia. Postoperative infectious complications were doubly increased in patients stented before operation compared to nonstented patients, while noninfectious complications were equal in both groups (38). *Enterococcus*, *Klebsiella*, *Streptococcus viridans*, and *Enterobacter aerogenes* were the most common organisms, and this spectrum of bacteria must be considered when administrating perioperative antibiotics; it is imperative to take intraoperative bile specimens for culture in order to guide selection of postoperative antibiotic therapy.

Diagnosis

The diagnosis of hilar cholangiocarcinoma is usually made on evaluation of obstructive jaundice or elevated liver enzymes. Biliary cancers may be clinically silent for long periods of time and it may be many months before a patient bearing such a tumor presents with overt clinical features. Progressive and unremitting jaundice is usually the predominant clinical feature, and diagnostic investigations are largely related to elucidation of the cause of biliary tract obstruction. A minority of patients will present with abdominal pain that may be mistakenly attributed to gallstone disease. While gallstones or even common bile duct stones may coexist with bile duct cancer, in the absence of certain predisposing conditions (e.g., PSC, oriental cholangiohepatitis), it is uncommon for choledocholithiasis to cause obstruction at the biliary confluence. It is therefore imperative to fully investigate and delineate the level and nature of any obstructing lesion causing jaundice to avoid missing the diagnosis of carcinoma.

Most patients are referred after having had some studies done elsewhere, usually a computed tomography (CT) scan and some form of direct cholangiography [percutaneous transhepatic cholangiography (PTC) or endoscopic retrograde cholangiopancreatography (ERCP)]. These studies are often inadequate for full assessment of the tumor extent. In addition, biopsies or brushings are frequently taken at the time of cholangiography (or even at the time of exploration in some cases) but are often nondiagnostic. In the authors' view, histologic confirmation of malignancy is not mandatory prior to exploration. With no prior suggestive history (i.e., prior biliary tract operation, PSC, hepatolithiasis), the finding of a focal stenotic lesion combined with the appropriate clinical presentation are sufficient for a presumptive diagnosis of hilar cholangiocarcinoma, which is correct in most instances (39). Once a diagnosis of cholangiocarcinoma is suggested, radiographic studies are crucial to determine the extent of the tumor to appropriately forge a therapeutic plan.

Radiographic Studies

Radiographic studies are pivotal in selecting patients for resection. In the past, CT, PTC, and angiography were considered standard investigations. While the preferred imaging studies may vary from center to center, the authors' current practice relies almost exclusively on noninvasive studies, specifically magnetic resonance cholangiopancreatography (MRCP) and duplex ultrasonography (US), which provide the same information with less risk to the patient.

Cholangiography

Cholangiography demonstrates the location of the tumor and the biliary extent of disease, both of which are critical in surgical planning. Although endoscopic retrograde cholangiography may provide some helpful information, PTC displays the intrahepatic bile ducts more reliably and has been the preferred approach. There is often an inappropriate knee-jerk reflex to proceed with some form of invasive cholangiography before complete radiographic assessment has been made, a situation that often results in unnecessary invasive procedures. Over the past several years, MRCP has emerged as a powerful noninvasive means of investigating the biliary tree, and can provide imaging detail that is comparable to that obtained with direct cholangiography (see below).

Computed Tomography

Cross-sectional imaging provided by CT remains an important study for evaluating patients with biliary obstruction and can provide valuable information regarding level of obstruction, vascular involvement, and liver atrophy (see below). Portal venous inflow and bile flow are important in the maintenance of liver cell size and mass (40). Segmental or lobar atrophy may result from a portal venous occlusion or biliary obstruction.

Duplex Ultrasonography

Ultrasonography is a noninvasive but operator-dependent study that often precisely delineates tumor extent (Fig. 2). US may not only demonstrate the level of biliary ductal obstruction but can also provide information regarding tumor extension within the bile duct and in the periductal tissues (41–43). Duplex US is firmly established as a highly accurate predictor of vascular involvement and resectability. In a series of 19 consecutive patients with malignant hilar obstruction, US with color spectral Doppler technique was equivalent to angiography and CT portography in diagnosing lobar atrophy, level of biliary obstruction, hepatic parenchymal involvement, and venous invasion (43). Duplex US is particularly useful for assessing portal venous invasion. In a series of 63 consecutive patients from Memorial Sloan-Kettering Cancer Center (MSKCC), duplex US predicted portal vein involvement in 93% of the cases with a specificity of 99% and a 97% positive predictive value. In the same series, angiography with CT angioportography had a 90% sensitivity, 99% specificity, and a 95% positive predictive value (44).

Magnetic Resonance Cholangiopancreatography

In the authors' practice, MRCP has largely replaced endoscopic and percutaneous cholangiography for diagnostic purposes in assessing hilar cholangiocarcinoma. Several studies have

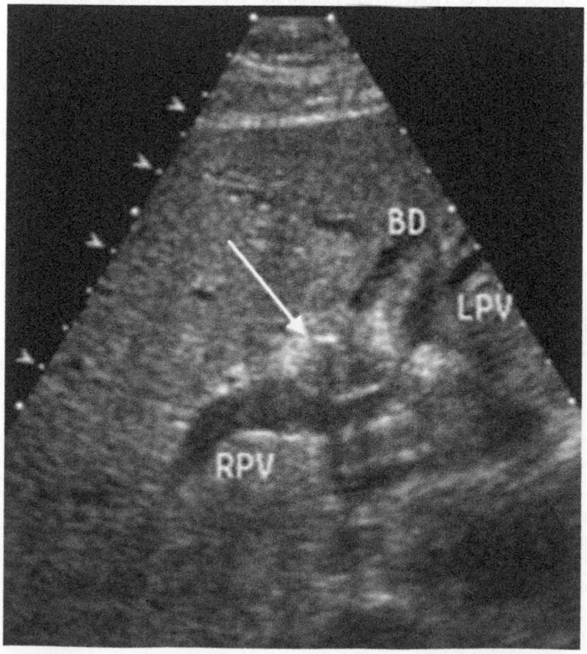

FIGURE 2 Ultrasonographic view of a hilar cholangiocarcinoma (*arrow*) with portal vein involvement. *Abbreviations*: RPV, right portal vein; BD, bile duct; LPV, left portal vein. *Source*: From Jarnagin WR et al., Seminars in Liver Disease 2004; 24:189–199.

demonstrated its utility in evaluating patients with biliary obstruction (45–48). MRCP may not only identify the tumor and the level of biliary obstruction but may also reveal obstructed and isolated ducts not appreciated at endoscopic or percutaneous study. MRCP also provides information regarding the patency of hilar vascular structures, the presence of nodal or distant metastases, and the presence of lobar atrophy (Fig. 3). Furthermore, unlike other modalities, MRCP does not require biliary intubation and its associated problems, not the least of which is bacterbilia, which may increase perioperative morbidity (38,49).

Alternative Diagnoses

The vast majority of patients with hilar strictures and jaundice have cholangiocarcinoma. However, alternative diagnoses are possible and can be expected in 10% to 15% of patients (40). The most common of these are gallbladder carcinoma, Mirizzi syndrome and idiopathic benign focal stenosis (malignant masquerade). Distinguishing gallbladder carcinoma from hilar cholangiocarcinoma can be difficult. A thickened, irregular gallbladder with infiltration into segments IV and V of the liver, selective involvement of the right portal pedicle, or obstruction of the common hepatic duct with occlusion of the cystic duct on endoscopic cholangiography or MRCP are all suggestive of gallbladder carcinoma. Mirizzi syndrome is a benign condition resulting from a large gallstone impacted in the neck of the gallbladder (Fig. 4). The ensuing pericholecystic and periductal inflammation and fibrosis can obstruct the proximal bile duct, which is often difficult to distinguish from a malignant cause (50–52). Benign focal strictures (malignant masquerade) can occur at the hepatic duct confluence but are uncommon (39,53–55).

The finding of a smooth, tapered stricture on cholangiography suggests a benign stricture, particularly with an antecedent history of choledocholithiasis. However, hilar cholangiocarcinoma remains the leading diagnosis until definitively disproved, which generally cannot be done short of an exploration. Furthermore, the alternative conditions that one may encounter are best assessed and treated at operation. It is dangerous to rely entirely on a negative result from a needle biopsy or biliary brush cytology, since they are often misleading, particularly in the face of compelling radiographic evidence of malignant disease (56).

Preoperative Evaluation and Assessment of Resectability

Evaluation of patients with hilar cholangiocarcinoma is principally an assessment of resectability, since resection is the only effective therapy. First and foremost, the surgeon must assess the patient's general condition and fitness for operation, which usually includes partial hepatectomy. The presence of significant comorbid conditions, chronic liver disease, and/or portal hypertension generally precludes resection. In these patients, biliary drainage is the most appropriate intervention, and the diagnosis should be confirmed histologically if chemotherapy or radiation therapy is anticipated. Patients with potentially resectable tumors occasionally present with biliary tract sepsis, frequently after intubation of the biliary tree. These patients require resuscitation and treatment of the infection before surgery can be considered.

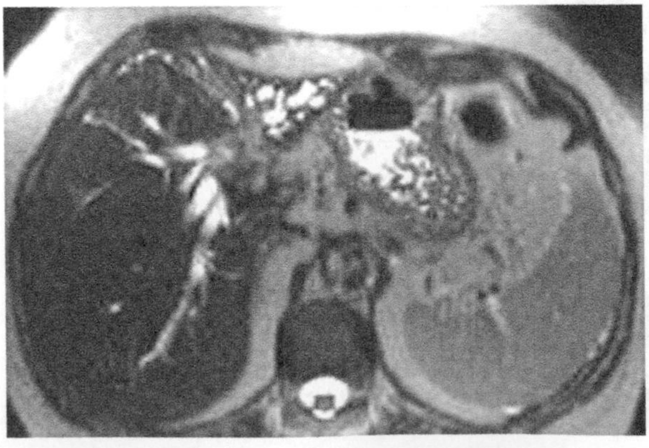

FIGURE 3 Axial MRCP view of a hilar cholangiocarcinoma. An irregular-appearing mass lesion is seen at the confluence of the proximal bile ducts, which appear white in this image. There is dilatation of the intrahepatic biliary radicles. Note the atrophy of the left liver, with dilated and crowded ducts. *Abbreviation*: MRCP, magnetic resonance cholangiopancreatography. *Source*: From Jarnagin WR et al., Seminars in Liver Disease 2004; 24: 189–199.

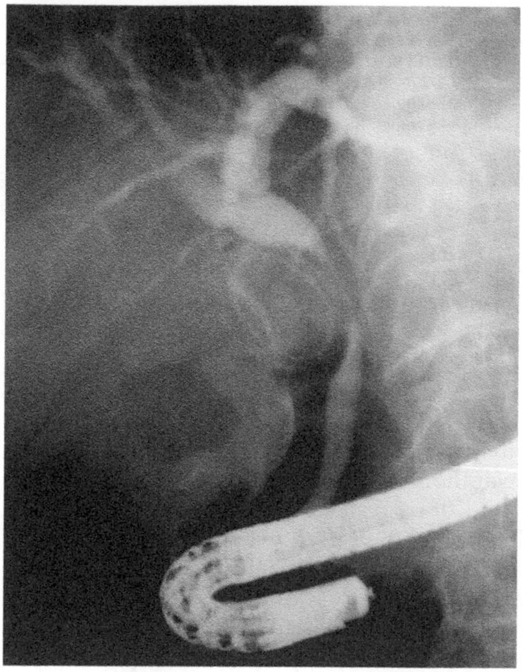

FIGURE 4 Mirizzi syndrome. ERCP view of a biliary stricture caused by a large stone impacted at the neck of the gallbladder. *Abbreviation*: ERCP, endoscopic retrograde cholangiopancreatography. *Source*: From Ref. 76.

The preoperative evaluation must address four critical determinants of resectability: extent of tumor within the biliary tree, vascular invasion, hepatic lobar atrophy, and the presence metastatic disease (4). Lobar atrophy is an often-overlooked finding in patients with hilar cholangiocarcinoma. However, its importance in determining resectability cannot be overemphasized, since it implies portal venous involvement and compels the surgeon to perform a partial hepatectomy, if the tumor is resectable (40). While longstanding biliary obstruction may cause moderate atrophy, concomitant portal venous compromise results in rapid and severe atrophy of the involved segments. Appreciation of gross atrophy on preoperative imaging is important, since it often influences both operative and nonoperative therapy (40). The resectional approach in such cases demands a concomitant partial hepatectomy. On the other hand, if resection is not an option, percutaneous biliary drainage through an atrophic lobe, unless necessary to control sepsis, should be avoided since it will not effect a reduction in bilirubin level. Atrophy is considered to be present if cross-sectional imaging demonstrates a small, often hypoperfused lobe with crowding of the dilated intrahepatic ducts (Fig. 3). Tumor involvement of the portal vein is usually present if there is compression/narrowing, encasement or occlusion seen on imaging studies. Portal vein involvement and/or lobar atrophy are common findings (4,57).

Until recently, there has been no clinical staging system that accounts fully for all of the tumor-related variables that influence resectability, namely biliary tumor extent, lobar atrophy, and vascular involvement. The modified Bismuth–Corlette classification stratifies patients based on the extent of biliary duct involvement by tumor (58). Although useful to some extent, it is not indicative of resectability or survival. The current American Joint Committee on Cancer (AJCC) T stage system is based largely on pathological criteria and has little applicability for preoperative staging. The ideal staging system should accurately predict resectability, the need for hepatic resection and correlate with survival. Such a system would assist the surgeon in formulating a treatment plan and help the patient understand the treatment options and outcome. The authors have proposed a preoperative staging system, using preoperative imaging studies, taking into account the extent of local tumor involvement (4,57). This staging system puts the finding of portal venous involvement and lobar atrophy into the proper context for determining resectability, especially when partial hepatectomy is viewed as an important component of the operative approach (Table 1). For example, a tumor with unilateral extension

TABLE 1 Proposed T Stage Criteria for Hilar Cholangiocarcinoma

Stage	Criteria
T1	Tumor involving biliary confluence +/– unilateral extension to second-order biliary radicles
T2	Tumor involving biliary confluence +/– unilateral extension to second-order biliary radicles AND *ipsilateral* portal vein involvement +/– *ipsilateral* hepatic lobar atrophy
T3	Tumor involving biliary confluence + bilateral extension to second-order biliary radicles OR unilateral extension to second-order biliary radicles with *contralateral* portal vein involvement OR unilateral extension to second-order biliary radicles with *contralateral* hepatic lobar atrophy OR main or bilateral portal venous involvement

Source: From Ref. 57.

into second-order bile ducts and associated with ipsilateral portal vein involvement and/or lobar atrophy would still be considered potentially resectable, while such involvement on the contralateral side would preclude a resection. The authors have found that this staging system correlated well with resectability and the likelihood of associated distant metastatic disease (57). The authors' criteria of unresectability are detailed in Table 2.

In many centers, primarily in Japan, a very detailed approach to definition of resectability is often used and is based on direct cholangiography of segmental ducts and cholangioscopy (59,60). This approach generally involves placement of multiple percutaneous biliary drainage catheters in order to allow complete access to the biliary tree. This approach to preoperative biliary drainage and cholangioscopy is often combined with preoperative portal vein embolization in an effort to lower the risk of postoperative hepatic failure (see below). Such an aggressive diagnostic evaluation appears to increase the resectability but requires a prolonged hospital stay and its true value is unclear (60,61).

Treatment Options

There are two objectives in the therapy of hilar cholangiocarcinoma: complete tumor excision with negative margins and subsequent restoration of biliary-enteric continuity. Multiple studies from several centers around the world have shown that complete resection is associated with five-year survival rates of approximately 25% to 40%, clearly better than can be achieved with nonoperative therapies. Clearly, patients treated nonoperatively typically have more advanced disease, and no comparative trials have been performed. Nevertheless, given the relatively poor response rates with chemotherapy and chemoradiation therapy, resection has emerged as the most effective treatment. Orthotopic liver transplantation has been attempted for unresectable hilar tumors. Klempnauer et al. reported four long-term survivors out of 32 patients submitted to transplantation for hilar cholangiocarcinoma (62). The same group also reported a 17.1% five-year survival for their overall transplant group (63). Comparable results

TABLE 2 Criteria of Unresectability

Patient factors
Medically unfit or otherwise unable to tolerate a major operation
Hepatic cirrhosis
Local tumor-related factors
Tumor extension to secondary biliary radicles bilaterally
Encasement or occlusion of the main portal vein proximal to its bifurcation
Atrophy of one hepatic lobe with contralateral portal vein branch encasement or occlusion
Atrophy of one hepatic lobe with contralateral tumor extension to secondary biliary radicles
Unilateral tumor extension to secondary biliary radicles with contralateral portal vein branch encasement or occlusion
Metastatic disease
Histologically proven metastases to N2 lymph nodes
Lung, liver, or peritoneal metastases

Source: From Ref. 57.

TABLE 3 Summary of Selected Studies Showing the Relationship Between the Rate of Partial Hepatectomy and Proportion of Negative Histologic Margins Achieved

Author	Complete gross resection (*N*)	Partial hepatectomy (%)	Negative margin (%)
Tsao (2000)	25	16	28
Cameron (1990)	39	20	15
Gerhards (2000)	112	29	14
Hadjis (1990)	27	60	56
Jarnagin (2001)	80	78	78
Klempnauer (1997)	147	79	79
Neuhaus (2000)	95	85	61
Nimura (1990)	55	98	83

were reported by Iwatsuki et al. (64). The results of transplantation have previously not been sufficiently adequate to justify its use, and most centers now do not perform liver transplantation for cholangiocarcinoma. More recently, data from the Mayo Clinic have emerged suggesting good results with transplantation in highly selected patients with low volume unresectable disease and combined with an intensive pretransplant treatment regimen (65,66). Although the data are compelling, this approach is applicable to a very small fraction of patients.

Resection

In patients with potentially resectable tumors based on preoperative imaging, the most effective therapy is resection, with the primary objective of complete removal of all gross disease with clear histologic margins (R0 resection). The importance of an R0 resection is clear from prior work showing that incomplete resections do not improve survival beyond that achievable with biliary drainage alone (4,57). There is now overwhelming evidence to support the argument that partial hepatectomy, combined with excision of the extrahepatic biliary apparatus, is usually required to achieve this goal (Table 3). A review of several series in the literature shows a close correlation between the proportion of patients submitted to concomitant partial hepatectomy and the proportion of R0 resections achieved. En bloc caudate lobectomy is also often necessary, particularly for tumors extending into the left hepatic duct (67). Since the principal biliary drainage of the caudate lobe is via the left hepatic duct, tumors extending into the left hepatic duct almost always involve the caudate duct and usually require caudate resection (68). A dilated caudate duct, suggesting tumor involvement, may occasionally be visualized on preoperative imaging (Fig. 5). In some cases, intraoperative frozen section of the caudate duct margin may

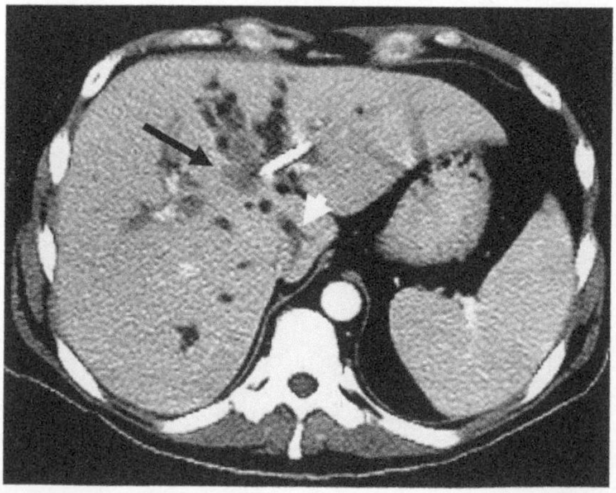

FIGURE 5 Axial CT scan view of a hilar cholangiocarcinoma (*black arrow*) arising primarily from the left hepatic duct. A percutaneous biliary drainage catheter can be seen traversing the tumor. A dilated caudate duct is indicated by the *white arrowhead*. *Abbreviation*: CT, computed tomography.

help the decision to proceed to caudate resection. Distinguishing resectable from unresectable tumors demands careful consideration of all available data, as discussed above. Even with high quality imaging, however, a significant proportion of patients are found to have unresectable disease only at the time of laparotomy. In a recent report from MSKCC, approximately 50% of patients with potentially resectable tumors had findings that precluded resection at the time of exploration (29). Staging laparoscopy has been used to in an effort to improve resectability rates, and appears to have a role. Two recent studies specifically analyzing patients with biliary cancer have shown that laparoscopy can identify a large proportion of patients with unresectable disease, primarily in the form of radiographically occult metastases (69,70). Weber et al. evaluated 56 patients with potentially resectable hilar cholangiocarcinomas; 33 were ultimately determined to have unresectable disease, of which 14% or 42% were identified at laparoscopy and spared an unnecessary laparotomy. The yield of laparoscopy was noted to be much higher in patients with more locally advanced tumors (T2 or T3 in the proposed staging system), which is consistent with other studies showing a direct correlation between AJCC T stage and the presence of metastases (71,72). Additionally, a number of recent reports have suggested a potential role for ^{18}F-deoxy glucose–positron emission tomography (FDG-PET) scanning as a means of identifying occult metastatic disease, however, most of these studies include small numbers of patients, and further evaluation is needed before PET can be recommended as a routine screening study for this disease (73–75).

Technical aspects of intraoperative tumor assessment, exposure, and resection are outside the scope of this chapter. The reader is referred to specialty texts for a detailed description of surgical techniques (76). The authors' general approach involves the liberal use of staging laparoscopy, followed by a full exploration of the abdomen and pelvis, including intraoperative US. Resection of the tumor involves, at a minimum, removal of the entire extrahepatic biliary apparatus from just above the pancreas distally to beyond the biliary confluence with a complete porta hepatis lymphadenectomy. Also, for the reasons cited above, en bloc partial hepatectomy is required in nearly every case in order to achieve complete tumor clearance. Tumor involvement of the main portal vein proximal to its bifurcation additionally requires a vascular resection and reconstruction if technically feasible.

The extent of lymphadenectomy that should be performed is an area of controversy, with some surgeons arguing for an extended nodal dissection (71,72). These studies have shown measurable five-year actuarial survival, even in the presence of metastatic disease to para-aortic nodal groups. However, an analysis of studies specifically reporting five-year survival in patients with any nodal involvement would suggest that very few patients benefit from such an aggressive approach (Table 4).

Results of Resection

Several studies have demonstrated long-term survival after resection of hilar cholangiocarcinoma (4,5,7,67,77,78). It is clear, however, that the results of resection depend critically on the status of the resection margins. Patients resected with negative histologic margins survive significantly longer than those with involved margins (4,77). Over the past 20 years, there has been

TABLE 4 Summary of Selected Series Showing Proportion of Number of Patients Surviving Five Years After Resection of Hilar Cholangiocarcinoma with Metastatic Disease to Regional Lymph Nodes

Author	Resections (*N*)	Node (+) (%)	Five-year survivors with (+) nodes (*N*)
Sugiura (1994)	83	51	3
Klempnauer (1997)	151	29	2
Nakeeb (1996)	109	–	0
Ogura (1998)	66	52	0
Iwatsuki (1998)	72	35	0
Kosuge (1999)	65	46	4
Jarnagin (2001)	80	24	3
Kitagawa (2001)	110	53	5
Total	802	–	17 (2.1%)

a steady increase in the use of hepatic resection in patients with hilar cholangiocarcinoma. The authors firmly believe that this is responsible for the increase in the percentage of R0 resections (negative histologic margins) and the observed improvement in survival after resection. This point is emphasized by the recently reported series of 269 patients accumulated over a 20-year interval (56). In this study, there was a progressive increase in the proportion of patients subjected to partial hepatectomy, with a corresponding increase in the incidence of negative histological margins and in survival. A more recent study from MSKCC reported results of resection in 106 consecutive patients and showed a median survival of 43 months in patients who underwent an R0 resection compared to 24 months in those with involved resection margins (29). Multivariate analysis showed that an R0 resection, a concomitant hepatic resection, well-differentiated histology, and papillary tumor phenotype were independent predictors of long-term survival; lymph node involvement had a significant adverse impact on survival only on univariate analysis.

Although improved survival is clearly achievable with an aggressive resectional approach, operative mortality rates have been high, even at the most experience centers. A major reason for this is the need to remove a substantial amount of functional hepatic parenchyma, often in the face of a contaminated biliary tree. Recently, preoperative portal vein embolization has been advocated as a means of potentially lowering operative risk. Advocated by Kinoshita et al. (79) and Makuuchi et al. (80), portal vein embolization occludes portal blood flow to the liver parenchyma that is to be resected in order to initiate compensatory hypertrophy of the future liver remnant. By reducing the amount of functioning liver parenchyma that is removed, postoperative hepatic dysfunction and hepatic failure may be minimized. In patients with hilar cholangiocarcinoma, this is typically undertaken after placement of multiple biliary drainage catheters to decompress the biliary tree. This preoperative strategy is particularly favored in Japanese centers, with a suggestion of improvement in perioperative results. Kondo et al. recently reported that, with this approach, consecutive resections were performed in 40 patients with no perioperative deaths. On the other hand, the recent study from MSKCC also showed a progressive improvement in operative mortality without using these adjunctive measures (29).

Adjuvant Therapy

Because cholangiocarcinoma are rare, meaningful clinical trials evaluating the use of adjuvant therapy have been difficult to perform. Several small, single center studies have attempted to investigate the benefit of postoperative adjuvant chemoradiation therapy in patients with hilar cholangiocarcinoma. In two separate reports from Johns Hopkins, Cameron et al. and Pitt et al. showed no benefit of adjuvant external beam and intraluminal radiation therapy (81,82). On the other hand, Kamada et al. suggested that radiation may improve survival in patients with histologically positive hepatic duct margins. Additionally, in a small series of patients, five with hilar cholangiocarcinoma, from Louisville, resectability was reportedly greater in patients given neoadjuvant radiation therapy prior to exploration (84). It must be remembered, however, that none of these studies was randomized and most consist of a small, heterogeneous group of patients. At the present time, there are no data to support the routine use of adjuvant or neoadjuvant radiation therapy, except in the context of a controlled trial.

The only phase III trial investigating adjuvant chemotherapy included 508 patients with resected bile duct tumors ($n = 139$), gallbladder cancers ($n = 140$), pancreatic cancers ($n = 173$), and ampullary tumors ($n = 56$) (85). These patients were randomized to surgery alone or surgery with MF [mitomycin/5-fluorouracil (5-FU)]. On subset analysis, there were no significant differences in survival or disease-free survival for bile duct tumors. As with radiation therapy, there are no data to support the routine use of chemotherapy in the adjuvant setting.

Palliation

The majority of patients with hilar cholangiocarcinoma are not suitable for resection. In this setting, the management options include some form of biliary decompression or supportive care. Jaundice alone is not necessarily an indication for biliary decompression, given the associated morbidity and mortality. The indications for biliary decompression in inoperable patients are intractable pruritus, cholangitis, the need for access to intraluminal radiotherapy, and finally to allow recovery of hepatic parenchymal function in patients receiving chemotherapeutic agents. Supportive care alone is probably the best approach for elderly patients with significant comorbid conditions, provided that pruritus is not a major feature. Patients who are found to be unresectable at operation represent a different group and operative biliary decompression can be performed successfully (4) and can be so constructed as to provide access to the biliary tree for postoperative irradiation (4,86).

Assessment of palliative biliary drainage procedures is difficult since the spectrum of patients ranges from the critically ill and unresectable to those in relatively good health with potentially resectable tumors. All patients should be properly assessed by experienced personnel with a view toward possible resection. This point cannot be over-emphasized. If the patient is deemed unresectable, the diagnosis should be confirmed with a biopsy. Biliary decompression can be obtained either by percutaneous transhepatic puncture or by endoscopic stent placement. It is important to realize that these patients have a short life expectancy and any periprocedural complication extends hospital stay and consumes time. Hilar tumors are more difficult to transverse with the endoscopic technique. Moreover, the failure rates and incidence of subsequent cholangitis are high (87). Thus, most patients with unresectable hilar tumors are not candidates for endoscopic biliary drainage.

Percutaneous Biliary Drainage

Percutaneous transhepatic biliary drainage and subsequent placement of a self-expandable metallic endoprosthesis (Wallstent®) can be successfully performed in most patients with hilar obstruction. However, satisfactory results, even by experienced interventional radiologists, are more difficult to achieve in patients with hilar tumors than in those with distal biliary obstruction (88–90). Frequently, hilar tumors isolate all three major hilar ducts (left hepatic, right anterior sectoral hepatic, and right posterior sectoral hepatic), and two or more stents must be placed for adequate drainage (91). One must also consider that jaundice may result from hepatic dysfunction secondary to portal vein occlusion. Jaundice in this setting, without intrahepatic biliary dilatation, is not correctable with biliary stents. In addition, lobar atrophy is an important factor when considering palliative biliary procedures. Our current indications for biliary decompression in inoperable patients are intractable pruritus, cholangitis, the need for access to intraluminal radiotherapy, and finally to allow recovery of hepatic parenchymal function in patients receiving chemotherapeutic agents.

The median patency of metallic endoprostheses at the hilus is approximately six months, significantly lower than that reported for similar stents placed in the distal bile duct (92). Becker et al. reported one-year patency rates of 46% and 89% for Wallstents placed at the hilus and the distal bile duct, respectively (88). Similarly, Stoker and Lameris documented occlusion in 36% of patients with Wallstents at the hilus compared with 6% of patients with Wallstents in the distal bile duct (93). In most series of Wallstents placed for hilar obstruction, documented stent occlusion requiring re-intervention occurs in 25% of patients (88,92–94). This concurs with our findings of a mean patency of 6.1 months in 35 patients palliated for malignant high biliary obstruction by placement of expandable metallic endoprostheses. The periprocedural mortality was 14% at 30 days and seven patients (24%) had documented stent occlusion requiring repeated intervention (92).

Intrahepatic Biliary-Enteric Bypass

Patients found to be unresectable at operation may be candidates for intrahepatic biliary-enteric bypass. The segment III duct is usually the most accessible and is our preferred approach, but the right anterior or posterior sectoral hepatic ducts can also be used (95). Typically, segment III bypass is used to restore biliary-enteric continuity after the bile duct has been divided and a locally invasive, unresectable tumor has been discovered. Segment III bypass provides excellent biliary drainage and is less prone to occlusion by tumor than are Wallstents since the anastomosis can be placed at some distance away from the tumor. Relief of jaundice will be achieved if at least one-third of the functioning hepatic parenchyma is adequately drained. Communication between the right and left hepatic ducts is not necessary, provided that the undrained lobe has not been percutaneously drained or otherwise contaminated (96). In this circumstance, there is a high risk of persistent biliary fistula and cholangitis. Bypass to an atrophic lobe or a lobe heavily involved with tumor is generally not effective. In a report of 55 consecutive bypasses in patients with malignant hilar obstruction, segment III bypass in patients with hilar cholangiocarcinoma ($n = 20$) yielded the best results. The one-year bypass patency in this group was 80% and there were no perioperative deaths (95). In general, patients known to have unresectable disease are probably best served with percutaneous drainage procedures, given the difficulty of performing an intrahepatic bypass.

Palliative Radiation Therapy

Patients with unresectable, locally advanced tumors but without evidence of widespread disease may be candidates for palliative radiation therapy. A combination of external beam radiation (5000–6000 cGy) and intraluminal iridium-192 (2000 cGy) delivered percutaneously is typically used. Several authors have demonstrated the feasibility of this approach but improved survival compared with biliary decompression alone has not been documented in a controlled study (81,86,97,98). In a group of 12 patients treated with this regimen over a three-year period at MSKCC, the median survival was 14.5 months. Episodes of cholangitis and intermittent jaundice were relatively common but the incidence of serious complications was low and there were no treatment-related deaths (86). Cameron et al. reported improved survival in irradiated patients compared to a group of patients not irradiated; however, the median survival in both groups was less than one year. Others have reported no benefit and question its routine use, given the increased incidence of complications and greater time spent in hospital (97). Radiation therapy is clearly not appropriate in patients with widespread disease. Systemic chemotherapy is the only option for these patients but response rates are low and no study has shown a significant survival benefit compared with biliary drainage alone.

Photodynamic Therapy

Ortner has recently evaluated the efficacy of photodynamic therapy in unresectable hilar cholangiocarcinoma (99,100). This method has previously been used in the treatment of tumors of the esophagus, colon, stomach, bronchus, bladder, and brain. It is a two-step procedure. First, a photosensitizer is injected, followed by direct illumination via cholangioscopy, which activates the compound causing tumor cell death. The authors treated nine patients in this fashion who had failed endoscopic stenting. They report no mortality for the procedure, however, there was a 25% mortality related to the initial endoscopic stenting, which must be considered. The authors do not mention their indication for biliary drainage. This information is important in order to assess the extent of disease prior to therapy. Detailed reasons for unresectability are not discussed, and the reported median survival of 439 days is therefore difficult to interpret. The data presented in this report, including decrease in bilirubin and some improved quality of life, do not suffice to advocate routine use of this method. Comparison in a randomized controlled fashion to other palliative modalities will be needed to define its real value.

Palliative Chemotherapy

In cases of advanced biliary tract cancers where curative surgical resection is not an option, palliative chemotherapy has been used to potentially improve quality of life, diminish symptoms, and increase survival. Only one randomized study has addressed such a role for chemotherapy in advanced biliary tract tumors (101). This study included 37 patients with advanced biliary tract cancers, who were randomized to receive chemotherapy 5-fluorouracil (5-FU/Leucovorin with or without etoposide) or best supportive care. Short-term improvements in survival (6.5 mo vs. 2.5 mo) were noted among the chemotherapy group. In addition, the treatment group also demonstrated improvement in quality of life as measured by the EORTC QLQ-C30 instrument.

Many agents (5-FU, gemcitabine, capecitabine, cisplatin, oxaliplatin, interferon) alone or in combination continue to be evaluated in multiple phase I and II trials. Partial disease responses consistently range for 10% to 30%. Although no consensus has been reached regarding the standard use of chemotherapy in cases of advanced biliary tract cancer, gemcitabine as a single agent has emerged given its more favorable profile in both toxicity and disease response (102). However, given the lack of randomized trial data to support the use of palliative chemotherapy in cases of advanced cholangiocarcinoma, it is best employed in the context of a clinical trial.

Summary

Treatment of perihilar cholangiocarcinomas, the most common and most challenging of biliary tract tumors, continues to evolve. Judicious use of preoperative imaging including duplex ultrasound, CT scan and especially MRCP along with improvements in surgical techniques have allowed better patient selection and the performance of appropriately radical operations with an acceptable mortality. Long-term survival and possible cure, rather than palliation, is now the primary aim. Recent postresection survival results justify an aggressive approach in attempting resection with negative margins. It should be recognized that partial hepatectomy is usually necessary to achieve this goal. The use of chemotherapy in the adjuvant setting has yet to be defined and awaits future clinical trials for direction. A few agents have shown some activity against biliary tract tumors in phase II studies involving patients with unresectable disease. No consensus has been reached regarding the use of palliative chemotherapy, however, gemcitabine is emerging as a reasonable choice. As with the adjuvant setting, further trials will hopefully define the role, if any that chemotherapy plays in palliating biliary tract cancer. All methods of biliary-enteric decompression, whether surgical or intubational, have considerable morbidity but allow reasonable palliation in some patients. Radiotherapy and photodynamic therapy may have a role in increasing stent patency and possibly survival. However, further study is required to establish their position within the current armamentarium. Hilar cholangiocarcinoma should not be approached with therapeutic nihilism. Diagnostic and therapeutic approaches to these lesions require special expertise and patients should be referred to centers where adequately trained teams are available.

Cholangiocarcinoma Involving the Distal Bile Duct

Tumors of the lower bile duct are classified according to their anatomical location, although there may be considerable overlap. Mid-bile duct tumors arise below the confluence in the common bile duct between the upper border of the duodenum and the cystic duct; distal bile duct tumors are those arising anywhere from the duodenum to the papilla of Vater (6). Tumors of the distal bile duct represent approximately 20% to 30% of all cholangiocarcinomas and 5% to 10% of all periampullary tumors (7,103–105). True mid-duct tumors are distinctly uncommon. Nakeeb et al. proposed an alternative classification scheme that divides cholangiocarcinomas into intrahepatic, perihilar, and distal subgroups, thus eliminating the mid-duct group which is often difficult to accurately classify (7). There are approximately 2000 new cases of distal bile duct cancer in the United States each year (103). As is true for hilar cholangiocarcinoma, adenocarcinoma is the principal histologic type in the lower bile duct; however, papillary tumors are more common in the distal bile duct than at the hilus (6).

Clinical Presentation and Diagnosis

The clinical presentation of distal bile duct cancer is generally indistinguishable from that of proximal cholangiocarcinoma or other periampullary malignancies. Progressive jaundice is seen in 75% to 90% of patients. Abdominal pain, weight loss, fever, or pruritus occur in one-third or fewer (7,103). Lesions in the periampullary region may mimic choledocholithiasis; the level of the serum bilirubin may provide a clue as to the etiology of the obstruction, with serum bilirubin >10 mg/dl more indicative of a malignant process (106).

Distal bile duct tumors are frequently mistaken for adenocarcinoma of the pancreas, the most common periampullary malignancy. In a series of 119 periampullary tumors, the site of origin was incorrectly diagnosed in 28% of patients preoperatively and in 20% of patients intraoperatively (107). Aside from diagnosis, ERCP can provide valuable information regarding the level of obstruction and may show clearly that the obstruction is arising from the bile duct without involvement of the pancreatic duct. ERCP may also be useful in cases where choledocholithiasis is suspected and may be therapeutic in these patients. PTC is generally less useful for tumors of the distal bile duct. A good quality cross-sectional imaging study is also required, usually a CT scan, to assess vascular involvement and/or metastatic disease. It is not uncommon that CT scan does not reveal a mass given the frequent small tumor size at presentation. Increasingly, MRCP is being used to evaluate periampullary tumors. As is true for hilar lesions, MRCP can provide information of the distal bile duct previously obtainable only with the combination of ERCP and CT (108).

In patients with a stricture of the distal bile duct and a clinical presentation consistent with cholangiocarcinoma, histologic confirmation of malignancy is generally unnecessary, unless nonoperative therapy is planned. Benign strictures do occur in the lower bile duct, but these are difficult to differentiate definitively from malignant strictures without resection. Percutaneous needle biopsy is difficult and often impossible because of the small size of these tumors. In addition, endoscopic brushings of the bile duct have an unacceptably low sensitivity, making a negative result virtually useless (109). Excessive reliance on the results of percutaneous or brush biopsies will only serve to delay therapy.

Staging and Assessment of Resectability

Carcinomas of the distal common bile duct are staged according to the AJCC system (sixth edition) for tumors of the extrahepatic bile ducts. This system is of limited clinical use, as it is based on pathological information and does not provide any information pertaining to factors that define resectability. The most important of these is the presence of tumor involvement of the portal vein, superior mesenteric artery, or common hepatic artery. Tumors involving a short segment of the portal vein (<2 cm) may be resected with reconstruction of the vein. Metastatic disease found within N2 lymph nodes (celiac, periportal, superior mesenteric) or the liver is a contraindication to resection. Unfortunately, much of the information regarding resectability is uncovered during exploration. In a series of 104 patients with distal bile duct cancer from Memorial Sloan Kettering, two-thirds of the patients found to have advanced/unresectable disease were discovered at surgical exploration (103).

Treatment Options

Complete resection is the only effective therapy for cancers of the lower bile duct (5–7,103–105). Meaningful experience with these relatively uncommon tumors has been limited to a few centers. Retrospective analysis containing significant number of patients reports five-year survival rates ranging from 14% to 40% after complete resection. In most studies, survival beyond one year was uncommon in patients subjected to palliative bypass or biliary intubation (6,34,103,104).

Resection of most distal bile duct cancers requires pancreaticoduodenectomy. In the series from MSKCC, only 13% of patients (6 of 45) were amenable to bile duct excision alone, while in the Veterans Hospital study this figure was 8% (3 of 34) (103,104). In comparison to pancreatic cancer, patients with distal bile duct cancer are more often amenable to resection, less often have microscopic disease at the resection margin and less frequently have spread of tumor to adjacent lymph nodes (7,103,105). In addition to an R0 resection, lymph node status is a critical determinant of outcome. Fong et al. found that lymph node status was the only independent predictor of long-term survival in resected patients, with positive nodes conferring a 6.7 times greater likelihood of recurrence and death (103). Similarly, Wade et al. identified no survivors beyond three years with involved regional lymph nodes (104).

The combined data from the literature would suggest that survival after resection of adenocarcinoma of the distal bile duct is at least as good and maybe better than that for pancreatic cancer (7,103,104). Moreover, it has long been assumed that survival after resection of distal bile duct tumors is greater than after resection of hilar cholangiocarcinomas (6). This assumption is almost certainly erroneous and likely evolved from older reports that did not take into account the status of resection margins in patients with hilar tumors. If adjusted for stage and completeness of resection, the survival rates appear to be comparable (5). Adjuvant therapy after resection (chemotherapy and radiation therapy) has not been proven to improve survival, although this issue has not been evaluated in a prospective fashion (7).

Palliating biliary obstruction in unresectable patients can be achieved with a surgical bypass (hepaticojejunostomy or choledochojejunostomy) or biliary endoprostheses. Endoprostheses for distal biliary obstruction are easier to place and have a greater long-term patency than those placed for hilar obstruction (88). Surgically created bypasses provide excellent relief of jaundice and can be done with an acceptably low morbidity and mortality. It has been suggested that surgical bypass is more appropriate for patients expected to survive more than six months (110). The authors generally use biliary endoprostheses in patients with clear-cut unresectable disease, discovered preoperatively or at staging laparoscopy, and in those unfit for operation.

Cholangiocarcinoma Involving the Intrahepatic Bile Ducts

IHC, also referred to as peripheral cholangiocarcinoma or cholangiolar carcinoma, originates from the intrahepatic biliary radicles. IHC accounts for approximately 10% of all cholangiocarcinomas. IHC is less frequently associated with underlying liver parenchymal disease than is hepatocellular carcinoma, although an association appears to exist. A recent study from the United States has demonstrated a 9% annual percentage increase and an overall 10-fold increase in mortality related to IHC since 1973 (111). Despite this observation, however, IHC remains a rare disease in Western countries.

The presenting symptoms of IHC are often subtle and many present with symptoms related to large lesions causing pain or compression of adjacent organs. Patients may also present with malaise and weight loss; fever may occur but is uncommon. Jaundice and pruritus may be seen in up to one-third of cases and is generally indicative of compression or invasion of the biliary confluence. Small lesions rarely yield significant findings on physical examination, and these tumors often present as incidental findings of imaging studies undertaken for nonspecific or even unrelated symptoms.

Differential Diagnosis

Patients usually present with radiological evidence of a solitary, intrahepatic tissue mass, often with satellite lesions. Percutaneous needle biopsy will demonstrate adenocarcinoma. Patients should be investigated for evidence of a primary tumor elsewhere [gastrointestinal (GI) tract, lung, breast], since the most common diagnosis for adenocarcinoma in the liver is metastatic disease. In addition, hepatitis serology panel and serum α-fetoprotein levels should be drawn to rule out a poorly differentiated hepatocellular carcinoma. In the absence of an extrahepatic primary site, patients with biopsy proven adenocarcinoma in the liver should be considered to have an IHC. Immunohistochemical staining of the biopsy specimen may suggest a lesion of pancreaticobiliary origin, further supporting this diagnosis.

Radiological Investigations

Radiographic studies generally show a large, relatively hypovascular soft tissue mass in the liver, usually without biliary dilatation. On magnetic resonance imaging (MRI) scans, these lesions are hypo- or isodense on T_1-weighted images and hyperdense on T_2-weighted images, while CT scan usually shows a hypodense mass. MRI and duplex ultrasound exams are also useful to evaluate extent of disease and involvement of hepatic vasculature.

Staging and Assessment of Resectability

Currently there is no useful clinical staging system for peripheral cholangiocarcinomas. The AJCC TNM (tumor node metastates) classification for primary liver cancers is applied both to hepatocellular carcinoma and IHC but is of little value clinically and not often utilized. Because peripheral cholangiocarcinomas tend to be relatively silent lesions, they are often large at presentation. In a recent review of 53 peripheral cholangiocarcinomas treated at MSKCC over a eight-year period, the median tumor diameter was 7.1 cm at presentation (114). Twenty patients were found to be unresectable at exploration for a 62% overall resectability rate. Operative findings precluding resection were intrahepatic metastases (35%), peritoneal metastases (30%), celiac lymph node metastases (25%), and portal vein involvement (10%). Staging laparoscopy was conducted in 22 patients, of which 6 were spared laparotomy secondary to findings of peritoneal and intrahepatic metastases.

Investigators from Japan have proposed a classification scheme based on tumor morphology that has undergone subsequent modification (112,113). According to this approach, tumors are classified as (*i*) mass forming type, (*ii*) periductal infiltrating type, (*iii*) mass forming plus periductal infiltrating, and (*iv*) intraductal papillary type. The mass forming and intraductal papillary types appear to have a more favorable outcome after resection.

Treatment Options

Hepatic resection with negative histological margins remains the only potentially curative treatment for this disease. In the absence of clear metastatic disease on imaging studies, otherwise fit patients should therefore be considered for operation with a goal of complete resection.

Only about 20% of patients with IHCs have resectable lesions at the time of presentation. Of the patients who appear respectable on preoperative imaging only two-thirds will be resectable at exploration (114). In the study by Weber et al., the authors not surprisingly found a significantly better median survival for resected versus explored, but unresectable, 37.4 months versus 11.6 months, respectively. Unfortunately, recurrence was seen in 60% of the resected patients and 75% of these recurrences were intrahepatic (114). Negative prognostic factors on univariate analysis from this series and others include positive resection margin, multiple hepatic tumors, vascular invasion, and perihepatic lymph node involvement (114–116). Three-year survival rates for resected patients range from 16% to 61%.

Orthotopic liver transplantation has been utilized in the management of some patients (117,118). Median survivals of up to 18 months have been achieved in node negative patients but no patient with involved perihepatic lymph nodes has survived beyond two years (32). For patients with small node negative tumors, a three-year survival rate of 64% has recently been reported (119). However, many of these lesions are suitable for resection, which would likely provide a comparable survival rate. Given the critical shortage of liver grafts, transplantation for IHC is not performed in most centers, unless it is done in the context of a clinical trial.

The use of chemotherapy, 5-FU or other agents, has not been shown to improve survival, either as adjuvant therapy following resection or in patients with unresectable lesions (120). External beam radiation therapy, intraoperative radiation, and intraluminal radiation therapy have all been evaluated in patients with peripheral cholangiocarcinoma. These studies are generally not well-controlled and involve small numbers of patients. No prospective trial or retrospective review has shown a significant survival benefit in patients with unresectable disease. In addition up to 10% have significant treatment-related complications with duodenal obstruction and bleeding (81). In an effort to target the radiation dose within the tumor, ^{31}I-labeled anti-CEA in conjunction with systemic chemotherapy has been used in patients with unresectable tumors (121). While a significant reduction in tumor volume was noted on CT scan in 27% of patients, there was no improvement in survival.

GALLBLADDER CANCER

Gallbladder cancer is an uncommon malignancy with approximately 5000 new cases per year in the United States (1). Historically, clinical attitudes toward gallbladder cancer have been based in pessimism and nihilism. These sentiments are reflected in a statement by Alfred Blalock in 1924 in which he states, "in malignancy of the gallbladder, when a diagnosis can be made without exploration, no operation should be performed, in as much as it only shortens the patient's life." This viewpoint gained further acceptance when a review of all cases of gallbladder cancer ($n = 6222$) reported in the English-language literature was undertaken by Piehler and Crichlow in 1978, demonstrating a cumulative median survival of five to eight months and five-year survivorship under 5% (122). The clinical frustration spawns from the usual late presentation, lack of effective therapy, and the resultant dismal prognosis. In fact, most older series reported a median survival of two to five months for untreated gallbladder cancers and less than 5% five-year survival for treated gallbladder cancers. However, improved understanding of the disease and its treatment has lead to prolonged survival and cure in selected patients. Currently, the only chance of cure is still complete surgical extirpation of the cancer. Recently, improved morbidity and mortality associated with radical resections involving the liver and biliary tract have led to a wider application of these therapies in selected patients, and thus more chances to cure this dreaded disease. Unfortunately, effective adjuvant therapy is still lacking. Many agents investigated with phase II trials in the palliative setting have demonstrated antitumor activity but randomized clinical trials are lacking to evaluate their true efficacy in this rare tumor.

Epidemiology

The highest incidence rates of gallbladder cancer worldwide are found in cultures indigenous to the Andes Mountains of South America. In North America, high incidence rates are found among native American Indians and Mexican Americans. Gallbladder cancer occurs in women almost three times more often than in men across all populations studied (123).

As with other biliary tract tumors, chronic inflammation is a common denominator of associated risk factors. The most common of these risk factors is cholelithiasis, especially large gallstones (123,124). Other conditions leading to gallbladder inflammation, such as cholecystoenteric fistula and chronic infection with typhoid bacillus bacteria, have also been noted as risk factors for the development of cancer. As with other GI malignancies, a progression from adenoma to carcinoma has been demonstrated within adenomatous polyps of the gallbladder (125). Gallbladder polyps have been noted in 3% to 6% of the population undergoing US. The vast majority are cholesterol polyps and have no malignant potential. However, about 1% of cholecystectomy specimens contain adenomatous polyps which have malignant potential (126). Yang et al. reviewed a series of 182 gallbladder polyps found in cholecystectomy specimens (127). Preoperative ultrasound was 93% sensitive in diagnosing a polypoid lesion of the wall of the gallbladder. Most of the polyps were non-neoplastic, benign cholesterol polyps (93%); however, 13 (7%) were discovered to harbor a malignancy. Furthermore, malignant potential appears to be proportional to size, among other risk factors. Yeh et al., in a series of 123 patients with polypoid lesions of the gallbladder, the likelihood of an associated malignancy correlated with size >1 cm, age >50 years, and the presence of multiple lesions (128). The conservative recommendation based on these studies is prophylactic cholecystectomy for polypoid lesions greater than 0.5 cm in size, although the likelihood of malignancy in polyps even up to 1 cm appears to be quite low. This is in contrast to gallbladder polyps arising in the setting of PSC, which are more often neoplastic (129). The authors' practice is to generally recommend cholecystectomy for polyps >1 cm; polypoid lesions <0.5 cm have a much lower likelihood of harboring a malignancy and should be followed with serial ultrasounds for evidence of growth or any change in character (125–127).

A gallbladder that demonstrates a calcified wall, otherwise known as "porcelain gallbladder" is also a condition associated with an increased risk of developing a gallbladder cancer (Fig. 6). The deposition of calcium into the wall is most likely the result of chronic inflammation. Porcelain gallbladder has been reported in approximately 0.5% to 1.0% of cholecystectomy specimens (130,131). The risk of malignancy in porcelain gallbladder has previously been considered extremely high (10–50%), although more recent studies have shown a much lower incidence (<10%) and that varies according to the type of mural calcification seen (131,132). Nevertheless, the current recommendations are for cholecystectomy for patients with porcelain gallbladder, which in most cases, can be done laparoscopically.

Histopathology and Staging

Gallbladder cancers are aggressive tumors with a propensity for local invasion, lymphatic metastasis, and peritoneal dissemination. The overwhelming majority of these neoplasms are adenocarcinomas. Papillary subtype has been associated with a relatively better prognosis compared to mucinous and adenosquamous subtypes (132). The AJCC staging is based on the familiar TMN system. T stage is dependent on the depth of invasion relative to the gallbladder wall and adjacent organs. The wall of the gallbladder consists of a mucosa and lamina propria, a thin muscular layer, perimuscular connective tissue, and a serosa. However, it should be noted that the gallbladder wall lacks a serosal covering along its border with the liver and the perimuscular connective tissue is continuous with the liver connective tissue. T1 tumors are confined to the mucosa. T2 tumors have invaded up to but not through the serosa. T3 tumors have penetrated the serosa and directly invaded an adjacent organ. This most likely involves local invasion into the liver and is limited to <2 cm in extent. T4 tumors are those that invade >2 cm into the liver or involve two or more adjacent organs via direct extension. The T-staging of gallbladder cancers is particularly important in postcholecystectomy patients, since depth of invasion dictates treatment recommendations and outcome. In considering N stage, at least three nodes must be evaluable to be considered adequate nodal staging. Nodal disease is classified as N0 for the absence of tumor within at least three resected lymph nodes. N1 disease is assigned to any positive cystic duct node or hepatoduodenal ligament nodes. N2 disease includes malignancy within celiac, superior mesenteric, or peripancreatic nodes. Metastatic

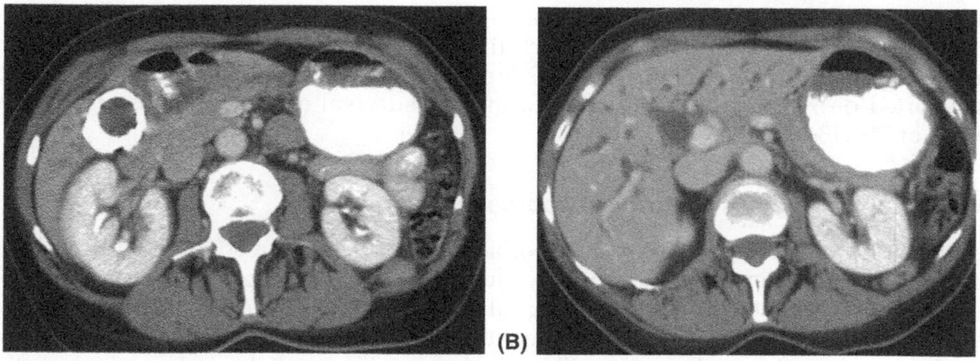

FIGURE 6 Axial CT images of a porcelain gallbladder. Note the marked, circumferential calcification of the gallbladder wall (**A**) and the intrahepatic biliary ductal dilatation (**B**). This patient had a gallbladder cancer arising in the setting of a porcelain gallbladder, which had progressed to involve the common hepatic duct. *Abbreviation*: CT, computed tomography.

disease refers to distant metastasis. It should be noted that most of the studies cited in this chapter refer to the TMN staging as outlined in the fifth edition system. These staging systems are designed to have the widest applicability in the multimodality treatment of gallbladder cancer. Changes made in the sixth edition are based on resectability. Stages I and II represent respectable disease versus unresectable disease, and stages III and IV represent locally unresectable and metastatic disease, respectively. The AJCC sixth edition restaging may allow for better stratification when constructing clinical trials.

The presence of jaundice is a relatively common (see below) and ominous associated finding in patients with gallbladder cancer. Given the proximity of the gallbladder with the major extrahepatic biliary ductal structures, concomitant biliary involvement should not be surprising and can take the form of direct extension or metastatic disease to the hepatoduodenal ligament. The typical finding is obstruction of the distal common hepatic duct or proximal common bile duct, although involvement at the hepatic duct confluence or at the ampullary level may be seen. Coexisting jaundice generally implies advanced disease that is beyond resectability. In an analysis of 240 patients with gallbladder cancer over a seven-year period, Hawkins et al. reported the presence of jaundice in 82 (34%), of which only 6 (7%) had disease amenable to a complete resection, and all of these patients had either recurred or died of disease by two years. Additionally, the median survival in jaundiced patients was 6 months compared to 16 months in patients presenting without jaundice (133).

Natural History

Most patients present late in the course of their disease. In fact, 75% of patients present with the cancer beyond the borders of resection (134). Two-thirds of the patients present with abdominal pain/biliary colic. Approximately one-third will present with jaundice and 10% will have significant weight loss (135). The majority of gallbladder cancers will be associated with cholelithiasis. The diagnosis is usually made for early-stage cancers upon pathologic examination of a cholecystectomy specimen resected under the pretense of a benign condition. Preoperative diagnosis should be suspected for any mass or irregularity of the gallbladder wall noted on radiologic exam (CT or ultrasound). In any patient suspected of having a gallbladder malignancy, a duplex ultrasound exam should be performed to evaluate the extent of disease and possible involvement of the portal vasculature. In addition, abdominal cross-sectional imaging (CT or MRI) should be performed to evaluate for nodal disease or M1 disease.

Given the rarity of this tumor, randomized clinical trials investigating different therapies have not been performed. However, many large series reviews have been reported and will necessarily serve as the natural history against which treatments are measured. In 1978, Piehler and Crichlow gathered data on 6222 cases of gallbladder cancer previously reported on in the English-language literature. Their results demonstrated a dismal five- to eight-month median survival and a cumulative five-year survivorship of 4%. Of note, 25% of these cases underwent a curative resection and experienced a 16.5% five-year survivorship (122). These results were mimicked by a large study conducted by the French Surgical Association by Cubertafond et al. that reported on 724 cases demonstrating a median survival of three months and five-year survival of 5% (136).

Evidence for an Aggressive Surgical Approach

Over the past three decades, decreasing morbidity and mortality associated with radical, en bloc resections including hepatectomy, bile duct resection, and regional lymphadenectomy have allowed for broader application of surgical resection in selected patients (135,137). Radical or extended cholecystectomy is the term used to describe en bloc resection of gallbladder with a rim of normal liver tissue adjacent to gallbladder fossa and associated portal lymphadenectomy thus distinguishing it from the standard cholecystectomy, open or laparoscopic, which is referred to as a "simple" cholecystectomy. The current surgical approaches generally employ segmental resections (segmentectomy 4/5) when possible or major resections (hemihepatectomy or extended hepatectomy) when necessary. In most cases, it is involvement of major hepatic vascular structures rather than depth of tumor invasion into the liver that dictates the extent of hepatic resection that must be performed.

In a series from MSKCC, Bartlett et al. report on 149 cases in which complete surgical radical resection yielded an actuarial five-year survival of 83% for stage II, 63% for stage III, 25% for stage IV (135). Of note, the long-term survivors with stage IV disease were T4, N0 disease. Many contemporary studies have reported similar results of significant long-term survival after complete resection, even for stages III and IV disease (138–141). The improved survival reported in these studies relative to historical studies demonstrates the importance of achieving negative margins in the treatment of gallbladder cancer. Further evidence in support that an aggressive surgical approach leads to improved survival was recently offered in a study by Dixon et al. from the University of Toronto (142). This study analyzed two time period cohorts that spanned a 12-year period. The latter half of the 12-year period included significantly more liver and bile duct resections indicative of the more aggressive surgical approach. These patients experienced a doubling of the median survival from nine months to 17 months and five-year survival rate increased to 35% from 7% when compared to the earlier time period. The authors attributed these results to a more aggressive surgical approach undertaken for patients in the more recent time period cohort.

Regional lymphadenectomy is currently employed as part of an aggressive surgical approach but evidence to support an associated survival benefit is controversial. The chance of nodal involvement increases with increasing T stage. Bartlett et al. found nodal disease associated with 46% of resected T2 tumors, 54% of resected T3 tumors (135). Node status was found to be the most powerful predictor of outcome and no patient with node positive disease experienced long-term survival. Poor outcome for node positive disease has been consistently reported throughout the Western literature. This is in contrast to Japanese studies in which node positive disease was found among long-term survivors (137,138,140). In fact, some authors have advocated the addition of a pancreaticoduodenectomy in order to eradicate node positive disease. Whether this discrepancy is the result of differences in surgical technique, disease biology, or staging, is controversial and is a matter for further study.

Surgical Therapy

The gallbladder cancer patient will present to the surgeon in three different clinical scenarios: (*i*) malignancy suspected preoperatively; (*ii*) malignancy found at the time of exploration; (*iii*) malignancy diagnosed after simple cholecystectomy. Contraindications to resection include distant spread (peritoneum, discontigous liver lesions), tumor involvement of the hepatic vasculature or biliary tree that would preclude a complete resection, and presence of disease in distant lymph node groups (N2 nodal disease as defined by AJCC fifth edition staging system: peripancreatic, periduodenal, periportal, celiac, and/or superior mesenteric). As discussed above, the presence of jaundice is a relative contraindication to resection.

The goal of resection should always be complete tumor extirpation with negative histologic margins (R0). The extent of surgical resection required to achieve this will vary, depending on several factors. In the most common situation, patients will present after a simple cholecystectomy, after which an incidental malignancy is identified. In such cases, the depth of tumor invasion into the gallbladder wall (T stage) will dictate subsequent treatment. Patients with cancer identified preoperatively typically have larger tumors than are seen in postcholecystectomy patients and usually require a radical resection. Gallbladder cancer identified intraoperatively is an uncommon but difficult situation, since one will have limited staging information; however, it would seem reasonable to err on the side of aggressive resection in these cases, since this is the only effective therapy.

It is important to remember that the incidence of lymph node and distant metastases is directly related to tumor depth of invasion into the gallbladder wall or T stage. In the study by Fong et al., distant and nodal metastases increased progressively from 16% to 79% and from 33% to 69%, respectively, in going from T2 to T4 tumors, and there was a corresponding and progressive decline in resectability, from 58% to 13% (143).

T1 Tumors

T1a tumors are most often discovered after laparoscopic cholecystectomy. This group of tumors is nearly always cured by simple cholecystectomy. The potential for nodal metastasis is small. The cure rate after simple cholecystectomy is 85% to 100% if negative margins are attained (144,145). T1b tumors, that is, those tumors that have extended into the muscle layer, in theory should be cured by a simple cholecystectomy, however, there have been reports in the literature documenting recurrence and death following a simple cholecystectomy for T1b tumors (146). Given the limited data regarding T1b gallbladder cancers in the literature, the decision to perform a simple cholecystectomy versus a more radical procedure should be made on case-by-case basis.

T2 Tumors

T2 lesions, tumors that extent into the perimuscular connective tissues/serosa but not into the liver, should be treated by aggressive resection, which should include removal of adjacent liver as well as a lymphadenectomy of the hepatoduodenal ligament with or without resection of the bile duct. As discussed above, the extent of hepatic resection required depends on whether or not there is tumor involvement of major hepatic vascular structures. In the absence of such involvement, the authors prefer to perform a segmental resection of segments IV and V, and most T2 tumors are amenable to such an approach. Similarly, a resection and reconstruction of the bile duct is performed only if necessary to clear tumor (135). It should be noted that the normal plane of dissection of simple cholecystectomy, open or laparoscopic, is within the perimuscular connective tissue intimately associated with the liver. Thus, a simple cholecystectomy will not achieve tumor clearance with certainty. A lymphadenectomy is performed in the treatment of T2 tumors given that approximately 50% of these lesions have associated lymph node metastases (135). The benefit of the extended resection over simple cholecystectomy is supported by data that demonstrate improved survival. de Aretxabal et al. reported five-year survival rates of 70% after radical cholecystectomy compared with 20% after simple cholecystectomy alone (147). Furthermore, in a study by Fong et al., a similar survival benefit was demonstrated in patients who were re-resected after simple cholecystectomy. Five-year survival rates of 61% were achieved in the patients who were re-resected compared to 19% of patients who did not undergo a radical second operation (143).

T3 Tumors

T3 tumors penetrate the serosa and may extend up to 2 cm into the liver parenchyma. None of these lesions would be cured by a simple cholecystectomy, which by definition would leave tumor behind in the gallbladder fossa. Tumors at this level of invasion require hepatic resection and porta hepatis lymphadenectomy at a minimum, and this often includes a major hepatectomy with bile duct resection and reconstruction. The same principles of management of T2 tumors applies to these tumors as well. When a complete resection is attained, five-year survival rates of 30% to 50% can be achieved in this patient population (135,140,143).

T4 Tumors

T4 lesions are grossly invasive of the liver, extending more than 2 cm into the parenchyma or invade two or more adjacent organs via local extension. Although systemic tumor dissemination is more likely in this patient population, studies have documented long-term survival after a complete resection, which usually requires a major partial hepatectomy. It should be noted that these rare cases of long-term survival usually do not have nodal disease (135,138).

Preoperative Suspicion of Malignancy

If gallbladder cancer is suspected preoperatively, an abdominal/pelvic CT scan and ultrasound are the studies of choice to define the extent of disease. MRI may also be employed. Ultrasound is particularly helpful to assess the gallbladder wall for evidence of invasiveness. The ultrasonographic finding of asymmetric thickening of the gallbladder wall is a worrisome finding and should not be disregarded as likely related to inflammation. Staging laparoscopy prior to laparotomy is helpful to assess the abdomen for evidence of peritoneal spread or discontiguous liver disease; however, laparoscopic cholecystectomy generally should be avoided when a preoperative cancer is suspected (52,69,70). In this situation, one is obliged to proceed with resection of an invasive malignancy, unless proven otherwise. It is not unreasonable to obtain frozen section histology to prove malignancy before proceeding with hepatic resection.

Unsuspected Malignancy at Exploration

It should be customary to inspect the gallbladder mucosa after simple cholecystectomy. Suspicious lesions should be sent immediately for frozen section. If a carcinoma is diagnosed, the need to perform additional surgery would be dictated by the T stage on frozen section. However, one will obtain limited information on frozen section histology, since a full histopathologic analysis is not possible. The authors would prefer to perform an oncologically correct resection, suitable for an invasive lesion, at the time it is discovered, unless there are extenuating circumstances that mandate otherwise. However, if the surgeon is not adept at radical cholecystectomy/hepatic resection the patient would be best served by transfer to a center/surgeon with experience in performing the appropriate operation. Such an approach is reasonable and does not negatively impact the patient's prognosis, provided that the definitive procedure is subsequently performed. Fong et al. showed that a prior noncurative cholecystectomy does not influence survival in patients who subsequently undergo re-operation and the appropriate resection (143).

Malignancy Diagnosed Post-Cholecystectomy

When the cancer is diagnosed by postoperative histology, the need for a more radical resection will be based on T stage as outlined above. Evidence for performing a second operation comes from a study by Shirai et al. in which they found a positive cystic duct node in 39/98 (40%) of gallbladder specimens in patients with undiagnosed gallbladder cancer. The data further demonstrated a significantly better long-term survival for those patients who were treated with a second resection (144). As mentioned above, a study by Fong et al. demonstrated a much improved five-year survival rate in patients undergoing a second operation compared to those who did not (143). Prior to undertaking a second operation, a high quality cross-sectional imaging (CT/MRI) should be obtained to appropriately stage the disease. Postoperative inflammatory changes may be indistinguishable from tumor and thus may necessitate bile duct resection or a more aggressive hepatic resection to ensure complete tumor eradication.

Postlaparoscopic cholecystectomy diagnosis of gallbladder cancer may predispose the patient to early peritoneal spread, especially if bile or stone spillage occurred (148). Given that inadvertent cholecystotomy during cholecystectomy is rarely documented, it is difficult to predict who is at increased risk for peritoneal dissemination and specifically, port site recurrence. Prior work has suggested that the risk of peritoneal recurrence is not necessarily greater in patients subjected to a noncurative laparoscopic cholecystectomy compared to open cholecystectomy (149). In the past, routine resection of laparoscopic port sites was recommended, in an effort to ensure clearance of microscopic disease that may have implanted during the laparoscopic procedure. However, there is little evidence to support the efficacy of routine resection of all port sites at re-operation (150). In the authors' experience, recurrence at the port sites is a harbinger of generalized peritoneal recurrence that would not have been prevented with resection of these areas.

Adjuvant Therapy

Adenocarcinomas of the gallbladder as illustrated above present a challenging clinical problem and only the minority (<25%) of patients who present are deemed eligible for radical resectional therapy. This is mostly due to the associated nonspecific symptoms occurring late in the course of a gallbladder cancer. Even for the patients who are able to undergo complete resection of their primary, relapse rates are high (149). In order to provide a rational framework upon which to develop adjuvant therapies for the resected patient, Jarnagin et al. at MSKCC investigated the initial pattern of recurrence after resection of biliary tract cancers. In considering only gallbladder cancers, their results demonstrated that in patients who underwent a potentially curative resection, 66% experienced a disease recurrence within a median follow-up of 24 months. In evaluating the pattern of recurrences, only 15% of patients developed a locoregional recurrence as the first site of failure, while the majority of patients (85%) had an initial recurrence that involved a distant site (149). The authors concluded that adjuvant therapies targeted at locoregional disease, such as radiotherapy, would be unlikely to significantly impact the course of this disease, further emphasizing the importance of developing effective systemic adjuvant therapies.

Most data for the use of adjuvant therapy in resected patients are derived from phase II trials in which treated patients are compared with historical controls. Most of these trials are limited by small numbers and are confounded by inclusion of patients with less than an R0 resection (151,152). Most of the phase II studies used some combination of chemoradiation. Given the small numbers in these studies, minimal conclusions can be drawn regarding the use of external beam radiation/chemotherapy in the adjuvant setting. In cases of incomplete resection, there remains a theoretical benefit in adding an additional locoregional therapy, such as external beam radiation therapy, for disease control.

One phase III multi-institutional trial of adjuvant chemotherapy was performed in Japan as reported by Takada et al. (85). It should be noted that this trial included 508 patients with biliary and pancreatic cancers. However, on subset analysis, this study included 140 gallbladder cancer patients who were randomized to receive surgical resection alone or resection plus adjuvant mitomycin and 5-FU. In considering only the gallbladder cancer patients, the actuarial five-year disease-free survival favored the adjuvant chemotherapy group, 20.3% versus 11.6% in comparison to the surgery alone group. From these data, it is reasonable to offer adjuvant chemotherapy with 5-FU and mitomycin to resected gallbladder patients, however, no consensus has been reached regarding routine use of adjuvant chemotherapy (102).

Palliation

Most gallbladder cancer patients present with advanced, incurable disease. Their symptoms may include pain, jaundice, or GI obstruction. Given the dismal prognosis of approximately two to five months, palliative therapies should be selected minimizing morbidity. Thus, palliative nonsurgical, endoscopic, or percutaneous methods of relieving both intestinal and biliary obstruction should be entertained first. If unresectable disease is discovered at the time of exploration, a segment III bypass can be performed to relieve jaundice but patients are best served by avoiding a major operative procedure and proceeding with percutaneous biliary drainage postoperatively (153). Intestinal bypass should be performed only in patients who have symptomatic obstruction. As in biliary obstruction, performing a less invasive endoscopic or percutaneous GI drainage procedure maybe the best option given the prognosis.

Summary

Despite the emergence over the past several years of safe en bloc radical resections, potentially curative resection is only possible in a minority of patients. In addition, the majority of patients will experience distant disease recurrence which remains a major obstacle in achieving long-term survival. The development of effective adjuvant therapy regimens is necessary if the mortality related to gallbladder cancer is to be reduced further. Currently, evidence for effective adjuvant therapy is lacking and cannot be considered standard of care.

REFERENCES

1. Landis SH, Murray T, Bolden S, Wingo PA. Cancer statistics, 1998. CA Cancer J Clin 1998; 48(1):6–29.
2. Kuwayti K, Baggenstoss AH, Stauffer MH, Priestly JI. Carcinoma of the major intrahepatic and the extrahepatic bile ducts exclusive of the papilla of Vater. Gynecol Obstet 1957; 104:357–366.
3. Carriaga MT, Henson DE. Liver, gallbladder, extrahepatic bile ducts, and pancreas. Cancer 1995; 75(suppl 1):171–190.
4. Burke EC, Jamagsin WR, Hochwald SN, Pisters PW, Fong Y, Blumgart LH. Hilar cholangiocarcinoma: patterns of spread, the importance of hepatic resection for curative operation, and a presurgical clinical staging system. Ann Surg 1998; 228(3):385–394.
5. Nagorney DM, Donohue JH, Farnell MB, Schleck CD, Ilstrup DM. Outcomes after curative resections of cholangiocarcinoma. Arch Surg 1993; 128(8):871–877; discussion 877–879.
6. Tompkins PK, Thomas D, Wile A, Longmire WP Jr. Prognostic factors in bile duct carcinoma: analysis of 96 cases. Ann Surg 1981; 194:447–457.
7. Nakeeb A, Pitt HA. Sohn TA, et al. Cholangiocarcinoma. A spectrum of intrahepatic, perihilar, and distal tumors. Ann Surg 1996; 224(4):463–473; discussion 473–475.
8. Berdah SV, Dclpcro JR, Garcia S, Hardwigsen J, Le Treut YP. A western surgical experience of peripheral cholangiocarcinoma. Br J Surg 1996; 83(11):1517–1521.
9. Chu KM, Lai EC, Al-Hadeedi S, et al. Intrahepatic cholangiocarcinoma. World J Surg 1997; 21(3): 301–305; discussion 305–306.
10. Harrison LE, Fong Y, Klimstra DS, Zee SY, Blumgart LH. Surgical treatment of 32 patients with peripheral intrahepatic cholangiocarcinoma. Br J Surg 1998; 85(8):1068–1070.
11. Saunders K, Longmire W Jr, Tompkins R, Chavez M, Cates J, Roslyn J. Diffuse bile duct tumors: guidelines for management. Am Surg 1991; 57(12):816–820.
12. Sako K, Seitzinger GL, Garside E. Carcinoma of the extrahepatic bile ducts: review of the literature and report of six cases. Surgery 1957; 41(3):416–437.
13. Okuda K, Kubo Y, Okazaki N, Arishima T, Hashimoto M. Clinical aspects of intrahepatic bile duct carcinoma including hilar carcinoma: a study of 57 autopsy-proven cases. Cancer 1977; 39(1):232–246.
14. Broome U, Olsson R, Loof L, et al. Natural history and prognostic factors in 305 Swedish patients with primary sclerosing cholangitis. Gut 1996; 38(4):610–615.
15. Katoh H, Shinbo T, Otagiri H, et al. Character of a human cholangiocarcinoma CHGS, serially transplanted to nude mice. Hum Cell 1988; 1(1):101–105.
16. Pitt HA, Dooley WC, Yeo CJ, Cameron JL. Malignancies of the biliary tree. Curr Probl Surg 1995; 32(1):1–90.
17. Broome U, Eriksson LS. Assessment for liver transplantation in patients with primary sclerosing cholangitis. J Hepatol 1994; 20(5):654–659.
18. Hewitt PM, Krige JE, Bornman PC, Terblanche J. Choledochal cysts in adults. Br J Surg 1995; 82(3):382–385.
19. Vogt DP. Current management of cholangiocarcinoma. Oncology (Williston Park), 1988; 2(6):37–44, 54.
20. Lipsett PA, Pitt HA, Colombani PM, Boitnott JK, Cameron JL. Choledochal cyst disease. A changing pattern of presentation. Ann Surg 1994; 220(5):644–652.
21. Tanaka K, Ikoma A, Hamada N, Nishida S, Kadono J, Taira A. Biliary tract cancer accompanied by anomalous junction of pancreaticobiliary ductal system in adults. Am J Surg 1998; 175(3):218–220.
22. Jeng KS, Ohta I, Yang FS, et al. Coexisting sharp ductal angulation with intrahepatic biliary strictures in right hepatolithiasis. Arch Surg 1994; 129(10):1097–1102.
23. Hakamada K, Sasaki M, Endoh M, Itoh T, Morita T, Konn M. Late development of bile duct cancer after sphincteroplasty: a ten- to twenty-two-year follow-up study. Surgery 1997; 121(5):488–492.
24. Chu KM, Lo CM, Liu CL, Fan ST. Malignancy associated with hepatolithiasis. Hepatogastroenterology 1997; 44(14):352–357.
25. Kubo S, Kinoshita H, Hirohashi K, Hamba H. Hepatolithiasis associated with cholangiocarcinoma. World J Surg 1995; 19(4):637–641.
26. Watanapa P. Cholangiocarcinoma in patients with opisthorchiasis. Br J Surg 1996; 83(8):1062–1064.
27. Weinbren K, Mutum SS. Pathological aspects of cholangiocarcinoma. J Pathol 1983; 139(2):217–238.
28. Rodgers CM, Adams JT, Schwartz SI. Carcinoma of the extrahepatic bile ducts. Surgery 1981; 90(4):596–601.
29. Jarnagin WR, Bowne W, Klimstra DS, et al. Papillary phenotype confers improved survival after resection of hilar cholangiocarcinoma. Ann Surg 2005; 241(5):703–712; discussion 712–714.

30. Tsuzuki T, Ogata Y, Iida S, Nakanishi I, Takenaka Y, Yoshii H. Carcinoma of the bifurcation of the hepatic ducts. Arch Surg 1983; 118(10):1147–1151.
31. Shimada H, Niimoto S, Matsuba A, Nakagawara G, Kobayashi M, Tsuchiya S. The infiltration of bile duct carcinoma along the bile duct wall. Int Surg 1988; 73(2):87–90.
32. The Liver Cancer Study Group of Japan. Primary liver cancer in Japan. Sixth report. Cancer 1987; 60(6):1400–1411.
33. Levi S, Urbano-Ispizua A, Gill R, et al. Multiple K-ras codon 12 mutations in cholangiocarcinomas demonstrated with a sensitive polymerase chain reaction technique. Cancer Res 1991; 51(13): 3497–3502.
34. Nakeeb A, Lipsett PA, Lillemoe KD, et al. Biliary carcinoembryonic antigen levels are a marker for cholangiocarcinoma. Am J Surg 1996; 171(1):147–152; discussion 152–153.
35. Farley DR, Weaver AL, Nagorney DM. "Natural history" of unresected cholangiocarcinoma: patient outcome after noncurative intervention. Mayo Clin Proc 1995; 70(5):425–429.
36. Vatanasapt V, Uttaravichien T, Mairiang EO, Pairojkul C, Chartbanchachai W, Haswell-Elkins M. Cholangiocarcinoma in north-east Thailand. Lancet 1990; 335(8681):116–117.
37. McPherson GA, Benjamin IS, Hodgson HJ, Bowley NB, Allison DJ, Blumgart LH. Pre-operative percutaneous transhepatic biliary drainage: the results of a controlled trial. Br J Surg 1984; 71(5): 371–375.
38. Heslin MJ, Brooks AD, Hochwald SN, Harrison LE, Blumgart LH, Brennan MF. A preoperative biliary stent is associated with increased complications after pancreatoduodenectomy. Arch Surg 1998; 133(2):149–154.
39. Wetter LA, Ring EJ, Pellegrini CA, Way LW. Differential diagnosis of sclerosing cholangiocarcinomas of the common hepatic duct (Klatskin tumors). Am J Surg 1991; 161(1):57–62; discussion 62–63.
40. Hadjis NS, Blumgart LH. Role of liver atrophy, hepatic resection and hepatocyte hyperplasia in the development of portal hypertension in biliary disease. Gut 1987; 28(8):1022–1028.
41. Gibson RN, Yeung E, Thompson JN, et al. Bile duct obstruction: radiologic evaluation of level, cause, and tumor resectability. Radiology 1986; 160(1):43–47.
42. Okuda K, Ohto M, Tsuchiya Y. The role of ultrasound, percutaneous transhepatic cholangiography, computed tomographic scanning, and magnetic resonance imaging in the preoperative assessment of bile duct cancer. World J Surg 1988; 12(1):18–26.
43. Hann LE, Greatrex KV, Bach AM, Fong Y, Blumgart LH. Cholangiocarcinoma at the hepatic hilus: sonographic findings. AJR Am J Roentgenol 1997; 168(4):985–989.
44. Bach AM, Hann LE, Brown KT, et al. Portal vein evaluation with US: comparison to angiography combined with CT arterial portography. Radiology 1996; 201(1):149–154.
45. Itoh K, Fujita N, Kubo K, et al. MR imaging of hilar cholangiocarcinoma—comparative study with CT. Nippon Igaku Hoshasen Gakkai Zasshi 1992; 52(4):443–451.
46. Guthrie JA, Ward J, Robinson PJ. Hilar cholangiocarcinomas: T^2-weighted spin-echo and gadolinium-enhanced FLASH MR imaging. Radiology 1996; 201(2):347–351.
47. Schwartz LH, Coakley FV, Sun Y, Blumgart LH, Fong Y, Panicek DM. Neoplastic pancreaticobiliary duct obstruction: evaluation with breath-hold MR cholangiopancreatography. AJR Am J Roentgenol 1998; 170(6):1491–1495.
48. Lee MG, Lee HJ, Kim MH, et al. Extrahepatic biliary diseases: 3D MR cholangiopancreatography compared with endoscopic retrograde cholangiopancreatography. Radiology 1997; 202(3):663–669.
49. Hochwald SN, Burke EC, Jamagin WE, Fong Y, Blumgart LH. Association of preoperative biliary stenting with increased postoperative infectious complications in proximal cholangiocarcinoma. Arch Surg 1999; 134(3):261–266.
50. Baer HU, Matthews SB, Schweizer WP, Gertsch P, Bluragart LH. Management of the Mirizzi syndrome and the surgical implications of cholecystcholedochal fistula. Br J Surg 1990; 77(7):743–745.
51. Cabooter M, Sas S, Laukens P. Mirizzi syndrome. Ned Tijdschr Geneeskd 1990; 134(14):708–711.
52. Gallery MP, Strasberg SM, Doherty GMP, Soper NJ, Norton JA. Staging laparoscopy with laparoscopic ultrasonography: optimizing resectability in hepatobiliary and pancreatic malignancy. J Am Coll Surg 1997; 185(1):33–39.
53. Hadjis NS, Adam A, Hatzis G, Blumgart LH. Mirizzi syndrome associated with liver atrophy. Diagnostic and management considerations. J Hepatol 1987; 4(2):245–249.
54. Verbeek PC, van Leeuwen DJ, de Wit LT, et al. Benign fibrosing disease at the hepatic confluence mimicking Klatskin tumors. Surgery 1992; 112(5):866–871.
55. Saldinger PF, Blumgart LH. Resection of hilar cholangiocarcinoma—a European and United States experience. J Hepatobiliary Pancreat Surg 2000; 7(2):111–114.
56. Rabinovitz M, Zajko AB, Hassanein T, et al. Diagnostic value of brush cytology in the diagnosis of bile duct carcinoma: a study in 65 patients with bile duct strictures. Hepatology 1990; 12(4 Pt 1):747–752.
57. Jamagin WR, Fong Y, DeMatteo RP, et al. Staging, resectability, and outcome in 225 patients with hilar cholangiocarcinoma. Ann Surg 2001; 234(4):507–517; discussion 517–519.
58. Bismuth H, Nakache R, Diamond T. Management strategies in resection for hilar cholangiocarcinoma. Ann Surg 1992; 215(1):31–38.

59. Nimura Y, Karniya J, Kondo Sn, Nagino M, Kanai M. Technique of inserting multiple biliary drains and management. Hepatogastroenterology 1995; 42(4):323–331.
60. Nimura Y, Kamiya J, Kondo S, et al. Aggressive preoperative management and extended surgery for hilar cholangiocarcinoma: Nagoya experience. J Hepatobiliary Pancreat Surg 2000; 7(2): 155–162.
61. Kondo S, Hirano S, Ambo Y, et al. Forty consecutive resections of hilar cholangiocarcinoma with no postoperative mortality and no positive ductal margins: results of a prospective study. Ann Surg 2004; 240(1):95–101.
62. Klempnauer J, Kridder GJ, Wemer M, Weimann A, Pichlmayr R. What constitutes long-term survival after surgery for hilar cholangiocarcinoma? Cancer 1997; 79(1):26–34.
63. Pichlmayr R, Weimahn A, Klempnauer J, et al. Surgical treatment in proximal bile duct cancer. A single-center experience. Ann Surg 1996; 224(5):628–638.
64. Iwatsuki S, Todo S, Marsh JW, et al. Treatment of hilar cholangiocarcinoma (Klatskin tumors) with hepatic resection or transplantation. J Am Coll Surg 1998; 187(4):358–364.
65. Heimbach JK, Haddock MG, Alberts SR, et al. Transplantation for hilar cholangiocarcinoma. Liver Transpl 2004; 10(10 suppl 2):S65–S68.
66. Lazaridis KN, Gores GJ. Cholangiocarcinoma. Gastroenterology 2005; 128(6):1655–1667.
67. Nimura Y, Hayakawa N, Kamiya J, Kondo S, Shionoya S. Hepatic segmentectomy with caudate lobe resection for bile duct carcinoma of the hepatic hilus. World J Surg 1990; 14(4):535–543; discussion 544.
68. Mizumoto R, Suzuki H. Surgical anatomy of the hepatic hilum with special reference to the caudate lobe. World J Surg 1988; 12(1):2–10.
69. Vollmer CM, Drebin JA, Middleton WD, et al. Utility of staging laparoscopy in subsets of peripancreatic and biliary malignancies. Ann Surg 2002; 235(1):1–7.
70. Weber SM, Dematteo RP, Fong Y, Blumgart LH, Jarnagin WR. Staging laparoscopy in patients with extrahepatic biliary carcinoma. Analysis of 100 patients. Ann Surg 2002; 235(3):392–399.
71. Kitagawa Y, Nagino M, Kamiya J, et al. Lymph node metastasis from hilar cholangiocarcinoma: audit of 110 patients who underwent regional and paraaortic node dissection. Ann Surg 2001; 233(3): 385–392.
72. Tojima Y, Nagino M, Ebata T, Uesaka K, Kamiya J, Nimura Y. Immunohistochemically demonstrated lymph node micrometastasis and prognosis in patients with otherwise node-negative hilar cholangiocarcinoma. Ann Surg 2003; 237(2):201–207.
73. Kluge R, Schmidt F, Caca K, et al. Positron emission tomography with [(18)F]fluoro-2-deoxy-D-glucose for diagnosis and staging of bile duct cancer. Hepatology 2001; 33(5):1029–1035.
74. Fritscher-Ravens A, Bohuslavizki KH, Broering DC, et al. FDG PET in the diagnosis of hilar cholangiocarcinoma. Nucl Med Commun 2001; 22(12):1277–1285.
75. Anderson CD, Rice MH, Pinson CW, Chapman WC, Chari RS, Delbeke D. Fluorodeoxyglucose PET imaging in the evaluation of gallbladder carcinoma and cholangiocarcinoma. J Gastrointest Surg 2004; 8(1):90–97.
76. Jarnagin WR, Blumgart LH, Saldinger P. Cancer of the bile ducts. In: Blumgart LH, Fong Y, eds. Surgery of the Liver and Biliary Tract. London: Saunders, 2000:1017.
77. Hadjis NS, Blenkham JI, Alexander N, Benjamin IS, Blugart LH. Outcome of radical surgery in hilar cholangiocarcinoma. Surgery 1990; 107(6): 597–604.
78. Baer HU, Stain SC, Dennison AR, Eggers B, Blumgart LH. Improvements in survival by aggressive resections of hilar cholangiocarcinoma. Ann Surg 1993; 217(1):20–27.
79. Kinoshita H, Sakai K, Hirohashi K, Igawa S, Yamasaki O, Kubo S. Preoperative portal vein embolization for hepatocellular carcinoma. World J Surg 1986; 10(5):803–808.
80. Makuuchi M, Thai BL, Takayasu K, et al. Preoperative portal embolization to increase safety of major hepatectomy for hilar bile duct carcinoma: a preliminary report. Surgery 1990; 107(5):521–527.
81. Cameron JL, Pitt HA, Zinner MJ, Kaufinan SL, Coleman J. Management of proximal cholangiocarcinomas by surgical resection and radiotherapy. Am J Surg 1990; 159(1):91–97; discussion 97–98.
82. Pitt HA, Nakeeb A, Abrams RA, et al. Perihilar cholangiocarcinoma. Postoperative radiotherapy does not improve survival. Ann Surg 1995; 221(6):788–797; discussion 797–798.
83. Kamada T, Saitou H, Takamura A, Nojima T, Okushiba SI. The role of radiotherapy in the management of extrahepatic bile duct cancer: an analysis of 145 consecutive patients treated with intraluminal and/or external beam radiotherapy. Int J Radiat Oncol Biol Phys 1996; 34(4):767–774.
84. McMasters KM, Tuttle TM, Leach SD, et al. Neoadjuvant chemoradiation for extrahepatic cholangiocarcinoma. Am J Surg 1997; 174(6):605–608; discussion 608–609.
85. Takada T, Amano H, Yasuda H, et al. Is postoperative adjuvant chemotherapy useful for gallbladder carcinoma? A phase III multicenter prospective randomized controlled trial in patients with resected pancreaticobiliary carcinoma. Cancer 2002; 95(8):1685–1695.
86. Kuvshinoff BW, Armstrong JG, Fong Y, et al. Palliation of irresectable hilar cholangiocarcinoma with biliary drainage and radiotherapy. Br J Surg 1995; 82(11):1522–1525.
87. Liu CL, Lo CM, Lai EC, Fan ST. Endoscopic retrograde cholangiopancreatography and endoscopic endoprosthesis insertion in patients with Klatskin tumors. Arch Surg 1998; 133(3):293–296.

88. Becker CD, Glatttli A, Maibach R, Baer HU. Percutaneous palliation of malignant obstructive jaundice with the Wallstent endoprosthesis: follow-up and reintervention in patients with hilar and non-hilar obstruction. J Vasc Interv Radiol 1993; 4(5):597–604.
89. Cheung KL, Lai EC. Endoscopic stenting for malignant biliary obstruction. Arch Surg 1995; 130(2): 204–207.
90. Miyazaki M, Ito H, Nakagawa K, et al. Aggressive surgical approaches to hilar cholangiocarcinoma: hepatic or local resection? Surgery 1998; 123(2):131–136.
91. Schima E. Surgery of the biliary tract in geriatric patients (author's transl). Zentralbl Chir 1977; 102(14):858–868.
92. Glattli A, Stain SC, Baer HU, Schweizer W, Triller J, Blumgart LH. Unresectable malignant biliary obstruction: treatment by self-expandable biliary endoprostheses. HPB Surg 1993; 6(3):175–184.
93. Stoker J, Lameris JS. Complications of percutaneously inserted biliary Wallstents. J Vasc Interv Radiol 1993; 4(6):767–772.
94. Rossi P, Bezzi M, Rossi M, et al. Metallic stents in malignant biliary obstruction: results of a multicenter European study of 240 patients. J Vasc Interv Radiol 1994; 5(2):279–285.
95. Jamagin WR, Burke E, Powers C, Fong Y, Blumgart LH. Intrahepatic biliary enteric bypass provides effective palliation in selected patients with malignant obstruction at the hepatic duct confluence. Am J Surg 1998; 175(6):453–460.
96. Baer HU, Rhyner M, Stain SC, et al. The effect of communication between the right and left liver on the outcome of surgical drainage for jaundice due to malignant obstruction at the hilus of the liver. HPB Surg 1994; 8(1):27–31.
97. Bowling TE, Galbraith SM, Hatfield AR, Solano J, Spittle MF. A retrospective comparison of endoscopic stenting alone with stenting and radiotherapy in non-resectable cholangiocarcinoma. Gut 1996; 39(96):852–855.
98. Vallis KA, Banjamin IS, Munro AJ, et al. External beam and intraluminal radiotherapy for locally advanced bile duct cancer: role and tolerability. Radiother Oncol 1996; 41(1):61–66.
99. Ortner M. Photodynamic therapy for cholangiocarcinoma. J Hepatobiliary Pancreat Surg 2001; 8(2):137–139.
100. Ortner M. Photodynamic therapy in the biliary tract. Curr Gastroenterol Rep 2001; 3(2):154–159.
101. Glimelius B, Hoffman K, Sjoden PO, et al. Chemotherapy improves survival and quality of life in advanced pancreatic and biliary cancer. Ann Oncol 1996; 7(6):593–600.
102. Daines WP, Rajagopalan V, Grossbard ML, Kozuch P. Gallbladder and biliary tract carcinoma: a comprehensive update, Part 2. Oncology (Williston Park) 2004; 18(8):1049–1059; discussion 1060, 1065–1066, 1068.
103. Fong Y, Blumgart LH, Lin E, Fortner JG, Brennan MF. Outcome of treatment for distal bile duct cancer. Br J Surg 1996; 83(12):1712–1715.
104. Wade TP, Prasad CN, Virgo KS, Johnson FE. Experience with distal bile duct cancers in U.S. Veterans Affairs hospitals: 1987–1991. J Surg Oncol 1997; 64(3):242–245.
105. Yeo CJ, Cameron JL, Sohn TA, et al. Six hundred fifty consecutive pancreaticoduodenectomies in the 1990s: pathology, complications, and outcomes. Ann Surg 1997; 226(3):248–257; discussion 257–260.
106. Way LW. Biliary Tract. In: Way LW, ed. Current Surgical Diagnosis and Treatment. 10th ed. McGraw-Hill, 1994:537–566.
107. Jones BA, Langer B, Taylor BR, Girotti M. Periampullary tumors: which ones should be resected? Am J Surg 1985; 149(1):46–52.
108. Georgopoulos SK, Schwartz LH, Jamagin WR, et al. Comparison of magnetic resonance and endoscopic retrograde cholangiopancreatography in malignant pancreaticobiliary obstruction. Arch Surg 1999; 134(9):1002–1007.
109. Ryan ME. Cytologic brushings of ductal lesions during ERCP. Gastrointest Endosc 1991; 37(2):139–142.
110. van den Bosch RP, van der Schelling GP, Klinkenbijil JH, Mulder PG, van Blankenstein M, Jeekel J. Guidelines for the application of surgery and endoprostheses in the palliation of obstructive jaundice in advanced cancer of the pancreas. Ann Surg 1994; 219(1):18–24.
111. Patel T. Increasing incidence and mortality of primary intrahepatic cholangiocarcinoma in the United States. Hepatology 2001; 33(6):1353–1357.
112. Nakanuma Y, Terada T, Tanaka Y, Ohta G. Are hepatolithiasis and cholangiocarcinoma aetiologically related? A morphological study of 12 cases of hepatolithiasis associated with cholangiocarcinoma. Virchows Arch A Pathol Anat Histopathol 1985; 406(l):45–48.
113. Hirohashi K, Uenishi T, Kubo S, Yamamoto T, Tanaka H, Shuto T, Kinoshita H. Macroscopic types of intrahepatic cholangiocarekioma: clinicopathologic features and surgical outcomes. Hepatogastroenterol 2002; 49(44):326–329.
114. Weber SM, Jamagin WR, Klimstra D, DeMatteo RP, Fong Y, Blomgart LH. Intrahepatic cholangiocarcinoma: resectability, recurrence pattern, and outcomes. J Am Coll Surg 2001; 193(4):384–391.
115. Valverde A, Bonhomme N, Farges O, Sauvanet A, Flejou JF, Belghiti J. Resection of intrahepatic cholangiocarcinoma: a Western experience. J Hepatobiliary Pancreat Surg 1999; 6(2):122–127.
116. El Rassi ZE, Partensky C, Scoazec JY, Henry L, Lombard-Bohas C, Maddem G. Peripheral cholangiocarcinoma: presentation, diagnosis, pathology and management. Eur J Surg Oncol 1999; 25(4):375–380.

117. Schlinkert RT, Nagomey DM, Van Heerden JA, Adson MA. Intrahepatic cholangiocarcinoma: clinical aspects, pathology and treatment. HPB Surg 1992; 5(2):95–101; discussion 101–102.
118. Ringe B, Canelo R, Lorf T. Liver transplantation for primary liver cancer. Transplant Proc 1996; 28(3):1174–1175.
119. Casavilla FA, Marsh JW, Iwatsuki S, et al. Hepatic resection and transplantation for peripheral cholangiocarcinoma. J Am Coll Surg 1997; 185(5):429–436.
120. Falkson G, MacIntyre JM, Moertel CG. Eastern Cooperative Oncology Group experience with chemotherapy for inoperable gallbladder and bile duct cancer. Cancer 1984; 54(6):965–969.
121. Stillwagon GB, Order BE, Haulk T, et al. Variable low dose rate irradiation (131I-anti-CEA) and integrated low dose chemotherapy in the treatment of nonresectable primary intrahepatic cholangiocarcinoma. Int J Radiat Oncol Biol Phys 1991; 21(6):1601–1605.
122. Piehler JM, Crichlow RW. Primary carcinoma of the gallbladder. Surg Gynecol Obstet 1978; 147(6): 929–942.
123. Lazcano-Ponce EC, Miquel JF, Munoz N, et al. Epidemiology and molecular pathology of gallbladder cancer. CA Cancer J Clin 2001; 51(6):349–364.
124. Serra I, Diehl AK. Number and size of stones in patients with asymptomatic and symptomatic gallstones and gallbladder carcinoma. J Gastrointest Surg 2002; 6(2):272–273; author reply 273.
125. Kozuka S, Tsubone N, Yasui A, Hachisuka K. Relation of adenoma to carcinoma in the gallbladder. Cancer 1982; 50(10):2226–2234.
126. Fong Y, Malhotra S. Gallbladder cancer: recent advances and current guidelines for surgical therapy. Adv Surg 2001; 35:1–20.
127. Yang HL, Sun YG, Wang Z. Polypoid lesions of the gallbladder: diagnosis and indications for surgery. Br J Surg 1992; 79(3):227–229.
128. Yeh CN, Jan YY, Chao TC, Chen MF. Laparoscopic cholecystectomy for polypoid lesions of the gallbladder: a clinicopathologic study. Surg Laparosc Endosc Percutan Tech 2001; 11(3):176–181.
129. Buckles DC, Lindor KD, Larusso NF, Petrovic LM, Gores GJ. In primary sclerosing cholangitis, gallbladder polyps are frequently malignant. Am J Gastroenterol 2002; 97(5):1138–1142.
130. Stephen AE, Berger DL. Carcinoma in the porcelain gallbladder: a relationship revisited. Surgery 2001; 129(6):699–703.
131. Kwon AH, Inui H, Matsui Y, Uchida Y, Hukui J, Kamiyama Y. Laparoscopic cholecystectomy in patients with porcelain gallbladder based on the preoperative ultrasound findings. Hepatogastroenterology 2004; 51(58):950–953.
132. Henson DE, Albores-Saavedra J, Corle D. Carcinoma of the gallbladder. Histologic types, stage of disease, grade, and survival rates. Cancer 1992; 70(6):1493–1497.
133. Hawkins WG, DeMatieo RP, Jamagin WR, Ben-Porat L, Blumgart LH, Fong Y. Jaundice predicts advanced disease and early mortality in patients with gallbladder cancer. Ann Surg Oncol 2004; 11(3):310–315.
134. Adson M. In: Moody F, ed. Advances in Diagnosis and Surgical Treatment of Biliary Tract Disease. Chicago: Year Book, 1983.
135. Bartlett DL, Fong Y, Fortner JG, Brennan MF, Blumgart LH. Long-term results after resection for gallbladder cancer. Implications for staging and management. Ann Surg 1996; 224(5):639–646.
136. Cubertafond P, Gainant A, Cucchiaro G. Surgical treatment of 724 carcinomas of the gallbladder. Results of the French Surgical Association Survey. Ann Surg 1994; 219(3):275–280.
137. Nakamura S, Sakaguchi S, Suzuki S, Muro H. Aggressive surgery for carcinoma of the gallbladder. Surgery 1989; 106(3):467–473.
138. Shirai Y, Yoshida K, Tsukada K, Muto T, Watanabe H. Radical surgery for gallbladder carcinoma. Long-term results. Ann Surg 1992; 216(5):565–568.
139. Donohue JH, Nagorney DM, Grant CS, Tsushima K, Ilstrup DM, Adson MA. Carcinoma of the gallbladder. Does radical resection improve outcome? Arch Surg 1990; 125(2):237–241.
140. Chijiiwa K, Tanaka M. Carcinoma of the gallbladder: an appraisal of surgical resection. Surgery 1994; 115(6):751–756.
141. Onoyama H, Yamamoto M, Tseng A, Ajiki T, Saitoh Y. Extended cholecystectomy for carcinoma of the gallbladder. World J Surg 1995; 19(5):758–763.
142. Dixon E, Vollmer CM Jr, Sahajpal A, et al. An aggressive surgical approach leads to improved survival in patients with gallbladder cancer: a 12-year study at a North American Center. Ann Surg 2005; 241(3):385–394.
143. Fong Y, Jarnagin W, Blumgart LH. Gallbladder cancer: comparison of patients presenting initially for definitive operation with those presenting after prior noncurative intervention. Ann Surg 2000; 232(4):557–569.
144. Shirai Y, Yoshida K,Tsukada K, Muto T. Inapparent carcinoma of the gallbladder. An appraisal of a radical second operation after simple cholecystectomy. Ann Surg 1992; 215(4):326–331.
145. Yamaguchi K, Tsuneyoshi M. Subclinical gallbladder carcinoma. Am J Surg 1992; 163(4):382–386.
146. Kimura W, Shimada H. A case of gallbladder carcinoma with infiltration into the muscular layer that resulted in relapse and death from metastasis to the liver and lymph nodes. Hepatogastroenterology 1990; 37(1):86–89.

147. de Aretxabala XA, Roa IS, Burgos LA, Araya JC, Villaseca MA, Silva JA. Curative resection in potentially resectable tumours of the gallbladder. Eur J Surg 1997; 163(6):419–426.
148. Fong Y, Brennan MF, Turnbull A, Colt DG, Blumgart LH. Gallbladder cancer discovered during laparoscopic surgery. Potential for iatrogenic tumor dissemination. Arch Surg 1993; 128(9): 1054–1056.
149. Jamagin WR, Ruo L, Little SA, et al. Patterns of initial disease recurrence after resection of gallbladder carcinoma and hilar cholangiocarcinoma: implications for adjuvant therapeutic strategies. Cancer 2003; 98(8):1689–1700.
150. Shoup M, Fong Y. Surgical indications and extent of resection in gallbladder cancer. Surg Oncol Clin N Am 2002; 11(4):985–994.
151. Kresl JJ, Schild SE, Henning GT, et al. Adjuvant external beam radiation therapy with concurrent chemotherapy in the management of gallbladder carcinoma. Int J Radiat Oncol Biol Phys 2002; 52(1):167–175.
152. Mahe M, Stampfli C, Romestaing P, Salerno N, Gerard JP. Primary carcinoma of the gall-bladder: potential for external radiation therapy. Radiother Oncol 1994; 33(3):204–208.
153. Kapoor VK, Pradeep R, Haribhakti SP, et al. Intrahepatic segment III cholangiojejunostomy in advanced carcinoma of the gallbladder. Br J Surg 1996; 83(12):1709–1711.

24 Bile Duct and Gallbladder Cancer: Chemotherapy and Radiotherapy

Michel Ducreux
Gastrointestinal Tract Oncology Service, Gustave Roussy Institute and Medical Oncology Service, Paul Brousse Hospital, Villejuif, France

Valérie Boige and David Malka
Gastrointestinal Tract Oncology Service, Gustave Roussy Institute, Villejuif, France

Biliary tract neoplasms account for 1% to 2% of all cases of cancer, with only approximately 7000 cases presenting in the United States annually. They include intrahepatic, perihilar, and distal cholangiocarcinomas (~20–25%, 50–60%, and 20–25% of cases, respectively), and gallbladder carcinomas, the more common of the two types (1). More than 95% of cases are adenocarcinomas, often well-differentiated and mucin-producing, with lymph node metastases, peritoneal and distant metastases, and multifocal or diffuse involvement of the biliary tree in 50%, 10% to 20%, and 5% of all patients at presentation, respectively (1,2). Poor prognosis and difficulties with clinical management are due to frequent late-stage diagnosis, advanced age at presentation [two-thirds of all cases occurring in patients older than 65 years (1,3)], the low diagnostic yield of biliary cytology, the technical demands of radical surgery (usually requiring hepatectomy or pancreaticoduodenectomy), and the lack of standard neoadjuvant, adjuvant, and palliative chemo-/radiotherapy. However, advances in imaging now allow for earlier diagnosis of biliary tract neoplasms and better surgical or palliative biliary stent planning, and newer combination chemotherapy regimens may improve patients' survival and quality-of-life.

WHAT IS THE EVIDENCE THAT ADJUVANT CHEMOTHERAPY INFLUENCES SURVIVAL FOLLOWING AN COMPLETE RESECTION OF CANCERS OF THE BILIARY TRACT?

Complete Resection

Complete resection is the only potentially curative therapy for all types of biliary tract neoplasms. Although reported five-year survival rates for intrahepatic and distal cholangiocarcinomas are generally better than those for perihilar cholangiocarcinomas [30–40, 20–30, and 9–18%, respectively (1,2)] stage-adjusted, five-year survival rates are seemingly comparable. Hepatic and/or portal vein resection are often needed; however, five-year survival rates drop if there is macroscopic (but not microscopic) vascular invasion, as recently pointed out in two retrospective series of patients with hilar cholangiocarcinoma (evidence level 4) (4,5).

Long-term survival is possible in early-stage gallbladder carcinomas. Tis and T1a gallbladder cancers can be treated with simple cholecystectomy only. However, in T stages 1b and beyond, agressive surgery (extended cholecystectomy) is important in improving the long-term prognosis (6,7).

An analysis of patterns of initial disease recurrence after resection in 177 patients with gallbladder carcinoma or hilar cholangiocarcinoma has shown that recurrent gallbladder carcinoma is much more likely than recurrent hilar cholangiocarcinoma to involve a distant site (evidence level 1b) (8). Gallbladder carcinoma was also associated with a much shorter time to recurrence and a shorter survival period after recurrence. These significant differences in clinical behavior should be considered for the determination of best adjuvant strategies in these patients.

Neoadjuvant Treatments

Given the small size of available studies and lack of randomized trials, there is no proven role for either adjuvant chemotherapy or external beam radiation therapy (EBRT), or both, either before or after complete resection of biliary tract neoplasms (1). However, postoperative EBRT in the range of 45 to 60 Gy (with the latter doses for positive margins), with or without systemic chemotherapy, is commonly administered, particularly in case of positive margins or metastases to lymph nodes. Indeed, surgery followed by adjuvant EBRT may be better than either surgery or EBRT alone in patients with extrahepatic cholangiocarcinomas, as suggested by a recent study of 118 patients (9). However, these results have not been supported by other studies emphasizing the urgent need of prospective randomized trial (10,11) (evidence level 4; all studies).

The benefit of a boost of intraluminal brachytherapy (ILB) also remains controversial (1). Gerhards et al. recently showed, in a retrospective study of 91 patients with resected hilar cholangiocarcinoma, that although overall median survival after treatment with adjuvant EBRT was longer than after resection alone (24 vs. 8 months, respectively), there was no significant benefit from the addition of ILB, which was associated with a significantly higher rate of cholangitis and bile leakage (12). In contrast, in the selected population of patients with microscopic tumor residue after surgical excision of Klatskin tumor, Todoroki et al. have shown that intraoperative radiotherapy combined with postoperative radiotherapy could improve the five-year survival rate to 34% versus 13% for the group of patients treated with resection alone (evidence level 4) (13).

Controversial results have also been reported in adjuvant therapy of gallbladder carcinoma. It did not have a significant effect on survival in a recent series of 42 patients who underwent extended resections for gallbladder cancer (14), a finding at variance from a (somewhat controversial) recent randomized trial assessing the efficacy of adjuvant chemotherapy with mitomycin C and 5-flourouracil (FU) in 508 patients with resected biliary or pancreatic cancer, which showed a better overall (26% vs. 14%; $P = 0.037$) and disease-free five-year survival (20% vs. 12%; $P = 0.02$) in the 140 patients with gallbladder carcinoma (evidence level 2b) (15). A more recent small retrospective study has given arguments in favor of radiochemotherapy with 37% and 33% of overall and disease-free survival, respectively in 22 patients with resected gallbladder carcinoma. These patients were treated with a rather homogeneous adjuvant treatment combining radiotherapy and concomitant 5-FU. However, the small number of patients included prevents any firm conclusion (evidence level 4) (16).

In ampullary carcinomas, a series has evaluated the efficacy of adjuvant radiochemotherapy (50 Gy + 5-FU) in 113 patients. Adjuvant radiochemotherapy did not improve the long-term survival (five-year survival rate 38% vs. 28%, NS) or decrease recurrence rate in patients with ampullary cancers who had undergone pancreatico-duodenectomy (6).

Adjuvant hepatic arterial chemotherapy with 5-FU has been given to 18 out of 37 patients after curative resection of biliary cancer. Nine of these 18 patients had bile duct cancer, seven had gallbladder cancer, and two had cancer of the papilla of Vater. The group of patients receiving hepatic arterial chemotherapy was well balanced with the group treated with surgery alone; the one-year survival rate was 76% in the adjuvant chemotherapy group versus 53% in the nonadjuvant chemotherapy group while the three-year survival rates were 48% and 40%, respectively ($P = 0.048$) (evidence level 2c) (17).

Photodynamic therapy (PDT) has shown interesting results in palliative treatment (see next). Some data are already available for this treatment in adjuvant setting: five patients with extrahepatic cholangiocarcinoma, two with intrahepatic disease, and one with ampullary carcinoma. Cancer cells were microscopically detected in the stump of the hepatic duct in six patients, and biliary stenosis caused by remnant tumor was observed in one patient; one patient had tumor recurrence with occlusion of the bile duct. In patients who underwent PDT for the stump, one patient had distant metastasis at 31 months and four patients did not show tumor recurrence. One patient died of an unrelated cause; the two patients with occlusion caused by tumor growth showed reocclusion at 20 and 8 months after initial successful result (18).

PDT could also be used as a neodadjuvant treatment. Seven patients with advanced proximal bile duct carcinoma were evaluated. Patients were treated with PDT at the area of infiltration and 2 cm beyond and underwent surgery after a median period of six weeks (range 3–44 weeks). In all patients, R0 resection was achieved, no viable tumor cells were found in the inner 4-mm layer of the surgical specimens. The PDT-pretreated epithelium of the tumor-free proximal resection margins exhibited only minimal inflammatory infiltration. The one-year recurrence-free survival rate was 83% (19).

Very aggressive neoadjuvant therapeutic approaches have been described, particularly in combination with liver transplantation. Seventeen patients were included in a study of brachytherapy with 60 Gy + 5-FU until transplantation. Eleven patients underwent transplantation at a median of 3.4 months (range 1–26) after diagnosis. Five of these patients (45%) are alive without evidence of tumor recurrence with a median follow-up of 7.5 years (range: 2.8–14.5) (evidence level 2b) (20). A study from the Mayo Clinic treated 38 patients with unresectable stage I/II perihilar cholangiocarcinoma and negative staging laparotomy with external beam irradiation, systemic 5-FU, and ILB plus oral capecitabine before liver transplantation. Of note, more than a third of the originally recruited patients ($n = 71$) were shown at staging laparotomy to have previously undetected regional lymphadenopathy, local disease extension, or perihilar implants and did not undergo transplantation. Of the 38 receiving a liver transplant, three died from surgical complications and five developed recurrent cholangiocarcinoma 22 to 64 months later. Overall five-year survival rate was 82% which is comparable to overall results of liver transplantation across the United States and was better than surgical resection survival rate which was 21% (21). Survival for all 71 patients enrolled in the transplant protocol was 79%, 61%, and 58% at one, three, and five years after enrolment in the protocol, respectively (evidence level 2b).

DOES CHEMOTHERAPY OR CHEMORADIOTHERAPY IMPROVE QUALITY-OF-LIFE IN PATIENTS WITH UNRESECTABLE CHOLANGIOCARCINOMA?

Chemotherapy

Systemic chemotherapy has not been clearly proven to prolong survival significantly in patients with unresectable biliary tract neoplasms (1). However, one small randomized study (22) has indicated that 5-FU, when compared to best supportive care, can add to both quantity and quality-of-life in advanced pancreatic and biliary cancer. Ninety-three patients were included in the study, but only 37 had biliary tract disease. In this subgroup of patients, overall survival was clearly superior in the treated group (six months vs. 2.5 months; evidence level 1b): this was significant in the study as a whole, but not in the biliary subgroup, probably because of lack of power due to small numbers. Many different chemotherapeutic regimens have been investigated in small, mostly uncontrolled studies, with generally poor results. Reported response rates for most single-agent regimens (e.g., 5-FU, mitomycin C, cisplatin, nitrosoureas, etoposide, methotrexate, adriamycin, irinotecan, and paclitaxel) did not consistently exceed 10% to 20% (Table 1) (1,23). Even when newer drugs are considered, results remain poor. Two phase II trials of tegafur-uracil plus leucovorin in 13 and 14 evaluable patients with advanced biliary tract neoplasms showed no objective tumor response (24,25). Two phase II trials of weekly irinotecan monotherapy in 25 and 36 evaluable patients with advanced biliary tract carcinomas, respectively showed a disappointing response rate of 8% (26,27). Raltitrexed showed very limited benefit in 41 patients with less than 7% of objective response rate (28).

TABLE 1 Response to Chemotherapy in Metastatic Cholangiocarcinoma. Heterogeneous Results When Using Recent Combination Therapy Schedules

Treatment	*n*	Percent OR	Progression-free survival months	Overall survival months
Gemcitabine + capecitabine (42)				
Gallbladder carcinoma	22	28	4.4	6.6
Other cholangiocarcinomas	23	34	9.0	19.0
Gemcitabine + oxaliplatin (41)				
Gallbladder carcinoma	25	4	1.8	6.2
Other cholangiocarcinomas	35	21	3.8	11.2
Capecitabine + oxaliplatin (53)				
Gallbladder carcinoma	27	23	—	12.8
Intrahepatic cholangiocarcinomas	18	0	—	5.8
Other cholangiocarcinomas	20	20	—	12.8

Abbreviation: OR, objective response.

Reported response rates of combination schedules are not very much better, except perhaps for infusional 5-FU–leucovorin–cisplatin combinations, with reported response rates of 19 (29) to 30% (30), however at the expense of increased toxicity. This increase in toxicity was clearly demonstrated in a randomized trial of European Organisation for Research and Treatment of Cancer (EORTC) with high-dose infusional 5-FU in one arm ($n = 27$ patients) and high-dose infusional 5-FU and leucovorin and cisplatin in the other arm ($n = 26$ patients). Overall response rate was 7% in the arm with 5-FU alone and 19% in the combined arm. However, there was one toxic death is this arm confirming that cisplatin in combination with 5-FU and leucovorin has a higher activity than 5-FU alone but is more toxic (31). A phase II trial of combined 5-FU, leucovorin, and oxaliplatin in 16 patients with advanced biliary tract adenocarcinomas showed a disease control rate of 56% and a median overall survival of 9.5 months (32,33). However, capecitabine-based combinations with cisplatin or oxaliplatin have given rather encouraging results with 21% and 23% response rates, respectively (33,34).

Extrapolating results obtained in pancreatic carcinoma, gemcitabine has been evaluated in different phase II trials, with a favorable toxicity profile, response rates of 8% to 60%, and overall survival times from 6.3 to 16.0 months (23). Possible options currently being investigated to further improve these results include modifications of the dose regimen (in particular, fixed dose rate infusion) as well as combinations with other potentially synergistic anticancer drugs (23). The combination of gemcitabine and irinotecan has given encouraging results in a very small phase II trial in 14 patients, with two objective responses (14%) (35). The combination of gemcitabine plus capecitabine has given interesting response rates of 24% in 16 patients with gallbladder carcinoma and 36% in 19 with cholangiocarcinoma (36). After these promising initial results, the same combination of gemcitabine plus cisplatin has recently given a somewhat disappointing response rate of 21% in a phase II trial of 42 patients, but an encouraging median overall survival exceeding nine months (34,37).

These results have been confirmed in a recent British randomized study: patients were randomized to receive either gemcitabine as a monotherapy or gemcitabine plus cisplatin. Eighty-six patients were included with metastatic or locally advanced diseases (38). Around 25% of the patients had gallbladder carcinoma in each arm. Severe lethargy was more frequently observed in the group of patients receiving gemcitabine plus cisplatin (29% vs. 9%). Seventy-six percent of tumor growth control was observed when combination therapy was given versus 58% with gemcitabine alone (evidence level 1b). Time to progression was also increased to eight months versus four months. An objective response rate of 27.5% has been previously observed with the same combination in a single-arm phase II trial including 40 assessable patients (I gallbladder carcinoma, 39 cholangiocarcinomas) (39).

However, the need for hyperhydration to prevent cisplatin nephrotoxicity and subsequent impairment of quality-of-life limits the use of this combination. At variance from cisplatin, oxaliplatin abrogates the need for such hyperhydration, has a more favorable safety profile, and can be administered to patients with hepatic dysfunction. In combination with gemcitabine, oxaliplatin has given very encouraging results in a phase II trial of 33 patients, with a response rate of 35%, and a remarkably long overall survival of 14.3 months (evidence level 2b) (40). An European multicentric evaluation of the same regimen has given less encouraging results with 12% of response in 70 patients (41).

Hepatic arterial chemotherapy is theoretically an attractive approach in patients with biliary tract neoplasms, as the biliary tree depends predominantly on the hepatic artery for its blood supply. However, high response rates (up to 44%) reported in the few short studies available are counterbalanced by short median survival times and durations of response, and because of the patterns of relapse, this approach is unlikely to replace systemic chemotherapy entirely (1).

Regarding results of recent phase II trials, it seems that gallbladder carcinomas and cholangiocarcinomas have different sensitivities to various drugs of chemotherapy. (Figs 1–3) Combination therapy with gemcitabine and capecitabine was more active in cholangiocarcinomas than in gallbladder tumors: 19 months of overall survival versus 6.6 months (42). The same was observed with combination of gemcitabine and oxaliplatin which gave 6.2 months of overall survival in 25 patients with gallbladder carcinoma, versus 11.2 months in 35 patients with other cholangiocarcinomas (41). On the other hand, combination chemotherapy with

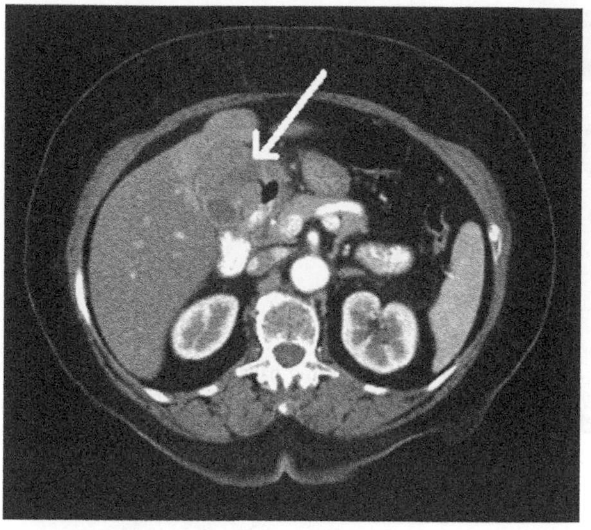

FIGURE 1 Gallbladder tumor with major heterogeneous thickening of the wall of gallbladder (*white arrow*).

capecitabine and oxaliplatin has given opposite results with 27% of objective response and 12.8 months of overall survival in 27 patients with gallbladder carcinoma, versus 0% of objective response and 5.8 months of overall survival in 18 patients with intrahepatic cholangiocarcinoma. Efficacy in extrahepatic cholangiocarcinoma was similar to that observed in gallbladder tumors. An innovative approach using percutaneous transhepatic biliary drainage tube coated with carboplatin has been evaluated. Five patients have been treated with these tubes for four months. Overall efficacy rate was 60%, but no confirmatory data have been published (43).

RADIOTHERAPY

To date, no randomized, controlled, trial study has clearly demonstrated long-term survival benefit for EBRT with or without ILB, or chemoradiation, over biliary drainage in patients with biliary tract neoplasms (1). A recent retrospective study showed that the combination of EBRT and ILB in 93 patients with unresectable extrahepatic bile duct carcinoma resulted in a median survival of 12 months, at the expense of mild-to-severe gastroduodenal complications in 32 patients (34%) (44). In another retrospective study, median time to tumor recurrence (nine months vs. five months; $P = 0.06$) and two-year survival rate (0% vs. 21%; $P = 0.015$) was significantly better with EBRT and ILB than with EBRT alone, without enhancement in treatment

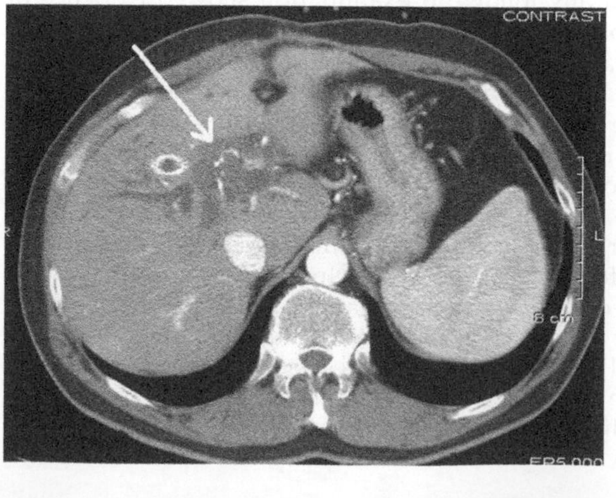

FIGURE 2 Hilar cholangiocarcinoma (Klatskin tumor) with infiltrative aspect of the hilar region and stent in the right part of the biliary tree (*white arrow*).

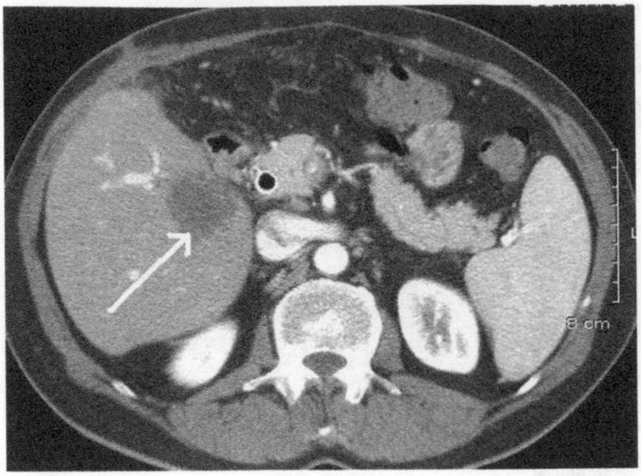

FIGURE 3 Same patient as in Figure 2 showing stent in the main bile duct and right liver metastasis (*white arrow*).

morbidity; however, no statistically significant difference was found in the recurrence rates between those who did and did not receive ILB (45) (evidence level 4).

A homogeneous systematic approach with metallic stent implantation followed by ILB was evaluated in 32 patients with various biliary malignancies. Mean survival was 457, 237, and 850 days in patients with Klatskin's tumor, gallbladder carcinoma, and carcinoma of the papilla of Vater, respectively. ILB appears to prolong survival in inoperable patients with Klatskin's tumor and carcinoma of the papilla compared with nontreated patients in previous studies. In contrast, no similar effect was noted in patients with gallbladder carcinoma (46) (evidence level 4).

PHOTODYNAMIC THERAPY

PDT involves the use of a nontoxic photosensitizer, which selectively accumulates in malignant tissue, and laser photoactivation to destroy malignant cells. Ortner et al. reported on the first randomized, controlled trial of biliary double stenting with and without Photofrin PDT in 39 patients with nonresectable, large (>3 cm diameter, ~80% tumor node metastases stage IV, bismuth type IV), proximal cholangiocarcinoma (47). Criteria of successful stenting had to be fulfilled before randomization, but successful biliary drainage (decrease in bilirubin levels >50% within one week) (Fig. 4) before randomization was obtained in only 21% of patients in both groups, as shown in earlier studies (48). Stent exchanges were performed every three months in both groups. PDT procedures necessitated initial stent removal, final insertion of a new set of endoprostheses, and confinement of patients in a darkened room for three to four days after injection. PDT was repeated if any follow-up examination showed evidence of residual tumor in the bile duct (70% of patients; mean number of PDT sessions, 2.4; range, 1–5). PDT resulted in improved biliary drainage (successful drainage, 72%), Karnofsky index ($P < 0.01$), and quality-of-life ($P < 0.001$), and prolongation of median survival (493 days vs. 98 days; relative hazard, 0.21 [confidence interval (CI), 0.12–0.35]; $P < 0.0001$, evidence level 1b). PDT was generally well tolerated (including mild, transient photosensitivity, 10% of patients), and burden of treatment was lower than with stenting alone ($P < 0.001$). Stenoses were seen in only two patients and were easily managed by further stenting. This trial was terminated prematurely because further randomization was deemed unethical. However, as patients successfully stented a month before screening were excluded, these results may be applicable only to those patients not helped by conventional biliary stenting, and the observed survival benefit may have been caused by relief of cholestasis rather than by tumor reduction. Indeed, patients in the PDT study arm did develop progressive disease and metastases, as previously reported (47). A recent phase II study in 24 patients with Bismuth type III/IV cholangiocarcinoma showed that the median survival after PDT was not statistically different significantly from a retrospectively analyzed historical control group of 20 patients treated

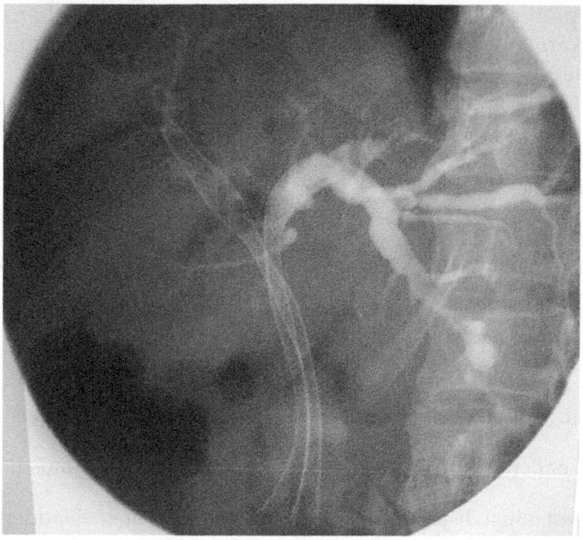

FIGURE 4 Bilateral stenting of hilar cholangiocarcinoma (metallic stents).

only with biliary drainage (9.9 months vs. 5.6 months; level 4 evidence) (49). Another phase II study investigated PDT as a neoadjuvant treatment in seven patients with advanced proximal bile duct carcinoma. In all patients, R0 resection was achieved. No viable tumor cells were found in the inner 4-mm layer of the surgical specimens. Biliary leakage did not occur, even though the bilio-enteric anastomoses were sewn to PDT-pretreated bile ducts. The one-year recurrence-free survival rate was 83% (19). A longer-term follow-up of an enlarged cohort of 23 patients showed less good results: median survival after treatment was 11.2 months for patients without distant metastases and 9.3 months for all patients. Four-year survival was less than 5% showing that although PDT appears effective for nonresectable hilar cholangiocarcinoma it does not prevent progression of the disease (50). In a recent randomized trial, 32 patients with nonresectable biliary duct carcinoma were treated with prostheses + PDT or with prostheses alone. The median survival after randomization was seven months for the control group and 21 months for the PDT group ($P = 0.0109$; evidence level 1b). However, four patients showed infectious complications after PDT versus one patient in the control group (51).

The assessment of the direct antitumor efficacy of PDT remains difficult due to the type of the tumor, which is essentially infiltrative. However, percutaneous transhepatic PDT was evaluated with monthly intraductal ultrasonography. At three months after PDT, the mean thickness of tumor mass had decreased from 8.7 ± 3.7 mm to 5.8 ± 2.0 mm ($P < 0.01$). At four months, the thickness of the mass had increased to 7.0 ± 3.7 mm. The median survival of the 24 patients was long: 19 ± 5.9 months (52).

CONCLUSION

Biliary, tract neoplasm remains a lethal malignancy. There are a few patients with resectable disease for which aggressive surgical resection should be considered. The high rate of distant metastases with this disease suggests that systemic chemotherapy could be useful. However, no standard adjuvant chemotherapy can be recommended at this moment. Improvements in the knowledge of pathogenesis of this disease, improvements in diagnostic tools, and surgical procedures suggest that a higher proportion of patients may be cured in the near future. In metastatic or locally advanced disease, gemcitabine-based chemotherapies could be used. Clear improvements are awaited from the development of targeted therapies using recently discovered knowledge of the pathogenetic pathways. Palliative radiotherapy may be suitable for patients with unresectable, locally advanced disease in the absence of distant metastases by contributing to biliary decompression and pain relief. Survival benefit is debatable, and there are no controlled studies. PDT has shown promising results, and recruitment to trials combining chemotherapy with PDT should be encouraged.

REFERENCES

1. Khan SA, Davidson BR, Goldin R, et al. Guidelines for the diagnosis and treatment of cholangiocarcinoma: consensus document. Gut 2002; 51(suppl 6):VI1–VI9.
2. Gores GJ. A spotlight on cholangiocarcinoma. Gastroenterology 2003; 125:1536–1538.
3. Michaud DS. The epidemiology of pancreatic, gallbladder, and other biliary tract cancers. Gastrointest Endosc 2002; 56:S195–S200.
4. Ebata T, Nagino M, Kamiya J, Uesaka K, Nagasaka T, Nimura Y. Hepatectomy with portal vein resection for hilar cholangiocarcinoma: audit of 52 consecutive cases. Ann Surg 2003; 238:720–727.
5. Uchiyama K, Nakai T, Tani M, et al. Indications for extended hepatectomy in the management of stage IV hilar cholangiocarcinoma. Arch Surg 2003; 138:1012–1016.
6. Sikora SS, Balachandran P, Dimri K, et al. Adjuvant chemoradiotherapy in ampullary cancers. Eur J Surg Oncol 2005; 31:158–163.
7. Sikora SS, Singh RK. Surgical strategies in patients with gallbladder cancer: nihilism to optimism. J Surg Oncol 2006; 93:670–681.
8. Jarnagin WR, Ruo L, Little SA, et al. Patterns of initial disease recurrence after resection of gallbladder carcinoma and hilar cholangiocarcinoma: implications for adjuvant therapeutic strategies. Cancer 2003; 98:1689–1700.
9. Heron DE, Stein DE, Eschelman DJ, et al. Cholangiocarcinoma: the impact of tumor location and treatment strategy on outcome. Am J Clin Oncol 2003; 26:422–428.
10. Gonzalez GD, Gouma DJ, Rauws EA, van Gulik TM, Bosma A, Koedooder C. Role of radiotherapy, in particular intraluminal brachytherapy, in the treatment of proximal bile duct carcinoma. Ann Oncol 1999; (10 suppl 4):215–220.
11. Pitt HA, Nakeeb A, Abrams RA, et al. Perihilar cholangiocarcinoma. Postoperative radiotherapy does not improve survival. Ann Surg 1995; 221:788–797.
12. Gerhards MF, van Gulik TM, Gonzalez GD, Rauws EA, Gouma DJ. Results of postoperative radiotherapy for resectable hilar cholangiocarcinoma. World J Surg 2003; 27:173–179.
13. Todoroki T, Ohara K, Kawamoto T, et al. Benefits of adjuvant radiotherapy after radical resection of locally advanced main hepatic duct carcinoma. Int J Radiat Oncol Biol Phys 2000; 46:581–587.
14. Behari A, Sikora SS, Wagholikar GD, Kumar A, Saxena R, Kapoor VK. Longterm survival after extended resections in patients with gallbladder cancer. J Am Coll Surg 2003; 196:82–88.
15. Takada T, Amano H, Yasuda H, et al. Is postoperative adjuvant chemotherapy useful for gallbladder carcinoma? A phase III multicenter prospective randomized controlled trial in patients with resected pancreaticobiliary carcinoma. Cancer 2002; 95:1685–1695.
16. Czito BG, Hurwitz HI, Clough RW, et al. Adjuvant external-beam radiotherapy with concurrent chemotherapy after resection of primary gallbladder carcinoma: a 23-year experience. Int J Radiat Oncol Biol Phys 2005; 62:1030–1034.
17. Takeda Y, Hasuike Y, Kashiwazaki M, Tsujinaka T. [Adjuvant arterial infusion chemotherapy for patients with biliary cancer]. Gan To Kagaku Ryoho 2004; 31:1835–1837.
18. Nanashima A, Yamaguchi H, Shibasaki S, et al. Adjuvant photodynamic therapy for bile duct carcinoma after surgery: a preliminary study. J Gastroenterol 2004; 39:1095–1101.
19. Wiedmann M, Caca K, Berr F, et al. Neoadjuvant photodynamic therapy as a new approach to treating hilar cholangiocarcinoma: a phase II pilot study. Cancer 2003; 97:2783–2790.
20. Sudan D, DeRoover A, Chinnakotla S, et al. Radiochemotherapy and transplantation allow long-term survival for nonresectable hilar cholangiocarcinoma. Am J Transplant 2002; 2:774–779.
21. Rea DJ, Heimbach JK, Rosen CB, et al. Liver transplantation with neoadjuvant chemoradiation is more effective than resection for hilar cholangiocarcinoma. Ann Surg 2005; 242:451–458.
22. Glimelius B, Hoffman K, Sjöden PO, et al. Chemotherapy improves survival and quality-of-life in advanced pancreatic and biliary cancer. Ann Oncol 1996; 7:593–600.
23. Scheithauer W. Review of gemcitabine in biliary tract carcinoma. Semin Oncol 2002; 29:40–45.
24. Mani S, Sciortino D, Samuels B, et al. Phase II trial of uracil/tegafur (UFT) plus leucovorin in patients with advanced biliary carcinoma. Invest New Drugs 1999; 17:97–101.
25. Chen JS, Yang TS, Lin YC, Jan YY. A phase II trial of tegafur-uracil plus leucovorin (LV) in the treatment of advanced biliary tract carcinomas. Jpn J Clin Oncol 2003; 33:353–356.
26. Sanz-Altamira PM, O'Reilly E, Stuart KE, et al. A phase II trial of irinotecan (CPT-11) for unresectable biliary tree carcinoma. Ann Oncol 2001; 12:501–504.
27. Alberts SR, Fishkin PA, Burgart LJ, et al. CPT-11 for bile-duct and gallbladder carcinoma: a phase II North Central Cancer Treatment Group (NCCTG) study. Int J Gastrointest Cancer 2002; 32:107–114.
28. Francois E, Hebbar M, Bennouna J, et al. A phase II trial of raltitrexed (Tomudex) in advanced pancreatic and biliary carcinoma. Oncology 2005; 68:299–305.

29. Taieb J, Mitry E, Boige V, et al. Optimization of 5-fluorouracil (5-FU)/cisplatin combination chemotherapy with a new schedule of leucovorin, 5-FU and cisplatin (LV5FU2-P regimen) in patients with biliary tract carcinoma. Ann Oncol 2002; 13:1192–1196.
30. Ducreux M, Rougier P, Fandi A, et al. Effective treatment of advanced biliary tract carcinoma using 5-fluorouracil continuous infusion with cisplatin. Ann Oncol 1998; 9:653–656.
31. Ducreux M, Van Cutsem E, Van Laethem JL, et al. A randomised phase II trial of weekly high-dose 5-fluorouracil with and without folinic acid and cisplatin in patients with advanced biliary tract carcinoma: results of the 40955 EORTC trial. Eur J Cancer 2005; 41:398–403.
32. Nehls O, Klump B, Arkenau HT, et al. Oxaliplatin, fluorouracil and leucovorin for advanced biliary system adenocarcinomas: a prospective phase II trial. Br J Cancer 2002; 87:702–704.
33. Nehls O, Oettle H, Hartmann J-T, et al. Oxaliplatin plus capecitabin in advanced biliary system adenocarcinomas: a multicenter phase II trial. Proc Am Soc Clin Oncol 2003; 22:280.
34. Kim TW, Chang HM, Kang HJ, et al. Phase II study of capecitabine plus cisplatin as first-line chemotherapy in advanced biliary cancer. Ann Oncol 2003; 14:1115–1120.
35. Bhargava P, Jani CR, Savarese DM, O'Donnell JL, Stuart KE, Rocha Lima CM. Gemcitabine and irinotecan in locally advanced or metastatic biliary cancer: preliminary report. Oncology (Huntington) 2003; 17:23–26.
36. Knox JJ, Hedley D, Oza A, et al. Phase II trial of gemcitabine plus capecitabine (GemCap) in patients with advanced or metastatic adenocarcinoma of the biliary tract. Proc Am Soc Clin Oncol 2003; 22:317.
37. Kim IH, Lee DH, Yoo JG, et al. The effect of intraluminal radiotherapy after metallic stent insertion in the malignant biliary tract obstruction (MBTO). Gastroenterology 2000; 116:A438.
38. Valle JW, Wasan H, Johnson P, et al. Gemcitabine, alone or in combination with cisplatin, in patients with advanced or metastatic cholangiocarcinoma (CC) and other biliary tract tumors: a multicenter, randomized, phase II (the UK ABC-01) study. 2006 Gastrointestinal Cancers Symposium (abs 98).
39. Thongprasert S, Napapan S, Charoentum C, Moonprakan S. Phase II study of gemcitabine and cisplatin as first-line chemotherapy in inoperable biliary tract carcinoma. Ann Oncol 2005; 16:279–281.
40. Maindrault-Goebel F, Selle F, Rosmorduc O, et al. A phase II study of gemcitabine and oxaliplatin (GEMOX) in advanced biliary adenocarcinoma (ABA). Final results. Proc Am Soc Clin Oncol 2003; 22:293.
41. André T, Reyes-Vidal JM, Fartoux L, et al. EXIBIT: An international multicenter phase II trial of gemcitabine and oxaliplatin (GEMOX) in patients with advanced biliary tract carcinoma. Proc Am Soc Clin Oncol 2006; 24 (abs 4135).
42. Knox JJ, Hedley D, Oza A, et al. Combining gemcitabine and capecitabine in patients with advanced biliary cancer: a phase II trial. J Clin Oncol 2005; 23:2332–2338.
43. Mezawa S, Homma H, Sato T, et al. A study of carboplatin-coated tube for the unresectable cholangiocarcinoma. Hepatology 2000; 32:916–923.
44. Takamura A, Saito H, Kamada T, et al. Intraluminal low-dose-rate 192Ir brachytherapy combined with external beam radiotherapy and biliary stenting for unresectable extrahepatic bile duct carcinoma. Int J Radiat Oncol Biol Phys 2003; 57:1357–1365.
45. Shin HS, Seong J, Kim WC, et al. Combination of external beam irradiation and high-dose-rate intraluminal brachytherapy for inoperable carcinoma of the extrahepatic bile ducts. Int J Radiat Oncol Biol Phys 2003; 57:105–112.
46. Bruha R, Petrtyl J, Kubecova M, et al. Intraluminal brachytherapy and selfexpandable stents in nonresectable biliary malignancies—the question of long-term palliation. Hepatogastroenterology 2001; 48:631–637.
47. Ortner ME, Caca K, Berr F, et al. Successful photodynamic therapy for nonresectable cholangiocarcinoma: a randomized prospective study. Gastroenterology 2003; 125:1355–1363.
48. Ducreux M, Liguory C, Lefebvre JF, et al. Management of malignant hilar biliary obstruction by endoscopy. Results and prognostic factors. Dig Dis Sci 1992; 37:778–783.
49. Dumoulin FL, Gerhardt T, Fuchs S, et al. Phase II study of photodynamic therapy and metal stent as palliative treatment for nonresectable hilar cholangiocarcinoma. Gastrointest Endosc 2003; 57: 860–867.
50. Wiedmann M, Berr F, Schiefke I, et al. Photodynamic therapy in patients with non-resectable hilar cholangiocarcinoma: 5-year follow-up of a prospective phase II study. Gastrointest Endosc 2004; 60:68–75.
51. Zoepf T, Jakobs R, Arnold JC, Apel D, Riemann JF. Palliation of nonresectable bile duct cancer: improved survival after photodynamic therapy. Am J Gastroenterol 2005; 100:2426–2430.
52. Shim CS, Cheon YK, Cha SW, et al. Prospective study of the effectiveness of percutaneous transhepatic photodynamic therapy for advanced bile duct cancer and the role of intraductal ultrasonography in response assessment. Endoscopy 2005; 37:425–433.
53. Nehls O, Oettle H, Hartmann J, et al. A prospective multicenter phase II trial of capecitabine plus oxaliplatin (CapOx) in advanced biliary system adenocarcinomas: the final results. Proc Am Soc Clin Oncol 2006; 24 [abs 4136].

25 Surgical Management of Hepatocellular Carcinoma

Norihiro Kokudo and Masatoshi Makuuchi
Hepatobiliary Pancreatic Surgery Division, Department of Surgery, University of Tokyo, Tokyo, Japan

This chapter provides an overview of recent findings on liver resection and liver transplantation for hepatocellular carcinoma (HCC). Surgery remains the only curative measure for HCC. Owing to recent progress in patient selection and perioperative care, both the short- and long-term outcomes of HCC patients have been dramatically improved. This review is based on the result of a literature search, which was systematically done to create clinical practice guidelines for hepatocellular carcinoma, the first evidence-based guidelines from Japan (1,2). Search strategies are documented in the appendix. The quality of available evidence was evaluated according to the classification of evidence created by the Centre for Evidence-Based Medicine at Oxford (3).

INDICATIONS FOR LIVER RESECTION IN HEPATOCELLULAR CARCINOMA PATIENTS

According to the 16th nationwide survey on HCC in Japan, a total of 19,920 new patients with HCC were registered between 2000 and 2001 (4) (evidence Level 2b). Of these patients, 5374 cases (27.0%) underwent hepatic resection, with an operative mortality rate of 0.9% (48/5374). This very low mortality rate can be largely attributed to recent progress in liver surgery, including careful patient selection and the adoption of safety criteria for determining the extent of the required hepatic resection.

The Child-Turcotte classification system was initially proposed for the prediction of patient outcome after undergoing a portocaval shunt; this system consists of a simple method for grading liver function and has been the gold standard for the assessment of liver function for almost four decades. The system was first published in 1964 (5) and was modified by Dr. Pugh in 1973 (6). For this reason, the Child-Turcotte classification system is also known as the Child-Pugh classification system. This scoring system includes five simple parameters: the presence or absence of encephalopathy and/or ascites, the serum total bilirubin level, the serum albumin level, and the prothrombin time. Although simple, this classification is quite useful for grading the severity of liver damage in cirrhotic patients. Generally, noncirrhotic patients and cirrhotic patients with Child-Pugh A liver function are considered candidates for hepatic resection (7). However, the safety limit for the extent of hepatic resection cannot be determined using this classification.

In 1993, Makuuchi et al. (8) proposed a surgical algorithm to solve the above problem (Fig. 1). The algorithm has only three parameters: the presence or absence of ascites, the serum total bilirubin level, and the indocyanine green (ICG) retention rate at 15 minutes. The extent of liver resection regarded as safe is shown at the bottom of the algorithm tree. The ICG test is one of the main parameters of this surgical decision tree, and most Japanese liver surgeons routinely perform this test prior to performing a liver resection. If one or more of the tumors can be removed by a hepatic resection within the safety limit indicated by this algorithm, the patient is considered operable. Use of this surgical algorithm has been shown to improve operative mortality and morbidity rates for the surgical treatment of HCC (9,10) (evidence Level 4). At the moment, the Makuuchi algorithm is the most popular algorithm for determining the extent of hepatic resections in Japan. However, the ICG test is not routinely performed in Western countries. In addition to the Child-Pugh score, some measure of portal pressure and the serum bilirubin level are usually used to select surgical candidates in Western countries (11).

Tumor number, size, and vascular invasion are the most important prognostic factors after liver resection (12,13). Patients with three or fewer HCC nodules are considered good

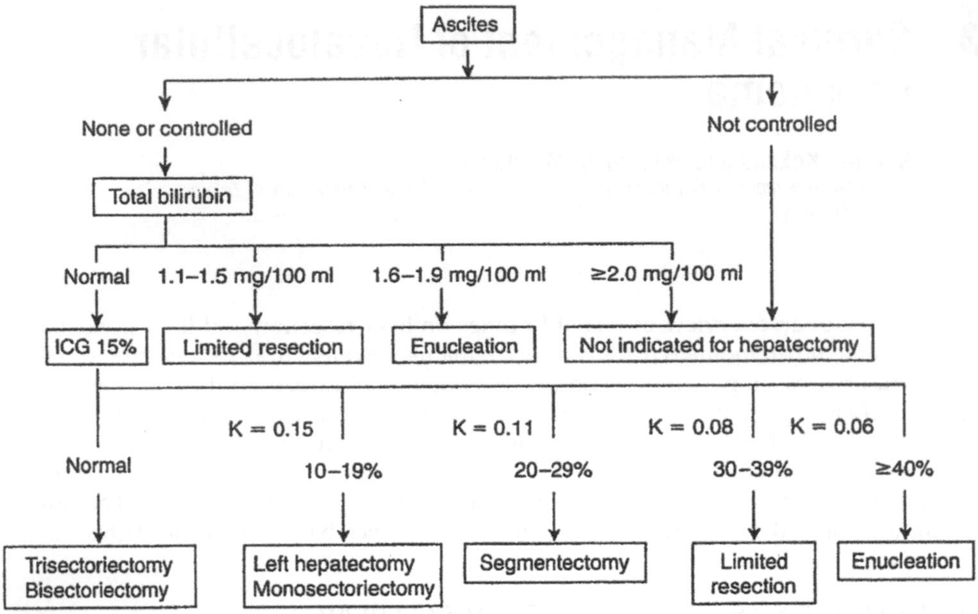

FIGURE 1 Decision tree for the selection of operative procedures in patients with hepatocellular carcinoma and liver cirrhosis. *Source*: From Ref. 8.

candidates for surgery. Although patients with large tumors (≥5 cm) often have an unfavorable outcome after resection, surgery provides the only chance for a cure.

Liver resection is sometimes attempted in patients with advanced disease. The prognosis of patients with HCC and a portal vein tumor thrombus is extremely poor (14). Chemotherapy or transarterial chemoembolization (TACE) have been used in patients with this condition, with unsatisfactory results (15,16). Minagawa et al. (17) proposed a combination of preoperative TACE and liver resection and reported a five-year survival rate of 42% (Fig. 2) (evidence Level 2b).

PREOPERATIVE IMAGING FOR CURATIVE RESECTION OF HEPATOCELLULAR CARCINOMAMM

Recent progress in imaging techniques has facilitated the recognition of early HCC as a principal tumor in at-risk subjects who undergo regular medical check-ups for chronic viral hepatitis or cirrhosis (18). Both dynamic CT and dynamic MRI are highly sensitive methods that are useful for detecting hypervascular HCC (19,20). The recent development of multi-detector-row CT may further increase the sensitivity of this modality.

For patients with confirmed HCC who have been scheduled for liver resection, CT imaging after the hepatic intra-arterial injection of iodized oil (lipiodol CT) is routinely performed to check for intrahepatic metastasis (Fig. 3). Lipiodol CT is superior to helical biphasic CT for the

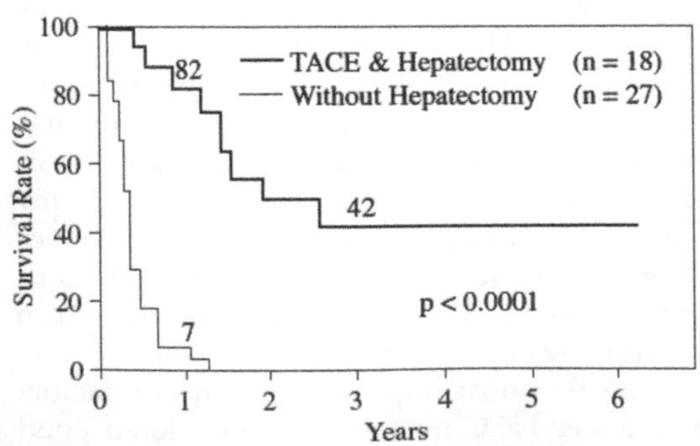

FIGURE 2 Overall survival of patients with hepatocellular carcinoma and gross portal vein tumor thrombus, grouped according to whether they underwent a hepatic resection. The difference in survival rates was statistically significant ($P < 0.0001$ for cirrhosis). *Abbreviation*: TACE, transarterial chemoembolization. *Source*: From Ref. 17.

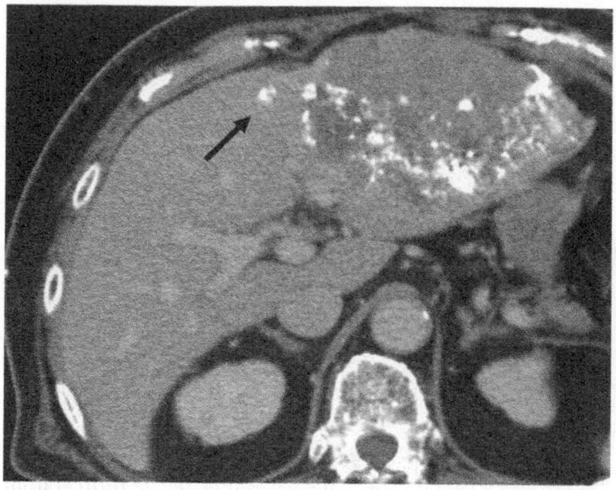

FIGURE 3 Intrahepatic metastasis in segment 4 (*arrow*) detected on a lipiodol-computed tomography image taken 2 weeks after the injection of lipiodol.

detection of small but moderately to poorly differentiated nodules (21) (evidence Level 2b). Intraoperative ultrasonography (IOUS) is also highly sensitive and should be routinely performed. It is not uncommon to detect new hepatic nodules using IOUS during a hepatic resection for HCC (22). IOUS is also sensitive in detecting vascular invasion, such as the presence of a tumor thrombus in the portal or hepatic veins (Fig. 4) (evidence Level 4).

The presence of extrahepatic lesions, including lung metastasis, bone metastasis, and lymph node metastasis, are generally contraindications for liver resection, and patients with advanced HCC should be examined for extrahepatic lesions prior to undergoing surgery. Full-body CT imaging is recommended to check for lung and lymph node metastases. When enlarged lymph nodes are visualized in the retropancreatic, diaphragmatic, or para-aortic regions, these lymph nodes should be biopsied before liver resection (Fig. 5).

The diagnostic accuracy of bone scintigraphy in patients with HCC has been questioned because bone scintigraphy has not been routinely performed in HCC patients with a low likelihood of bone metastasis. Maillefert et al. reported a bone-metastasis detection rate of 67% using ^{99m}Tc-MDP (methylene diphosphonate) scintigraphy and suggested that other agents taken up specifically by hepatocytes, like technetium 99m pyridoxyl-methyltryptophan (23) might also be useful. Lee et al. recently reported that ^{99m}Tc-MDP scintigraphy was highly sensitive in detecting bone metastasis in high-risk patients who were symptomatic or who had an elevated serum alpha-fetoprotein level (Fig. 6) (24) (evidence Level 4).

Preliminary reports have suggested that positron emission tomography (PET) is not useful for the detection of occult HCC in high-risk patients, such as those with hepatitis

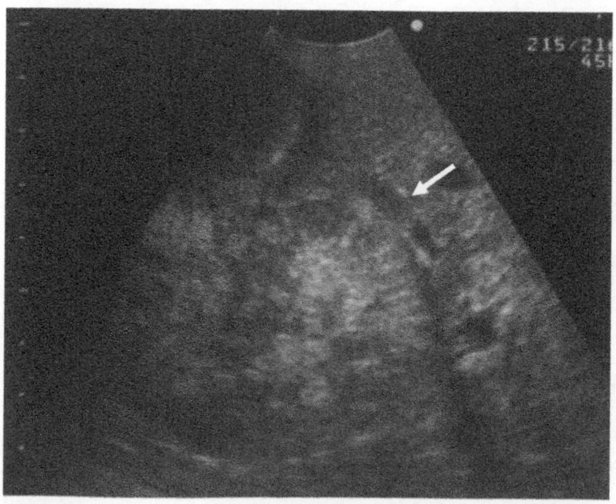

FIGURE 4 Tumor thrombus in the right hepatic vein (*arrow*) visualized by intraoperative ultrasonography.

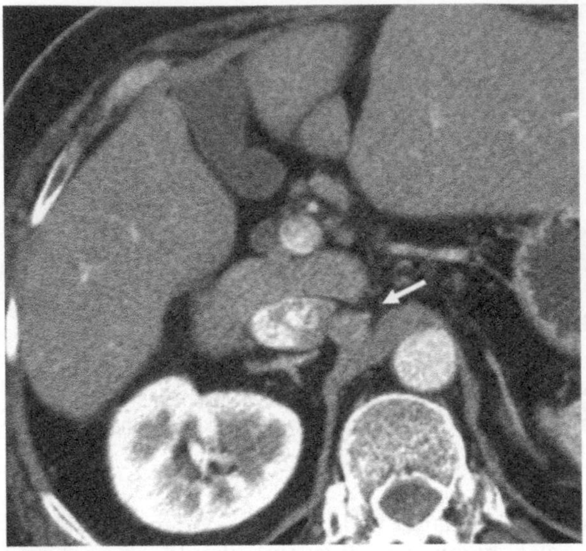

FIGURE 5 A histologically confirmed metastatic lymph node in the para-aortic region (*arrow*) from a hepatocellular carcinoma in segment 7. A round node, 16 mm in diameter, was slightly enhanced in the periphery.

C cirrhosis (25). Fluorine 18 fluorodeoxyglucose (FDG) PET has a high average false-negative rate of 40% to 50% for the detection of HCC. The accumulation of FDG in HCC varies and depends on the activity of glucose-6-phosphatase, an enzyme that dephosphorylates intracellular FDG and allows it to be removed from the liver (26) (evidence Level 2b). The degree of FDG uptake in HCCs has also been shown to reflect tumor differentiation; well-differentiated HCCs have a low FDG uptake, which is distinguishable from that of benign lesions, while moderately or poorly differentiated HCCs have a high FDG uptake (27). FDG-PET is not commonly used as a screening tool for the detection of intrahepatic or extrahepatic HCC. Ho et al. reported that ^{11}C-acetate, another radiotracer used for PET, had a high sensitivity and specificity for the detection of HCC when used in combination with FDG (28). Although the sensitivity of ^{11}C-acetate does not appear to be as high as that of FDG, it may play a complementary role for the detection of HCC lesions that do not easily take up FDG (26).

PREOPERATIVE PORTAL VEIN EMBOLIZATION FOR HEPATOCELLULAR CARCINOMA

Preoperative hemihepatic portal vein embolization (PVE) has been introduced in an attempt to extend the indications for major hepatic resections and increase the safety of this procedure.

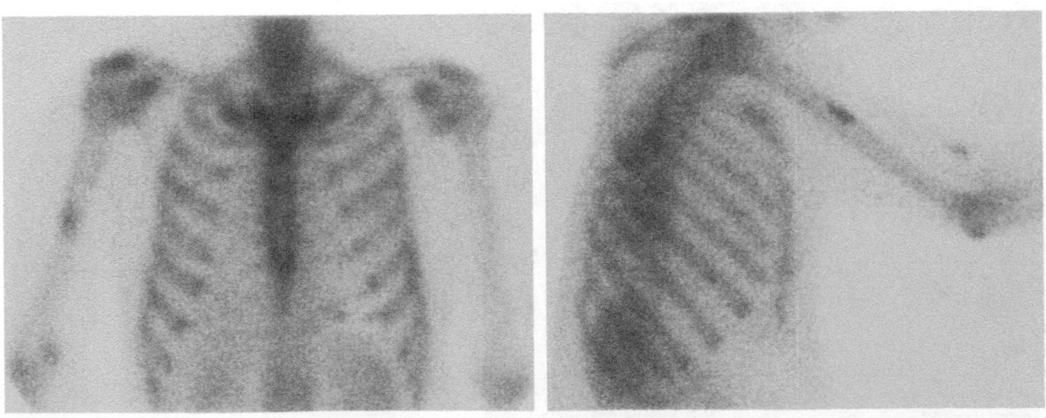

FIGURE 6 Bone metastasis in the right humerus detected by ^{99m}Tc-MDP scintigraphy. *Abbreviation*: MDP, methylene diphosphonate.

PVE was first developed by Makuuchi et al. in 1990 (29) for the treatment of hilar cholangiocarcinoma. PVE induces homolateral atrophy of the portion of the liver scheduled for resection and contralateral compensatory hypertrophy in the remnant liver, thereby decreasing the risk of postoperative liver failure. In 1986, Kinoshita began applying this technique in HCC patients scheduled to undergo hepatic resection (30).

Generally, PVE is indicated when the remnant liver is expected to be less than 40% of the preoperative liver volume in patients with normal liver function [no jaundice, 15-min retention rate of indocyanine green (ICG-R15) <10%], or less than 50% in patients with liver dysfunction (obstructive jaundice or an ICG-R15 of 10–19%) (31). PVE is not recommended for patients with moderate or severe liver dysfunction (ICG-R15 ≥ 20%) because the hypertrophy of the unembolized lobe may be retarded, placing the patient at risk for hepatic failure after the PVE.

Tanaka et al. (32) compared the long-term outcomes of HCC patients who underwent a right hepatectomy with or without preoperative PVE. Although the tumor-free survival rates were similar in the two groups, the cumulative survival rate was significantly higher in the PVE group. They speculated that the improved survival rate in the PVE group was attributable to the better residual hepatic function in this group, which enhanced the patients' tolerance to further treatment, including second hepatic resections. Azoulay et al. (33) and Wakabayashi et al. (34) reported comparable long-term results in PVE and non-PVE groups (evidence Level 2b).

The indications for PVE in patients with HCC are controversial for several reasons: (1) the livers of most HCC patients are compromised by an underlying liver disease, and the capacity for liver regeneration after hepatic resection is thought to be impaired under such conditions, making it difficult to predict whether sufficient hypertrophy of the future remnant liver segments can be achieved after PVE; (2) most HCCs are hypervascular tumors fed mainly by arterial blood flow, and the cessation of the portal flow induces a compensatory increase in arterial flow in the embolized segments (35), resulting in the rapid progress of the tumors after PVE (34); and (3) arterioportal shunts are frequently found in cirrhotic livers and HCC tumors, and these shunts may attenuate the effect of PVE (36) (evidence Level 4). To overcome the above concerns, Aoki et al. combined selective TACE with PVE before performing major hepatic resections in HCC patients. This double preparation was aimed at (1) using TACE to prevent tumor progression during the period between the PVE and the planned hepatectomy and (2) strengthening the effect of the PVE by first embolizing any arterioportal shunt that may exist using TACE. They applied sequential TACE and PVE in 17 patients with HCC, and 16 of these patients (94%) actually underwent a subsequent major hepatectomy; no postoperative mortalities were experienced in this series, and the five-year overall survival rate was 55.6% (Fig. 7).

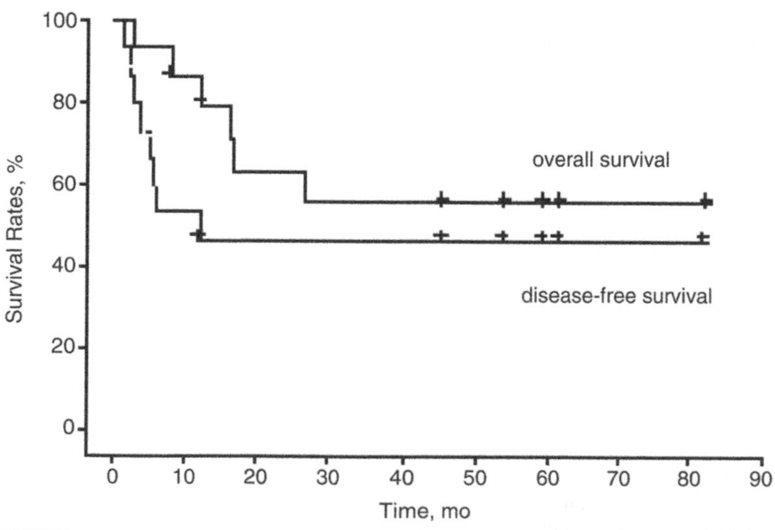

FIGURE 7 Disease-free and overall survival rates after curative resections with preoperative sequential transarterial chemoembolization and portal vein embolization ($n = 15$). *Source*: From Ref. 36.

SELECTION CRITERIA FOR LIVER TRANSPLANTATION IN HEPATOCELLULAR CARCINOMA PATIENTS

Total hepatectomy with transplantation has been regarded as a solution to HCC in patients with cirrhotic livers when hepatic resection is not feasible (37). The careful selection of patients with smaller HCC lesions and without vascular invasion or extrahepatic disease may lead to a post-transplant survival rate similar to that observed for non-HCC indications. In 1996, Mazzaferro et al. (38) reported excellent survival and recurrence outcomes using defined criteria for the selection of HCC candidates for liver transplantation (evidence Level 4). These criteria are now referred to as the Milan criteria (Table 1A). Specifically, cadaveric liver transplantations were performed in patients with a single (≤5 cm) HCC nodule or less than three (≤3 cm) HCC nodules. The recurrence rate was 8%, and the four-year, recurrence-free survival rate was 83%. To extend the indications for liver transplantation in HCC patients, the UCSF group modified the above criteria as follows: the solitary tumor ≤ 6.5 cm, or three or fewer nodules with the largest lesion ≤4.5 cm, and the total tumor diameter ≤ 8 cm. These modified criteria are known as the UCSF criteria. According to Yao et al. (39), the UCSF criteria liberalized the Milan criteria for selecting HCC candidates for transplantation, enabling an additional 23% of HCC candidates to undergo transplantation and obtain an outcome very similar to that of patients who fit the Milan criteria (evidence Level 4).

In living-donor liver transplantation (LDLT), where concerns regarding organ sharing are minimal, the criteria for transplantation have been expanded in Japanese and Western countries (Table 1B) (11). LDLT trials for patients with HCC are now ongoing at Japanese centers. According to a nationwide survey by the Japanese Study Group for Liver Transplantation, 208 patients with HCC had undergone an LDLT as of the end of 2002. So far, the long-term results appear favorable, with a five-year survival rate of 62.0% (40) (evidence Level 4).

LIVER RESECTION VS. TRANSPLANTATION FOR HEPATOCELLULAR CARCINOMA

Liver transplantation is the optimal treatment for HCC because it provides the widest possible resection margins for the cancer, removes the underlying cirrhotic liver tissue that is at risk for the development of de novo HCC, and restores normal hepatic function (41). With the refinement of the selection criteria mentioned in the previous section, several studies have shown

TABLE 1 Proposed Criteria for Selection of Hepatocellular Carcinoma Candidates for Liver Transplantation

Criteria for cadaveric liver transplantation
Milan criteria [35]
Solitary lesion ≤5 cm
2 or 3 lesions; none >3 cm
No gross vascular invasion
UCSF criteria [36]
Solitary lesion ≤6.5 cm
2 or 3 lesions; none >4.5 cm and total diameter ≤8 cm
No gross vascular invasion
Extended criteria for living-donor liver transplantation
University of Tokyo criteria
No. of tumor ≤5
Maximal diameter ≤5 cm
No gross vascular invasion
Barcellona criteria [8]
Solitary lesion ≤7 cm
3 lesions ≤5 cm or 5 lesions ≤3 cm
Downstaging: partial response to any treatment lasting <6 mo that meets the conventional criteria for liver transplantation

Abbreviation: UCSF, University of California, San Francisco.

that liver transplantation for early-stage HCC yields excellent results that are superior to those for resection and equal to those of transplantation candidates with nonmalignant diseases (38,42–44) (evidence Level 2b).

While the superiority of liver transplantation for early-stage HCC patients with poor liver function is unquestioned, the selection of transplantation as a first-line treatment for HCC patients with adequate liver function remains controversial. Owing to an organ shortage, liver resection is routinely performed in patients with small HCC and good liver function. Cha et al. (45) analyzed the long-term outcome after liver resection in 180 patients with HCC who met the Milano criteria and were eligible to receive a transplantation. The perioperative morbidity and mortality rates of this series were low (25% and 2.8%, respectively), and the five-year survival rate was 69%, which was comparable to that reported for patients who underwent a liver transplantation (evidence Level 4). They concluded that resection should be considered as the standard therapy for patients with HCC who have an adequate liver reserve. On the other hand, Adam et al. (41) questioned whether liver resection should be used as a possible bridge to transplantation because transplantation after resection was associated with a higher operative mortality, an increased risk of recurrence, and a poorer outcome than primary liver transplantation. The availability of a liver graft and the mortality and morbidity rates for liver resection and liver transplantation should be carefully weighed when deciding between a liver resection and a liver transplantation. A large, randomized controlled trial directly comparing liver transplantation and liver resection has yet to be performed.

REFERENCES

1. Group formed to establish "Guidelines for evidence-based clinical practice for the treatment of liver cancer." Clinical practice guidelines for hepatocellular carcinoma. Kanehara & Co. Ltd., Tokyo, 2005 [in Japanese].
2. Makuuchi M, Kokudo N. Clinical practice guidelines for hepatocellular carcinoma: the first evidence based guidelines from Japan. World J Gastroenterol 2006; 12:828–829.
3. http://www.cebm.net/levels_of_evidence.asp.
4. The Liver Cancer Study Group of Japan. Report of 16th nation wide survey of primary liver cancer in Japan (2000–2001). The Liver Cancer Study Group of Japan, Kyoto, 2004 [in Japanese].
5. Child CG, Turcotte JG. Surgery and portal hypertension. Major Probl Clin Surg 1964; 1:1–85.
6. Pugh RNH, Murray-Lyon IM, Dawson JL, Pietroni MC, Williams R. Transection of the oesophagus for bleeding oesophageal varices. Br J Surg 1973; 60:646–649.
7. Ryder SD. Guidelines for the diagnosis and treatment of hepatocellular carcinoma (HCC) in adults. Gut 2003; 52(suppl III):iii1–iii8.
8. Makuuchi M, Kosuge T, Takayama T, et al. Surgery for small liver cancers. Semin Surg Oncol 1993; 9:298–304.
9. Torzilli G, Makuuchi M, Inoue K, et al. No-mortality liver resection for hepatocellular carcinoma in cirrhotic and noncirrhotic patients. Is there a way? A prospective analysis of our approach. Arch Surg 1999; 134:984–992.
10. Imamura H, Seyama Y, Kokudo N, et al. One thousand fifty six hepatectomies without mortality in an eight-year period. Arch Surg 2003; 138:1198–1206.
11. Bruix J, Llovet JM. Prognostic prediction and treatment strategy in hepatocellular carcinoma. Hepatology 2002; 35:519–524.
12. The Liver Cancer Study Group of Japan. Predictive factors for long-term prognosis after partial hepatectomy for patients with hepatocellular carcinoma in Japan. Cancer 1994; 74:2772–2780.
13. Poon RT, Fan ST, Lo CM, Liu CL, Wong J. Intrahepatic recurrence after curative resection of hepatocellular carcinoma: long-term results of treatment and prognostic factors. Ann Surg 1999; 229: 216–222.
14. Llovet JM, Bustamante J, Castells, et al. Natural history of untreated nonsurgical hepatocellular carcinoma: rationale for the design and evaluation of therapeutic trials. Hepatology 1999; 29:62–67.
15. Ando E, Yamashita F, Tanaka M, Tanikawa K. A novel chemotherapy for advanced hepatocellular carcinoma with tumor thrombosis of the main trunk of the portal vein. Cancer 1997; 79:1890–1896.
16. Chung JW, Park JH, Han JK, Choi BI, Han MC. Hepatocellular carcinoma and portal vein invasion: results of treatment with transcatheter oily chemoembolization. Am J Roentgenol 1995; 165:315–321.
17. Minagawa M, Makuuchi M, Takayama T, Ohtomo K. Selection criteria for hepatectomy in patients with hepatocellular carcinoma and portal vein tumor thrombus. Ann Surg 2001; 233:379–384.
18. Okuda K. Early recognition of hepatocellular carcinoma. Hepatology 1986; 6:729–738.

19. Peterson MS, Baron RL, Marsh JW Jr, Oliver JH 3rd, Confer SR, Hunt LE. Pretransplantation surveillance for possible hepatocellular carcinoma in patients with cirrhosis: epidemiology and CT-based tumor detection rate in 430 cases with surgical pathologic correlation. Radiology 2000; 217:743–749.
20. Rode A, Bancel B, Douek P, et al. Small nodule detection in cirrhotic livers: evaluation with US, spiral CT, and MRI and correlation with pathologic examination of explanted liver. J Comput Assist Tomogr 2001; 25:327–336.
21. Nakayama A, Imamura H, Matsuyama Y, et al. Value of lipiodol computed tomography and digital subtraction angiography in the era of helical biphasic computed tomography as preoperative assessment of hepatocellular carcinoma. Ann Surg 2001; 234:56–62.
22. Kokudo N, Bandai Y, Imanishi H, et al. Management of new hepatic nodules detected by intraoperative ultrasonography during hepatic resection for hepatocellular carcinoma. Surgery 1996; 119:634–640.
23. Maillefert JF, Tebib J, Quipourt V, et al. Normal technetium-99m diphosphonate bone scintigraphy in skeletal metastases from hepatocellular carcinoma. J Hepatol 1994; 21:684.
24. Lee KH, Park JM, Yoon JK, Koh KC, Paik SW, Kim BT. Bone scintigraphy of skeletal metastasis in hepatoma patients treated by TAE. Hepatogastroenterology 2003; 50(54):1983–1986.
25. Liangpunsakul S, Agarwal D, Horlander JC, Kieff B, Chalasani N. Positron emission tomography for detecting occult hepatocellular carcinoma in hepatitis C cirrhotics awaiting for liver transplantation. Transpl Proc 2003; 35:2995–2997.
26. Delbeke D, Pinson CW. 11C-acetate: a new tracer for the evaluation of hepatocellular carcinoma. J Nucl Med 2003; 44:222–223.
27. Khan MA, Combs CS, Brunt EM, et al. Positron emission tomography scanning in the evaluation of hepatocellular carcinoma. J Hepatol 2000; 32:792–797.
28. Ho CL, Yu SC, Yeung DW. 11C-acetate PET imaging in hepatocellular carcinoma and other liver masses. J Nucl Med 2003; 44:213–221.
29. Makuuchi M, Thai BL, Takayasu K, et al. Preoperative portal embolization to increase safety of major hepatectomy for hilar bile duct carcinoma: a preliminary report. Surgery 1990; 107:521–527.
30. Kinoshita H, Sakai K, Hirohashi K, Igawa S, Yamasaki O, Kubo S. Preoperative portal vein embolization for hepatocellular carcinoma. World J Surg 1986; 10:803–808.
31. Kubota K, Makuuchi M, Kusaka K, et al. Measurement of liver volume and hepatic functional reserve as a guide to decision-making in resectional surgery for hepatic tumors. Hepatology 1997; 26: 1176–1181.
32. Tanaka H, Hirohashi K, Kubo S, Shuto T, Higaki I, Kinoshita H. Preoperative portal vein embolization improves prognosis after right hepatectomy for hepatocellular carcinoma in patients with impaired hepatic function. Br J Surg 2000; 87:879–882.
33. Azoulay D, Castaing D, Krissat J, et al. Percutaneous portal vein embolization increases the feasibility and safety of major liver resection for hepatocellular carcinoma in injured liver. Ann Surg 2000; 232:665–672.
34. Wakabayashi H, Ishimura K, Okano K, et al. Is preoperative portal vein embolization effective in improving prognosis after major hepatic resection in patients with advanced-stage hepatocellular carcinoma? Cancer 2001; 92:2384–2390.
35. Nagino M, Nimura Y, Kamiya J, Kanai M, Hayakawa N, Yamamoto H. Immediate increase in arterial blood flow in embolized hepatic segments after portal vein embolization: CT demonstration. Am J Roentgenol 1998; 171:1037–1039.
36. Aoki T, Imamura H, Hasegawa K, et al. Sequential preoperative arterial and portal venous embolizations in patients with hepatocellular carcinoma. Arch Surg 2004; 139(7):766–774.
37. Wall WJ, Marotta PJ. Surgery and transplantation for hepatocellular cancer. Liver Transpl 2000; 6:S16–S22.
38. Mazzaferro V, Regalia E, Doci R, et al. Liver transplantation for the treatment of small hepatocellular carcinoma in patients with cirrhosis. N Engl J Med 1996; 334:693–699.
39. Yao FY, Ferrel L, Bass NM, Bacchetti P, Ascher NL, Roberts JP. Liver transplantation for hepatocellular carcinoma: comparison of the proposed UCSF criteria with the Milan criteria and the Pittsburgh modified TNM criteria. Liver Transpl 2002; 8:765–774.
40. The Japanese Liver Transplantation Society. Liver transplantation in Japan. Registry by the Japanese Liver Transplantation Society. Ishoku 2003; 38:401–408 [in Japanese].
41. Adam R, Azoulay D, Castaing D, et al. Liver resection as a bridge to transplantation for hepatocellular carcinoma on cirrhosis. A reasonable strategy? Ann Surg 2003; 238:508–519.
42. Bismuth H, Chiche L, Adam R, Castaing D, Diamond T, Dennison A. Liver resection versus transplantation for hepatocellular carcinoma in cirrhotic patients. Ann Surg 1993; 218:145–151.
43. Michel J, Suc B, Montpeyroux F, et al. Liver resection or transplantation for hepatocellular carcinoma? Retrospective analysis of 215 patients with cirrhosis. J Hepatol 1997; 26:1274–4180.
44. Yao FY, Ferrell L, Bass NM, et al. Liver transplantation for hepatocellular carcinoma: expansion of tumor size limits does not adversely impact survival. Hepatology 2001; 33:1394–1403.
45. Cha CH, Ruo L, Fong Y, et al. Resection of hepatocellular carcinoma in patients otherwise eligible for transplantation. Ann Surg 2003; 238:315–323.

APPENDIX

Search strategies for surgical management of hepatocellular carcinoma (cited from Ref. 1 with permission)
[Treatment: Surgery (Resection Transplantation)]

File 155: MEDLINE (R) 1966–2002/Sep W4

Set	Description
S1	Carcinoma, Hepatocellular/DE
S2	(Hepatocell? or Liver ( ) Cell) (1N) Carcinoma? or Hepatoma?
S3	HCC and Liver Neoplasms!
S4	S1:S3
S5	S4/Human or (S4 not animal/GS)
S6	S5/ENG
S7	S6 and PY = 1980:2001
S8	S7 not case report/GS
S9	S8 not (DT = review? or review literature/DE)
S10	S8 and systematic (1W) (review? + overview?)/TI or S9
S11	S1 (L) SU
S12	Liver neoplasms! (L) SU or liver! (L) SU
S13	Surgical procedures, operative! not transplantation!
S14	(Hepatectom? or resect? or surg? or operat?
S15	S10 and (S11 or S12 or S13 or S14)
S16	S15 and S1/MAJ or S15 and (HCC or hepatocell? or hepatoma?)/TI
S17	S15 and (S11/MAJ or S12/MAJ or S13/MAJ or S14/TI)
S18	S16 and S17
S19	S18 not DT = (comment or letter or news or editorial)
S20	Liver transplantation or liver! (L) TR
S21	Hepat? or liver or HCC) (3N) (transplant? or graft?)
S22	S10 and (S20 or S21)
S23	S22 and S1/MAJ or S22 and (HCC or hepatocell? or hepatoma?)/TI
S24	S23 and (S20/MAJ or S21/TI)
S25	S23 and S24
S26	S25 not DT = (comment or letter or news or editorial) 200

[Diagnosis: Diagnostic imaging (except US)]

File 155: MEDLINE (R) 1966–2002/Oct W4

Set	Description
S1	Carcinoma, hepatocellular/DE
S2	(Hepatocell? or liver ( ) cell) (1N) carcinoma? or hepatoma?
S3	HCC and liver neoplasms!
S4	S1:S3
S5	S4/human or (S4 not animal/GS)
S6	S5/ENG or S5 and LA = Japanese
S7	S6 and PY=>1982
S8	S7 and (S1 (L) (RA or RI) or liver! (L) (RA or RI)
S9	S7 and diagnostic imaging!
S10	S7 and image processing, computer-assisted!
S11	S7 and radiology! and S1 (L) DI
S12	S7 and (CT or tomograph? or MRI or IMAG? or angiogra? or scint?)/TI
S13	S8:S12
S14	DT = guideline + practice guideline + consensus development conference? (Guidelines + practice guidelines)/DE + guideline?/TI + recommendation?/TI + evidence? (W) based/TI
S15	Clinical protocols/DE + patient care planning! + (clinical + critical) (1W) (path + paths + pathway?)/TI + (clinical + treatment?) (2N) protocol?/TI + care (1N) planning?/TI + (good (1W) clinical (1W) practice?)/TI

S16	S14 OR S15
S17	Systematic (1W) (review? + overview?) + peer review!
S18	JN = (Cochrane Database Syst Rev + ACP Journal Club + ACP J Club + Health Technol Assess + Evid Rep Technol Assess?)
S19	S17 or S18
S20	DT = meta-analysis + meta-analysis/DE + (METAANALY? + META (W) ANALY?/TI
S21	DT = randomized controlled trial + randomized controlled trials/DE + random allocation/DE + random? + double-blind method/DE + single-blind method/DE + (Singl? + Double? + Trebl? + Tripl?) (W) (Blind? + Mask?)
S22	DT = controlled clinical trial + controlled clinical trials! + placebos/DE + single-blind method/DE + cross-over studies/DE + placebo? + comparative study/GS + control? (1W) (trial? + stud?)
S23	DT = clinical trial? + clinical trials!/DE + (clinical (1W) trial?)/TI
S24	DT = multicenter study + multicenter studies/DE + (Multicent? + Multi (W) Cent?)/TI
S25	Cohort studies!
S26	Case-control studies! + matched-pair analysis/DE
S27	DT = review of reported cases + case (W) series/TI
S28	S16 or S19:S27
S29	S13 and S28 1,075
S30	S29 not case report/GS 941
S31	S30 not DT = (letter or news or comment or editorial) 937

[Diagnosis: Ultrasonic wave (US)]

File 155:MEDLINE (R) 1966–2002/Oct W3

Set	Description
S1	Carcinoma, hepatocellular/DE
S2	(Hepatocell? or liver cell) (1N) carcinoma? or hepatoma?
S3	HCC and liver neoplasms!
S4	S1:S3
S5	S4/human or (S4 not animal/GS)
S6	S5/ENG or S5 and LA = Japanese
S7	S6 and PY=>1982
S8	S7 and (S1 (L) US or liver! (L) US)
S9	S7 and (ultrasonography! or ultrasonics!)
S10	S7 and (ultrasound? or endosonogr? or sonogr?)/TI
S11	S8:S10 1,022

26 Chemotherapy and Radiotherapy for the Treatment of Hepatocellular Carcinoma

Pierre Chan, Ching Lung Lai, and Man Fung Yuen
Department of Medicine, Queen Mary Hospital, University of Hong Kong, Hong Kong, China

Hepatocellular carcinoma (HCC) can be treated by surgical and nonsurgical means. However, only around 20% to 30% of patients with HCC are resectable on presentation because of advanced disease or impaired liver reserve secondary to underlying cirrhosis (1). Patients usually present late because HCC smaller than 8 cm is usually asymptomatic. The tumors are also often multifocal. Recurrence after "complete" resection is common, either due to micrometastases undetected during operation or to the development of new foci of tumors. Therefore, most HCC are managed by nonsurgical means.

Nonsurgical methods include transarterial chemoembolization (TACE), systemic chemotherapy, hormonal therapy, immunotherapy, various local ablative therapies and radiotherapy. This chapter will focus on the use of chemotherapy and radiotherapy in the management of advanced HCC, as well as review their roles in adjuvant and neoadjuvant therapies.

TRANSARTERIAL CHEMOEMBOLIZATION

Over the past 20 years, TACE has become the treatment of choice for patients with inoperable HCC. As the name suggests, "transarterial" (TA) means accessing the hepatic artery via the femoral artery under fluoroscopic guidance. Chemotherapeutic agents (C) used include cisplatin, doxorubicin, and mitomycin. They are mixed and emulsified with lipiodol, which is an oily contrast agent (iodized oil) that allows drugs to remain selectively in tumors for long periods. Embolization (E) of hepatic artery will result in tumor necrosis, thus enhancing antitumor efficacy. Substances used in embolization include gelatin sponge (gelfoam), starch, glass microspheres or polyvinyl alcohol. The rationale of TACE depends on the fact that the liver has two major blood supplies: the hepatic artery and the portal vein. Normal liver cells receive 60% to 70% of their blood supply from the portal vein, while liver tumor cells are solely supplied by the hepatic artery. TACE can also achieve high local chemotherapy concentrations, both by targeting the drug intra-arterially into the tumor and through retention of the drug with lipiodol. This will also result in low systemic toxicity.

The efficacy of TACE in reducing tumor growth and in prolonging survival has been reported in nonrandomized studies from 1985 to 1996 (2–11). However, three randomized controlled trials from 1995 to 1998 failed to show any significant benefit in survival (12–14). Two meta-analyses in 2003 show differing results, with one showing survival benefit at two years and the other demonstrating no survival benefit (15,16).

Most recently, three randomized controlled trials show survival advantage for TACE compared with conservative management, when only patients with relatively preserved liver function are considered for therapy (17–19). In these three randomized controlled trials, the patients were chosen according to strict criteria, with relatively normal bilirubin and prothrombin time, and no evidence of gastrointestinal bleeding or portal vein thrombosis. In the study of Yuen et al., the cumulative survival rates at six-months, one-year, two-years, three-years, and four-years of patient receiving TACE are 93.8%, 86.3%, 78.8%, 57.5%, and 51.3%, respectively, when compared to patient receiving no active treatment 62.5%, 62.5%, 50%, 50%, and 43.8% ($P = 0.02$, $P = 0.023$, $P = 0.017$, $P =$ ns, $P =$ ns), respectively. Tumor response was observed in 28% of patients receiving TACE (19).

TACE should be given every two to three months until there is no evidence of residual tumors. It should be withheld whenever complications, progression of disease or contraindications to TACE occur. This may be the reason for the failure to demonstrate survival benefit in some trials in which TACE was given only for limited sessions (12–14). Tumors size of >10 cm in diameter and serum albumin levels of <35 g/L are independent poor prognostic factors. TACE in patients who have these factors results in a treatment mortality rate of 20% and poor survival (20).

TACE is indicated for inoperable hepatocellular carcinoma and can also be used as neoadjuvant therapy prior to other forms of treatment, including surgical resection, radiofrequency ablation, and liver transplantation. Contraindications include extrahepatic metastases, vascular complications (portal vein thrombosis, hepatic artery thrombosis, and severe arteriovenous shunting) and poor hepatic function (Child's C liver cirrhosis, Okuda stage III, serum bilirubin level >50 μmol/L, severe ascites, history of hepatic encephalopathy, and recent variceal bleeding).

Complications include fever, nausea and vomiting, abdominal pain, gastrointestinal bleeding due to ischemia to the gastrointestinal tract, liver or spleen abscess, acalculous cholecystitis, and, most importantly, liver failure. Postembolization syndrome, including fever and elevated transaminases, is described in a prospective study (21), with 41% of patients having a fever >38.5°C and 93% of patients developing elevated transaminases. Rise in transaminases is often due to tumor necrosis and is therefore considered to indicate successful embolization. However, the study of Wigmore et al. does not show any survival benefit in patients with postembolization syndrome (21). In another prospective study investigating the complications after TACE, fever (74%), nausea and/or vomiting (59%), and abdominal pain (45%) are the most common side effects (22). Acute hepatic decompensation (with raised bilirubin, prolonged prothrombin time, development of ascites and/or hepatic encephalopathy) occurs in 20% of patients receiving TACE but most of the episodes of liver failure are temporary and reversible. Irreversible liver failure occurs after TACE in about 1.5% to 3% of patients (22,23). The factors that appear to predispose patients to the development of irreversible acute hepatic decompensation after TACE are: high dosage of cisplatin, high basal levels of bilirubin, prolonged prothrombin time, and advanced liver cirrhosis. Pretreatment liver function and the stage of cirrhosis always should be the chief considerations for patients receiving TACE. The results of the recent study demonstrated that when a strict entry criterion of a bilirubin level <50 μmol/L is used, only a very small proportion of patients will develop in irreversible liver failure (22). A pilot study of transcatheter arterial interferon embolization (TAIE) has been in performed recently in 18 patients with inoperable HCC. They were given interferon-alpha-2b intra-arterially. Complete responses and partial responses (>50% tumor reduction) were observed in 28.6% and 35.7% of patients, respectively. The median survival was 15.9 months. Transient fever and rigor were the most common side effects observed. Five patients (27.8%) developed hypothyroidism. No significant liver decompensation was observed (24). While the results are encouraging, more large-scale randomized studies are required before any firm conclusions can be drawn concerning the efficacy of TAIE.

In conclusion, TACE given in repeated sessions is shown to have survival benefit in one meta-analysis and three recent randomized controlled trials in patients with preserved liver function. However, the chances of complete remission are remote and the prolongation of survival modest.

Level 1b evidence, Grade A recommendation: In patients with relatively good liver function, selected according to strict criteria, TACE performed repeatedly until tumor disappearance, progression, or complications prolong survival in inoperable HCC.

RADIOTHERAPY

Treatment of inoperable HCC by radiotherapy (RT) has been widely studied (25–32). Several studies show positive results (25–32), with doses of >50 Gray (Gy) resulting in improved tumor response rate and prolonged median survival (33,34). External RT is performed in the following situations: in patients after failure of TACE (26), when TACE is contraindicated because of portal vein thrombosis (27,28), and when RT is given together with TACE (29–31). In a Korean study of 27 patients, RT was effective in patients failing TACE, with a mean tumor dose of 51.8 ± 7.9 Gy, in daily 1.8-Gy fractions. An objective response was observed in 66.7% of patients. The median survival was 26 months from the diagnosis and 14 months after starting RT (26).

RT is also shown to be effective in two Japanese studies in patients with portal vein thrombosis and not considered suitable for surgery or TACE. A total dose of 50 Gy to 60 Gy was given. The median survival was seven months. An objective response was observed in 11 of 19 cases (57.9%) (27,28).

A combination of RT and TACE is shown to be effective in a retrospective study in China and a prospective study in Korea (29,30). In the Chinese study, a total of 107 patients with large unresectable HCC were treated with TACE followed by external beam irradiation, achieving an objective response in 48.6% of patients and a median survival of 18 months (29). The 30 patients in the Korean study were given TACE together with RT with a mean tumor dose of 44.0 ± 9.3 Gy in daily 1.8 Gy fractions. The objective response rate was 63.3% and the median survival was 17 months (30).

There have been two controlled studies comparing RT combined with TACE and RT/TACE given alone (31,32). One study of 42 patients finds that the two-year survival rate for the combination of TACE and RT (58%) was similar to TACE alone (56%) but better than RT alone (11%) (TACE + RT vs. RT, $P = 0.0007$; TACE versus RT $P = 0.01$). However, the poor results for patients receiving RT alone might be due to the selection bias of patients with more advanced disease and compromised condition (31). The other study involving 76 patients with large unresectable HCC shows that the objective response rate of TACE plus irradiation was higher than TACE alone (47.4 % vs. 28.1%, $P < 0.05$). The overall survival rates in the TACE plus irradiation group (64.0%, 28.6%, and 19.3% at one, three and five years, respectively) were significantly better than those receiving TACE alone (39.9%, 9.5%, and 7.2%, respectively) ($P = 0.0001$) (32). Further studies with larger patient populations are required to elucidate the benefit or otherwise of RT in combination with TACE.

Evidence level 2b, no recommendation: Two small RCTs differ as to whether external beam RT adds to the survival benefit of TACE.

RT has quite significant side effects, including abnormal liver function tests, ascites, hepatomegaly, thrombocytopenia, and gastritis (25,26,35). The occurrence of radiation-induced liver disease is related to the dose of radiation and the proportion of the liver exposed to radiation. There is a 5% to 10% chance of developing radiation-induced liver disease after doses of 30 Gy to 35 Gy, while the risk increases to 50% after whole liver exposure to 40 Gy to 50 Gy (35). When less than a third of the liver is exposed to radiation, doses as high as 100 Gy may be safely delivered (36).

There are recent attempts to reduce the adverse effects of radiation. These include three dimensional conformal radiation techniques (3D-CRT) (25,37), intensity modulated radiation therapy (IMRT) (38) and image-guided radiation therapy (IGRT) (35). Prospective controlled trials are required to investigate their clinical use in the future.

Another method developed to deliver local radiation is the use of radioactive isotopes given to the tumor via the hepatic artery. The radioactive isotopes studied are iodine-131 (39) and yttrium-90 microspheres (40). Iodine-131 emits mainly gamma radiation and its half life is eight days, while yttrium-90 emits beta radiation with a half life of 64 hours. Injections of radiolabeled iodine-131 to 27 patients with HCC and portal vein thrombosis yielded survival rates at three, six, and nine months of 71%, 48%, 7%, respectively (39). Selective internal radiation therapy using 90Y microspheres is effective and well tolerated for selected cases of unresectable HCC. In one study, the response rate in terms of decline in tumor marker levels was higher than that based on reduction in tumor volume as measured by computed tomography. The median survival of 71 patients was 9.4 months. The treatment is well tolerated, with no bone marrow toxicity or clinical evidence of radiation hepatitis or pneumonitis (40).

In conclusion, RT may have some benefits for advanced HCC in terms of improved median survival. Further larger prospective randomized trials are required to confirm its efficacy. RT may be an option in a patient having advanced HCC with portal vein thrombosis in which operation and TACE are contraindicated. New developments of radiation techniques and intra-arterial radioactive isotopes have reduced the side effects of radiation.

SYSTEMIC CHEMOTHERAPY

Systemic chemotherapy is not used routinely for advanced HCC. There are factors related to the tumors. HCC is relatively chemoresistant, partly due to the presence of drug-resistant genes, including *p-glycoprotein*, *glutathione-S-transferase*, heat shock proteins and mutations in p53. There are also factors related to the patients. Patients often do not tolerate chemotherapy well because of the underlying liver dysfunction and liver cirrhosis.

Several chemotherapy agents, including doxorubicin, epirubicin, 5-fluorouracil and leucovorin, gemcitabine, thalidomide, and capecitabine, have been studied in the treatment of advanced HCC either as single agents (41–46) or in combination (47–49). The response rates vary from 20% to 50%, but no improvement in overall survival has been reported. A number of small uncontrolled studies report an overall response to doxorubicin monotherapy to be less than 20%. The only controlled trial involving 104 patients showed a modest improvement in median survival (10.6 weeks vs. 7.5 weeks with doxorubicin and conservative treatment respectively, $P = 0.036$). However, doxorubicin caused fatal complications (septicemia and cardiotoxicity) in 25% of patients (41). Cardiotoxicity can occur even in patients receiving less than the recommended "cardiotoxic" dose of 500 mg/m^2. Doxorubicin is not an ideal agent for treatment of HCC.

The response rate to epirubicin is also low at 20% and there is no proven survival benefit (42). 5-Fluorouracil has been evaluated in many studies of unresectable HCC. As a single agent, its efficacy is low. However, when given in combination with leucovorin, the response rate has been reported as 28% (43). A phase II trial of gemcitabine shows no objective responses in 30 patients (44).

Many combination cytotoxic regimes have been tested in patients with advanced HCC. Cisplatin-based combination regimes usually result in higher objective response rates than non-cisplatin-containing regimes. The response rates to cisplatin and doxorubicin (47), 5-fluorouracil; mitoxantrone, and cisplatin (48); and epirubicin, cisplatin and infusion 5-fluorouracil (49) are 18% to 49%, 47%, and 15%, respectively.

Interferon alfa has also used in treating advanced HCC. Two controlled trials by Lai et al. involving 75 and 71 patients, and using very high doses of interferon of 50×10^6 IU/m^2 three times weekly, showed a 30% response rate and improvement in median survival compared with no treatment ($P < 0.0001$ and $P = 0.0471$, respectively) (50,51). Another study of 58 patients using a much lower dose of interferon 3×10^6 IU/m^2, three times weekly did not show any survival advantage (52). It appears that for interferon to be effective in HCC, a much higher dose than that used for treatment of chronic hepatitis B and C is required. However the side effects of interferon are severe, especially with high dose regimes. Giving interferon intra-arterially (TAIE mentioned above) reduces the side effects to a marked extent.

Evidence level 2b, no recommendation: High dose alpha interferon improves survival in advanced HCC, but at the cost of severe side effects.

Several hormonal agents have also been studied. These include tamoxifen, megestrol, octreotide, and lanreotide. In theory, HCC with the presence of hormone receptors at varying concentrations on the malignant cells may benefit from hormone receptor blockade such as tamoxifen. However several prospective randomized trials and a meta-analysis of tamoxifen in patients with advanced HCC fail to show any survival benefits (53–56). A few small trials suggest some possible effects with megestrol (57), octreotide (58), and lanreotide (59). But these have either not been confirmed (60) or are awaiting larger confirmatory studies.

Immunotherapy and gene therapy have the potential for the treatment of HCC. Immunotherapies including cytokines, lymphocyte-activated killer cells, and interleukin-2 are being tested but the final results are still pending.

Finally, combinations of different modalities in systemic therapy for HCC have been investigated. They include the combination of the hormone tamoxifen and doxorubicin (61), and combination of chemotherapy and interferon (62–64), with response rate of 32% and 26% to 50%, respectively. However the good response rate does not result in significant improvement of overall survival.

In summary, because of low tumor response rates, an absence of unequivocal improvement in survival, and severe side effects in cirrhotic patients, systemic chemotherapy is not recommended for routine use in patients with advanced HCC, particularly in patients with impaired liver function.

NEOADJUVANT AND ADJUVANT THERAPY

There are many studies evaluating the use of TACE as a neoadjuvant therapy. A meta-analysis of preoperative transarterial chemotherapy fails to show any positive effects on survival or recurrence (65). Other case series describe the use of intra-arterial Iodine-131 lipiodol (66), systemic chemoimmunotherapy (67), and radiotherapy (68,69) as neoadjuvant therapies. Although they can decrease the size of the tumors before surgery there has been no resultant survival benefit in most studies. In addition, the sample sizes of most of the studies so far reported are small, with only a limited number of randomized trials. No concrete conclusions of benefit can be drawn.

The benefit of adjuvant therapy for patient with HCC after operation also remains unclear. The adjuvant therapies investigated include systemic chemotherapy, intra-arterial therapy and radiotherapy. Although one trial of adjuvant chemotherapy shows an improvement in disease-free survival (70), several randomized controlled trials do not show any definite survival benefit (70–72). Adjuvant TACE is associated with a significant improvement in disease-free survival (32% vs. 12% at three-year) and median disease-free interval (852 days vs. 485 days) in the treatment and control groups, respectively (73). However no improvement in overall survival is noted (73,74). Controlled trials of intra-arterial lipiodol iodine-131 show beneficial effect in reducing tumor recurrence (29% vs. 59%) and increased median disease-free survival (57 months vs. 14 months) (75), while other trials show reduction in recurrence by using interferon alfa (76), interferon beta (77), and oral polyprenoic acid (78) as adjuvant therapy.

Because of the small sample sizes, the heterogeneous patient population, the non-standardized endpoints and the lack of confirmation studies, the benefit of adjuvant therapy for HCC is still controversial.

Evidence level 2b, recommendation Grade C: Adjuvant intra-arterial lipiodol iodine-131 therapy may improve survival after resection for HCC other forms of adjuvant therapy have yet to demonstrate consistent benefits in overall survival.

CONCLUSIONS

Among the chemotherapy and radiotherapy regimes used in the treatment of advanced HCC, only TACE has been shown to have significant overall survival benefit in one meta-analysis and three randomized controlled trials in patients with relatively preserved liver function. As for radiotherapy, systemic chemotherapy, adjuvant, and neoadjuvant therapies, more prospective controlled studies are required to justify their use and benefit in advanced HCC.

REFERENCES

1. Yuen MF, Lai CL. Screening for hepatocellular carcinoma: survival benefit and cost-effectiveness. Ann Oncol 2003; 14(10):1463–1467. Review.
2. Okuda K, Ohtsuki T, Obata H, et al. Natural history of hepatocellular carcinoma and prognosis in relation to treatment. Study of 850 patients. Cancer 1985; 56:918–928.
3. Sasaki Y, Imaoka S, Kasugai H, et al. A new approach to chemoembolization therapy for hepatoma using ethiodized oil, cisplatin, and gelatin sponge. Cancer 1987; 60:1194–1203.
4. Lin DY, Liaw YF, Lee TY, Lai CM. Hepatic arterial embolization in patients with unresectable hepatocellular carcinoma—a randomized controlled trial. Gastroenterology 1988; 94:453–456.
5. Kasugai H, Kojima J, Tatsuta M, et al. Treatment of hepatocellular carcinoma by transcatheter arterial embolization combined with intraarterial infusion of a mixture of cisplatin and ethiodized oil. Gastroenterology 1989; 97:965–971.
6. Liaw YF, Lin DY. Transcatheter hepatic arterial embolization in the treatment of hepatocellular carcinoma. Hepatogastroenterology 1990; 37:484–488.
7. Vetter D, Wenger JJ, Bergier JM, et al. Transcatheter oily chemoembolization in the management of advanced hepatocellular carcinoma in cirrhosis: Results of a Western comparative study in 60 patients. Hepatology 1991; 13:427–433.
8. Ngan H, Lai CL, Fan ST, et al. Treatment of inoperable hepatocellular carcinoma by transcatheter arterial chemoembolization using an emulsion of cisplatin in iodized oil and gelfoam. Clin Radiol 1993; 47:315–320.
9. Stuart K, Stokes K, Jenkins R, et al. Treatment of hepatocellular carcinoma using doxorubicin/ethiodized oil/gelatin powder chemoembolization. Cancer 1993; 72:3202–3209.
10. Stefanini GF, Amorati P, Biselli M, et al. Efficacy of transarterial targeted treatments on survival of patients with hepatocellular carcinoma. Cancer 1995; 75:2427–2434.
11. Bayraktar Y, Balkanci F, Kayhan B, et al. A comparison of chemoembolization with conventional chemotherapy and symptomatic treatment in cirrhotic patients with hepatocellular carcinoma. Hepatogastroenterology 1996; 43:681–687.

12. Groupe d'Etude et de Traitement du Carcinome Hepatocellulaire. A comparison of lipiodol chemoembolization and conservative treatment for unresectable hepatocellular carcinoma. N Engl J Med 1995; 332:1256–1261.
13. Bruix J, Llovet JM, Castells A, et al. Transarterial embolization versus symptomatic treatment in patients with advanced hepatocellular carcinoma: results of a randomized, controlled trial in a single institution. Hepatology 1998; 27:1578.
14. Pelletier G, Ducreux M, Gay F, et al. Treatment of unresectable hepatocellular carcinoma with lipiodol chemoembolization—a multicenter randomized trial. J Hepatol 1998; 29:129.
15. Llovet JM, Bruix J. Systematic review of randomized trials for unresectable hepatocellular carcinoma: Chemoembolization improves survival. Hepatology 2003; 37:429.
16. Geschwind JF, Ramsey DE, Choti MA, et al. Chemoembolization of hepatocellular carcinoma: Results of a metaanalysis. Am J Clin Oncol 2003; 26:344.
17. Llovet JM, Real MI, Montana X, et al. Arterial embolisation or chemoembolisation versus symptomatic treatment in patients with unresectable hepatocellular carcinoma: A randomized controlled trial. Lancet 2002; 359:1734.
18. Lo CM, Ngan H, Tso WK, et al. Randomized controlled trial of transarterial lipiodol chemoembolization for unresectable hepatocellular carcinoma. Hepatology 2002; 35:1164.
19. Yuen MF, Chan AO, Wong BC, et al. Transarterial chemoembolization for inoperable, early stage hepatocellular carcinoma in patients with Child-Pugh grade A and B: Results of a comparative study in 96 Chinese patients. Am J Gastroenterol 2003; 98(5):1181–1185.
20. Poon RT, Ngan H, Lo CM, et al. Transarterial chemoembolization for inoperable hepatocellular carcinoma and postresection intrahepatic recurrence. J Surg Oncol 2000; 73(2):109–114.
21. Wigmore SJ, Redhead DN, Thomson BN, et al. Postchemoembolisation syndrome-tumor necrosis or hepatocyte injury? Br J Cancer 2003; 89:1423.
22. Chan OO, Yuen MF, Hui CK, et al. A prospective study regarding the complications of transcatheter intraarterial lipiodol chemoembolization in patients with hepatocellular carcinoma. Cancer 2002; 94:1747.
23. Ngan H, Lai CL, Fan ST, et al. Transcatheter arterial chemoembolisation in inoperable hepatocellular carcinoma: four-year follow-up. J Vascu Interv Radiol 1996; 7:419–425.
24. Yuen MF, Ooi CG, Hui CK, et al. A pilot study of transcatheter arterial interferon embolization for patients with hepatocellular carcinoma. Cancer 2003; 97(11):2776–2782.
25. Robertson JM, Lawrence TS, Dworzanin LM, et al. Treatment of primary hepatobiliary cancers with conformal radiation therapy and regional chemotherapy. J Clin Oncol 1993; 11:1286.
26. Seong J, Park HC, Han KH, et al. Local radiotherapy for unresectable hepatocellular carcinoma patients who failed with transcatheter arterial chemoembolization. Int J Radiat Oncol Biol Phys 2000; 47:1331.
27. Tazawa J, Maeda M, Sakai Y, et al. Radiation therapy in combination with transcatheter arterial chemoembolization for hepatocellular carcinoma with extensive portal vein involvement. J Gastroenterol Hepatol 2001; 16:660.
28. Yamada K, Izaki K, Sugimoto K, et al. Prospective trial of combined transcatheter arterial chemoembolization and three-dimensional conformal radiotherapy for portal vein tumor thrombus in patients with unresectable hepatocellular carcinoma. Int J Radiat Oncol Biol Phys 2003; 57:113.
29. Guo WJ, Yu EX. Evaluation of combined therapy with chemoembolization and irradiation for large hepatocellular carcinoma. Br J Radiol 2000; 73:1091.
30. Seong J, Keum KC, Han KH, et al. Combined transcatheter arterial chemoembolization and local radiotherapy of unresectable hepatocellular carcinoma. Int J Radiat Oncol Biol Phys 1999; 43:393.
31. Chia-Hsien Cheng J, Chuang VP, Cheng SH, et al. Unresectable hepatocellular carcinoma treated with radiotherapy and/or chemoembolization. Int J Cancer 2001; 96:243.
32. Guo WJ, Yu EX, Liu LM, et al. Comparison between chemoembolization combined with radiotherapy and chemoembolization alone for large hepatocellular carcinoma. World J Gastroenterol 2003; 9(8):1697–1701.
33. Robertson JM, Lawrence TS, Dworzanin LM, et al. Treatment of primary hepatobiliary cancers with conformal radiation therapy and regional chemotherapy. J Clin Oncol 1993; 11:1286–1293.
34. Park HC, Seong J, Han KH, et al. Suh, Dose-response relationship in local radiotherapy for hepatocellular carcinoma. Int J Radiat Oncol Biol Phys 2002; 54:150–155.
35. Fuss M, Salter BJ, Herman TS, et al. External beam radiation therapy for hepatocellular carcinoma: potential of intensity-modulated and image-guided radiation therapy. Gastroenterology 2004; 127(5 suppl 1):S206–S217. Review.
36. Dawson LA, Ten Haken RK, Lawrence TS. Partial irradiation of the liver. Semin Radiat Oncol 2001; 11:240–246.
37. Cheng SH, Lin YM, Chuang VP, et al. A pilot study of three-dimensional conformal radiotherapy in unresectable hepatocellular carcinoma. J Gastroenterol Hepatol 1999; 14:1025.
38. Cheng JC, Wu JK, Huang CM, et al. Dosimetric analysis and comparison of three-dimensional conformal radiotherapy and intensity-modulated radiation therapy for patients with hepatocellular carcinoma and radiation-induced liver disease. Int J Radiat Oncol Biol Phys 2003; 56:229–234.

39. Raoul JL, Guyader D, Bretagne JF, et al. Randomized controlled trial for hepatocellular carcinoma with portal vein thrombosis: Intra-arterial iodine-131-iodized oil versus medical support. J Nucl Med 1994; 35:1782.
40. Lau WY, Ho S, Leung TW, et al. Selective internal radiation therapy for nonresectable hepatocellular carcinoma with intraarterial infusion of 90yttrium microspheres. Int J Radiat Oncol Biol Phys 1998; 40:583.
41. Lai CL, Wu PC, Chan GC, et al. Doxorubicin versus no antitumor therapy in inoperable hepatocellular carcinoma. A prospective randomized trial. Cancer 1988; 62:479.
42. Hochster HS, Green MD, Speyer J, et al. 4′Epidoxorubicin (epirubicin): Activity in hepatocellular carcinoma. J Clin Oncol 1985; 3:1535.
43. Porta C, Moroni M, Nastasi G, Arcangeli G. 5-Fluorouracil and d,l-leucovorin calcium are active to treat unresectable hepatocellular carcinoma patients: Preliminary results of a phase II study. Oncology 1995; 52:487.
44. Fuchs CS, Clark JW, Ryan DP, et al. A phase II trial of gemcitabine in patients with advanced hepatocellular carcinoma. Cancer 2002; 94:3186.
45. Patt YZ, Hassan MM, Aguayo A, et al. Oral capecitabine for the treatment of hepatocellular carcinoma, cholangiocarcinoma, and gallbladder carcinoma. Cancer 2004; 101:578.
46. Lin AY, Brophy N, Fisher GA, et al. Phase II study of thalidomide in patients with unresectable hepatocellular carcinoma. Cancer 2005; 103:119.
47. Lee J, Park JO, Kim WS, et al. Phase II study of doxorubicin and cisplatin in patients with metastatic hepatocellular carcinoma. Cancer Chemother Pharmacol 2004; 54:385.
48. Ikeda M, Okusaka T, Ueno H, et al. A phase II trial of continuous infusion of 5-fluorouracil, mitoxantrone, and cisplatin for metastatic hepatocellular carcinoma. Cancer 2005; 103:756.
49. Boucher E, Corbinais S, Brissot P, et al. Treatment of hepatocellular carcinoma (HCC) with systemic chemotherapy combining epirubicin, cisplatinum and infusional 5-fluorouracil (ECF regimen). Cancer Chemother Pharmacol 2002; 50:305.
50. Lai CL, Wu PC, Lok AS, et al. Recombinant alpha 2 interferon is superior to doxorubicin for inoperable hepatocellular carcinoma: a prospective randomised trial. Br J Cancer 1989; 60:928.
51. Lai CL, Lau JY, Wu PC, et al. Recombinant interferon-alpha in inoperable hepatocellular carcinoma: a randomized controlled trial. Hepatology 1993; 17:389.
52. Llovet JM, Sala M, Castells L, et al. Randomized controlled trial of interferon treatment for advanced hepatocellular carcinoma. Hepatology 2000; 31:54.
53. Castells A, Bruix J, Bru C, et al. Treatment of hepatocellular carcinoma with tamoxifen: A double-blind placebo-controlled trial in 120 patients. Gastroenterology 1995; 109:917.
54. Tamoxifen in treatment of hepatocellular carcinoma: a randomised controlled trial. CLIP Group (Cancer of the Liver Italian Programme). Lancet 1998; 352:17.
55. Chow PK, Tai BC, Tan CK, et al. High-dose tamoxifen in the treatment of inoperable hepatocellular carcinoma: a multicenter randomized controlled trial. Hepatology 2002; 36:1221.
56. Nowak A, Findlay M, Culjak G, Stockler M. Tamoxifen for hepatocellular carcinoma. Cochrane Database Syst Rev 2004.
57. Villa E, Ferretti I, Grottola A, et al. Hormonal therapy with megestrol in inoperable hepatocellular carcinoma characterized by variant oestrogen receptors. Br J Cancer 2001; 84:881–885.
58. Kouroumalis, E, Skordilis, P, Thermos, K, et al. Treatment of hepatocellular carcinoma with octreotide: A randomised controlled study. Gut 1998; 42:442.
59. Raderer M, Hejna MH, Muller C, et al. Treatment of hepatocellular cancer with the long acting somatostatin analog lanreotide in vitro and in vivo. Int J Oncol 2000; 16:1197.
60. Yuen MF, Poon RT, Lai CL, Fan ST. A randomized placebo-controlled study of long-acting octreotide for the treatment of advanced hepatocellular carcinoma. Hepatology 2002; 36:687.
61. Cheng AL, Yeh KH, Fine RL, et al. Biochemical modulation of doxorubicin by high-dose tamoxifen in the treatment of advanced hepatocellular carcinoma. Hepatogastroenterology 1998; 45:1955.
62. Leung TW, Tang AM, Zee B, et al. Factors predicting response and survival in 149 patients with unresectable hepatocellular carcinoma treated by combination cisplatin, interferon-alpha, doxorubicin and 5-fluorouracil chemotherapy. Cancer 2002; 94:421.
63. Patt YZ, Hassan MM, Lozano RD, et al. Phase II trial of systemic continuous fluorouracil and subcutaneous recombinant interferon alfa-2b for treatment of hepatocellular carcinoma. J Clin Oncol 2003; 21:421.
64. Sakon M, Nagano H, Dono K, et al. Combined intraarterial 5-fluorouracil and subcutaneous interferon-alpha therapy for advanced hepatocellular carcinoma with tumor thrombi in the major portal branches. Cancer 2002; 94:435.
65. Mathurin P, Raynard B, Dharancy S, et al. Meta-analysis: Evaluation of adjuvant therapy after curative liver resection for hepatocellular carcinoma. Aliment Pharmacol Ther 2003; 17(10): 1247–1261.
66. Brans B, De Winter F, Defreyne L, et al. The anti-tumoral activity of neoadjuvant intra-arterial 131I-lipiodol treatment for hepatocellular carcinoma: a pilot study. Cancer Biother Radiopharm 2001; 16:333.

67. Lau WY, Ho SK, Yu SC, et al. Salvage surgery following downstaging of unresectable hepatocellular carcinoma. Ann Surg 2004; 240:299.
68. Sitzmann, JV. Conversion of unresectable to resectable liver cancer: an approach and follow-up study. World J Surg 1995; 19:790.
69. Tang ZY, Uy YQ, Zhou XD, et al. Cytoreduction and sequential resection for surgically verified unresectable hepatocellular carcinoma: evaluation with analysis of 72 patients. World J Surg 1995; 19:784.
70. Yamamoto M, Arii S, Sugahara K, Tobe T. Adjuvant oral chemotherapy to prevent recurrence after curative resection for hepatocellular carcinoma. Br J Surg 1996; 83:336–340.
71. Ono T, Nagasue N Kohno H, et al. Adjuvant chemotherapy with epirubicin and carmofur after radical resection of hepatocellular carcinoma: a prospective randomized study. Semin Oncol 1997; 24(suppl 6):S6-18–S6-25.
72. Kohno H, Nagasue N, Hayashi T, et al. Postoperative adjuvant chemotherapy after radical hepatic resection for hepatocellular carcinoma (HCC). Hepatogastroenterology 1996; 43:1405–1409.
73. Izumi R, Shimizu K, Iyobe T, et al. Postoperative adjuvant hepatic arterial infusion of lipiodol containing anticancer drugs in patients with hepatocellular carcinoma. Hepatology 1994; 20:295–301.
74. Yamasaki S, Hasegawa H, Kinoshita H, et al. A prospective randomized trial of the preventive effect of pre-operative transcatheter arterial embolization against recurrence of hepatocellular carcinoma. Jpn J Cancer Res 1996; 87:206–211.
75. Lau WY, Leung TW, Ho SK, et al. Adjuvant intra-arterial iodine-131-labelled lipiodol for resectable hepatocellular carcinoma: a prospective randomised trial. Lancet 1999; 353:797.
76. Kubo S, Nishiguichi S, Hirohashi K, et al. Effects of long-term postoperative interferon alfa therapy on intrahepatic recurrence after resection of hepatitis C virus-related hepatocellular carcinoma. Ann Intern Med 2001; 134:963.
77. Ikeda K, Arase Y, Saitoh S, et al. Interferon beta prevents recurrence of hepatocellular carcinoma after complete resection or ablation of the primary tumor—a prospective randomized study of hepatitis C virus-related liver cancer. Hepatology 2000; 32:228.
78. Muto Y, Moriwaki H, Ninomiya M, et al. Prevention of second primary tumors by an acyclic retinoid, polyprenoic acid, in patients with hepatocellular carcinoma. Hepatoma Prevention Study Group. N Engl J Med 1996; 334:1561.

27 Carcinoid Tumors

27a. Primary Disease

Graeme J. Poston and Louise E. Jones
Department of Surgery, University Hospital Aintree, Liverpool, U.K.

Carcinoid tumors were first described by Lubarsch in 1888 (1), who found multiple tumors in the distal small bowel of two patients at postmortem examination. However, the term *karzinoide* was not adopted until proposed by Obendorfer in 1907 when he described small bowel tumors that behaved in a more indolent fashion than conventional gastrointestinal carcinomas (2). Carcinoid tumors can arise in any gut-related organ, including the lungs and bronchus (3). Carcinoid tumors arise from neuroendocrine cells, and are characterized by positive reactions to silver stains and neuroendocrine markers including neuron-specific enolase, synaptophysin, and chromogranin (3). Histologically, carcinoid cells contain numerous membrane-bound secretory granules which contain a number of peptide hormones and biogenic amines. These substances include serotonin, which is metabolized to 5-hydroxyindole acetic acid (5-HIAA) and excreted in the urine. Carcinoid tumors have been found to also secrete corticotrophin, histamine, dopamine, substance P, neurotensin, prostaglandins, kallikrein, vasoactive intestinal polypeptide (VIP), gastrin releasing polypeptide (GRP), calcitonin, gastrin, and pancreastatin (3,4).

BIOLOGY

Secretion of these various gastrointestinal hormones varies widely between the anatomical sites of the primary tumor (5). Patients with midgut tumors having significantly higher levels of serotonin, correspond to higher metastatic tumor burden (3,5). Although measurement of daily urinary excretion of 5-HIAA is a universally adopted measurement for both detecting and following metastatic carcinoid disease (3), there are wide variations in daily urinary secretion within individual patients (6). Presently, chromogranin A is considered the best general neuroendocrine serum or plasma marker available for both diagnosis and therapeutic evaluation and is increased in 50% to 100% of patients with various neuroendocrine tumors (7–10). In both the laboratory setting (11) and following surgical resection in patients (12), serum chromogranin A levels relate directly to tumor volume. However, caution must be exercised when assaying for serum levels of chromogranin A since antibodies have been raised to several different and specific regions of the molecule, and only the mid-portion fragment CgA 176–195 (chromacin) is expressed in all tumors (13). Furthermore, there are different analytical properties between the commercially available kits for chromogranin A measurements, giving rise to different performances (14). This fact must be taken into consideration when comparing results from different clinical studies.

As with all neuroendocrine tumors, carcinoid cells express somatostatin receptors (3). Activation of these receptors results in inhibition of adenyl cyclase, so decreasing conductance in voltage-sensitive calcium channels with activation of potassium channels, and stimulation of tyrosine phosphatase activity (15). Somatostatin is an inhibitory neuropeptide, which acts on various targets throughout the body to regulate a variety of physiological functions including inhibition of endocrine and exocrine secretions, modulation of neurotransmission, motor and cognitive functions, inhibition of intestinal motility, absorption of nutrients and ions, vascular contractility, and inhibition of normal and tumor cell proliferation (16). It exerts its effects through interactions with five somatostatin receptor subtypes (sst1–sst5), which belong to the family of G-protein-coupled receptors with seven transmembrane spanning domains and are variably expressed in a variety of tumors including gastro-entero-pancreatic tumors, pituitary adenomas, and carcinoid tumors (16). There are data to show that the sst2 receptor acts as a tumor suppressor (16–18). The clinical significance of these somatostatin receptors on carcinoid tumors will be discussed later.

EPIDEMIOLOGY

The overall age-adjusted incidence rates for carcinoid in Sweden are 2.0 for men and 2.4/100,000 for women in 1983–1998 (19) with similar rates seen in Holland (20). Although one small study reported incidence rates four times higher (21), these large-scale population rates are nearly twice those previously reported (3), and probably reflect better detection of the disease rather than a true increase in prevalence (19). Some have proposed that the higher rates seen in women may reflect a hormonal influence on etiology (19,20). However, U.S. population-based studies, while showing similar overall age-adjusted incidence rates (22,23), have suggested a 3% estimated annual increase in prevalence which may be real (23), rather than better use of diagnostic techniques (19,20,22).

Historically, the appendix has been considered to be the commonest site for primary carcinoid tumors (3). With the improving diagnosis rates, more recent data from the U.S. National Cancer Institute Surveillance Epidemiology and End Results (SEER) Program showed that 24% of carcinoid patients had more than one tumor (22). Within the gastrointestinal tract (which accounts for 54.4% of all carcinoid tumors), the small intestine is the most common site (44.7%), followed by the rectum (19.6%), appendix (16.7%), colon (10.6%), and stomach (7.2%) (23). Furthermore, while earlier reports have suggested good outcomes following surgical resection of appendix carcinoid tumors (24–27), the outlook for such patients is deteriorating with five-year survival as low as 76% (23). This finding may relate to signet ring cell carcinomas being previously diagnosed as carcinoid tumors (28). The overall relative five-year survival was 82% (22), but for site-specific disease five-year survival was stomach 75.1%, small intestine 76.1%, appendix 76.3% and rectum 87.5% (23).

Other anatomic sites include the ovary (which is the single most affected extra-gastrointestinal site) (29,30). Primary organs in which carcinoids are commonly mistaken for some of the more conspicuous endemic tumors, include the oesophagus, pancreas, liver, biliary tract, gallbladder, Meckel's diverticulum, nasopharynx, middle ear, and breast (29,30). Carcinoid tumors with the worst prognosis include those arising in the pancreas (37% five-year survival) and cervix (12–33% three-year survival) (29,30).

GENETICS

Unlike the hereditary multiple endocrine neoplasia (MEN) syndromes, carcinoid has traditionally been considered a sporadic nonhereditary condition (31). However, there have been long-established clinical observations to suggest genetic factors in its etiology. These factors include increased risk of second cancers of colon and rectum, small bowel, oesophagus, and stomach, lung/bronchus, urinary tract, and prostate (32). Furthermore, blacks have almost double the incidence of carcinoid tumors when compared to whites (33). Chromosome 18 deletions are common events in classical midgut carcinoid tumors, with deletions found in 88% (34). Bronchopulmonary carcinoid is more prevalent in patients with MEN-1 (autosomal dominant syndrome associated with neoplasia of pituitary, pancreas, parathyroid, and foregut lineage neuroendocrine tissue), but its occurrence does not portend a poorer prognosis in the majority of those affected (35,36). There are sporadic reports of familial carcinoids (37), and studies in Sweden have suggested that the standardized incidence ratios (SIRs) for carcinoid in the offspring of carcinoid parents were 4.35 for small intestinal and 4.65 for colorectal carcinoids (compared to the age-adjusted incidence rates of carcinoid in Sweden which were 0.76 for men and 1.29/100,000 for women) (38). If both offspring and parents presented with small intestinal carcinoids, then the SIR increased to 12.31 (38). Offspring carcinoids were also increased if parents presented with bladder and other endocrine tumors, the latter association probably due to MEN-1 (38). Risks for secondary cancers were also increased, particularly at sites where familial risks (including small bowel carcinoids) were found (38).

NATURAL HISTORY

It is clear to those who treat carcinoid patients on a regular basis that many patients will live for years with incurable disease, but there is an assumption that this is a relatively low-grade malignancy (39). In contrast to appendix carcinoids, which usually run a relatively benign course, other midgut carcinoids exhibit early mural invasion, early metastases to lymph nodes and liver, and symptoms from hormone oversecretion (39,40). Even minute carcinoids (<5 mm) have a 6% metastasis rate (ranging from 3.7% in the rectum to 17.2% in the jejunum and ileum) (40). Although there is good evidence of significant delays (of up to five years) in determining the correct diagnosis in symptomatic patients (3,41), and extent of disease at diagnosis does impact upon survival, extent is not mitigated by early diagnosis (41). This observation indicates that outcome is dictated more by the biology of the disease, than the timing of diagnosis in the course of the tumor (39–41). The two clinical factors that predominantly predict long-term survival are symptomatic presentation and site of origin (foregut and midgut carcinoids having lower five-year survivals than those with hindgut tumors) (42).

Histochemical markers of a poorer prognosis remain controversial. Some argue that the degree of expression of the proliferation protein Ki-67 and the p53 tumor suppression protein are indicative of a worse prognosis (43,44), while this has not been borne out in other studies (45). Other putative markers of poorer prognosis include the p21 oncoprotein (45) and human chorionic gonadotrophin free-beta chain (46). Of perhaps more therapeutic interest is the observation that c-kit proto-oncogene, a tyrosine kinase inhibitor, is overexpressed in a subset of small cell lung cancers (47) and colonic (48) and other (49,50) neuroendocrine carcinomas. This finding raises the possibility of future therapeutic strategies employing the newly available tyrosine kinase inhibitors (47–50).

Carcinoid tumors are notorious for their association with fibrosis (51), which occurs in peritumoral tissues, heart, and lungs (3,51). Carcinoid heart disease occurs in two-thirds of patients with the carcinoid syndrome (52). Tricuspid valvular disease is a common manifestation of the midgut carcinoid syndrome and advanced changes are associated with poorer long-term survival (53–56). Echocardiography is now a standard investigation in the work-up of patients with carcinoid syndrome and has a high predictive value when assessing prognosis (53,57). The tricuspid valve is most frequently affected, and the most common dysfunctional state is regurgitation (58). The pulmonary valve is the second most frequently affected, but in contrast carcinoid tends to cause stenosis rather than regurgitation (58). In all cases, valve dysfunction is due to the presence of thickened carcinoid plaques, composed of myofibroblast proliferation and collagen deposition (58). However, the results of timely surgical valve replacement can improve both quality and length of life significantly (level 4 evidence) (3,59,60).

Factors associated with progression of carcinoid heart disease include higher elevations of serum serotonin levels (and therefore increased 24-hour urinary 5-HIAA excretion) (61). The exact causal relationship between elevated serotonin and carcinoid heart disease remains unclear but may be due to increased transforming growth factor-1 (TGF-1) expression and activity within the interstitial cells of the heart valves, mediated indirectly by increased phospholipase C activity (62,63). An alternate putative pathway for the effect of serotonin on fibroblasts of the right side heart valves is indirectly through elevated levels of atrial natriuretic peptide, which in turn leads to increased TGF-beta and fibroblast growth factor (FGF) (64). It is more likely that the mechanism that drives fibrosis in carcinoid mesenteric sclerosis and angiopathy is more complex, probably working through a host of agents including TGF-beta-3, nerve growth factor (NGF)-2, FGF-2, insulin-like growth factor (IGF), and other factors including bone morphogenic protein (BMP)-4 (65), and the epidermal growth factor (EGF)/ErbB1 receptor (66).

PRIMARY CARCINOID TUMORS

Bronchial Carcinoid

True bronchial carcinoids account for approximately 2% of primary lung tumors (67,68), and represent the best differentiated form of a spectrum of pulmonary neuroendocrine tumors (small cell being the least differentiated) (69). They probably arise in the neuroendocrine Kulchitzky cells found within the bronchial mucosa (70). Most patients present in the fifth decade of life (68) with atypical chest symptoms or incidental finding on a routine chest X-ray (69,71). Classical carcinoid syndrome is rare in these patients and only seen with established liver metastases (69,72). If anatomically feasible, then conservative resection (wedge or segmental) is the treatment of choice (69,73). Factors associated with a decreased disease-free (and overall) survival include atypical histological appearance, presence of multicentric tumorlets, and lymph node involvement (69,74,75). While patients whose lymphatic spread is confined to the N1 basin have a small chance of cure after surgical resection, those patients with N2 nodal involvement face a dismal prognosis (22% survival at five years, evidence level 4) (75).

Gastric Carcinoid

Gastric carcinoid neoplasms are uncommon and make up approximately 1% of all gastric tumors (76). However, data are emerging that show that the true incidence has been increasing over the last 50 years from 0.3% to 1.7%, with the greatest increase seen in white females (3,77). Interestingly, the five-year survival from the SEER data for gastric carcinoids has risen from 51% to 63% over the same five decades (77). Clearly, there are multifactorial influences on these changes, including greater endoscopic surveillance and more sophisticated pathological evaluation (3,77). Sixty percent are <2 cm at the time of presentation and these smaller tumors are usually multiple and frequently associated with chronic gastritis type A (CAG-A) (78,79). Metastases are uncommon (15%) and usually associated with larger, solitary, sporadic tumors (78,79). Similarly, elevated serotonin levels are found in 22%, with true carcinoid syndrome reported in only 4% (78).

Gastric carcinoid tumors can be separated into three distinct groups on the basis of clinical and histopathological findings, and these groupings will determine subsequent management. These groupings are: those associated with CAG-A; those linked with the Zollinger-Ellison (ZE) syndrome; and those arising as solitary, usually large, sporadic tumors (3). It is likely that up to 75% of gastric carcinoid tumors are associated with CAG-A, usually linked to pernicious anaemia (80–87). This condition, because of the link to pernicious anaemia, is more frequently found in women, with a peak incidence in the sixth and seventh decades (80,84,85). These CAG-A-related carcinoids are frequently an incidental finding during gastroscopic investigation of indigestion, frequently <1 cm in size and multiple, and nearly always located in the gastric body and fundus (80,84,85). CAG-A is associated with hypochlorhydria which results in hypergastrinemia (86), and this resulting oversecretion of gastrin then causes hyperplasia of the enterochromaffin-like cells of the gastric mucosa (3,86). There are a number of reports of CAG-A-associated carcinoids being surrounded by areas of enterochromaffin-like cell hyperplasia (80,82,88,89). Interestingly, there are as yet no reports of proton pump inhibitor-induced hypergastrinemia linked to gastric carcinoid formation in humans. Although some have advocated endoscopic resection of these gastric microcarcinoids (3), patients with this condition can be managed safely using a conservative approach (90). These tumors do not metastasize, and the only long-term problem is the potential for chronic blood loss, compounding the potential iron deficiency anemia to which they are already prone. Were this to occur, then simple antrectomy (removing the source of gastrin production) will lead to regression of the fundic carcinoids within a year of surgery (evidence level 4) (3,90,91).

Less than 10% of gastric carcinoid tumors are associated with the ZE syndrome, occurring exclusively in patients with MEN-1 (80). The appropriate treatment of gastric carcinoids in this condition mirrors that of those seen in CAG-A (3,91). If the gastrinoma(s) are excised surgically (bearing in mind their malignant potential), then the carcinoids will regress spontaneously (91). Up to 15% of gastric carcinoids occur sporadically (3). These tumors are more common in men and arise in normally appearing mucosa (80). They are usually solitary, have a higher propensity to metastasize (the majority already metastatic at diagnosis), more frequently associated with the carcinoid syndrome, and so the prognosis is poorer at presentation (3). If the disease is confined to the stomach and adjacent lymph nodes, then radical gastrectomy (as for any other gastric carcinoma), is the appropriate treatment strategy (92). Data are emerging that suggest survival benefit following liver resection in patients with metastatic sporadic gastric carcinoid (93), but presently we must await the outcome of this approach from other centers.

Pancreato-Duodenal Carcinoids

Pancreatic carcinoids account for just over 1% of all cases (94), and exhibit a far higher metastatic rate than all other carcinoids apart from those arising in the ileo-cecal region (94). Five-year survival is extremely less (29%) when compared to other sites of carcinoid tumors (23–27,94). Since these tumors behave more like noncarcinoid pancreatic neuroendocrine tumors, the surgical management should therefore be analogous to that for exocrine pancreatic carcinoma (95). Lymph node metastases and distant metastases predict poorer outcome by univariate analysis, but only distant metastases retain significance on multivariate analysis (95). On the other hand, duodenal carcinoids are relatively indolent, low-grade malignancies (96). Many are detected as incidental microscopic findings within random duodenal biopsies, and these should simply be monitored by regular endoscopic review. The average macrotumor size is <2 cm, and is accompanied by a relatively low metastatic rate (27%) and high five-year survival rate (83%) (96). Carcinoid syndrome developing from duodenal carcinoids is extremely uncommon (96).

Small Bowel Carcinoid

The commonest site for carcinoid tumors is in the small bowel, and these account for roughly one-third of all small bowel tumors (3,23,97–99). These tumors are most frequently located in the terminal ileum and are usually multicentric (100). Patients with these tumors are most frequently diagnosed in their sixth and seventh decades (97,101), and usually after a history of long-standing symptoms, frequently misdiagnosed as irritable bowel syndrome (101). Metastases to mesenteric lymph nodes occur early in the course of the disease, and may be extremely large at presentation (101). Mesenteric lymphatic metastases are associated with marked mesenteric fibrosis and varices which may preclude safe surgical resection, so necessitating enteric by-pass surgery to relieve intestinal obstruction (101,102). These mesenteric metastases may be of sufficient mass to cause flushing and even the full carcinoid syndrome, without overt evidence of metastatic disease to the liver (103,104).

Five- and 10-year survival following diagnosis of small bowel carcinoid tumors are 67% and 54%, respectively (105), although median survival is better (7.4 years) for those who are able to undergo resection rather than by-pass (four years) of their primary tumors (106). Whenever possible, radical surgical resection should be attempted, and in the absence of liver metastases can be potentially curative in up to 90% of cases (evidence level 4) (107,108).

Appendix Carcinoids

Unlike small bowel carcinoids which arise from serotonin-producing intraepithelial neuroendocrine cells (100,109), appendix carcinoids appear to arise from subepithelial neuroendocrine cells within the lamina propria (110,111). Although carcinoids are the most common tumor to involve the appendix (112), the appendix is not the most frequent site for the development of carcinoids (vide supra). However, they are the most frequently occurring carcinoid tumors in children (113). Most (75%) tumors are located in the distal third of the appendix, and less than 10% are found near the base (112).

The most important prognostic factor is tumor size (3,112–118). Metastases from tumors <1 cm in size are extremely rare (116). Additional factors include vascular and lymphatic invasion, and tumors adjacent to the base of the appendix (117,118). Those with tumors <1 cm away from the base of the appendix (usually a coincidental finding following appendicectomy for appendicitis) should be considered cured by appendicectomy (3,114,117,118). In younger patients, consideration should be given to subsequent right hemicolectomy in patients with tumors between 1 and 2 cm, those with lymphatic and/or vascular invasion, and those with tumors close to the base of the appendix (3,114,117,118). All patients found to have a carcinoid tumor >2 cm in size, or involving the appendix base resection margin, should be managed as carcinoma of the appendix, and offered right hemicolectomy to reduce the risk of disease progression (3,113–118) (grade C recommendation based on level 4 evidence). Five-year survival is 94% for those with disease confined microscopically to the appendix, 85% for those with N1 lymph node metastases, but only 35% for those with distant (peritoneal and liver) disease (76).

Colorectal Carcinoids

Carcinoids constitute 1% of colorectal tumors (76), and arise from serotonin-producing neuroendocrine epithelial cells (3,76). Interestingly, in contrast to small bowel and colonic carcinoids, rectal carcinoids usually contain glucagons and glycentin-related peptides, instead of serotonin (119). Colorectal carcinoids are a disease of later life, with most of them presenting in the sixth and seventh decades of life (76,120). More carcinoids arising in the large bowel are benign adenomatous polyps at presentation (120–122), in contrast to noncarcinoid colorectal tumors where the majority are nearly all carcinomas at the time of detection (123). Size (>2 cm) is the single most important predictive determinant of metastatic disease (121,124,125).

Small (<1 cm), benign polypoid colorectal carcinoid tumors can be managed safely by endoscopic snaring (3,121,126). Tumors greater than 2 cm in size should be regarded as carcinomas until proven otherwise, and managed accordingly (124,125). However, the management of colorectal carcinoids between 1 and 2 cm in size, remains controversial, and although several authors have advocated local excision, others advise caution (3,124–127). Factors associated with poorer prognosis (and therefore advocating a more radical approach to treatment) include muscular invasion, symptomatic at presentation, and tumor ulceration (124–127). Five-year survival rates are 81% for those with local disease, 47% with lymph node metastases, but only 18% for those with distant disease (76).

REFERENCES

1. Lubarsch O. Ueber den primaren Krebs des Ileum, nebst Bemerkungen uber das gleichzeitige Vorkommen von Krebs und Tuberkolose. Virchows Arch 1888; 111:280–317.
2. Obendorfer S. Karzinoide Tumoren des Dunndarms. Frank Z Pathol 1907; 1:425–429.
3. Kulke MH, Mayer RJ. Carcinoid tumors. New Engl J Med 1999; 340:858–867.
4. Calhoun K, Toth-Fejel S, Cheek J, Pommier R. Serum peptide profiles in patients with carcinoid tumors. Am J Surg 2003; 186:28–31.
5. Onaitis MW, Kirshbom PM, Hayward TZ, et al. Gastrointestinal carcinoids: characterization by site of origin and hormone production. Ann Surg 2000; 232:549–556.
6. Zuetenhorst JM, Korse CM, Bonfrer JM, et al. Daily cyclic changes in the urinary excretion of 5-hydroxyindoleacetic acid in patients with carcinoid tumors. Clin Chem 2004; 50:1634–1639.
7. Eriksson B, Oberg K, Stridsberg M. Tumor markers in neuroendocrine tumors. Digestion 2000; 62(S1):33–38.
8. Tomassetti P, Migliori M, Simoni P, et al. Diagnostic value of plasma chromogranin A in neuroendocrine tumours. Eur J Gastroenterol Hepatol 2001; 13:55–58.
9. Seregni E, Ferrari L, Bajetta E, et al. Clinical significance of blood chromogranin A measurement in neuroendocrine tumours. Ann Oncol 2001; 12(S2):S69–S72.
10. Nehar D, Lombard-Bohas C, Olivieri S, et al. Interest of chromogranin A for diagnosis and follow-up of endocrine tumours. Clin Endocrinol 2004; 60:644–652.
11. Kolby L, Bernhardt P, Sward C, et al. Chromogranin A as a determinant of midgut carcinoid tumour volume. Regul Pept 2004; 120:269–273.
12. Sondenaa K, Sen J, Heinle F, et al. Chromogranin A, a marker of the therapeutic success of resection of neuroendocrine liver metastases: preliminary report. World J Surg 2004; 28:890–895.
13. Portel-Gomes GM, Grimelius L, Johansson H, et al. Chromogranin A in human neuroendocrine tumors: an immunohistochemical study with region-specific antibodies. Am J Surg Pathol 2001; 25:1261–1267.
14. Stridsberg M, Eriksson B, Oberg K, Janson ET. A comparison between three commercial kits for chromogranin A measurements. J Endocrinol 2003; 177:337–341.
15. Reisine T, Bell G. Molecular biology of somatostatin receptors. Endocrinol Rev 1995; 16:427–442.
16. Bousquet C, Guillermet J, Vernejoul F, et al. Somatostatin receptors and regulation of cell proliferation. Dig Liver Dis 2004; 36(S1):S2–S7.
17. Hofland LJ, lamberts SW. Somatostatin receptor subtype expression in human tumors. Ann Oncol 2001; 12(S2):S31–S36.

18. Kulaksiz H, Eissele R, Rossler D, et al. Identification of somatostatin receptor subtypes 1, 2A, 3 and 5 in neuroendocrine tumours with specific antibodies. Gut 2002; 50:52–60.
19. Hemminki K, Li X. Incidence trends and risk factors of carcinoid tumors: a nationwide epidemiologic study from Sweden. Cancer 2001; 92:2204–2210.
20. Quaedvlieg PF, Visser O, Lamers CB, et al. Epidemiology and survival with carcinoid disease in The Netherlands. An epidemiological study with 2391 patients. Ann Oncol 2001; 12:1295–1300.
21. Berge T, Linnell F. Carcinoid tumours: frequency in a defined population during a 12-year period. Acta Pathol Microbiol Scand (A) 1976; 84:322–330.
22. Crocetti E, Paci E. Malignant carcinoids in the USA, SEER 1992–1999. An epidemiological study with 6830 cases. Eur J Cancer Prev 2003; 12:191–194.
23. Maggard MA, O'Connell JB, Ko CY. Updated population-based review of carcinoid tumors. Ann Surg 2004; 240:117–122.
24. Anderson JR, Wilson BG. Carcinoid tumours of the appendix. Br J Surg 1985; 72:545–546.
25. MacGillivray DC, Heaton RB, Rushin JM, Cruess DF. Distant metastasis from a carcinoid tumor of the appendix less than one centimetre in size. Surgery 1992; 111:466–471.
26. Parkes SE, Muir KR, Al Sheyyab M, et al. Carcinoid tumours of the appendix in children 1957–1986: incidence, treatment and outcomes. Br J Surg 1993; 80:502–504.
27. Modlin IM, Kidd M, Latich I, et al. Current status of gastrointestinal carcinoids. Gastroenterology 2005; 128:1717–1751.
28. McCusker ME, Cote TR, Clegg LX, Sobin LH. Primary malignant neoplasms of the appendix: a population-based study from the surveillance, epidemiology and end-results program, 1973–1998. Cancer 2002; 94:3307–3312.
29. Modlin IM, Lye KD, Kidd M. A 5-decade analysis of 13,715 carcinoid tumors. Cancer 2003; 97:934–959.
30. Modlin IM, Shapiro MD, Kidd M. An anaysis of rare carcinoid tumors: clarifying these clinical conumdrums. World J Surg 2005; 29:92–101.
31. Loetlela PD, Jauch A, Holtgreve-Grez H, Thakker RV. Genetics of neuroendocrine and carcinoid tumours. Endocr Relat Cancer 2003; 10:437–450.
32. Tichansky DS, Cagir B, Borrazzo F, et al. Risk of second cancers in patients with colorectal carcinoids. Dis Colon Rectum 2002; 45:91–97.
33. Haselkorn T, Whittemore AS, Lilienfield DE. Incidence of small bowel cancer in the United States and worldwide: geographic, temporal, and racial differences. Cancer Causes Control 2005; 16:781–787.
34. Lollgen RM, Hessman O, Szabo E, et al. Chromosome 18 deletions are common events in classical midgut carcinoid tumors. Int J Cancer 2001; 92:812–815.
35. Sachithanandan N, Harle RS, Burgess JR. Bronchopulmonary carcinoid in multiple endocrine neoplasia type 1. Cancer 2005; 103:509–515.
36. Oliviera AM, Tazelaar HD, Wentzlaff KA, et al. Familial pulmonary carcinoid tumors. Cancer 2001; 91:2104–2109.
37. Pal T, Liede A, Mitchell M, et al. Intestinal carcinoid tumours in a father and a daughter. Can J Gastroenterol 2001; 15:405–409.
38. Hemminki K, Li X. Familial carcinoid tumors and subsequent cancers: a nationwide epidemiologic study from Sweden. Int J Cancer 2001; 94:444–448.
39. Mignon M. Natural history of neuroendocrine enteropancreatic tumors. Digestion 2000; 62:51–58.
40. Soga J. Early-stage carcinoids of the gastrointestinal tract: an analysis of 1914 reported cases. Cancer 2005; 103:1587–1595.
41. Toth-Fejel S, Pommier RF. Relationship among delay of diagnosis, extent of disease, and survival in patients with abdominal carcinoid tumors. Am J Surg 2004; 187:575–579.
42. Van Gompel JJ, Sipplel RS, Warner TF, Chen H. Gastrointestinal carcinoid tumors: factors that predict outcome. World J Surg 2004; 28:387–392.
43. Rorstad O. Prognostic indicators for carcinoid neuroendocrine tumors of the gastrointestinal tract. J Surg Oncol 2005; 89:151–160.
44. Sokmensuer C, Gedikoglu G, Uzunalimoglu B. Importance of proliferation markers in gastrointestinal carcinoid tumors: a clinicopathologic study. Hepatogastroenterology 2001; 48:720–723.
45. Kawahara M, Kammori M, Kanauchi H, et al. Immunohistochemical prognostic indicators of gastrointestinal carcinoid tumours. Eur J Surg Oncol 2002; 28:140–146.
46. Rock E, Levy D, Stuart K, et al. Human chorionic gonadotrophin free beta chain is a negative prognostic indicator in malignant carcinoid. J Clin Oncol 2005; 23(16S):875s.
47. Butnor KJ, Burchette JL, Sporn TA, et al. The spectrum of kit (CD117) immunoreactivity in lung and pleural tumors: a study of 96 cases using a single-source antibody with a review of the literature. Arch Pathol Lab Med 2004; 128:538–553.
48. Akintola-Ogunremi O, Pfeifer JD, Tan BR, et al. Analysis of protein expression and gene mutation of c-kit in colorectal neuroendocrine carcinomas. Am J Surg Pathol 2003; 27:1551–1558.
49. Della-Torre S, Bajetta E, Ferrari L, et al. Immunostaining for c-kit (CD117) in well differentiated and poorly differentiated neuroendocrine tumors. Proc ASCO 2004; 23:889.
50. Erler B, Finch M, Hodges A, et al. cd117 overexpression in neuroendocrine carcinomas. Proc ASCO 2004; 23:854.

51. Modlin IM, Shapiro MD, Kidd M. Carcinoid tumors and fibrosis: an association with no explanation. Am J Gastroenterol 2004; 99:2466–2478.
52. Lundin L, Norheim I, Landelius J, et al. Carcinoid heart disease: relationship of circulating vasoactive substances to ultrasound detectable cardiac abnormalities. Circulation 1988; 77:264–269.
53. Westberg G, Wangberg B, Ahlman H, et al. Prediction of prognosis by echocardiography in patients with midgut carcinoid syndrome. Br J Surg 2001; 88:865–872.
54. Thatipelli MR, Uber PA, Mehra MR. Isolated tricuspid stenosis and heart failure: a focus on carcinoid heart disease. Congest Heart Fail 2003; 9:294–296.
55. Quaedvlieg PF, Lamers CB, Taal BG. Carcinoid heart disease: an update. Scand J Gastroenterol Suppl 2002; 236:66–71.
56. Meijer WC, van Veldhuisen DJ, Kema IP, et al. Cardiovascular abnormalities in patients with a carcinoid syndrome. Neth J Med 2002; 60:10–16.
57. Di Luzio S, Rigolin VH. Carcinoid heart disease. Curr Treat Options Cardiovasc Med 2000; 2:399–406.
58. Simula DV, Edwards WD, Tazelaar HD, et al. Surgical pathology of carcinoid heart disease: a study of 139 valves from 75 patients spanning 20 years. Mayo Clin Proc 2002; 77:139–147.
59. Connolly HM, Schaff HV, Mullany CJ, et al. Surgical management of left-sided carcinoid heart disease. Circulation 2001; 104:136–140.
60. Connolly HM, Schaff HV, Mullany CJ, et al. Carcinoid heart disease: impact of pulmonary valve replacement in right ventricular function and remodelling. Circulation 2002; 106:151–156.
61. Moller JE, Connolly HM, Rubin J, et al. Factors associated with progression of carcinoid heart disease. N Engl J Med 2003; 348:1005–4015.
62. Jian B, Xu J, Connolly J, et al. Serotonin mechanisms in heart valve disease I: serotonin-induced up-regulation of transforming growth factor-beta 1 via G-protein signal transduction in aortic valve interstitial cells. Am J Pathol 2002; 161:2111–2121.
63. Xu J, Jian B, Chu R, et al. Serotonin mechanisms in heart valve disease II: the 5-HT2 receptor and its signalling pathway in aortic valve interstitial cells. Am J Pathol 2002; 161:2209–2218.
64. Zuetenhorst JM, Bonfrer JM, Korse CM, et al. Carcinoid heart disease: the role of urinary 5-hydroxyindoleacetic acid excretion and plasma levels of atrial natriuretic peptide, transforming growth factor-beta and fibroblast growth factor. Cancer 2003; 97:1609–1615.
65. Zhang PJ, Furth EE, Cai X, et al. The role of beta-catenin, TGF beta 3, NGF2, FGF2, IGFR2 and BMP4 in the pathogenesis of mesenteric sclerosis and angiopathy in midgut carcinoids. Hum Pathol 2004; 35:670–674.
66. Shworak NM. Angiogenic modulators in valve development and disease: does valvular disease recapitulate developmental signalling pathways? Curr Opin Cardiol 2004; 19:140–146.
67. Harpole DH Jr, Feldman JM, Buchanan S, et al. Bronchial carcinoid tumors: a retrospective analysis of 126 patients. Ann Thorac Surg 1992; 54:50–55.
68. Vadasz P, Palffy G, Egervary M, Schaff Z. Diagnosis and treatment of bronchial casrcinoid tumors: clinical and pathological review of 120 operated patients. Eur J Cardiothorac Surg 1993; 7:8–11.
69. Chughtai TS, Morin JE, Sheiner NM, et al. Bronchial carcinoid: twenty years' experience defines a selective surgical approach. Surgery 1997; 122:801–808.
70. Paladagu RR, Benfield JR, Pak HY, et al. Broncho-pulmonary Kulchitzky cell carcinomas: a new classification scheme for typical and atypical carcinoids. Cancer 1985; 55:1303–1311.
71. Okike N, Bernatz PE, Woolner LB. Carcinoid tumors of the lung. Ann Thorac Surg 1976; 22: 270–277.
72. McCaughan BC, Martini N, Bains MS. Bronchial carcinoids: review of 124 cases. J Thorac Cardiovasc Surg 1985; 89:8–17.
73. Dusmet ME, McKneally MF. Pulmonary and thymic carcinoid tumors. World J Surg 1996; 20:189–195.
74. Daddi N, Ferolla P, Urbani M, et al. Surgical treatment of neuroendocrine tumors of the lung. Eur J Cardiothorac Surg 2004; 26:813–817.
75. Cardillo G, Sera F, Di Martino M, et al. Bronchial carcinoid tumors: nodal status and long-term survival after resection. Ann Thorac Surg 2004; 77:1781–1785.
76. Modlin IM, Sandor A. An analysis of 8305 cases of carcinoid tumors. Cancer 1997; 79:813–829.
77. Modlin IM, Lye KD, Kidd M. A 50-year analysis of 562 gastric carcinoids: small tumor or larger problem? Am J Gastroenterol 2004; 99:23–32.
78. Soga J. Gastric carcinoids: a statistical evaluation of 1,094 cases collected from the literature. Surg Today 1997; 27:892–901.
79. Gencosmanoglu R, Sen-Oran E, Kurtkaya-Yapicier O, et al. Gastric polypoid lesions: analysis of 150 endoscopic polypectomy specimens from 91 patients. World J Gastroenterol 2003; 9:2236–2239.
80. Rindi G, Bordi C, Rappel S, et al. Gastric carcinoids and neuroendocrine carcinomas: pathogenesis, pathology, and behaviour. World J Surg 1996; 20:168–172.
81. Modlin IM, Gilligan CJ, Lawton GP, et al. Gastric carcinoids: the Yale experience. Arch Surg 1995; 130:255–256.
82. Bordi C, Yu JY, Baggi MT, et al. Gastric carcinoids and their precursor lesions: a histologic and immunohistochemical study of 23 cases. Cancer 1991; 67:663–672.

83. Rindi G, Luinetti O, Cornaggia M, et al. Three sub-types of gastric argyrophil carcinoid and the gastric neuroendocrine carcinoma: a clinico-pathologic study. Gastroentology 1993; 104: 994–1006.
84. Thomas RM, Baybick JH, El-Sayed AM, Sobin LH. Gastric carcinoids: an immunohistochemical and clinicopathologic study of 104 patients. Cancer 1994; 73:2053–2058.
85. Gough DB, Thompson GB, Crotty TB, et al. Diverse clinical and pathologic features of hypergastrinemia. World J Surg 1994; 18:473–479.
86. Moses RE, Frank BB, Leavitt M, Miller R. The syndrome of type A chronic atrophic gastritis, pernicious anemia, and multiple gastric carcinoids. J Clin Gastroenterol 1986; 8:61–65.
87. Jordan PH Jr, Barroso A, Sweeney J. Gastric carcinoids in patients with hypergastrinemia. J Am Coll Surg 2004; 199:552–555.
88. Sjoblom SM, Sipponnen P, Karonen SL, Jarvinen HJ. Mucosal argyrophil endocrine cells in pernicious anaemia and upper gastrointestinal carcinoid tumours. J Clin Pathol 1989; 42:371–377.
89. Solcia E, Fiocca R, Villani L, et al. Morphology and pathogenesis of endocrine hyperplasia, precarcinoid lesions, and carcinoids arising in chronic atrophic gastritis. Scand J Gastroenterol Suppl 1991; 180:146–159.
90. Hosokawa O, Kaizaki Y, Hattori M, et al. Long-term follow up of patients with multiple gastric carcinoids associated with type A gastritis. Gastric Cancer 2005; 8:42–46.
91. Richards ML, Gauger P, Thompson NW, Giordano TJ. Regression of type II gastric carcinoids in multiple endocrine neoplasia type 1 patients with Zollinger-Ellison syndrome after surgical excision of all gastrinomas. World J Surg 2004; 28:652–658.
92. Boudreaux JP, Putty B, Frey DJ, et al. Surgical treatment of advanced-stage carcinoid tumours: lessons learned. Ann Surg 2005; 241:845–846.
93. Wu FS, Yu XF, Teng LS, Ma ZM. Malignant gastric carcinoids with liver metastasis. Hepatobiliary Pancreat Dis Int 2004; 3:406–410.
94. Soga J. Carcinoids of the pancreas. Cancer 2005; 104:1180–1187.
95. Jarufe NP, Coldham C, Orug T, et al. Neuroendocrine tumours of the pancreas: predictors of survival after surgical treatment. Dig Surg 2005; 22:157–162.
96. Soga J. Endocrinocarcinokas (carcinoids and their variants) of the duodenum. An evaluation of 927 cases. J Exp Clin Cancer Res 2003; 22:349–363.
97. Barclay TH, Schapira DV. Malignant tumors of the small intestine. Cancer 1983; 51:878–881.
98. Ito H, Perez A, Brooks DC, et al. Surgical treatment of small bowel cancer: a 20-year single institution experience. J Gastrointest Surg 2003; 7:925–930.
99. Rangiah DS, Cox M, Richardson M, et al. Small bowel tumours: a 10 year experience in four Sydney teaching hospitals. ANZ J Surg 2004; 74:788–792.
100. Lundqvist M, Wilander E. A study of the histpopathogenesis of carcinoid tumors of the small intestine and appendix. Cancer 1987; 60:201–216.
101. Makridis C, Oberg K, Juhlin C, et al. Surgical treatment of midgut carcinoid tumors. World J Surg 1990; 14:377–385.
102. Akerstrom G, Hellman P, Hessman O, Osmak L. Management of midgut carcinoids. J Surg Oncol 2005; 89:161–169.
103. Sonnet S, Wiesner W. Flush symptoms caused by a mesenteric carcinoid without liver metastases. JBR-BTR 2002; 85:254–256.
104. Cooper MA, Smith A, Khalifa M. Carcinoid syndrome from gastrointestinal carcinoid tumour without distant metastases. J Clin Gastroenterol 2002; 35:106–107.
105. Zar N, Garmo H, Holmberg L, et al. Long-term survival of patients with small intestinal carcinoid tumors. World J Surg 2004; 28:1163–1168.
106. Hellman P, Lundstrom T, Ohrvall U, et al. Effect of surgery on the outcome of midgut carcinoid disease with lymph node and liver metastases. World J Surg 2002; 26:991–997.
107. Schindl M, Kaczirek K, Passler C, et al. Treatment of small intestinal neuroendocrine tumors: is an extended multimodal approach justified? World J Surg 2002; 26:976–984.
108. Talamonti MS, Goetz LH, Rao S, Joehl RJ. Primary cancers of the small bowel: analysis of prognostic factors and results of surgical management. Arch Surg 2002; 137:564–570.
109. Moyana TN, Satkunam N. A comparative immunohistochemical study of jejunoileal and appendiceal carcinoids: implications for histogenesis and pathogenesis. Cancer 1992; 70:1081–1088.
110. Lundqvist M, Wilander E. Subepithelial neuroendocrine cells and carcinoid tumours of the human small intestine and appendix: a comparative immunohistochemical study with regard to serotonin, neuron-specific enolase and S-100 protein reactivity. J Pathol 1986; 148:141–147.
111. Shaw PA. Carcinoid tumours of the appendix are different. J Pathol 1990; 612:189–190.
112. Moertel CG, Dockerty MB, Judd ES. Carcinoid tumors of the vermiform appendix. Cancer 1968; 21:270–278.
113. Parkes SE, Muir KR, Al Sheyyab M, et al. Carcinoid tumours of the appendix in children 1957–1986: incidence, treatment and outcome. Br J Surg 1993; 80:502–504.
114. Anderson JR, Wilson BG. Carcinoid tumours of the appendix. Br J Surg 1985; 72:545–546.

115. Thirlby R, Kasper CS, Jones RC. Metastatic carcinoid of the appendix: report of a case and review of the literature. Dis Colon Rectum 1984; 27:42–46.
116. MacGillivray DC, Heaton RB, Rushin JM, Cruess DF. Distant metastases from a carcinoid tumor of the appendix less than one centimetre in size. Surgery 1992; 111:466–471.
117. Varisco B, McAlvin B, Dias J, Franga D. Adenocarcinoid of the appendix: is right hemicolectomy necessary? A meta-analysis of retrospective chart reviews. Am J Surg 2004; 70:593–599.
118. Bucher P, Gervaz P, Ris F, et al. Surgical treatment of appendiceal adenocarcnoid (goblet cell carcinoid). World J Surg 2005; pub online on Sept 8, 2005.
119. Capella C, Heitz PU, Hofler H, et al. Revised classification of neuroendocrine tumours of the lung, pancreas and gut. Virchows Arch 1995; 425:457–460.
120. Rosenberg JM, Welch JP. Carcinoid tumors of the colon: a study of 72 patients. Am J Surg 1985; 149:775–779.
121. Burke M, Shepherd N, Mann CV. Carcinoid tumours of the rectum and anus. Br J Surg 1987; 74: 358–361.
122. Ballantyne GH, Savoca PE, Flannery JT, et al. Incidence and mortality of carcinoids of the colon: data from the Connecticut Tumor Registry. Cancer 1992; 69:2400–2405.
123. Bernick PE, Klimstra DS, Shia J, et al. Neuroendocrine carcinomas of the colon and rectum. Dis Colon Rectum 2004; 47:163–169.
124. Soga J. Carcinoids of the rectum: tumors of the carcinod family. Acta Med Biol 1982; 29:157–201.
125. Naunheim KS, Zeitels J, Kaplan EL, et al. Rectal carcinoid tumors—treatment and prognosis. Surgery 1983; 94:670–676.
126. Kobayashi K, Katsumata T, Yoshizawa S, et al. Indications for endoscopic polypectomy for rectal carcinoids and clinical usefulness of endoscopic ultrasonography. Dis Colon Rectum 2005; 48:285–291.
127. Jetmore AB, Ray JE, Gathright JB Jr, et al. Rectal carcinoids: the most frequent carcinoid tumor. Dis Colon Rectum 1992; 35:717–725.

27b. Carcinoid Syndrome

Graeme J. Poston and Louise E. Jones
Department of Surgery, University Hospital Aintree, Liverpool, U.K.

The clinical course of patients with nonresectable metastatic carcinoid is highly variable and largely unpredictable (1–4). Patients with high tumor burden can remain relatively asymptomatic for years, totally oblivious to their disease. Others with minimal residual (but nonresectable) disease in the small-bowel mesentery can suffer all the symptoms of the carcinoid syndrome without having disease in the liver (vide supra). However, the majority of patients with carcinoid metastatic to the liver will exhibit at least some, if not all of the symptoms of the carcinoid syndrome (1–4). These symptoms include facial and sometimes torso flushing which may progress to rosacea and scleroderma (5), and may include the cutaneous manifestations of pellagra (5). Other symptoms include diarrhea, breathlessness, and wheezing and may be precipitated by certain foods including alcohol and chocolate. The exact hormonal mechanism of these symptoms remains unknown.

Advanced carcinoid syndrome is characterized by the manifestation of fibrosis (6). This fibrosis affects the small bowel mesentery (where it can cause intestinal obstruction), the lungs (exacerbating carcinoid lung disease) and most importantly the heart, and in particular right side valves (6). As patients with carcinoid now live longer than heretofore (vide infra), cardiac manifestations now affect two-thirds of patients and are proving to cause the terminal events (1,4,6–9). Although historically, valve replacement surgery in symptomatic carcinoid patients has been associated with a relatively higher operative mortality than that seen in noncarcinoid patients (10–16), those who do survive gain significant symptom improvement and quality-of- life (QOL) (17,18).

DETECTING METASTATIC DISEASE

In many cases, metastatic disease will be overt at presentation (1,4). Patients with known primary carcinoid tumors will develop symptoms of the carcinoid syndrome, or are found to have metastases at investigation or laparotomy for their primary tumor. Following apparently curative surgery for primary carcinoid tumor(s), it is good practice to establish radiologic and biochemical baseline parameters with which comparisons can be made as symptoms evolve in the future. We would advocate a full fasting gut-hormone screen (including chromogranin A), 24-hour urine for 5-hydroxyindoleacetic acid (5-HIAA), liver ultrasound scan, and, if economically feasible, radiolabeled somatostatin analog scintigraphy (vide infra).

Ultrasound scanning is relatively cheap, noninvasive, and widely available but operator-dependent. Endoscopic ultrasound is useful in planning treatment for primary luminal gut carcinoids (19) and locating pancreatic neuroendocrine tumors (20). Recent technological advances in computerized tomography (CT) and magnetic resonance imaging (MRI), coupled with developments in scintigraphy using somatostatin analogs, meta-iodobenzylguanidine (MIBG) and positron emission tomography (PET), now allow better radiologic evaluation of disease staging (21). MRI is particularly useful in characterizing lesions in the liver (21) and lungs (22).

Radio-labeled somatostatin analog scintigraphy remains presently the gold standard in confirming the location of functioning neuroendocrine tumor tissue (23–26) (evidence level 3b). All neuroendocrine tumors possess the ability to express functioning somatostatin receptors of the various receptor subgroups (27–30), and radiolabeled identification of such functioning tissue will predict response to treatment using somatostatin analogs (25) (vide infra). Midgut carcinoids (by far the commonest) predominantly express somatostatin receptors from subgroup 2 (sst2) (31). Traditionally, somatostatin analogs have been labeled using indium-111 (23–26), but this has several drawbacks, including limited availability, suboptimal gamma energy, and high radiation burden to the patient (32). Data now exist to show at least equivalence of technetium-99 (32,33)—and yttrium-86 (34) labeled somatostatin analogs in localization and treatment planning in advanced carcinoid disease. Nearly 70% of carcinoid tumors will also take up ^{131}I-MIBG (35). MIBG is a biogenic amine precursor, which is actively taken up by tumors derived from the neural crest and stored in neurosecretory granules (36). Administration of MIBG labeled with radioactive iodine (^{131}I-MIBG) causes targeted irradiation of these tumors and can be used in therapy (37). In direct scintigraphy comparisons, MIBG is inferior to radiolabeled octreotide in localization of carcinoid tumors (evidence level 1b) (38).

PET-CT is now playing an ever increasing role in both localizing disseminated cancer, and also in monitoring the disease response to systemic therapies (39–41). While initial reports attempted to use ^{18}F-labeled deoxyglucose (FDG) (39–41), more recent studies have used more carcinoid-specific agents in an attempt to improve specificity. These agents included: 5-hydroxy-L-tryptophan (5-HTP) (39–42); ^{64}Cu-1,4,8,11-tetra-azacyclo-tetradecane-*N,N′,N″,N‴*-tera-acetic acid (TETA-OC) (43); and ^{18}F-DOPA (44). However, in direct comparisons, none as yet appear superior to somatostatin analog scintigraphy in tumor localization (45,46).

RESECTION OF CARCINOID LIVER METASTASES

In most instances, advanced neuroendocrine tumors follow an indolent course (47). Hepatic metastases are common, and although they may cause incapacitating endocrinopathies, pain, and even death, they may frequently remain asymptomatic for much of their course (47). Therefore, the appropriate timing and efficacy of interventions remain controversial and should always remain within the domain of the multidisciplinary team (47–49). Operative mortality is higher than that seen after resection of colorectal metastases because of the associated endocrinopathy (and in particular cardiac comorbidity) (47–50). The risk of perioperative complications can be reduced by the routine administration of continuous octreotide infusion (evidence level 4) (50).

Five-year survival after liver resection for carcinoid ranges between 47% and 82% (47,51–58). Factors influencing long-term survival after hepatectomy in these patients include size of metastases, radicality of resection, localization of primary tumor, and extent of liver replacement (47,51–55). Cytoreductive (R2 resection) surgery [using either resectional (57–61) or ablative (62–70) techniques] has been advocated for both liver (59–70) and peritoneal disease (71) where resection with curative intent is not possible. Median symptom-free survival of up to five years has been reported following cytoreductive surgery (60,61), but it is still too early to interpret objectively survival data from the reports of ablative treatment (62–70).

Liver transplantation continues to be advocated as a treatment for liver only carcinoid metastases (72–77). There has been some recent improvement in operative mortality for this procedure in these patients (72–77). Bearing in mind the relatively good prognosis of these patients (even with large volume liver replacement), there is no evidence that this approach confers any survival benefit over nonsurgical techniques. When one considers the never-decreasing demand on the limited donor pool of suitable livers, one is reminded of the words of the philosopher Abraham Maslow, "if the only tool you have is a hammer, then you tend to see every problem as a nail!"

Finally, remains the question of the management of the very rare primary carcinoids of the liver and biliary tract. If technically feasible, then resection with curative intent remains the object of treatment (54,78,79). When not feasible, there are anecdotal case reports of long-term survival following orthotopic liver transplantation (79).

CHEMOEMBOLIZATION

As with all established hepatic metastases, carcinoid deposits derive their blood supply exclusively from the hepatic artery. Hepatic artery embolization (HAI), especially when complemented by the addition of regional chemotherapy [transarterial chemoembolization (TACE)], therefore offers a theoretically attractive therapeutic treatment strategy. When compared directly to surgical resection in the same center, outcomes after HAI, although improving symptoms (80), do not compare favorably for survival (evidence level 4) (58).

Chemotherapy agents employed during TACE include streptozotocin (81), doxorubicin (82), or various combinations of cytotoxic regimens (83–85). The largest single-center report to date of 125 patients from Pittsburgh, reports one-, five-, and ten-year survivals of 59%, 35%, and 19%, respectively with a mean follow-up of 3.2 years (85). When TACE is compared directly with HAI, the addition of chemotherapy to the procedure does not confer any significant survival benefit over HAI alone in carcinoid patients (86,87).

SOMATOSTATIN ANALOGS

Somatostatin analogs now form the bedrock of the medical management of patients with symptomatic carcinoid syndrome whose disease is beyond resection with curative intent (88). Two analogs, octreotide and lanreotide, are widely available commercially, and both can be administered as depot long-acting preparations (obviating the need for regular self-injection several times each day) (89).

Symptomatic response to long-term octreotide correlates closely with radiolabeled octreotide scintigraphy positivity (90). There are now a number of reports of good long-term (up to five-year) compliance (with good symptomatic improvement) of patients on long-acting (LAR) octreotide (91,92), although patients need to be monitored regularly to confirm their ongoing dosage requirements (93). Interestingly, patients with gastric type-1 carcinoids associated with chronic gastritis type A (CAG-A) do show a decrease in gastric enterochromaffin-like cell (ECL) hyperplasia (which predisposes to type-1 gastric carcinoid) with commensurate falls in serum chromogranin A, despite no fall in the putative driving force of the ECL hyperplasia, elevated serum gastrin levels (94).

Similar results with good symptom control are seen with lanreotide therapy (95–99). In prospective cross-over evaluations to compare efficacy, patient acceptability, and tolerance no differences were found between octreotide and lanreotide (100). Although there have been reports of carcinoid tumor regression while on long-term somatostatin analog therapy (98,101–103), these must be regarded as anecdotal and treated with caution (evidence level 4) (104).

TARGETED NUCLEAR TREATMENTS

The holy grail of the treatment of inoperable solid cancers is a cytotoxic treatment that selectively targets the tumor cells, while having little or no effect on the surrounding normal host tissue. Because of their unique behavior, neuroendocrine tumors, carcinoid in particular, lend themselves perhaps more than any other to this approach. Two approaches are now being evaluated which find their way into the therapeutic armamentarium: MIBG (36,37) and radiolabeled somatostatin analogs (34,35).

Between 50% and 70% of carcinoid patients have tumors that will actively take up (therefore positive to) MIBG (34,35,37,105–107). The exact mechanism of MIBG therapy effects in the treatment of carcinoids remains unclear. Guanidine is a precursor of DOPA in the adrenergic catecholamine synthetic pathway (34). The uptake of MIBG by neuroendocrine tumors is probably mediated by vesicular monoamine transporters into the tumor cells (108), and interestingly the response to ^{131}I-labeled MIBG is enhanced by pretreatment with nonlabeled MIBG (105,106). Good long-term symptomatic control, with decreased demand for somatostatin analog treatment has now been reported in a number of series (37,105–107,109,110), and this improvement is reportedly cost-effective (37). Toxicities include: pancytopenia, thrombocytopenia, nausea, emesis, and hypothyroidism (as a consequence of ^{131}I treatment) (37,105–107,109,110).

There is less experience in the use of targeted, labeled, somatostatin-analog therapy because for many years it was difficult to achieve a stable association between the analogs and isotopes which would be effective therapeutically. Early studies attempted to employ ^{111}In-pentreotide but the benefit appeared limited (111–115). We may be close to an advance in therapy using octreotide labeled with either ^{90}Y (116–120) or ^{177}Lu (119). These formulations, based on DOTA-D-Phe1-Tyr3-octreotide (DOTATOC) appear to be much more stable in clinical use, and early reports indicate a higher response rate than that seen after MIBG therapy (116–120). Toxicities include: lymphocytopenia, anemia, and renal impairment (117,118).

SYSTEMIC THERAPIES

By and large, systemic therapies (chemotherapy and biological therapies other than somatostatin analogs) have not proven worthwhile in the carcinoid syndrome. Early studies have demonstrated no benefit for the use of conventional cytotoxic chemotherapy (121–124). Earlier optimism for the use of interferon treatment (1) has not been borne out in clinical practice (125,126), even when added to other treatments including MIBG (127,128). Despite anecdotal reports to support the use of interferon in carcinoid disease (129), there is no evidence from large-scale studies to support this therapeutic strategy (level 2b evidence) (130,131).

Outcomes following conventional cytotoxic chemotherapy regimens are limited to phase II studies showing little survival benefit from conventional chemotherapy (132,133) or taxol derivatives (level 2b evidence) (134–137).

Recently, interest has returned to the use of the newer targeted biological therapies. Gefitinib [an inhibitor of epidermal growth factor receptor (EGFR)]-sensitive tyrosine kinase inhibits the growth of human carcinoid cells in vitro (138) and along with SU11248 (139), another tyrosine kinase inhibitor, has been demonstrated to stabilize advanced carcinoid tumors in small phase II clinical trials (140). Preliminary phase II studies of bevacizumab (a human monoclonal antibody to vascular endothelial growth factor) look promising (141,142), but side effects include increased rates of hypertension (143). Finally, there are preliminary data on the use of imatinib (gleevec), an inhibitor of platelet-derived growth factor (144), bortezomib, a proteosome inhibitor (145), and temsirolimus, a small-molecule inhibitor of the mammalian target of rapamycin (mTOR) (146).

QUALITY-OF-LIFE

QOL is a multidimensional concept that is being used more and more as an outcome variable in the evaluation of cancer treatments. There is no single agreed definition; however, most researchers agree that it is a multidimensional concept and assessment should be based on subjective evaluation by the patient (147,148). It has been difficult to show significant survival benefits of carcinoid treatments, and those that do prolong life may actually reduce QOL. It is now widely accepted that quality of survival is as important as quantity of survival and both these factors have to be considered when deciding on treatment management.

Improved treatments have probably prolonged life for many patients with carcinoid disease, and the use of somatostatin analogs can control the symptoms of disease for long periods of time (89–92). However, it is important that life is not just prolonged but also has good quality. The relatively long survival associated with carcinoid tumors, together with complex symptoms and use of multiple treatment modalities reinforce the need to address QOL in this patient group. The aim of many treatments is to palliate symptoms, or prolong time without symptoms and so comprehensive assessment of QOL is often as important as evaluation of symptoms. The absence of a large evidence base of treatment outcomes and resulting side effects specific for this disease indicates the importance of the contribution of QOL data in aiding decision-making.

The involvement of patients in the decision-making process has emphasized the need to address QOL in order for patients to make informed decisions. Patients are now being encouraged to assume an active role in treatment decision-making, yet it poses difficulty if this process is to be performed on survival figures alone. An understanding of how patients perceive symptoms and how treatment choices and disease progression will affect their QOL will greatly assist in the holistic management of this disease.

There is currently no disease-specific QOL-score questionnaire for patients with carcinoid disease. Few reports have been published examining this specific patient group and QOL (149–155). It is difficult to draw a general conclusion from those reports identified before as different health-related QOL instruments were used and the questionnaires were not specific enough for patients with neuroendocrine tumors, including carcinoid. The majority of QOL research originates from the Uppsala Akademiska Hopsital, Sweden. Larsson (149–155) examined this subject using the European Organisation for Research and Trials in Cancer, QOL core questionnaire (EORTC QLQ-C30) and discovered that patients with carcinoid disease rated life as relatively good. The results showed that the symptoms which mostly affected the patients' quality of the life where: fatigue, dyspnea, and diarrhea. The symptom of fatigue was also discovered to affect all dimensions of QOL in a qualitative study which focussed on patients diagnosed with metastatic carcinoid disease (156).

The only cancer-specific questionnaire used in some of the aforementioned studies is the EORTC QLQ-C30 but it is limited by the fact that it does not cover specific carcinoid disease issues like flushing (157). Current core cancer QOL questionnaires such as the EORTC QLQ-C30 (147) and FACT-G (158) do not address symptoms that are specific and problematic to patients with carcinoid and neuroendocrine tumors. To address this deficit, a disease-specific QOL score questionnaire for patients with neuroendocrine tumors is currently under development by the EORTC QOL group. This study is aimed to develop a module for patients with neuroendocrine tumors of the gastrointestinal tract in adherence with the modular approach to QOL assessment and guidelines proposed by the EORTC QOL group (147,159–162). The module will consist of QOL issues that are important to patients with carcinoid or a neuroendocrine tumor and will supplement the generic core questionnaire, the EORTC QLQ-C30. Once validated, the module will be an extremely useful tool in measuring QOL for this patient group and will play a valuable part in the future management of carcinoid disease.

REFERENCES

1. Kulke MH, Mayer RJ. Carcinoid tumors. New Engl J Med 1999; 858–867.
2. Modlin IM, Sandor A. An analysis of 8305 cases of carcinoid tumors. Cancer 1997; 79:813–829.
3. Williams ED, Sandler M. The classification of carcinoid tumours. Lancet 1963; 1:238–239.
4. Ramage JK, Catnach SM, Williams R. Overview: the management of metastatic carcinoid tumors. Liver Transplant Surg 1995; 1:107–110.
5. Bell HK, Poston GJ, Vora J, Wilson NJE. Cutaneous manifestations of the malignant carcinoid syndrome. Br J Dermatol 2005; 152:71–75.
6. Modlin IM, Shapiro MD, Kidd M. Carcinoid tumors and fibrosis: an association with no explanation. Am J Gastroenterol 2004; 99:2466–2478.
7. Lundin L, Norheim I, Landelius J, et al. Carcinoid heart disease: relationship of circulating vasoactive substances to ultrasound detectable cardiac abnormalities. Circulation 1988; 77:264–269.
8. Robiolio PA, Rigolin VH, Wilson JS, et al. Carcinoid heart disease: correlation of high serotonin levels with valvular abnormalities detected by cardiac catheterisation and echocardiography. Circulation 1995; 92:790–795.
9. Pellikka PA, Tajik AJ, Khandheria BK, et al. Carcinoid heart disease: clinical and echocardiographic spectrum in 74 patients. Circulation 1993; 87:1188–1196.

10. Thatipelli MR, Uber PA, Mehra MR. Isolated tricuspid stenosis and heart failure: a focus on carcinoid heart disease. Congest Heart Fail 2003; 9:294–296.
11. Quaedvlieg PF, Lamers CB, Taal BG. Carcinoid heart disease: an update. Scand J Gastroenterol Suppl 2002; 236:66–71.
12. Meijer WC, van Veldhuisen DJ, Kema IP, et al. Cardiovascular abnormalities in patients with a carcinoid syndrome. Neth J Med 2002; 60:10–16.
13. Di Luzio S, Rigolin VH. Carcinoid heart disease. Curr Treat Options Cardiovasc Med 2000; 2:399–406.
14. Simula DV, Edwards WD, Tazelaar HD, et al. Surgical pathology of carcinoid heart disease: a study of 139 valves from 75 patients spanning 20 years. Mayo Clin Proc 2002; 77:139–147.
15. Connolly HM, Schaff HV, Mullany CJ, et al. Surgical management of left-sided carcinoid heart disease. Circulation 2001; 104:136–140.
16. Connolly HM, Schaff HV, Mullany CJ, et al. Carcinoid heart disease: impact of pulmonary valve replacement in right ventricular function and remodelling. Circulation 2002; 106:151–156.
17. Robiolio PA, Rigolin VH, Harrison JK, et al. Predictors of outcome of tricuspid valve replacement in carcinoid heart disease. Am J Cardiol 1995; 75:485–488.
18. Connolly HM, Nishimura RA, Smith HC, et al. Outcomes of cardiac surgery for carcinoid disease. J Am Coll Cardiol 1995; 25:410–416.
19. Kobayashi K, Katsumata T, Yoshizawa S, et al. Indications for endoscopic polypectomy for rectal carcinoids and clinical usefulness of endoscopic ultrasonography. Dis Colon Rectum 2005; 48:285–291.
20. Anderson MA, Carpenter S, Thompson NW, et al. Endoscopic ultrasound is highly accurate and directs management in patients with neuroendocrine tumors of the pancreas. Am J Gastroenterol 2000; 96:2271–2277.
21. Kaltsas G, Rockall A, Papdogias D, et al. Recent advances in radiological and radionuclide imaging and therapy of neuroendocrine tumours. Eur J Endocrinol 2004; 151:15–27.
22. Schaefer JF, Vollmar J, Schick F, et al. Solitary pulmonary nodules: dynamic contrast-enhanced MR imaging—perfusion differences in malignant and benign lesions. Radiology 2004; 232:544–553.
23. Lamberts SWJ, Bakker WH, Reubi JC, Krenning EP. Somatostatin-receptor imaging in the localization of neuroendocrine tumors. N Engl J Med 1990; 323:1246–1249.
24. Krenning EP, Kwekkeboom DJ, Oei HY, et al. Somatostatin-receptor scintigraphy in gastroenteropancreatic tumors: an overview of European results. Ann N Y Acad Sci 1994; 733:416–424.
25. Janson ET, Westlin JE, Eriksson B, et al. [^{111}In-DTPA-D-Phe1] octreotide scintigraphy in patients with carcinoid tumours: the predictive value for somatostatin analogue treatment. Eur J Endocrinol 1994; 131:577–581.
26. Savelli G, Lucignani G, Seregni E, et al. Feasibility of somatostatin receptor scintigraphy in the detection of occult primary gastro-entero-pancreatic (GEP) neuroendocrine tumours. Nucl Med Commun 2004; 25:445–449.
27. Reisine T, Bell G. Molecular biology of somatostatin receptors. Endocrinol Rev 1995; 16:427–442.
28. Bousquet C, Guillermet J, Vernejoul F, et al. Somatostatin receptors and regulation of cell proliferation. Dig Liver Dis 2004; 36(S1):S2–S7.
29. Hofland LJ, lamberts SW. Somatostatin receptor subtype expression in human tumors. Ann Oncol 2001; 12(S2):S31–S36.
30. Kulaksiz H, Eissele R, Rossler D, et al. Identification of somatostatin receptor subtypes 1, 2A, 3, and 5 in neuroendocrine tumours with specific antibodies. Gut 2002; 50:52–60.
31. Hashemi SH, Benjegard SA, Ahlman H, et al. ^{111}In-labelled octreotide binding by the somatostatin receptor subtype 2 in neuroendocrine tumours. Br J Surg 2003; 90:549–554.
32. Decristoforo C, Mather SJ, Cholewinski W, et al. 99mTc-EDDA/HYNAC-TOC: a new 99mTc-labelled radiopharmaceutical for imaging somatostatin receptor-positive tumours; first clinical results and intra-patient comparison with ^{111}In-labelled octreotide derivatives. Eur J Nucl Med 2000; 27:1318–1325.
33. Gabriel M, Decristoforo C, Maina T, et al. 99mTc-N4-[Tyr3]octreotate versus 99mTc-EDDA/HYNIC-[Tyr3]octreotide: an interpatient comparison of two novel technetium-99m labelled tracers for somatostatin receptor scintigraphy. Cancer Biother Radiopharm 2004; 19:73–79.
34. Forster GJ, Engelbach MJ, Brockmann JJ, et al. Preliminary data on biodistribution and dosimetry for therapy planning of somatostatin receptor positive tumours: comparison of (86)Y-DOTATOC and (111)In-DTPA-octreotide. Eur J Nucl Med 2001; 28:1743–1750.
35. Otte A, Mueller-Brand J, Dellas S, et al. Yttrium-90-labelled somatostatin analogue for cancer treatment. Lancet 1998; 351:417–418.
36. Hoefnagel CA, Lewington VJ. MIBG therapy. In: Murray IPC, Ell PJ, eds. Nuclear Medicine. Vol. 2. Edinburgh: Churchill Livingstone, 1994:851–864.
37. Pathirana AA, Vinjamuri S, Byrne C, et al. ^{131}I-MIBG radionuclide therapy is safe and cost-effective in the control of symptoms of the carcinoid syndrome. Eur J Surg Oncol 2001; 27:404–408.
38. Kaltsas G, Korbonits M, Heintz E, et al. Comparison of somatostatin analog and meta-iodobenzylguanidine radionuclides in the diagnosis and localization of advanced neuroendocrine tumors. J Clin Endocrinol Metab 2001; 86:895–902.

39. Eriksson B, Bergstrom M, Orlefors H, et al. Use of PET in neuroendocrine tumors. In vivo applications and in vitro studies. Q J Nucl med 2000; 44:68–76.
40. Sundin A, Eriksson B, bergstrom M, et al. PET in the diagnosis of neuroendocrine tumors. Ann NY Acad Sci 2004; 1014:246–257.
41. Eriksson B, Bergstrom M, Sundin A, et al. The role of PET in localization of neuroendocrine and adrenocortical tumors. Ann N Y Acad Sci 2002; 970:159–169.
42. Orlefors H, Sundin A, Garske U, et al. Whole-body (11)C-5-hydroxytryptophan positron emission tomography as a universal imaging technique for neuroendocrine tumors: comparison with somatostatin receptor scintigraphy and computed tomography. J Clin Endocrinol Metab 2005; 90:3392–3400.
43. Anderson CJ, Dehdashti F, Cutler PD, et al. ^{64}Cu-TETA-octreotide as a PET imaging agent for patients with neuroendocrine tumors. J Nucl Med 2001; 42:213–221.
44. Hoegerle S, Altehoefer C, Ghanem N, et al. Whole-body ^{18}F dopa PET for detection of gastrointestinal carcinoid tumors. Radiology 2001; 220:373–380.
45. Virgolini I, Patri P, Novotny C, et al. Comparative somatostatin receptor scintigraphy using In-111-DOTA-lanreotide and In-111-DOTA-Tyr3-octreotide versus F-18-FDG-PET for evaluation of somatostatin receptor-mediated radionuclide therapy. Ann Oncol 2001; 12(2):S41–S45.
46. Kowalski J, Henze M, Schuhmacher J, et al. Evaluation of positron emission tomography imaging using [^{68}Ga]-DOTA-D Phe(1)-Tyr(3)-octreotide in comparison to [^{111}In]-DTPAOC SPECT. First results in patients with neuroendocrine tumors. Mol Imag Biol 2003; 5:42–48.
47. Chamberlain RS, Canes D, Brown KT, et al. Hepatic neuroendocrine metastases: does intervention alter outcomes? J Am Coll Surg 2000; 190:432–445.
48. Sutcliffe R, Maguire D, Ramage J, et al. Management of neuroendocrine liver metastases. Am J Surg 2004; 187:39–46.
49. Sarmiento JM, Que FG. Hepatic surgery for metastases from neuroendocrine tumors. Surg Oncol Clin N Am 2003; 12:321–342.
50. Kinney MA, Warner ME, Nagorney DM, et al. Perianaesthetic risks and outcomes of abdominal surgery for metastatic carcinoid tumours. Br J Anaesth 2001; 87:447–452.
51. Nave H, Mossinger E, Feist H, et al. Surgery as primary treatment in patients with liver metastases from carcinoid tumors: a retrospective, unicentric study over 13 years. Surgery 2001; 129: 170–175.
52. Touzios JG, Kiely JM, Pitt SC, et al. Neuroendocrine hepatic metastases: does aggressive management improve survival? Ann Surg 2005; 241:776–783.
53. Norton JA, Warren RS, Kelly MG, et al. Aggressive surgery for metastatic liver neuroendocrine tumors. Surgery 2003; 134:1057–1063.
54. el Rassi ZS, Ferdinand L, Mohsine RM, et al. Primary and secondary liver endocrine tumors: clinical presentation, surgical approach and outcome. Hepatogastroenterology 2002; 49:1340–1346.
55. Sarmiento JM, Heywood G, Rubin J, et al. Surgical treatment of neuroendocrine metastases to the liver: a plea for resection to increase survival. J Am Coll Surg 2003; 197:29–37.
56. Knox CD, Feurer ID, Wise PE, et al. Survival and functional quality of life after resection for hepatic carcinoid metastases. J Gastrointest Surg 2004; 8:653–659.
57. Soreide JA, van Heerden JA, Thompson GB, et al. Gastrointestinal carcinoid tumors: long-term prognosis for surgically treated patients. World J Surg 2000; 24:1431–1436.
58. Yao KA, Talamonti MS, Nemcek A, et al. Indications and results of liver resection and hepatic chemoembolization for metastatic gastrointestinal neuroendocrine tumors. Surgery 2001; 130:677–682.
59. McEntee GP, Nagorney DM, Kvols LK, et al. Cytoreductive hepatic surgery for neuroendocrine tumors. Surgery 1990; 108:1091–1096.
60. Chung MH, Pisegna J, Spirt M, et al. Hepatic cytoreduction followed by a novel long-acting somatostatin analog: a paradigm for intractable neuroendocrine tumors metastatic to the liver. Surgery 2001; 130:954–962.
61. Gulec SA, Mountcastle TS, Frey D, et al. Cytoreductive surgery in patients with advanced-stage carcinoid tumors. Am Surg 2002; 68:667–671.
62. Cozzi PJ, Englund R, Morris DL. Cryotherapy treatment of patients with hepatic metastases from neuroendocrine tumors. Cancer 1995; 76:501–509.
63. Wessels FJ, Schell SR. Radiofrequency ablation treatment of refractory carcinoid hepatic metastases. J Surg Res 2001; 95:8–12.
64. Hellmann P, Ladjevardis S, Skogseid B, et al. Radiofrequency tissue ablation using cooled tip for liver metastases of endocrine tumors. World J Surg 2002; 26:1052–1056.
65. Dick EA, Joarder R, de Jode M, et al. MR-guided laser thermal ablation of primary and secondary liver tumours. Clin Radiol 2003; 58:112–120.
66. Henn AR, Levine EA, McNulty W, Zagoria RJ. Percutaneous radiofrequency ablation of hepatic metastases for symptomatic relief of neuroendocrine symptoms. Am J Roentgenol 2003; 181:1005–1010.
67. O'Toole D, Maire F, Ruszniewski P. Ablative therapies for liver metastases of digestive endocrine tumours. Endoc Relat Cancer 2003; 10:463–468.
68. Gillams A, Cassoni A, Conway G, Lees W. Radiofrequency ablation of neuroendocrine liver metastases—the Middlesex experience. Abdom Imag 2005; 30:435–441.

69. Navarra G, Ayav A, Weber JC, et al. Short- and long-term results of intraoperative radiofrequency ablation of liver metastases. Int J Colorectal Dis 2005; 20:521–528.
70. Atwell TD, Charboneau JW, Que FG, et al. Treatment of neuroendocrine cancer metastatic to the liver: the role of ablative techniques. Cardiovasc Intervent Radiol 2005; 28:409–421.
71. Elias D, Sideris L, Liberale G, et al. Surgical treatment of peritoneal carcinomatosis from well-differentiated digestive endocrine carcinomas. Surgery 2005; 137:411–416.
72. Bechstein WO, Neuhaus P. Liver transplantation for hepatic metastases of neuroendocrine tumors. NY Acad Sci 1994; 733:507–514.
73. Lang H, Oldhafer KJ, Weimann A, et al. Liver transplantation for metastatic neuroendocrine tumors. Ann Surg 1997; 225:347–354.
74. Le Treut YP, Delpero JR, Dousset B, et al. Results of liver transplantation in the treatment of metastatic neuroendocrine tumors: a 31-case French multicentric report. Ann Surg 1997; 225:355–364.
75. Fernandez JA, Robles R, Marin C, et al. Role of liver transplantation in the management of metastatic neuroendocrine tumors. Transplant Proc 2003; 35:1832–1833.
76. Ahlman H, Friman S, Cahlin C, et al. Liver transplantation for treatment of metastatic neuroendocrine tumors. Ann NY Acad Sci 2004; 1014:265–269.
77. Florman S, Toure B, Kim L, et al. Liver transplantation for neuroendocrine tumors. J Gastrointest Surg 2004; 8:208–212.
78. Knox CD, Anderson CD, Lamps LW, et al. Long-term survival after resection for primary hepatic carcinoid tumor. Ann Surg Oncol 2003; 10:1171–1175.
79. Fenwick SW, Wyatt JI, Toogood GJ, Lodge JP. Hepatic resection and transplantation for primary carcinoid tumors of the liver. Ann Surg 2004; 239:210–219.
80. Schell SR, Camp ER, Caridi JG, Hawkins IF Jr. Hepatic artery embolization for control of symptoms, octreotide requirements, and tumor progression in metastatic carcinoid tumors. J Gastrointest Surg 2002; 6:664–670.
81. Dominguez S, Denys A, Madeira I, et al. Hepatic arterial chemoembolization with streptozotocin in patients with metastatic digestive endocrine tumours. Eur J Gastroenterol Hepatol 2000; 12:151–157.
82. Roche A, Girish BV, de Baere T, et al. Trans-catheter arterial chemoembolization as first-line treatment for hepatic metastases from endocrine tumors. Eur Radiol 2003; 13:136–140.
83. Kress O, Wagner HJ, Wied M, et al. Transarterial chemoembolization of advanced liver metastases of neuroendocrine tumors—a retrospective single-center analysis. Digestion 2003; 68:94–101.
84. Fiorentini G, Rossi S, Bonechi F, et al. Intra-arterial chemoembolization in liver metastases from neuroendocrine tumors: a phase II study. J Chemother 2004; 16:293–297.
85. Dong XD, Yin X, Zeh HJ, et al. Long-term outcome in patients with liver metastases from neuroendocrine tumors treated with chemoembolization. Proc ASCO 2005; 23:349S (abstract 4167).
86. Gupta S, Yao JC, Ahrar K, et al. Hepatic artery embolization and chemoembolization for treatment of patients with metastatic carcinoid tumors: the MD Anderson experience. Cancer J 2003; 9:261–267.
87. Gupta S, Johnson MM, Murthy R, et al. Hepatic arterial embolization and chemoembolization for the treatment of patients with metastatic neuroendocrine tumors. Cancer 2005; 104(8):1590–1602.
88. Oberg K, Kvols L, Caplin M, et al. Consensus report on the use of somatostatin analogs for the management of neuroendocrine tumors of the gastrointestinal system. Ann Oncol 2004; 15:966–973.
89. Rubin J, Ajani J, Schirmer W, et al. Octretide acetate long-acting formulation versus open-labelled subcutaneous octreotide acetate in malignant carcinoid syndrome. J Clin Oncol 1999; 17:600–606.
90. Filosso PL, Ruffini E, Oliaro A, et al. Long-term survival of atypical bronchial carcinoids with liver metastases, treated with octreotide. Eur J Cardiothorac Surg 2002; 21:913–917.
91. Garland J, Buscombe JR, Bouvier C, et al. Sandostatin LAR (long-acting octreotide acetate) for malignant carcinoid syndrome: a 3-year experience. Aliment Pharmacol Ther 2003; 17:437–444.
92. Welin SV, Janson ET, Sundin A, et al. High-dose treatment with a long-acting somatostatin analogue in patients with advanced midgut carcinoid tumours. Eur J Endocrinol 2004; 151:107–112.
93. Woltering E, Mamikunian PM, Zeitz S, et al. Octreotide acetate (LAR) dose effect on plasma octreotide levels: impact on neuroendocrine tumor management. Proc ASCO 2005; 23:235S (abstract 3177).
94. Fykse V, Sandvik AK, Qvigstad G, et al. Treatment of ECL cell carcinoids with octreotide LAR. Scand J Gastroenterol 2004; 39:621–628.
95. Tomassetti P, Migliori M, Gullo L. Slow-release lanreotide treatment in endocrine gastrointestinal tumors. Am J Gastroenterol 1998; 93:1468–1471.
96. Wymenga ANM, Eriksson B, Salmela PI, et al. Efficacy and safety of prolonged-release lanreotide in patients with gastrointestinal neuroendocrine tumors and hormone-related symptoms. J Clin Oncol 1999; 17:1111–1117.
97. Ricci S, Antonuzzo A, Galli L, et al. Octreotide acetate long-acting release in patients with metastatic neuroendocrine tumors pretreated with lanreotide. Ann Oncol 2000; 11:1127–130.
98. Ducreux M, Ruszniewski P, Chayvialle JA, et al. The antitumoral effect of the long-acting somatostatin analog lanreotide in neuroendocrine tumors. Am J Gastroenterol 2000; 95:3276–3281.
99. Ricci S, Antonuzzo A, Galli L, et al. Long-acting depot lanreotide in the treatment of patients with advanced neuroendocrine tumors. Am J Clin Oncol 2000; 23:412–415.

100. O'Toole D, Ducreux M, Bommelaer G, et al. Treatment of carcinoid syndrome: a prospective crossover evaluation of lanreotide versus octreotide in terms of efficacy, patient acceptability, and tolerance. Cancer 2000; 88:770–776.
101. Imtiaz KE, Monteith P, Khaleeli A. Complete histological regression of metastatic carcinoid tumour after treatment with octreotide. Clin Endocrinol 2000; 53:755–758.
102. Leong WL, Pasieka JL. Regression of metastatic carcinoid tumors with octreotide therapy: two case reports and a review of the literature. J Surg Oncol 2002; 79:180–187.
103. Bondanelli M, Ambrosio MR, Zatelli MC, et al. Regression of liver metastases of occult carcinoid tumour with slow release lanreotide therapy. World J Gastroenterol 2005; 11:2041–2044.
104. Granberg D, Eriksson B, Wilander E, et al. Experience in treatment of metastatic pulmonary carcinoid tumors. Ann Oncol 2001; 12:1383–1391.
105. Taal BG, Hoefnagel C, Boot H, et al. Improved effect of ^{131}I-MIBG treatment by predosing with non-radiolabeled MIBG in carcinoid patients, and studies in xenografted mice. Ann Oncol 2000; 11:1437–1443.
106. Hoefnagel CA, Taal BG, Sivro F, et al. Enhancement of ^{131}I-MIBG uptake in carcinoid tumours by administration of unlabelled MIBG. Nucl Med Commun 2000; 21:755–761.
107. Mukherjee JJ, Kaltsas GA, Islam N, et al. Treatment of metastatic carcinoid tumours, phaeochromocytomas, paraganglionoma and medullary carcinoma of the thyroid with (131)I-meta-iodobenzylguanidine [(131)I-mIBG]. Clin Endocrinol 2001; 55:47–60.
108. Kolby L, Bernhardt P, Levin-Jakobsen AM, et al. Uptake of meta-iodobenzylguanidine in neuroendocrine tumours is mediated by vesicular monoamine transporters. Br J Cancer 2003; 89:1383–1388.
109. Sywak MS, Pasieka JL, McEwan A, et al. ^{131}I-meta-iodobenzylguanidine in the management of midgut carcinoid tumors. World J Surg 2004; 28:1157–1162.
110. Safford SD, Coleman RE, Gockerman JP, et al. Iodine-131 metaiodobenzylguanidine treatment for metastatic carcinoid. Results in 98 patients. Cancer 2004; 101:1987–1993.
111. van Eijck CHJ. Treatment of advanced endocrine gastroenteropancreatic tumours using radiolabelled somatostatin analogues. Br J Surg 2005; 92:1333–1334.
112. Slooter GD, Breeman WA, Marquet RL, et al. Anti-proliferative effect of radiolebelled octreotide in a metastases model in rat liver. Int J Cancer 1999; 81:767–771.
113. McCarthy KE, Woltering EA, Anthony LB. In situ radiotherapy with ^{111}In-pentetreotide. State of the art perspectives. Q J Nucl Med 2000; 44:88–95.
114. Meyers MO, Anthony LB, McCarthy KE, et al. High-dose indium ^{111}In pentetreotide radiotherapy for metastatic atypical carcinoid tumor. South Med J 2000; 93:809–811.
115. Buscombe JR, Caplin ME, Hilson AJ. Long-term efficacy of high-activity ^{111}In-pentetreotide therapy in patients with disseminated neuroendocrine tumors. J Nucl Med 2003; 44:1–6.
116. Waldherr C, Pless M, Maecke HR, et al. The clinical value of [^{90}Y-DOTA]-D-Phe1-Tyr3-octreotide (^{90}Y-DOTATOC) in the treatment of neuroendocrine tumours: a clinical phase II study. Ann Oncol 2001; 12:941–945.
117. Waldherr C, Pless M, Maecke HR, et al. Tumor response and clinical benefit in neuroendocrine tumors after 7.4 GBq (90)Y-DOTATOC. J Nucl Med 2002; 43:610–616.
118. Valkema R, Kvols LK, Pawels S, et al. Peptide receptor radiotherapy (PRRT) with [Y-90-DOTA, Tyr3]octreotide: toxicity and efficacy of 4-cycle and single-cycle regimens. Proc ASCO 2004; 23:206 (abstract 3046).
119. Kwekkeboom DJ, Teunissen JJ, Bakker WH, et al. Radiolabelled somatostatin analog [^{177}Lu-DOTA0,Tyr3] octreotate in patients with endocrine gastroenteropancreatic tumors. J Clin Oncol 2005; 23:2754–2762.
120. Kwekkeboom DJ, Mueller-Brand J, Paganelli G, et al. Overview of results of peptide receptor radionuclide therapy with 3 radiolabelled somatostatin analogs. J Nucl Med 2005; 46:62S–66S.
121. Bajetta E, Bichisao E, Artale S, et al. New clinical trials for the treatment of neuroendocrine tumors. Q J Nucl Med 2000; 44:96–101.
122. Kaltsas GA, Mukherjee JJ, Isidori A, et al. Treatment of advanced neuroendocrine tumours using combination chemotherapy with lomustine and 5-fluorouracil. Clin Endocrinol 2002; 57:169–183.
123. Oberg K. Chemotherapy and biotherapy in the treatment of neuroendocrine tumours. Ann Oncol 2001; 12(S2):S111–S114.
124. Rougier P, Mitry E. Chemotherapy in the treatment of neuroendocrine malignant tumors. Digestion 2000; 62(S1):73–78.
125. Nillson A, Janson GT, Eziksson B, Larsso A. Levels of angiogenic peptides in sera from patients with carcinoid tumours during alpha-interferon treatment. Anticancer Res 2001; 21:4087–4090.
126. Kolby L, Persson G, Franzen S, Ahren B. Randomized clinical trial of the effect of interferon alpha on survival in patients with disseminated carcinoid tumours. Br J Surg 2003; 90:687–693.
127. Hopfner M, Sutter AP, Huether A, et al. A novel approach in the treatment of neuroendocrine gastrointestinal tumors: additive antiproliferative effects of interferon-gamma and meta-iodobenzylguanidine. BMC Cancer 2004; 4:23.
128. Zuetenhorst JM, Valdes Olmos RA, Muller M, et al. Interferon and meta-iodobenzylguanidin combinations in the treatment of metastatic carcinoid tumours. Endocr Relat Cancer 2004; 11:553–561.

129. Pape UF, Wiedenmann B. Adding interferon-alpha to octreotide slows tumour progression compared with octreotide alone but evidence is lacking for improved survival in people with disseminated midgut carcinoid tumours. Cancer Treat Rev 2003; 29:565–569.
130. Stuart K, Levy DE, Anderson T, et al. Phase II study of interferon gamma in malignant carcinoid tumors (E9292): a trial of the Eastern Cooperative Oncology Group. Invest New Drugs 2004; 22:75–81.
131. Wirth LJ, Carter MR, Janne PA, Johnson BE. Outcome of patients with pulmonary carcinoid tumors receiving chemotherapy or chemoradiotherapy. Lung Cancer 2004; 44:213–220.
132. Sun W, Lipsitz S, Catalano P, et al. Phase II/III study of doxorubacin with fluorouracil compared with streptozotocin with fluorouracil or dacarbazine in the treatment of advanced carcinoid tumors: Eastern Cooperative Oncology Group study E1281. J Clin Oncol 2005; 23:4897–4904.
133. Fine RL, Fogelman DR, Schreibman SM, et al. Effective treatment of neuroendocrine tumors with temozolomide and capecitobine. Proc ASCO 2005; 23:361S [abstract 4216].
134. Ansell SM, Pitot HC, Burch PA, et al. A phase II study of high-dose paclitaxel with advanced neuroendocrine tumors. Cancer 2001; 91:1543–1548.
135. Kulke MH, Kim H, Stuart K, et al. A phase II study of decetaxel in patients with metastatic carcinoid tumors. Cancer Invest 2004; 22:353–359.
136. Kegel T, Grothe A, Jordan M, et al. Paclitaxel, carboplatin and etoposid (TCE) in the treatment of advanced neuroendocrine tumours. Proc ASCO 2005; 23:373S [abstract 4263].
137. Miranda FT, Spigel DR, Hainsworth JD, et al. Paclitaxel/carboplatin/ etoposide (PCE) therapy for advanced poorly differentiated neuroendocrine (PDNE) carcinoma: a Minnie Pearl Cancer Network phase II trial. Proc ASCO 2005; 23:322S (abstract 4058).
138. Hopfner M, Sutter AP, Berst B, et al. A novel approach in the treatment of neuroendocrine gastrointestinal tumours. Targeting the epidermal growth factor receptor by gefitinib (ZD1839). Br J Cancer 2003; 89:1766–1775.
139. Kulke M, Lenz HJ, Meropol NJ, et al. A phase 2 study to evaluate the efficacy and safety of SU11248 in patients with unresectable neuroendocrine tumors. Proc ASCO 2005; 23:310S (abstract 4008).
140. Hobday TJ, Mahoney M, Erlichman C, et al. Preliminary results of a phase II trial of gefitinib in progressive metastatic neuroendocrine tumors (NET): a phase II Consortium (P2C) study. Proc ASCO 2005; 23:328S (abstract 4084).
141. Yao JC, Charnsangavej S, Faria SC, et al. Rapid decrease in blood flow, blood volume and vascular permeability in carcinoid patients treated with bezacizumab. Proc ASCO 2004; 23:198 (abstract 3013).
142. Yao JC, Ng C, Hoff PM, et al. Improved progression free survival, and rapid, sustained decrease in tumor perfusion among patients with advanced carcinoid treated with bevacizumab. Proc ASCO 2005; 23:309S (abstract 4007).
143. Mares JE, Worah S, Mathew SV, et al. Increased rate of hypertension among patients with advanced carcinoid treated with bevacizumab. Oroc ASCO 2005; 23:329S (abstract 4087).
144. Carr K, Yao JC, Rashid A, et al. A phase II trial of imatinib in patients with advanced carcinoid tumor. Proc ASCO 2005; 23:343 (abstract 4124).
145. Shah MH, Young D, Kindler HL, et al. Phase II study of the proteasome inhibitor bortezomib (PS-341) in patients with metastatic neuroendocrine tumors. Clin Cancer Res 2004; 10:6111–6118.
146. Duran I, Le L, Saltman D, et al. A phase II trial of temsirolimus in metastatic neuroendocrine carcinomas. Proc ASCO 2005; 23:215S (abstract 3096).
147. Aaronson NK, Cull A, Kaasa S, Sprangers M. The EORTC modular approach to quality of life assessment in oncology. Int J Mental Health 1994; 23:75–96.
148. Shumaker SA, Naughton MJ. The international assessment of health-related quality of life: a theoretical perspective. In: Schumaker SA, Bernzon R, eds. The International Assessment of Health-Related Quality of Life: Theory, Translation, Measurement and Analysis. Oxford: Rapid Communications of Oxford, 1995:3–10.
149. Larsson G, Haglund K, Von Essen L. Distress, quality of life and strategies to "keep a good" mood in patients with carcinoid tumours: patient and staff perceptions. Eur J Cancer Care (Engl) 2003; 12:46–57.
150. Larsson G, Sjoden PO, Oberg K, Eriksson B, Von Essen L. Health-related quality of life, anxiety and depression in patients with midgut carcinoid tumours. Acta Oncol 2001; 40:825–831.
151. Larsson G, Sjoden PO, Oberg K, Von Essen L. Importance-satisfaction discrepancies are associated with health-related quality of life in five-year survivors of endocrine gastrointestinal tumours. Ann Oncol 1999; 10:1321–1327.
152. Larsson G, Von Essen L, Sjoden PO. Health-related quality of life in patients with endocrine tumours of the gastrointestinal tract. Acta Oncol 1999; 38:481–490.
153. Jacobsen MB, Hanssen LE. Clinical effects of octreotide compared to placebo in patients with gastrointestinal neuroendocrine tumours. Report on a double-blind, randomized trial. J Intern Med 1995; 237:269–275.
154. Wymenga AN, Eriksson B, Salmela PI, et al. Efficacy and safety of prolonged-release lanreotide in patients with gastrointestinal neuroendocrine tumors and hormone-related symptoms. J Clin Oncol 1999; 17:1111.

155. O'Toole D, Ducreux M, Bommelaer G, et al. Treatment of carcinoid syndrome: a prospective crossover evaluation of lanreotide versus octreotide in terms of efficacy, patient acceptability, and tolerance. Cancer 2000; 88:770–776.
156. Jones LE. Patient perceptions and experiences of fatigue with metastatic carcinoid disease. MSc thesis. University of Liverpool, 2005.
157. Davies AHG, Friend L, Jones L, et al. Development of a disease-specific EORTC quality of life score questionnaire for patients with gastrointestinal tumours. Gut 2005.
158. Cella DF, Tulsky DS, Gray G, et al. The functional assessment of cancer therapy scale: development and validation of the general measure. J Clin Oncol 1993; 11:570–579.
159. Aaronson NK, Bullinger M, Ahmedzai S. A modular approach to quality of life assessment in cancer clinical trials. Recent Results Cancer Res 1998; 111:231–249.
160. Aaronson, NK, Cull A, Kassa S, Sprangers MAG. The EORTC modular approach to quality of life. Int J Ment Health 1994; 23(2):75–96.
161. Sprangers MA, Cull A, Bjordal K, Groenvold M, Aaronson NK. The European Organisation for research and treatment of cancer approach to quality of life assessment: guidelines for developing questionnaire modules. EORTC study group on quality of life. Qual Life Res 1993; 2(4):287–295.
162. Sprangers MA, Cull A, Groenvold M, Bjordal K, Blazeby J, Aaronson NK. The European Organisation for research and treatment of cancer approach to developing questionnaire modules: an update and overview. EORTC Quality of Life Study Group. Qual Life Res 1998; 7(4):291–300.

28 Gastrointestinal Stromal Tumor: Surgery

Y. Nancy You
Department of Surgery, Mayo Clinic, Rochester, Minnesota, U.S.A.

Ronald DeMatteo
Department of Surgery, Memorial Sloan-Kettering Cancer Center, New York, New York, U.S.A.

The management of gastrointestinal stromal tumors (GISTs) represents one of the most exciting and rapidly advancing fields in gastrointestinal oncology. Although GISTs were declared a distinctive clinico-pathological entity in 1983, their clinical management has been recently revolutionized by the introduction of effective molecularly targeted therapy. The tyrosine kinase KIT, recognized to be essential in the pathogenesis of GISTs, has become not only a marker for diagnosis but also a target for drug therapy. While surgical resection previously offered the only hope for patients with GISTs, their optimal management today integrates surgery with drug therapy in a multidisciplinary approach. It is important to realize that much of the evidence basis for the clinical management of GIST has not matured. As the current diagnostic criteria for GISTs were not formally defined until the National Institute of Health (NIH) consensus meeting in 2001, most retrospective studies are contaminated by non-GIST tumors (1). Prospective studies, mostly initiated after 2000, have limited follow-up or are ongoing or emerging. This chapter aims to review the available literature surrounding the molecular pathology of GISTs, their clinical characteristics, as well as the current role of surgery for patients presenting with primary disease or with metastatic/recurrent disease. The development and the clinical efficacy of targeted drug therapy are discussed in detail in the following chapter and will not constitute the main focus of this chapter.

PATHOLOGICAL AND MOLECULAR CHARACTERIZATION OF GISTS

Pathology and Immunohistochemistry

GISTs are the most common mesenchymal tumors of the gastrointestinal tract, but they were not recognized as a distinctive entity until the early 1980s. With the availability of electron microscopy, features of both smooth muscle and neuronal differentiation were found in GISTs. This duality distinguished them from other neoplasms derived solely from smooth muscle cells (e.g., leiomyoma, leiomyoblastomas, or leiomyosarcomas) or nerve cells (e.g., neurofibrosarcomas, schwannomas, or gastrointestinal autonomic nerve tumors (GANTs) (2). GISTs occur most commonly as a single tumor mass but, rarely, can occur as multifocal primary tumor nodules. They vary greatly in size and in histological appearance. Three distinct subtypes have been described: (*i*) spindle cell type (70%), containing uniform oval-shaped spindle cells in short fascicles with a storiform growth pattern; (*ii*) epitheliod cell type (20%), containing round cells with a nested growth pattern; and (*iii*) mixed cell type (10%) (1,3,4).

While most expert pathologists can diagnose GISTs by histomorphology, immunohistochemical profiling is currently indicated to confirm the diagnosis (1). Ninety-five percent of GISTs are positive for the immunophenotype marker KIT (or CD117) and 70% are positive for CD34. Additional markers such as smooth muscle actin (SMA), S100 and desmin are positive in 40%, 5%, and 2% of GISTs, respectively. These aid in the differential diagnosis of GISTs: positive SMA and desmin in the absence of CD117 point to other sarcomas of myogenic origin, while S100 positivity is more consistent with tumors of neurogenic origin (1,3). Additionally, approximately 5% of otherwise morphologically typical GISTs are KIT-negative. These tumors have only been recently recognized, and the small numbers analyzed to date preclude differentiating their behavior from KIT-positive GISTs (5,6).

The putative cells of origin for GISTs are mesenchymal progenitors that normally differentiate into the interstitial cells of Cajal (ICC). These are pacemaker cells interfacing between the smooth muscle cells and the autonomic nerve cells in the walls of the gastrointestinal tract. It has been postulated that other mesenchymal cells derived from the same progenitor may be present in the omentum, mesentery, and retroperitoneum, and therefore may account for the minority of GISTs arising at those locations outside of the gastrointestinal tract (7).

Genotype and Mutation Analysis

The pathogenesis of GISTs has been scrutinized on a molecular level. Oncogenic mutations cluster on the *KIT* gene and the *PDGFRA* gene. These encode for two homologous transmembrane tyrosine kinase receptors, KIT and platelet-derived growth factor receptor-alpha (PDGFRA), respectively. In the normal cell, binding of the specific ligand [stem-cell factor (SCF) or PDGF] to the extramembrane domain of the receptor leads to receptor homodimerization, kinase activation, and receptor autophosphorylation. All these result in controlled activation of the downstream cellular cascade involving proteins from the STAT, MAP, RAS, and JAK families (8,9). In GIST cells, receptor activation becomes ligand-independent, and downstream pathways for cell proliferation and apoptosis inhibition are activated.

The majority (80%) of GISTs are classified as *KIT*-mutant/*PDGFRA*-wild type (4). *KIT* mutation is necessary and sufficient for GIST tumorogenesis. Mutant *KIT* DNA was able to constitutively activate the KIT receptor when introduced into cell lines and into nude mice (10). The mutant receptor lacked normal inhibition of receptor dimerization or autoactivated receptor kinases, thereby activating the downstream signaling cascade independent of the ligand (2,10,11). On the other hand, approximately 3% to 5% of GISTs are *KIT*-wild type/*PDGFRA*-mutant (4). The *PDGFRA* mutation plays an independent oncogenic role, as the introduction of mutant *PDGFRA* cDNA to cells also resulted in ligand-independent tyrosine phosphorylation (12). Although one study suggested that these *KIT*-wild type/*PDGFR*-mutant GISTs are found in a higher proportion in KIT-negative GISTs (5), this observation awaits confirmation in larger studies. An additional 10% to 15% of GISTs are *KIT*-wild type/*PDGFRA*-wild type (4). And finally, no *KIT*-mutant/*PDGFRA*-mutant primary GIST has been identified to date. Mutations in these two genes are currently thought to be mutually exclusive in the primary tumor, although they may coexist after tumors acquire secondary mutations as they develop resistance to drug therapy (5,8,13).

Imatinib mesylate (STI571, Gleevac, Novartis, Basel, Switzerland) is an inhibitor of specific protein tyrosine kinases including ABL (Abelson proto-oncogene), KIT, and PDGFR (14). By competing with ATP for the kinase-binding site, the drug inhibits receptor activation and disables downstream cascades (15,16). Imatinib is thought to be active in both *KIT*-mutant and *PDGFRA*-mutant GISTs, although its efficacy in *PDGFRA*-mutant GISTs has not been widely studied (4,11). Furthermore, emerging evidence suggests that the precise location of mutation influences the response to imatinib. Several isoforms of mutants have been identified by mutation analysis. For *KIT*, these include exon 11 in the juxta-membrane domain (mutated in 67% of GISTs), exon 9 in the extracellular domain (18%), and exons 13 and 17 in the kinase domain (1–4%). For *PDGFR*, the clusters are located on exon 12 in the juxtamembrane domain (0.8%) and exon 18 in the kinase domain (3.9%) (11,12). Patients with GISTs harboring exon 11 *KIT* mutations experienced significantly higher partial response rate and longer overall survival (OS) than those with tumors containing an exon 9 *KIT* mutation or no detectable mutation of *KIT* or *PDGFRA* (11).

Prognostic Factors for Clinical Behavior

Numerous pathological and molecular factors have been assessed to predict the biological behavior of GISTs. It is now recognized that the majority of GISTs have malignant potential (4,7). Therefore, GISTs are classified according to their risk of malignant progression rather than as benign or malignant. A risk assessment scale (Table 1) was developed after an NIH consensus meeting in 2001 based on the two most consistent prognostic factors: tumor size and mitotic rate (1). Tumor recurrence and metastases were observed in over 50% of high-risk tumors but

TABLE 1 Risk Assessment Classification for Malignant Behavior in GISTs According to the 2001 NIH Consensus

Risk category	Size	Mitotic count per HPF
Very low	<2 cm	<5
Low	2–5 cm	<5
Intermediate	<5 cm	6–10
	5–10 cm	<5
High	>5 cm	>5
	>10 cm	Any
	Any	>10

Abbreviations: GISTs, gastrointestinal stromal tumors; HPF, high-powered field; NIH, National Institutes of Health.
Source: From Ref. 83.

only <5% of the low-risk ones. Additionally, tumor specific deaths occurred in 83% of patients with high-risk tumors but only 1% of those with low- and intermediate-risk ones (17).

The site of tumor origin has been advocated as an additional factor in risk stratification. Several studies have described the pathological features of GISTs arising from different sites. In a series of 1765 gastric GISTs, most (>80%) of the tumors followed an indolent course, with 48% of patients being alive without evidence of disease for a median time of 14.1 years. Survival outcomes strongly correlated with tumor size and mitotic activity (18). In contrast, among 50 patients with small bowel GISTs, 59% developed distant metastases and the actuarial disease-free survival at five years was only 18% (19). GISTs of the colon are relatively rare, but mitotic activity, infiltrative growth through muscularis propria, and mucosal invasion have been identified as poor prognostic factors in a study of 20 colonic GISTs (20). Lastly, the behavior of GISTs of the rectum and the anus can also be predicted by tumor size and mitotic rate in a series of 144 GISTs. While tumor recurrence and metastases were observed in only 5% of the small (<2cm) and less mitotically active (≤5 mitoses/50 HPF) GISTs, they occurred in 55% to 86% of the large (>5cm) and mitotically active (>5 mitoses/50HPF) tumors (21,22). Although these detailed pathological studies provide insight into the natural history of GISTs, their results are difficult to compare. The only large study which directly compared outcomes of tumors from different sites demonstrated worse long-term overall survival for GISTs arising from the esophagus and small bowel than those from the stomach (23). However, this early study suffered from the drawback of basing the diagnosis of GIST on histology alone and did not employ immunochemistry. Additionally, most pathological series lack details regarding the surgical resections these patients underwent. It is therefore impossible to determine whether the reported survival outcomes were influenced by less than adequate surgical therapy or other non-tumor factors. Thus the natural history of GISTs arising from different anatomic sites remains to be further defined.

Several other prognostic factors for survival and recurrence outcomes have been analyzed. Factors commonly identified in multivariate models in various studies have included: tumor size >5 cm (24–27), intermediate-or-high grade (26), mixed histology (28), >5 mitotic count/50 HPF(29) or 3 mitotic count/10 HPF (25), MIB-1 proliferation index >10% (30,31), Ki67 labeling index > 5% (29), or the presence of a deletion or insertion exon 11 *KIT* mutation (28).

CLINICAL MANIFESTATION OF GISTS
Epidemiology

Although GISTs are the most common sarcoma of the gastrointestinal tract, they remain a rare entity, accounting for only 5% of all sarcomas and 1% of all gastrointestinal tract cancers. The true epidemiology of GISTs has been difficult to determine. Available registry-based studies are summarized in Table 2. The larger studies may contain a heterogeneous cohort of both GISTs and non-GIST sarcomas, as tumors previously coded as "stromal sarcoma," "leiomyosarcomas," or other mesenchymal tumors were assumed to be GISTs (32). Conclusions and survival figures

TABLE 2 Summary of Large Registry-Based Studies on GISTs

	N (years)	Database	Study cohort definition	Median age	Gender (male/ female)	Annual incidence
Emory et al. 1999 (23)	1004 (1954–1997)	Armed Forces Institute of Pathology	Histology	59 (8–93)	NR	NR
Nilsson et al. 2004 (17)	288 (1993–2000)	Western Sweden registry	Histology, KIT+	69 (10–92)	144/144 (50%/50%)	14.5 per million
Mucciarini et al. 2004 (33)	113 (1988–2002)	Northern Italy registry	Histology, KIT+ or PDGFRA+	67	57/56 (50%/50%)	13 per million
Tran et al. 2005 (32)	1458 (1992–2000)	SEER	Diagnosis codes including stromal sarcoma, leiomyosarcoma, mesenchymoma, fibrosarcoma, schwannoma/ neurofibroma, angiosarcoma	62.9 (20–98)	54%/46%	0.68 per million

Abbreviations: GISTs, gastrointestinal stromal tumors; NR, not reported; PDGFRA, platelet-derived growth factor receptor-alpha; SEER, Surveillance, Epidemiology and End Results Registry, National Cancer Institute.

based on such studies must be interpreted with caution since the non-GIST sarcomas have a different natural history. Only the two smaller studies confirmed the diagnosis of GIST by the current immunohistochemistry criteria (17,33). The Italian registry study where tumors were confirmed to be either *KIT*-mutant or *PDGFRA*-mutant estimated the annual incidence of GISTs to be 13 per million, while the estimate was 14.5 per million in the Swedish study containing *KIT*-mutant tumors (17,33). Assuming minimal variation based on geography and race, this translates to approximately 5000 new cases per year in the Uunited States (2). The annual prevalence of GISTs may be as high as 129 per million as many patients have a prolonged clinical course ranging from five to 15 years (17,34). Although a slight male predominance has been reported in some studies, others have reported equal sexual predilection. The median age of patients affected by GISTs ranges between 59 and 69 years (Table 2), but it has been reported in all ages.

Pediatric GISTs are rare and have been described in only 16 isolated case reports and a few small case series (35). The diagnosis is typically made early in the second decade of life. Affected children are commonly female and present with chronic anemia, pain, and an abdominal mass (36). In addition, the patients tend to lack *KIT* or *PDGFRA* mutations, have a unique gene expression profile, and have an indolent clinical course (37). Complete surgical resection is an important prognostic factor, though the limited number of patients analyzed to date precludes formal comparison with adult tumors.

Familial GISTs develop in kindreds of patients harboring germ-line *KIT* mutations. These patients commonly develop multiple GISTs, particularly in the stomach and the small bowel, during their teenage years (2). Additionally, they may manifest heritable pigmented macules on the skin of the face, hands, axilla, and perineum, and demonstrate mastocytosis on skin biopsy. Based on the small number of patients reported to date, the prognosis of familial GISTs seems more favorable than sporadic GISTs.

In another rare subset of patients, GISTs occur as a part of a genetic syndrome. Multiple small bowel GISTs have been described in up to 25% of the patients with neurofibromatosis 1 (NF 1), though the molecular mechanism linking the NF1 gene to pathogenesis of GIST is unknown (34). Additionally, gastric GISTs may occur as a component of Carney's triad, a syndrome of unknown etiology comprised of gastric GISTs, pulmonary chondromas, and extra-adrenal paragangliomas. These patients may face a more benign clinical course than those with sporadic GISTs, as the disease-specific mortality was only 13% in 79 patients after 20 years of follow-up (38).

Clinical Presentation

GISTs can arise anywhere along the gastrointestinal tract, most commonly from the stomach (50–60%) and the small bowel (20–30%), but also from the esophagus (5%) and the colon and rectum (10–15%). Extra-gastrointestinal tract sites of origin include mesentery, omentum, and retroperitoneum (1). The clinical presentation of patients with GIST tumors ranges widely and may depend on tumor location. Symptomatic patients typically present with pain, bleeding, perforation, and/or localized mass effect. Vague abdominal discomfort develops in most patients, particularly when the tumor becomes sizable. Gastrointestinal bleeding may occur in 25% of all patients, and tumor ulceration into the bowel lumen may be visualized on endoscopy. While frank tumor perforation through a hollow viscous, and hemorrhagic tumor rupture into the peritoneal cavity, occur infrequently, such patients may present in distress requiring emergent intervention. Symptoms of local compression may include dysphagia, early satiety, bowel intussusception or obstruction, or rarely obstructive jaundice, depending on the location of the tumor mass (34,39). Nonetheless, a substantial proportion of patients remain asymptomatic. Their tumors are diagnosed incidentally during radiological evaluation, endoscopy or exploratory laparotomy. In Japan, where screening endoscopy for gastric adenocarcinoma is commonly performed, the majority (62%) of reported GISTs were discovered incidentally (40).

Imaging of GISTs

Imaging of GISTs is indicated to define disease burden, assess resectability, monitor response to therapy and survey for disease metastasis. Currently, the imaging modality of choice is contrast-enhanced computer tomography (CT). At diagnosis, GISTs typically appear as well-circumscribed, predominantly extra-luminal tumors. Contrast enhancement is usually homogeneous within the tumor, though large tumors may exhibit necrotic centers. An enhancing soft-tissue rim may be seen (41,42). The burden of metastatic disease is most frequently found in the liver, omentum and the peritoneum (4,42). In monitoring response to therapy, criteria for objective response is commonly defined by the Response Evaluation Criteria in Solid Tumors (RECIST) (43) criteria or the Southwestern Oncology Group (SWOG) criteria (44). However, these traditional criteria can be very misleading because they depend on tumor size. Frequently, a GIST tumor may stay the same size for a while even though it is responding. What can be seen is that the tumor becomes hypodense and hypovascular (45). CT may show these changes within a month, although the maximal response may not be reached until 6 to 8 months. Assessing treatment response may be particularly important in a subgroup of patients when the decision to pursue surgical resection is dependent on tumor response to imatinib. Functional imaging with PET scan detects tumor response much earlier than CT (46). It may therefore be considered for the select patient who requires a prompt decision for adjunctive surgery based on early tumor response. The use of PET is currently limited by its cost and relative inaccessibility, but its two additional indications include detection of unrecognized metastatic disease in high-risk patients, and resolution of inconsistent or inconclusive findings from other imaging modalities (4).

THE ROLE OF SURGERY IN THE CLINICAL MANAGEMENT OF GISTs

The surgical management of GISTs depends on the extent of disease at presentation. For patients who present with localized and potentially resectable disease, surgical resection is the primary therapy. On the other hand, for patients presenting with disease that is marginally resectable, metastatic, or progressive or recurrent, the currently recommended first-line therapy is imatinib drug therapy. Surgery plays an adjunctive or salvage role in these patients.

Patients Presenting with Localized and Resectable Disease

Outcomes of Resection

Surgical resection is the first-line therapy for patients presenting with a localized and resectable primary tumor. However, the oncologic outcomes of surgery in this specific group of patients remain poorly understood. Large registry-based studies often lack detailed information regarding the type of surgery and margin status, making it difficult to correlate surgical therapy to

TABLE 3 Summary of Oncological Outcomes After Surgical Resection of Gross Disease

	N	Study cohort definition	Site of origin	Follow-up (median)	Survival outcomes
Aparicio, 2004 (25)	59	Histology	All	3.8 yrs	OS (5 yr) 54% DFS (5 yr) 15%
Bucher, 2004 (30)	17	Histology & KIT +	Small bowel	5.8 yrs	OS (5 yr) 74% DFS (2 yr) 88%
Langer, 2003 (54)	37	Histology & KIT +	All	2.2 yrs	OS (2 yr) 87%
Fujimoto, 2003 (47)	129	Histology & KIT +	Stomach	NR	[a]OS (5 yr) 93% (10 yr) 88%
Wu, 2003 (62)	22	Histology & KIT +	All	1.2 yrs	OS (2 yr) 86% DFS (2 yr) 64%
Crosby, 2001 (19)	35	Histology	Small bowel	2 yrs	Median 50 mo DFS (5 yr) 42%
Pierie, 2001 (26)	39	Histology	All	3.2 yrs	OS (5 yr) 42%
DeMatteo, 2000 (24)	80	Histology	All	2 yrs	[a]Median 66 mo DSS (5 yr) 54%

[a]Representing survival outcomes in the subgroup of patients presenting with localized primary GIST.
Abbreviations: DFS, disease-free survival; DSS, disease-specific survival; GIST, gastrointestinal stromal tumor; NR, not reported; OS, overall survival.

oncologic outcome (18,32). Recent institutional series which provide surgical details are summarized in Tables 3 and 4. These studies often compensate for their smaller sample sizes by including a heterogeneous mixture of GISTs in the study cohort. The specific subgroup of patients who present with localized and resectable primary disease is either analyzed with all other patients of varying disease burdens, or may comprise only 40% to 50% of the total sample (24,47). Although anatomical site of origin is known to influence both gene expression patterns (48) as well as clinical outcomes (23), most studies contain tumors from a variety of sites and report oncologic outcomes for the entire cohort. These studies also lack uniformity in the use of immunohistochemical criteria for diagnosis and post-operative chemoradiation and they have different types of follow-up. Thus, oncologic outcomes summarized in Table 3 should be interpreted with caution. Overall, survival is approximately 85% at 2 years and 42% to 93% at 5 years. In the specific subgroup of patients with localized disease, oncologic outcomes after gross tumor resection, achieved in 86% to 97% of the patients, have only been separately reported in two studies (24,47). The largest U.S. study reported a five-year disease-specific survival of 54% with a median survival exceeding five years (24), while the Japanese study reported superior survival of 93% at five years (47). This discrepancy may be explained by the fewer large (>10 cm) and non-gastric (known to be more malignant) GISTs in the Japanese series (47). However, even after total gross tumor resection, long-term tumor recurrence, both local and systemic, has been reported at substantial rates. As summarized in Table 4, 13% to 83% of patients develop recurrent GISTs at a median of 16 to 25 months after complete surgical resection. The recurrence rate remains impressive at 40% even in the series of 80 patients presenting with

TABLE 4 Summary of Tumor Recurrence After Surgical Resection of Gross Disease

	N	Site of origin	Follow-up (median)	Recurrence	Time to recurrence (median)
Aparicio, 2004 (25)	59	All	3.8 yrs	49 (83%)	NR
Samiian, 2004 (55)	28	All	2.8 yrs	10 (36%)	16 mo
Mochizuki, 2004 (31)	70	Stomach	5 yrs	8 (13%)	20 mo
Langer, 2003 (54)	37	All	2.2 yrs	10 (26%)	23 mo
Fujimoto, 2003 (47)	135	Stomach	NR	20 (15%)	NR
Crosby, 2001 (19)	35	Small bowel	2 yrs	Local: 15 (43%) Distant: 24/41 (59%)	Local: 25 mos Distant: 21 mos
Pierie, 2001 (26)	39	All	3.2 yrs	16 (41%)	19 mo
DeMatteo, 2000 (24)	80	All	2 yrs	32 (40%)	NR

Abbreviation: NR, not reported.

localized and resectable primary tumors (24). In summary, gross total surgical resection should be the first-line therapy in patients presenting with localized primary disease. However, the long-term oncological outcomes of surgical therapy have not been robustly established. Future studies dedicated to this specific patient population, defining the study cohort by the current immunochemical criteria, and stratifying outcome by pathological features and anatomical sites of origin, would be valuable.

Surgical Factors of Prognostic Importance

Oncological outcomes have been consistently superior among patients who underwent complete gross tumor resection (R0 or R1 resection) than those who underwent tumor debulking only (R2 resection). Incomplete gross tumor resection independently curtailed median survival to 22 months (vs. 66 months with complete resection) in a series of 200 GISTs (24). And five-year survival rates were only 8% to 9% after incomplete resection (*vs.* 42% with complete resection) (19,26). Furthermore, gross tumor rupture leads to similar oncologic consequences as incomplete gross resection. A study of 191 leiomyosarcomas (most of which can be assumed to be GIST) reported that the median survival in patients with tumor rupture was 17 months, compared to 22 months with those with incomplete resection (49).

In view of these findings, expert panels recommend that tumor dissemination, tumor hemorrhage, or frank rupture should be avoided whenever feasible. By this principle, when surgical resection is anticipated, preoperative percutaneous biopsy of the tumor mass for the purpose of obtaining a definitive diagnosis is not warranted given the high risk of tumor shedding, bleeding, or rupture. Additionally, intraoperative surgical manipulation should be done with care so as to avoid tearing the pseudocapsules of these often soft and fleshy tumors. Wedge and segmental resections are preferred over submucosal enucleation procedures which carry a higher risk of tumor dissemination. Lastly, laparoscopic resection of GISTs remains investigational and is currently not recommended, except for very small tumors (3,4). Despite its technical safety and feasibility, the oncological adequacy and long-term outcomes of laparoscopic resection have not been proven (50,51). The largest experience is limited to only 14 gastric GISTs showing no recurrence after 3.5 years of follow-up (50).

The adequacy of resection margin remains undefined for GISTs. In an early study of 53 gastric leiomyosarcomas, radical resection with wide gross margins beyond 2 to 3 cm did not impact on survival or recurrence rates (52). Assuming most of the leiomyosarcomas were in fact GISTs, and in the absence of evidence to the contrary, limited resection with gross margins of 1 to 2 cm is currently regarded as adequate therapy (4). Most GISTs tend to displace and compress adjacent organs rather than frankly invade them (53). However, when dense adhesions surround larger tumors, en-bloc resection of the tumor along with adherent organs is required (39). In addition to resection of gross disease, achieving negative microscopic margins is preferred. Although microscopic margin status did not influence disease-specific survival for the 80 patients presenting with localized tumor (24), a small study comparing R0 to R1/R2 resection demonstrated shortened OS after a non-R0 resection (10.8 vs. 48.2 months) (27), and another study found higher disease-specific mortality (54). However, the management of a patient found to have a positive microscopic margin on final pathology remains controversial and is determined after balancing the risks of re-exploration and watchful waiting (3).

Experts currently agree that extended lymphadenectomy offers no oncological advantage in the surgical management of GISTs. Akin to other sarcomas, GISTs are thought to spread hematogenously rather than lymphatically. Nodal involvement is exceedingly rare (24,26), and no nodal metastasis was observed in a study where systematic nodal dissection was performed in 62 GISTs (47). Routine lymphadenectomy is therefore not warranted, unless clinically enlarged nodes are evident (3,4,39).

Adjuvant Drug Therapy

One frontier of active research involves adjuvant therapy in the form of imatinib. The impetus for adjuvant therapy is several-fold. First, complete surgical resection alone is likely inadequate therapy for GISTs, given the high rates of both local and systemic tumor recurrence. Second, recurrent disease is highly morbid, curtailing three-year survival to 20% from 64% (24,26,55). Third, while previous conventional chemotherapy and radiotherapy lacked efficacy (56), imatinib, with its proven activity against measurable metastatic disease and relatively favorable toxicity profile, is an attractive candidate for adjuvant therapy (3). The rationale for adjuvant use of imatinib is that systemic therapy administered after resection of gross tumor may eradicate any residual microscopic disease and impact on survival. However, these proposed benefits are balanced against the concern that adjuvant therapy may compromise the efficacy of therapy when GISTs do recur by facilitating the development of imatinib resistance (3). Therefore, four multi-institutional clinical trials are underway to elucidate the benefit and risks of adjuvant imatinib. Two phase II studies focus on high-risk GISTs. The American College of Surgeons Oncology Group (ACOSOG) has completed accrual to a single-arm phase II trial (Z9000) using imatinib (400 mg daily for 12 months) after R0/R1 resection of high risk (size >10cm, ruptured, or multifocal) primary GIST. Early results showed tolerable toxicity and good protocol compliance rates, indicating the feasibility of administering imatinib in the adjuvant setting (57). Efficacy data await longer follow-up. A parallel phase II trial of the Scandinavian Sarcoma Group randomizes patients to either 12 or 36 months of imatinib therapy. Two additional phase III trials aim to define the benefit of adjuvant imatinib. The U.S. trial (ACOSOG Z9001) randomizes patients to either imatinib (400 mg daily for 12 months) or placebo. Patients who develop recurrence on the placebo arm may be unblinded and crossed over to the imatinib arm. The trial has enjoyed rapid accrual, and its end points of overall and recurrence-free survival are projected to mature before 2010 (Fig. 1). The European Organization for Research and Treatment of Cancer (EORTC) Soft Tissue and Bone Sarcoma Group is conducting a parallel open-label trial randomizing patients to adjuvant imatinib (400 mg daily for 24 months) or observation. Currently, adjuvant use of imatinib should take place in the context of a clinical trial whenever possible (3).

Marginally Resectable Disease

A subgroup of patients with GIST, present with disease best characterized as "marginally resectable." Complete gross resection of these tumors typically requires either radically extensive surgery or highly morbid procedures that severely compromise organ function or quality of life. Common locations for these tumors may be the gastroesophageal junction, first and second portions of the duodenum, or the low rectum (4). Recently, imatinib has been advocated in the neoadjuvant setting with the goals of either allowing function-sparing resections in marginally resectable patients, or converting unresectable tumors. The feasibility of major surgical resection after imatinib was reported in a series of 17 patients. Ninety-four percent underwent complete gross tumor resection after a median of 10 months of imatinib therapy (58). Anecdotally, 12 weeks of preoperative imatinib allowed for a more limited resection in a patient with a previously locally advanced pelvic GIST. After seven months of follow-up, the patient remained free of disease (59). Lastly, neoadjuvant drug therapy is being tested in a phase II trial for patients with potentially resectable primary or recurrent GISTs sponsored by the Radiation

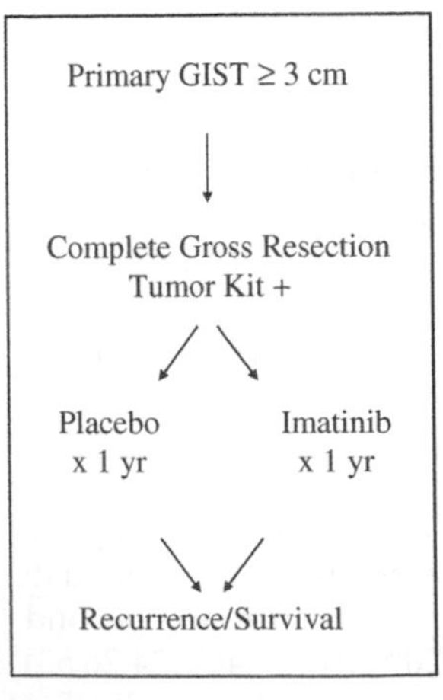

FIGURE 1 The Intergroup ACOSOG Z 9001 trial: A phase III randomized double-blinded study of adjuvant imatinib mesylate versus placebo in patients following the resection of primary GIST. Patients who develop tumor recurrence on the placebo arm may cross over to imatinib therapy. *Abbreviations*: ASOCOG, American College of Surgeons Oncology Group; GIST, gastrointestinal stromal tumor.

Therapy Oncology Group (RTOG S0132). Surgical resection is undertaken after 8 weeks of imatinib with the goal of improving progression free survival (60). Currently, using imatinib in the neoadjuvant setting for patients with marginally resectable or unresectable disease remains investigational and should be performed in the setting of a clinical trial whenever possible (3).

Patients Presenting with Recurrent or Metastatic GIST

Patients with GIST may present with synchronous metastases at initial diagnosis or develop metachronous metastases after initial surgical resection. The main patterns of metastases include peritoneal dissemination and/or hepatic metastases (18,24). Lung, bone, and lymph nodes are late sites of spread. Metastatic disease may be completely resectable, able to be debulked, or unresectable. Currently, the first-line therapy is the same for all these subgroups of patients and consists of systemic drug therapy, such as imatinib (4). However, surgery still may play an adjunctive role in these patients.

Metastatic Disease

Historically, patients underwent surgical debulking of their metastatic disease in the absence of alternative therapeutic options. From early studies, these patients faced a median survival of less than 18 to 22 months (24,60), while their response rate to doxorubin-based and other conventional chemotherapies only ranged from 0% to 15% (56). A more recent phase II trial reported a median survival of 16.7 months for GISTs and a dismal objective tumor response rate of 1.8% (61). Thus, patients who presented with technically resectable metastatic disease often underwent surgical debulking, as reported in several of the surgical series summarized in Table 3 (24,26,62). Oncologic outcome has only been reported anecdotally, but prolongation of survival was suggested with one study reporting a median survival of 16 months after complete resection of metachronous metastases (24). However, most patients developed subsequent recurrence and then died. Thus, the long-term benefit of surgical resection in this patient population remains largely unproven.

In the current era, therapy for metastatic disease is imatinib, and surgical resection is only indicated in select patients as an adjunct to drug therapy. The success of imatinib has been remarkable. Since the first clinical use of imatinib in a 50-year-old woman who had a 52% reduction in tumor volume sustained over 11 months (63), a series of clinical trials have taken place, as summarized in Table 5 and discussed in more detail in the next chapter. After the maximal tolerated dose was defined in the initial phase I trial (64,65), phase II trials have reported sustained partial response (PR)/stable disease (SD) rates, while disease progression and death occurred in only 14% of the 147 patients (66). These results were confirmed in two large phase III trials, observing a complete response (CR) rate of 5% along with a PR/SD rate of 79% (67), as well as favorable two-year OS estimates of 69% to 78% (67,68). Despite these remarkable outcomes, however, imatinib does not completely supplant surgical resection. It does not eradicate disease, and CR remains rare while PR ranges between 60% and 80% at best. When residual tumor masses were resected in 17 patients with demonstrated radiological response to imatinib, only 12% were found to have no evidence of viable tumor cells on pathology (58). In our experience in over 45 patients who have undergone resection after imatinib therapy, almost all patients were found to have residual disease (unpublished data). Therefore, when complete gross resection of the residual tumor mass is technically feasible, resection may be indicated in patients who partially respond or at least do not progress after imatinib therapy (3,4).

A subset of patients present with metastatic disease confined to one organ, typically the liver or the peritoneum, and surgical resection may play a larger role in their management. Metastatic disease confined to the liver occurs in 25% to 50 % of all patients (60,69). Limited evidence suggests that select patients, particularly those with a favorable (>2 years) interval from the primary tumor to hepatic metastases, may benefit after complete surgical resection of hepatic metastases (69). A five-year disease-free survival of 30% with a median survival of 39 months was observed in 34 patients with GISTs or leiomyosarcomas (70), In another study, hepatic metastasectomy resulted in a five-year disease-free survival of 11% with a medians urvival of 39 months among 10 patients with immunohistochemically confirmed GISTs (71).

TABLE 5 Summary of Clinical Trials in Patients with Metastatic GIST: Response Rates to Imatinib

Triale	N	Dosage (mg)	CR	PR	SD	PD	Followup, months (median)
EORTC phase I (64,65)[a]	32	400 qd/ 300 bid/ 400 bid/ 500 bid	0	51%	31%	9%	>10
US Finland, CSTIB2222 phase II (83)[b]	140	400 qd/ 600 qd	0	54%	28%	14%	9.6
EORTC phase III (67)[a]	897	400 qd/ 400 bid	5%	47%	32%	22%	25
Intergroup S0033 phase III (68)[b]	746	400 qd/ 800 qd	43% 41%		32% 32%	18%	14

[a]— the RECIST criteria; [b]— the SWOG criteria.
Abbreviations: CR, complete response; EORTC, European Organization for Research and Treatment of Cancer; GIST, gastrointestinal stromal tumor; PD, progressive disease; PR, partial response; RECIST, Response Evaluation Criteria in Solid Tumors; SD, stable disease; SWOG, Southwestern Oncology Group.

When complete surgical resection of hepatic metastases is not feasible, or when recurrent disease develop, other local therapies in the forms of radiofrequency ablation (RFA), transcatheter arterial chemoembolization (TACE), or hepatic artery pump may be considered (56). Outcomes of these therapies have mostly only been reported for sarcomas and not GISTs specifically (72,73). For disseminated peritoneal metastases, complete gross debulking has been considered, though most published studies pertain to sarcomas (74). Intraperitoneal chemotherapy has had limited success for sarcomatosis (4,75,76).

Recurrent, Resistant, or Progressive Disease

Surgery may play a role in the management of patients whose disease progresses despite imatinib and in others who develop resistance to imatinib. Resistance to imatinib may emerge as primary (occurring within the first 6 months) or secondary (occurring after the first 6 months), and may be widespread or clonal. Secondary clonal resistance manifests as a focally enlarged or metabolically active nodule within a larger tumor mass (77). The underlying molecular basis may be acquisition of additional specific *KIT* mutations, genomic amplification or activation of alternative cellular signaling (13,78,79). Currently, surgical resection for clonal resistance is indicated (3,4), particularly when other sites of metastatic disease are adequately controlled by imatinib. Alternatively, percutaneous RFA has been shown to be safe and feasible in this patient population (80). For multifocal resistant or progressive disease, new systemic agents active against imatnib-resistant GISTs are being developed. SU11248 targets multiple receptor kinases and has shown clinical benefit in 54% of patients in a phase I/II trial (81). Additionally, everolimus, a potent anti-proliferative agent, has been used in combination with imatinib, based on an observed close association between KIT and mTOR (mammalian target of rapamycin) in clonal resistance (82). Finally, palliative debulking of GISTs may be indicated for patients with tumor perforation or hemorrhage, or in those who are poor risk surgical candidates.

CONCLUSION

The surgical management of GISTs has evolved substantially over the past five years, concurrent with the development of molecularly targeted drug therapy. The optimal care of patients with GIST in the current era demands a multidisciplinary approach. For patients presenting with localized resectable disease, complete surgical resection of the tumor remains the primary therapy, but drug therapy is being considered in the adjuvant or neoadjuvant settings. While patients with non-localized disease largely benefit from systemic drug therapy, surgical resection continues to play an adjunctive or salvage role. Currently available evidence from retrospective studies is limited. While the results of ongoing prospective trials are maturing, more retrospective and population-based studies are needed to better document the oncological outcomes and prognostic factors in different subsets of patients.

REFERENCES

1. Fletcher CD, Berman JJ, Corless C, et al. Diagnosis of gastrointestinal stromal tumors: a consensus approach. Hum Pathol 2002; 33(5):459–465.
2. Corless CL, Fletcher JA, Heinrich MC. Biology of gastrointestinal stromal tumors. J Clin Oncol 2004; 22(18):3813–3825.
3. Blay JY, Bonvalot S, Casali P, et al. Consensus meeting for the management of gastrointestinal stromal tumors: report of the GIST Consensus Conference of 20–21 March 2004, under the auspices of ESMO. Ann Oncol 2005; 16(4):566–578.
4. Demetri GD, Benjamin RS, Blanke CD, et al. Optimal management of patients with gastrointestinal stromal tumors (GISTs). JNCCN 2004; 2(suppl 1):3.
5. Medeiros F, Corless CL, Duensing A, et al. KIT-negative gastrointestinal stromal tumors: proof of concept and therapeutic implications. Am J Surg Pathol 2004; 28(7):889–894.
6. Tzen CY, Mau BL. Analysis of CD117-negative gastrointestinal stromal tumors. World J Gastroenterol 2005; 11(7):1052–1055.
7. Joensuu H, Fletcher C, Dimitrijevic S, Silberman S, Roberts P, Demetri G. Management of malignant gastrointestinal stromal tumours. Lancet Oncol 2002; 3(11):655–664.
8. Heinrich MC, Rubin BP, Longley BJ, Fletcher JA. Biology and genetic aspects of gastrointestinal stromal tumors: KIT activation and cytogenetic alterations. Hum Pathol 2002; 33(5):484–495.
9. Duensing A, Medeiros F, McConarty B, et al. Mechanisms of oncogenic KIT signal transduction in primary gastrointestinal stromal tumors (GISTs). Oncogene 2004; 23(22):3999–4006.
10. Hirota S, Isozaki K, Moriyama Y, et al. Gain-of-function mutations of c-kit in human gastrointestinal stromal tumors. Science 1998; 279(5350):577–580.
11. Heinrich MC, Corless CL, Demetri GD, et al. Kinase mutations and imatinib response in patients with metastatic gastrointestinal stromal tumor. J Clin Oncol 2003; 21(23):4342–4349.
12. Heinrich MC, Corless CL, Duensing A, et al. PDGFRA activating mutations in gastrointestinal stromal tumors. Science 2003; 299(5607):708–710.
13. Antonescu CR, Arkun K, Besmer P, et al. Acquired resistance to imatinib in gastrointestinal stromal tumor occurs through secondary gene mutation. Clin Cancer Res 2005; 11(11):4182–4190.
14. Savage DG, Antman KH. Imatinib mesylate—a new oral targeted therapy. N Engl J Med 2002; 346(9):683–693.
15. Tuveson DA, Willis NA, Jacks T, et al. STI571 inactivation of the gastrointestinal stromal tumor c-KIT oncoprotein: biological and clinical implications. Oncogene 2001; 20(36):5054–5058.
16. Heinrich MC, Griffith DJ, Druker BJ, Wait CL, Ott KA, Zigler AJ. Inhibition of c-kit receptor tyrosine kinase activity by STI 571, a selective tyrosine kinase inhibitor. Blood 2000; 96(3):925–932.
17. Nilsson B, Bumming P, Meis-Kindblom JM, et al. Gastrointestinal stromal tumors: the incidence, prevalence, clinical course, and prognostication in the preimatinib mesylate era—a population-based study in western Sweden. Cancer 2005; 103(4):821–829.
18. Miettinen M, Sobin LH, Lasota J. Gastrointestinal stromal tumors of the stomach: a clinicopathologic, immunohistochemical, and molecular genetic study of 1765 cases with long-term follow-up. Am J Surg Pathol 2005; 29(1):52–68.
19. Crosby JA, Catton CN, Davis A, et al. Malignant gastrointestinal stromal tumors of the small intestine: a review of 50 cases from a prospective database. Ann Surg Oncol 2001; 8(1):50–59.
20. Tworek JA, Goldblum JR, Weiss SW, Greenson JK, Appelman HD. Stromal tumors of the abdominal colon: a clinicopathologic study of 20 cases. Am J Surg Pathol 1999; 23(8):937–945.
21. Miettinen M, Furlong M, Sarlomo-Rikala M, Burke A, Sobin LH, Lasota J. Gastrointestinal stromal tumors, intramural leiomyomas, and leiomyosarcomas in the rectum and anus: a clinicopathologic, immunohistochemical, and molecular genetic study of 144 cases. Am J Surg Pathol 2001; 25(9):1121–1133.
22. Tworek JA, Goldblum JR, Weiss SW, Greenson JK, Appelman HD. Stromal tumors of the anorectum: a clinicopathologic study of 22 cases. Am J Surg Pathol 1999; 23(8):946–954.
23. Emory TS, Sobin LH, Lukes L, Lee DH, O'Leary TJ. Prognosis of gastrointestinal smooth-muscle (stromal) tumors: dependence on anatomic site. Am J Surg Pathol 1999; 23(1):82–87.
24. DeMatteo RP, Lewis JJ, Leung D, Mudan SS, Woodruff JM, Brennan MF. Two hundred gastrointestinal stromal tumors: recurrence patterns and prognostic factors for survival. Ann Surg 2000; 231(1):51–58.
25. Aparicio T, Boige V, Sabourin JC, et al. Prognostic factors after surgery of primary resectable gastrointestinal stromal tumours. Eur J Surg Oncol 2004; 30(10):1098–1103.
26. Pierie JP, Choudry U, Muzikansky A, Yeap BY, Souba WW, Ott MJ. The effect of surgery and grade on outcome of gastrointestinal stromal tumors. Arch Surg 2001; 136(4):383–389.
27. Ozguc H, Yilmazlar T, Yerci O, et al. Analysis of prognostic and immunohistochemical factors in gastrointestinal stromal tumors with malignant potential. J Gastrointest Surg 2005; 9(3): 418–429.
28. Singer S, Rubin BP, Lux ML, et al. Prognostic value of KIT mutation type, mitotic activity, and histologic subtype in gastrointestinal stromal tumors. J Clin Oncol 2002; 20(18):3898–3905.

29. Wong NA, Young R, Malcomson RD, et al. Prognostic indicators for gastrointestinal stromal tumours: a clinicopathological and immunohistochemical study of 108 resected cases of the stomach. Histopathology 2003; 43(2):118–126.
30. Bucher P, Taylor S, Villiger P, Morel P, Brundler MA. Are there any prognostic factors for small intestinal stromal tumors? Am J Surg 2004; 187(6):761–766.
31. Mochizuki Y, Kodera Y, Ito S, et al. Treatment and risk factors for recurrence after curative resection of gastrointestinal stromal tumors of the stomach. World J Surg 2004; 28(9):870–875.
32. Tran T, Davila JA, El-Serag HB. The epidemiology of malignant gastrointestinal stromal tumors: an analysis of 1,458 cases from 1992 to 2000. Am J Gastroenterol 2005; 100(1):162–168.
33. Mucciarini C, Bertolini F, Cirilli C, et al. Gastrointestinal stromal tumors (GIST): evaluation of malignancy and prognosis in 113 cases retrieved from a population based cancer registry of Northern Italy. Proc Am Soc Clin Oncol 2004; 22(14S):Abstract No. 4232.
34. Miettinen M, Majidi M, Lasota J. Pathology and diagnostic criteria of gastrointestinal stromal tumors (GISTs): a review. Eur J Cancer 2002; 38 (suppl 5):S39–S51.
35. Cypriano MS, Jenkins JJ, Pappo AS, Rao BN, Daw NC. Pediatric gastrointestinal stromal tumors and leiomyosarcoma. Cancer 2004; 101(1):39–50.
36. Price V, Chilton-Maceneill S, Malkin D, Pappo A, Smith C, Zielenska M. Clinical and molecular characteristics of pediatric gastrointestinal stromal tumors (GISTs). Proc Am Soc Clin Oncol 2004; 22(14S (July 15 suppl)):Abstract No. 8537.
37. Prakash S, Sarran L, Socci N, et al. Gastrointestinal stromal tumors in children and young adults: a clinicopathologic, molecular, and genomic study of 15 cases and review of the literature. J Pediatr Hematol Oncol 2005; 27(4):179–187.
38. Carney JA. Gastric stromal sarcoma, pulmonary chondroma, and extra-adrenal paraganglioma (Carney triad): natural history, adrenocortical component, and possible familial occurrence. Mayo Clin Proc 1999; 74(6):543–552.
39. DeMatteo RP, Brennan MF. Gastrointestinal stromal tumors. In: Cameron J, ed. Current Surgical Therapy. 8th ed. St. Louis: Mosby; 2004:100–103.
40. Fletcher CD. Clinicopathologic correlations in gastrointestinal stromal tumors. Hum Pathol 2002; 33(5):455.
41. Lee CM, Chen HC, Leung TK, Chen YY. Gastrointestinal stromal tumor: computed tomographic features. World J Gastroenterol 2004; 10(16):2417–2418.
42. Burkill GJ, Badran M, Al-Muderis O, et al. Malignant gastrointestinal stromal tumor: distribution, imaging features, and pattern of metastatic spread. Radiology 2003; 226(2):527–532.
43. Therasse P, Arbuck SG, Eisenhauer EA, et al. New guidelines to evaluate the response to treatment in solid tumors. European Organization for Research and Treatment of Cancer, National Cancer Institute of the United States, National Cancer Institute of Canada. J Natl Cancer Inst 2000; 92(3):205–216.
44. Green S, Weiss GR. Southwest Oncology Group standard response criteria, endpoint definitions and toxicity criteria. Invest New Drugs 1992; 10(4):239–253.
45. Chen MY, Bechtold RE, Savage PD. Cystic changes in hepatic metastases from gastrointestinal stromal tumors (GISTs) treated with Gleevec (imatinib mesylate). Am J Roentgenol 2002; 179(4):1059–1062.
46. Bauer S, Corless CL, Heinrich MC, et al. Response to imatinib mesylate of a gastrointestinal stromal tumor with very low expression of KIT. Cancer Chemother Pharmacol 2003; 51(3):261–265.
47. Fujimoto Y, Nakanishi Y, Yoshimura K, Shimoda T. Clinicopathologic study of primary malignant gastrointestinal stromal tumor of the stomach, with special reference to prognostic factors: analysis of results in 140 surgically resected patients. Gastric Cancer 2003; 6(1):39–48.
48. Antonescu CR, Viale A, Sarran L, et al. Gene expression in gastrointestinal stromal tumors is distinguished by KIT genotype and anatomic site. Clin Cancer Res 2004; 10(10):3282–3290.
49. Ng EH, Pollock RE, Munsell MF, Atkinson EN, Romsdahl MM. Prognostic factors influencing survival in gastrointestinal leiomyosarcomas. Implications for surgical management and staging. Ann Surg 1992; 215(1):68–77.
50. Otani Y, Ohgami M, Igarashi N, et al. Laparoscopic wedge resection of gastric submucosal tumors. Surg Laparosc Endosc Percutan Tech 2000; 10(1):19–23.
51. Dempsey DT, Kelberman IA, Dabezies MA. Laparoscopic resection of gastric leiomyosarcoma. J Laparoendosc Adv Surg Tech A 1997; 7(6):357–362.
52. Grant CS, Kim CH, Farrugia G, Zinsmeister A, Goellner JR. Gastric leiomyosarcoma. Prognostic factors and surgical management. Arch Surg 1991; 126(8):985–989.
53. Yantiss RK, Spiro IJ, Compton CC, Rosenberg AE. Gastrointestinal stromal tumor versus intra-abdominal fibromatosis of the bowel wall: a clinically important differential diagnosis. Am J Surg Pathol 2000; 24(7):947–957.
54. Langer C, Gunawan B, Schuler P, Huber W, Fuzesi L, Becker H. Prognostic factors influencing surgical management and outcome of gastrointestinal stromal tumours. Br J Surg 2003; 90(3):332–339.
55. Samiian L, Weaver M, Velanovich V. Evaluation of gastrointestinal stromal tumors for recurrence rates and patterns of long-term follow-up. Am Surg 2004; 70(3):187–191; discussion 191–192.
56. Dematteo RP, Heinrich MC, El-Rifai WM, Demetri G. Clinical management of gastrointestinal stromal tumors: before and after STI-571. Hum Pathol 2002; 33(5):466–477.

57. DeMatteo RP, Antonescu CR, Chadaram V, et al. Adjuvant imatinib mesylate in patients with primary high risk gastrointestinal stromal tumor (GIST) following complete resection: safety results from the U.S. Intergroup Phase II trial ACOSOG Z9000. J Clin Oncol 2005; 23(16S):Abstract No. 9009.
58. Scaife CL, Hunt KK, Patel SR, et al. Is there a role for surgery in patients with "unresectable" cKIT+ gastrointestinal stromal tumors treated with imatinib mesylate? Am J Surg 2003; 186(6): 665–669.
59. Bumming P, Andersson J, Meis-Kindblom JM, et al. Neoadjuvant, adjuvant and palliative treatment of gastrointestinal stromal tumours (GIST) with imatinib: a centre-based study of 17 patients. Br J Cancer 2003; 89(3):460–464.
60. Eisenberg BL, Judson I. Surgery and imatinib in the management of GIST: emerging approaches to adjuvant and neoadjuvant therapy. Ann Surg Oncol 2004; 11(5):465–475.
61. Edmonson JH, Marks RS, Buckner JC, Mahoney MR. Contrast of response to dacarbazine, mitomycin, doxorubicin, and cisplatin (DMAP) plus GM-CSF between patients with advanced malignant gastrointestinal stromal tumors and patients with other advanced leiomyosarcomas. Cancer Invest 2002; 20(5–6):605–612.
62. Wu PC, Langerman A, Ryan CW, Hart J, Swiger S, Posner MC. Surgical treatment of gastrointestinal stromal tumors in the imatinib (STI-571) era. Surgery 2003; 134(4):656–665; discussion 665–666.
63. Joensuu H, Roberts PJ, Sarlomo-Rikala M, et al. Effect of the tyrosine kinase inhibitor STI571 in a patient with a metastatic gastrointestinal stromal tumor. N Engl J Med 2001; 344(14): 1052–1056.
64. van Oosterom AT, Judson I, Verweij J, et al. Safety and efficacy of imatinib (STI571) in metastatic gastrointestinal stromal tumours: a phase I study. Lancet 2001; 358(9291):1421–1423.
65. van Oosterom AT, Judson IR, Verweij J, et al. Update of phase I study of imatinib (STI571) in advanced soft tissue sarcomas and gastrointestinal stromal tumors: a report of the EORTC Soft Tissue and Bone Sarcoma Group. Eur J Cancer 2002; 38 (suppl 5):S83–S87.
66. Blanke CD, Corless CL, Demetri GD, et al. Long-term follow-up of advanced gastrointestinal stromal tumor (GIST) patients treated with imatinib mesylate. Gastrointestinal Cancer Symposium, The American Society of Clinical Oncology, 2004. Abstract No. 20.
67. Verweij J, Casali PG, Zalcberg J, et al. Progression-free survival in gastrointestinal stromal tumours with high-dose imatinib: randomised trial. Lancet 2004; 364(9440):1127–1134.
68. Benjamin RS, Fletcher CD, Blanke CD, et al. Phase III dose—randomized study of imatinib mesylate (STI571) for GIST: intergroup S0033 early results. Proc Am Soc Clin Oncol 2003; 22(Abstract No. 3271.):814.
69. Mudan SS, Conlon KC, Woodruff JM, Lewis JJ, Brennan MF. Salvage surgery for patients with recurrent gastrointestinal sarcoma: prognostic factors to guide patient selection. Cancer 2000; 88(1):66–74.
70. DeMatteo RP, Shah A, Fong Y, Jarnagin WR, Blumgart LH, Brennan MF. Results of hepatic resection for sarcoma metastatic to liver. Ann Surg 2001; 234(4):540–547.
71. Shima Y, Horimi T, Ishikawa T, et al. Aggressive surgery for liver metastases from gastrointestinal stromal tumors. J Hepatobiliary Pancreat Surg 2003; 10(1):77–80.
72. Lang H, Nussbaum KT, Kaudel P, Fruhauf N, Flemming P, Raab R. Hepatic metastases from leiomyosarcoma: a single-center experience with 34 liver resections during a 15-year period. Ann Surg 2000; 231(4):500–505.
73. Mavligit GM, Zukwiski AA, Ellis LM, Chuang VP, Wallace S. Gastrointestinal leiomyosarcoma metastatic to the liver. Durable tumor regression by hepatic chemoembolization infusion with cisplatin and vinblastine. Cancer 1995; 75(8):2083–2088.
74. Karakousis CP, Blumenson LE, Canavese G, Rao U. Surgery for disseminated abdominal sarcoma. Am J Surg 1992; 163(6):560–564.
75. Sugarbaker PH. Intraperitoneal chemotherapy and cytoreductive surgery for the prevention and treatment of peritoneal carcinomatosis and sarcomatosis. Semin Surg Oncol 1998; 14(3): 254–261.
76. Eilber FC, Rosen G, Forscher C, Nelson SD, Dorey F, Eilber FR. Recurrent gastrointestinal stromal sarcomas. Surg Oncol 2000; 9(2):71–75.
77. Shankar S, Vansonnenberg E, Desai J, Dipiro PJ, Van Den Abbeele A, Demetri GD. Gastrointestinal stromal tumor: new nodule-within-a-mass pattern of recurrence after partial response to imatinib mesylate. Radiology 2005; 235(3):892–898.
78. Chen LL, Trent JC, Wu EF, et al. A missense mutation in KIT kinase domain 1 correlates with imatinib resistance in gastrointestinal stromal tumors. Cancer Res 2004; 64(17):5913–5919.
79. Fletcher JA, Corless CL, Dimitrijevic S, et al. Mechanisms of resistance to imatinib mesylate (IM) in advanced gastrointestinal stromal tumor (GIST). Proc Am Soc Clin Oncol 2003; 22:Abstract No. 3275.
80. Dileo P, Randhawa R, Vansonnenberg E, et al. Safety and efficacy of percutaneous radio-frequency ablation (RFA) in patients with metastatic gastrointestinal stromal tumor with clonal elevation of lesions refractory to imatinib mesylate (IM). J Clin Oncol 2004; 22(14S):Abstract No. 9024.

81. Demetri GD, Desai J, Fletcher JA, et al. SU11248, a multi-targeted tyrosine kinase inhibitor, can overcome imatinib resistance caused by diverse genomic mechanisms in patients with metastatic gastrointestinal stromal tumor. J Clin Oncol 2004; 22(14S):Abstract No. 3001.
82. van Oosterom AT, Dumez H, Desai J, et al. Combination signal transduction inhibition: a phase I/II trial of the oral mTOR-inihibitor everolimus and imatinib mesylate(IM) in patients with gastrointestinal stromal tumor refractory to IM. J Clin Oncol 2004; 22(14S):Abstract No. 3002.
83. Fletcher C, Berman J, Corless C, et al. Diagnosis of gastrointestinal stromal tumors: a consensus approach. Hum Pathol 2002; 33:459–465.

29 Chemotherapy and Other Nonsurgical Approaches for Gastrointestinal Lymphomas

Dorothy C. Pan and Carol S. Portlock
Department of Medicine, Memorial Sloan-Kettering Cancer Center, New York, New York, U.S.A.

INTRODUCTION

Gastrointestinal (GI) tract lymphomas are a heterogeneous group of disorders comprising ~10% of all non-Hodgkin's lymphomas (NHL). Much interest is focused on these lymphomas, particularly mucosa-associated lymphoid tissue (MALT) lymphomas as it represents a model through which antigen mediated lymphomagenesis can be studied. For GI tract lymphomas as a whole, therapeutic options other than surgery have become the mainstay of treatment. This chapter will examine the different subtypes of NHL involving the GI tract; define the underlying pathogenesis of MALT lymphomas; and consider the options of chemotherapy, radiotherapy, and antibiotics as definitive treatment approaches for the common histologic subtypes of NHL involving the GI tract.

CLINICAL FEATURES AND STAGING OF EXTRANODAL LYMPHOMAS

The typical sites of GI tract involvement by corresponding histologic subtype of NHL, as defined by the World Health Organization (WHO) classification (1), are shown in Figure 1. While NHL can arise in any GI tract locale, the more common entities include gastric MALT lymphoma, diffuse large B-cell lymphoma (DLBCL) of the stomach, and diffuse colonic involvement by mantle-cell lymphoma, known as multiple lymphomatous polyposis (MLP). Other histologies that involve the GI tract include follicular lymphomas which frequently affect the duodenum (2,3) and which sometimes mimic MLP, immunoproliferative small intestinal disease (IPSID), a MALT precursor which has been associated with antigen-drive phenomena (4,5), and Burkitt's lymphoma of the ileocecal valve, which can cause intussusception.

The limitations of the Ann Arbor staging classification (6) exist when applied to staging extranodal NHL. Hence, the staging classification that is commonly adopted to assess GI tract involvement is a modification of the Blackledge staging system reported by Rohatiner et al. for the International Extranodal Lymphoma Study Group (IELSG) (7). The three stages of this system and their substages are described in Table 1. Stage I comprises disease confined to the GI tract, while stage II is stratified according to the degree of nodal involvement and extension into adjacent organs. Stage IV represents disseminated disease or disease distant from the primary GI tumor (e.g., supra-diaphragmatic involvement).

The typical initial staging procedures for extranodal lymphomas include endoscopy, computerized tomography (CT) imaging, and positron-emission tomography (PET) scans as indicated by histologic subtype. Endoscopic ultrasound has also been evaluated in a number of series to assess the depth of mucosal infiltration and regional node involvement with better accuracy (8,9).

INDOLENT NON-HODGKIN'S LYMPHOMAS

Mucosa-Associated Lymphoid-Tissue Lymphoma

The most common indolent NHL involving the GI tract is extranodal marginal zone lymphoma of MALT type (1), now referred to as MALT lymphoma. It harbors features that are distinct from its nodal counterpart with characteristic favorable five-year overall survival (OS) (81% vs. 56%, $p = 0.09$) and localized disease presentation (10).

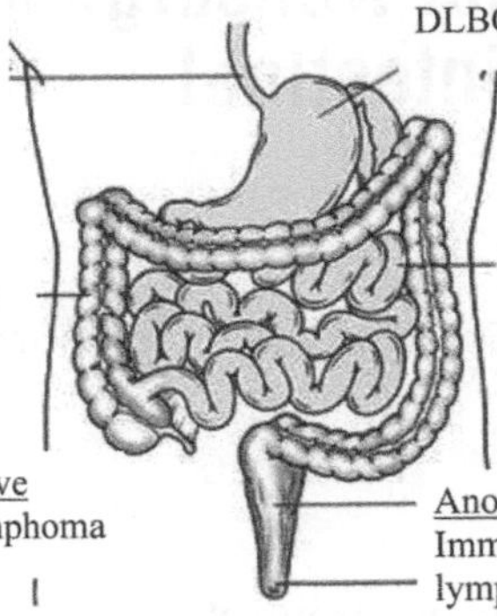

FIGURE 1 Types of lymphoma found in the gastrointestinal tract and their distribution. *Abbreviations*: DLBCL, diffuse large b-cell lymphoma; IPSID, immunoproliferative small intestinal disease; MALT lymphoma, mucosa-associated lymphoid tissue lymphoma.

The term MALT lymphoma was first coined in 1983 by Isaacson and Wright (11) after recognizing this lymphoma subtype as a distinct entity found in the mucosal epithelium of various organ systems. The prototypic MALT lymphoma arises in the stomach, an organ that does not normally harbor lymphoid tissue. Histopathology studies have demonstrated that neoplastic, marginal zone B-cell infiltrates surround reactive B-cell follicles which invade glandular epithelium, known as lymphoepithelial lesions (LEL). This abnormal lymphoproliferation recapitulates the features of Peyer's patches in the terminal ileum (12). Immunohistochemical staining have characterized this monotypic B-cell proliferation as expressing CD20 antigen and IgM and lacking expression of CD5, CD10, and CD23 cell-surface markers (13).

The earliest observation of an inflammatory stimulus inciting lymphoproliferation was reported by Isaacson's group (14), who showed that the development of gastric lymphoid tissue and MALT lymphoma was associated with chronic infection with *Helicobacter pylori*, a microaerophilic bacteria representing common GI flora and residing in the protective mucous layer of the stomach. Several lines of evidence corroborate an association between *H. pylori* and the development of MALT lymphoma. Epidemiologic studies demonstrate a correlation between *H. pylori* and both low- and high-grade MALT lymphomas (15,16). In addition, molecular analyses of gastric biopsy specimens preceding the development of MALT lymphoma have been shown to harbor *H. pylori* (17).

These studies have generated the hypothesis that *H. pylori* is the antigen stimulus for the development of gastric MALT lymphoma. In the earlier phases of disease development, both inflammatory and immune cells are recruited to the mucosa by the *H. pylori* stimulus, resulting in the formation of acquired MALT. Cag-A-positive strains of *H. pylori* are more virulent, and have been shown to incite an inflammatory response causing oxidative damage (18). while this inflammatory response occurs, a parallel host immunologic response stimulates the proliferation of neoplastic B-lymphocytes through *H. pylori*-specific T-cells (19) or by direct autoantigens

TABLE 1 Staging Classification of Gastrointestinal Lymphomas

Stage	Definition	Sites
Stage I	Single primary site, or multiple noncontiguous sites	
Stage II	Tumor extension within the intra-abdominal cavity	
II_1	Local nodal involvement	Paragastric or paraintestinal
II_2	Distant nodal involvement	Mesenteric, retroperitoneal, inguinal
IIE	Extension to adjacent organs or tissue	
Stage IV	Disseminated disease, or GI tract disease with supra-diaphragmatic disease	

Abbreviation: GI, Gastrointestinal.
Source: From Ref. 7.

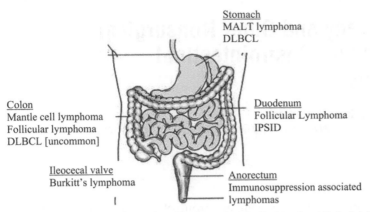

(20). Ongoing somatic immunoglobulin gene mutations suggest that continued antigen stimulation plays a role in clonal expansion (21). As genetic events occur, MALT lymphoma can acquire autonomous growth that is *H. pylori* independent.

Several genetic aberrations are associated with MALT lymphomas, including the translocations t(11;18)(q21;q21), t(1;14)(p23;q32), t(14;18)(q32;q21) which occur more frequently in non-GI MALT lymphomas (22), and trisomy 3 (23), 12, and 18, respectively. This discussion will focus on the two well-described genetic abnormalities associated with GI lymphomas—t(11;18)(q21;q21) and t(1;14)(p23;q32). The translocation t(11;18)(q21;q21) fuses the *N*-terminus of the apoptosis inhibitor gene API2 with the *C*-terminus of the MALT1 gene on chromosome 18q (24), resulting in constitutive activation of nuclear factor-kappaB (NF-κB) and modulation of cellular activation, proliferation, and survival signaling. This translocation has been found in 30% to 60% of low-grade MALT lymphomas (25), but has been identified in virtually no cases of high-grade DLBCL (26). In MALT lymphoma that harbors t(11;18) (q21;q21), the translocation is usually the sole genetic abnormality; these tumors do not typically transform into DLBCL. The t(11;18)(q21;q21) translocation has been associated with infection with the more virulent CagA-positive strains of *H. pylori* (27). In contrast, MALT lymphoma without t(11;18)(q21;q21) has been shown to develop multiple other genetic aberrations, such as allelic imbalances and loss of heterozygosity that are similar to those found in high-grade DLBCL of the stomach, implicating the development of multiple genetic events in progression to DLBCL (28).

The t(1;14)(p23;q32) gene mutation is identified in ~5% of MALT lymphomas. This translocation deregulates BCL10 protein expression by juxtaposing the BCL10 gene under control of the immunoglobulin-heavy chain (IgH) gene promoter (29,30). Dysregulation of BCL10 by this translocation links antigen-receptor signaling to nuclear translocation and constitutive activation of NF-κB, which transactivates genes that regulate the proliferation and survival of B-lymphocytes (31–35).

Numerous therapeutic studies demonstrate that eradication of *H. pylori* with combination antibiotic regimens result in regression of MALT lymphoma with typical overall response rates (ORR) of ~75%, and study findings ranging between 60% and 92% (36–40). The earliest study of antibiotic intervention was reported by Wotherspoon et al. (36), who observed complete eradication *of H. pylori* with antimicrobial therapy in six patients and corresponding regression of MALT lymphoma in five of these patients. This finding was subsequently confirmed in several larger series (37–40). In a prospective trial of 34 patients with stage IE or II_2E gastric MALT treated with antibiotic doublets, 79% of *H. pylori*-positive patients achieved an objective regression to antibiotics [complete response (CR) 50%], although half of partial responders eventually failed therapy. None of the *H. pylori*-negative patients achieved a response to antibiotics (39). In addition to *H. pylori* status, other factors predictive of regression of gastric MALT lymphoma to antimicrobial therapy include the depth of mucosal involvement and regional lymph-node status evaluated by endoscopic ultrasound (9).

Between 20% and 30% of *H. pylori*-positive gastric MALT are refractory to antibiotic therapy. Several studies indicate that the t(11;18)(q21;q21) translocation is identified in higher frequencies (60–75%) in patients resistant to *H. pylori* eradication (41,42). This finding suggests that the API2-MALT1 fusion may confer a *H. pylori*-independent growth advantage of MALT lymphoma. In *H. pylori*-negative patients, t(11;18)(q21;q21) was also found in frequencies >50%, and were correlated with disease in advanced presentation (stage IIE and above) (43). Recent findings suggest that BCL-10 and NF-κB can also predict *H.-pylori*-independent status of gastric MALT lymphoma either with or without t(11;18)(q21;q21) (44).

Eradication of *H. pylori* and regression of MALT lymphoma has traditionally been evaluated by both histopathology review and polymerase chain reaction (PCR) (45). When LEL lesions are not identified on histologic examination, PCR analysis may detect monoclonal bands for the immunoglobulin heavy chain variable (IgV_H) region representing the lymphoma clone (45). Thiede et al. (46) reported that 45% of patients achieving a CR to antibiotic therapy harbored monoclonal bands on PCR analysis with persistence of monoclonality often for years. These persisting monoclonal cells were identified as basal lymphoid cell clusters on microdissection studies, and speculated to be the B-cell lymphoma in a quiescent state (46). The finding of ongoing somatic mutation and clonal evolution after eradication of *H. pylori* supports the concept of continuing autoreactivity (47). Thus, while the clinical significance of these monoclonal PCR products remains unclear, this may be an indicator of patients predisposed to disease relapse. These findings suggest that antibiotics suppress rather than eradicate the neoplastic clone, and that long-term follow up of MALT lymphoma is required particularly in patients with PCR evidence of disease.

Small series demonstrate the favorable natural history of patients with *H. pylori*-associated MALT lymphoma, initially treated with antibiotics and who were then managed expectantly despite persistent clonality (48). Long-term follow up of MALT lymphomas indicate that late relapses do occur despite high CR rates requiring ongoing surveillance (49). Anecdotal cases of gastric adenocarcinoma arising in previously treated *H. pylori*-positive MALT lymphoma have also been described (50).

Both local and systemic treatment strategies have been employed for antibiotic-refractory MALT lymphoma. While no prospective data comparing surgery, systemic chemotherapy, or combined modality therapy is available, favorable outcomes have been reported with all types of treatment (51,52). In one retrospective series of stages IE and IIE, gastric MALT lymphoma treated with different therapies, freedom from progression (FFP) (81% chemotherapy, 86% surgery, 95% combination) and OS were similar in all treatment groups irrespective of the therapeutic approach (52).

Local therapy remains an effective option for MALT lymphoma that is refractory to antibiotics. The role of definitive radiotherapy was assessed in a prospective single institutional study from Memorial Sloan-Kettering Cancer Center (53). Seventeen patients with stage IE or II_2E gastric MALT lymphoma refractory to antibiotics were treated with radiotherapy (median dose, 30 Gy) to the stomach and adjacent lymph nodes. All patients achieved a CR with 100% event-free survival (EFS) at 27 months median follow up. A correlative molecular study in this patient cohort revealed that the majority of these patients remained positive by clonotypic PCR despite sustained biopsy-proven remissions, suggesting that persisting monoclonal cells may lack additional intra- or intercellular signaling required to exert a malignant phenotype (54). The favorable outcomes with radiotherapy for localized MALT lymphoma are corroborated by a series of 103 patients from Princess Margaret Hospital (55), which included stage IE or IIE MALT of various anatomic sites with the findings of an aggregate five-year disease-free survival (DFS) of 77% and OS of 98%. All gastric MALT lymphomas achieved a CR and remained in continuous remission. Treatment was well tolerated with minimal adverse effects.

Cytotoxic chemotherapy for MALT lymphomas has not been evaluated extensively, but established active agents include alkylators as single agents (56) or in combination (57). Alkylator therapy (cyclophosphamide or chlorambucil) given as protracted oral treatment has been reported in the literature to achieve CR rates of 75% in patients with stage I and IV MALT lymphomas (56). The combination of mitoxantrone, chlorambucil, and prednisone (MCP) yielded an ORR of 93% (CR 53%) in a small series of patients with all types of MALT lymphoma of both limited and advanced stages (57). More recent data from the LY03 cooperative group study from the IELSG, Groupe d'Etude des Lymphomes de l'Adulte (GELA), and the United Kingdom Lymphoma Group assessed the benefit of chlorambucil consolidation following antibiotic therapy for *H. pylori*-associated MALT lymphoma. Patients with a histologic CR after antibiotic therapy were randomized to receive chlorambucil or observation. A preliminary report of the molecular results of this study shows that 74% of patients achieved a histologic CR, while 56% had a molecular CR by PCR analysis (58). The activity of cladribine, a purine analog, was reported in a prospective phase II study of 25 assessable patients with an aggregate CR rate of 84%. All patients with gastric MALT presentation achieved a CR (59). The t(11;18)(q21;q21) translocation did not adversely affect the response of gastric MALT lymphoma to cladribine (60).

Rituximab is a chimeric monoclonal antibody that recognizes the pan B-cell antigen CD20 and has significant clinical activity in MALT lymphomas (61–63). The IELSG conducted a phase II study of rituximab for four weekly doses in 34 evaluable patients with untreated or relapsed MALT lymphoma of all stages and various primary sites. Of 15 patients with gastric MALT lymphoma, 13 patients received prior treatment with antibiotics for *H. pylori* but subsequently relapsed. The ORR for primary gastric disease was 64% with chemotherapy-naïve patients achieving more favorable responses. Results were notable for a high relapse rate (36%) in the entire study cohort (62). In 26 assessable patients with gastric MALT lymphoma, who were ineligible for or resistant to antibiotic therapy, single-agent rituximab yielded an

ORR of 77% with 46% complete responders. The t(11;18)(q21;q21) translocation was evaluated by fluorescence in situ hybridization in this study, but did not correlate with disease response (63).

Taken together, the literature supports the use of antibiotics as first-line therapy for *H. pylori*-positive patients through epidemiologic data and clinical treatment results from multiple single-arm studies. For relapsed patients or *H. pylori*-negative disease, radiotherapy represents an acceptable treatment for localized MALT lymphoma, although evidence is present only in the form of single cohort studies. Systemic therapy with either conventional cytotoxic chemotherapy and/or immunotherapy may be utilized for patients with more advanced presentation of disease, while less commonly used to treat localized disease.

Immunoproliferative Small Intestinal Disease

First described in 1962, primary intestinal lymphoma of the Mediterranean basin has been renamed IPSID by the WHO classification. It is recognized as a specific type of MALT lymphoma, and is associated with alpha heavy chain production although both nonsecretory and gamma heavy chain variants have also been described. This disease preferentially involves the duodenum and proximal jejunum, in addition to the mesenteric and retroperitoneal lymph nodes. The clinical hallmarks of this disease are a protein-losing enteropathy and malabsorptive state (64).

Unlike MALT lymphomas, IPSID is not known to harbor a t(11;18)(q21;q21) translocation or other specific chromosomal aberrations. Anecdotal reports demonstrate regression of IPSID after eradication of *H. pylori* (4), although larger series do not corroborate a causal role of *H. pylori* infection (65). Likewise, no correlation with Epstein–Barr virus infection has been identified (66). Recent evidence implicating an antigen stimulus in the pathogenesis of IPSID suggests an association with *Campylobacter jejuni* infection. This correlation was detected molecularly through a PCR-based assay in an index patient, and substantiated by a retrospective analysis of archival intestinal-biopsy specimens in several additional patients (5). Other pertinent observations implicating *C. jejuni* as a bacterial species that may provide an antigen stimulus for the development of IPSID include epidemiologic data showing an overlapping prevalence of IPSID and hyperendemic *C. jejuni* infection in developing countries and shared sensitivity to antimicrobial therapy used to treat *H. pylori* (64).

IPSID that is confined to the intestinal mucosa, may be treated effectively with antibiotics, such as tetracycline, and aggressive supportive management of clinical symptoms (67). Some debate has arisen over whether to suppress the antigenic stimulus on a chronic basis (68). Systemic chemotherapy has been evaluated for patients with symptomatic and advanced presentations of disease (69,70), with improved CR rates using anthracycline-based regimens compared with non-anthracycline containing chemotherapy (62% vs. 40%) in a single retrospective analysis (69).

AGGRESSIVE NON-HODGKIN'S LYMPHOMA

Diffuse Large B-Cell Lymphoma

DLBCL is the most common aggressive B-cell histology accounting for ~30% of all subtypes of NHL (71). The typical site of GI disease is the stomach (72,73), although involvement of the small bowel and ileocecal valve has also been observed (74). DLBCL of the stomach may arise de novo or represent transformation of low-grade MALT lymphoma. Molecular analysis of tumor specimens that are t(11;18)-negative, demonstrate progressive accumulation of other genetic aberrations correlating with transformation to DLBCL (28).

The International Prognostic Index (IPI) stratifies DLBCL into four risk categories based on five prognostic factors: age, stage, performance status, number of extranodal sites involved, and serum lactate dehydrogenase (75). Based on this scoring system, the IELSG formulated a stage-modified IPI to assess risk in localized DLBCL of the stomach (76). In this model, five variables were evaluated with special consideration to define stage II into subsets based on regional node involvement according to the International Workshop Staging System (7), and extranodal sites to include sites other than the primary GI tumor. Risk categories revealed favorable OS and EFS for patients with 0-1 adverse prognostic factors, compared to those with three or more adverse risk features [OS 90% vs. 40%; EFS 82% vs. 35%; $p = 0.00001$] underscoring the heterogeneity of limited stage patients. The multiplicity of treatments administered in this study speaks on the controversies in management that persist in this field. Molecular classifications using genome-wide evaluation has defined subsets of DLBCL based on the stage of cell differentiation, showing differential survival patterns in germinal center B-like DLBCL and activated B-like DLBCL phenotypes (77). These newer classification schemes may supplement, or eventually supplant, the IPI by improving the precision with which diseases within a given histologic subtype can be distinguished.

For advanced stage DLBCL and other aggressive histologic subtypes, systemic cyclophosphamide, doxorubicin, vincristine, prednisone (CHOP) chemotherapy has remained the standard chemotherapy backbone with historically similar three-year OS (52%) compared to second-generation regimens (78). In a comparison of CHOP and rituximab to CHOP alone for advanced DLBCL in elderly patients, chemo-immunotherapy resulted in significant improvement in ORR (76% vs. 63%, $p = 0.005$) (79) with statistically significant improvement of progression-free survival (PFS) and OS at five-year median follow up (80). For DLBCL confined to the stomach, multiple single-arm studies assessing standard CHOP chemotherapy have resulted in CR rates in the range of 87–100% (81,82). Treatment was well tolerated without significant GI events of hemorrhage or perforation as previously reported in the literature (83). The relative contribution of rituximab to CHOP in the localized disease setting is unclear as excellent results are achieved with standard chemotherapy alone (82).

The use of chemotherapy with radiotherapy in GI-tract lymphomas is based on prospective randomized clinical trial results for limited-stage DLBCL and other aggressive histologies of NHL (84,85). Miller et al. (84) compared eight cycles of CHOP with short-course CHOP for three cycles followed by involved-field radiotherapy (40–55 Gy) in a prospective randomized multicenter study [Southwest Oncology Group (SWOG) 8736] of 401 patients with stage I or II intermediate or high-grade NHL as classified in the International Working Formulation (86). Patients in the combined modality treatment arm achieved favorable five-year estimates of PFS (77% vs. 64%; $p = 0.03$) and OS (82% vs. 72%; $p = 0.02$) compared to the chemotherapy arm (84), although no significant difference in OS or failure-free survival (FFS) was noted between the two arms at 10-year follow-up (87). The addition of rituximab to three cycles of CHOP plus involved-field radiotherapy demonstrates improved two-year PFS (94% vs. 85%) compared to matched controls on the basis of preliminary results of SWOG 0014 (88). In limited-stage aggressive NHL of the stomach, chemotherapy and radiation were assessed in 24 patients with stages IE and IIE disease with four cycles of combination chemotherapy followed by radiotherapy. Results revealed the feasibility of stomach preservation with combined modality therapy (89). PCR analysis in a small series of patients with predominantly transformed or de novo gastric DLBCL reveals more effective clearance of monoclonal cells with chemoradiotherapy in contrast to findings after *H. pylori* eradication with antimicrobial therapy (90). The premise of ECOG 1484 was to assess the relative benefit of low-dose radiotherapy (30 Gy) to six cycles of CHOP chemotherapy in patients with selected stage I (with adverse risk)and stage II disease. While the radiotherapy arm achieved an improved six-year DFS (73% vs. 56%; $p = 0.05$), no OS benefit was detected (85).

Surgical resection has had a long-established historical role in the management of aggressive lymphomas of the stomach (91), with combination surgical-based approaches described in the literature dating back more than two decades ago (92). Since then, multiple comparisons of surgery combined with radiotherapy and/or chemotherapy versus chemotherapy alone have been reported. Binn et al. (93) compared a surgical approach used by the Groupe D'etude des Lymphomes Digestifs (GELD) versus systemic chemotherapy as given by the GELA. This study compared surgical resection followed by anthracycline-based chemotherapy for three to four cycles versus full-course CHOP or a CHOP-like regimen for stages IE or IIE gastric DLBCL. Findings revealed similar estimates of five-year OS (90.5% vs. 91.1%; $p = 0.303$) and EFS (85.9% vs. 91.6%; $p = 0.187$), suggesting that chemotherapy alone affords outcomes comparable to surgical combinations (93). A prospective, nonrandomized German Multicenter Study (94) evaluated surgery with radiotherapy +/− chemotherapy versus radiotherapy

+/− chemotherapy in limited stage low- or intermediate-grade gastric lymphomas. The aggregate results of surgical versus nonsurgical management revealed comparable five-year OS (82.0% vs. 84.4%). Important caveats of this study were its nonrandomized study design reflected in nonidentical study cohorts, and inclusion of heterogeneous histologies in a singular survival analysis.

Aviles et al. (95) conducted a prospective randomized four-arm trial of surgery alone (S); surgery followed by radiotherapy (S + R); surgery followed by chemotherapy (S + CT) versus chemotherapy alone (CT) in 589 patients with stage IE or IIE DLBCL. Results showed similar responses in all four arms. However, patients in either chemotherapy arm (S + CT or CT) achieved significantly improved EFS at 10 years (S, 28%; S + R, 23%; S + CT, 82%; CT, 92%) and OS at 10 years (S, 54%; S + R, 53%; S + CT, 91%; CT, 96%) compared to those receiving regional therapy only. These findings corroborate prior nonrandomized study results that chemotherapy alone is at least comparable to chemotherapy and surgery, obviating the need for surgical intervention as front-line therapy.

Emerging data suggests that combination antimicrobial therapy is feasible as initial management of selected *H. pylori*-positive patients with high-grade gastric MALT, and results in successful eradication of *H. pylori* in virtually all treated patients (9,96–97). Sixty-two to 87% of responding patients also achieved complete histologic regression of MALT lymphoma, with at least half remaining in complete remission for extended periods of time. These results suggest that the presence of high-grade histology is not necessarily indicative of loss of *H. pylori* dependence (97). Both nuclear expression of BCL10 and NF-κB were shown to predict *H. pylori*-independent status in high-grade gastric MALT, which may have implications in selecting appropriate first-line treatment for the future (98). The t(11;18)(q21;q21) gene translocation is not frequently identified in gastric DLBCL, and has not been shown to have prognostic value in this setting.

In summary, when chemotherapy alone is compared to surgical-based approaches in gastric DLBCL, the outcomes of single- and combined-modality studies yield comparable results. These findings suggest that systemic chemotherapy can supplant surgical-based approaches with the advantages of organ preservation. Short-course CHOP for three to four cycles followed by involved-field radiotherapy has gained wide acceptance as an initial treatment strategy for limited-stage disease; six cycles of chemotherapy alone remains another option as well. The additive effect of rituximab to CHOP in combined-modality therapy demonstrates preliminary benefit. These results indicate that surgical intervention need not be routinely employed as initial therapy for DLBCL, but rather reserved for emergent complications, such as GI hemorrhage or visceral perforation.

Mantle-Cell Lymphoma

Mantle-cell lymphoma is an uncommon aggressive subtype of NHL accounting for <10% of all lymphomas, and has characteristic features of poor OS and FFS, with a median survival of approximately three years (71). Mantle-cell lymphoma has been reported to involve the GI tract in 15% to 30% of cases in the historical literature, typically in a diffuse polypoid pattern of colonic involvement termed MLP (99,100) as is demonstrated in Figure 2. Individual case reports of non-MLP forms of GI tract involvement (101) and polypoid involvement of the stomach (102) have also been reported. Intussusception is a rare complication (103).

Romaguera et al. (104) detected a significantly increased incidence of GI tract involvement when complete endoscopic assessment was performed in a series of 60 patients with mantle-cell lymphoma. While only a quarter of these patients presented with GI symptoms, 88% of patients harbored microscopic disease in the lower GI tract and 43% displayed abnormalities in the upper tract. Aggressive endoscopic staging did not result in treatment changes despite the higher frequencies of GI-tract involvement. PET scans may now be utilized to assess the GI tract (105).

Few series (106,107) have evaluated treatment of MLP as a separate entity. The largest series of MLP has been reported by the GELD. In 31 patients, anthracycline-based chemotherapy with AVmCP (doxorubicin, teniposide, cyclophosphamide, prednisolone) resulted in superior

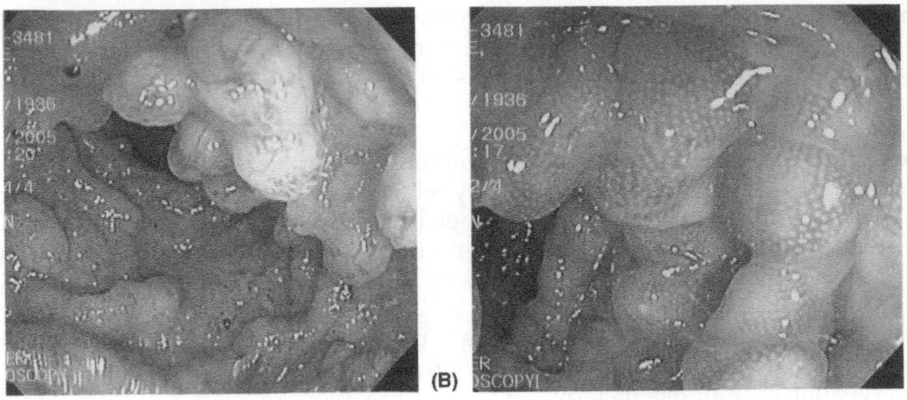

(A) (B)

FIGURE 2 Lymphomatous polyposis of the colon.

ORR compared to cyclophosphamide, vincristine, prednisolone (COP) (80% vs. 30%) with a projected five-year survival of 59% in the anthracycline-containing chemotherapy arm. High-dose therapy was an effective regimen for relapsing or partially responding patients (106).

The clinical series of MLP parallel results of standard and dose-intensified combination chemotherapy for mantle-cell lymphoma in general. The addition of rituximab to CHOP chemotherapy has been evaluated in two series, which resulted in improved ORR but did not impact PFS (108,109). Dose-intense chemotherapy without stem-cell rescue (110,111) has been evaluated to improve results achieved with conventional CHOP chemotherapy. The hyper-CVAD (fractionated cyclophosphamide, doxorubicin, vincristine, and dexamethasone) regimen alternating with high-dose methotrexate and cytarabine (MA) without autologous stem-cell transplantation (ASCT) was originally reported in elderly patients and yielded an ORR of 92% (CR 68%) and median FFS of 15 months (110). Preliminary results of a prospective phase II trial of hyper-CVAD alternating with MA without ASCT in all age groups demonstrate a CR rate of 87% after six cycles with a three-year FFS of 67% and OS of 81% at 40 month's median follow up. Complete endoscopic assessment was performed in all patients with 70% harboring GI tract involvement (111).

Superior treatment results have also been demonstrated with high-dose therapy and ASCT in comparison to conventional chemotherapy (112–118). In a matched-pair analysis of patients with advanced-stage mantle-cell lymphoma treated with rituximab and ASCT versus historical controls who received standard chemotherapy, a statistically significant improvement in three-year PFS (89% vs. 29%; $p < 0.00001$) and a trend toward better OS (88% vs. 65%, $p = 0.052$) were detected (113). Myeloablative regimens using a radiolabeled anti-CD20 antibody, $_{131}$I tositumomab, result in CR rates in excess of 90% and an estimated three-year PFS of 62% (117). Mini-allogeneic transplantation is a promising treatment strategy for relapsed mantle-cell lymphoma (118).

Collectively, these clinical series highlight the role of combination chemotherapy as the standard treatment for mantle-cell lymphoma. The presence of GI-tract involvement does not generally alter treatment, and few adverse GI complications have been reported with systemic therapy, as patients usually present with diffuse polyps rather than ulcerative or hemorrhagic disease. Different forms of dose-intense therapy, either with or without stem-cell transplantation, demonstrate considerable improvements in response rates and intermediate survival endpoints reflecting significant progress in this field.

CONCLUSIONS AND FUTURE DIRECTIONS

GI lymphomas represent a paradigm for studying infection-induced neoplasia, as much has been accomplished in understanding the histopathologic and molecular events of antigen-driven inflammation and lymphomagenesis. As the molecular features of MALT lymphomas are more clearly elucidated, key events in oncogenic transformation may be identified as targets for pharmacologic intervention.

Nonsurgical approaches for the management of NHL in general remain appealing because of favorable results achieved in single-arm and randomized studies, and preservation of organ function. Attractive options for the future include the addition of immunotherapy to existing chemotherapy regimens, as well as the development of targeted agents that may inactivate events necessary to promote disease pathogenesis.

REFERENCES

1. Harris NL, Jaffe ES, Diebold J, et al. The World Health Organization classification of neoplasms of the hematopoietic and lymphoid tissues: report of the Clinical Advisory Committee meeting—Airlie House, Virginia, November, 1997. Hematol J 2000; 1(1):53–66.
2. Lebrun DP, Kamel OW, Cleary ML, Dorfman RF, Warnke RA. Follicular lymphomas of the gastrointestinal tract. Pathologic features in 31 cases and bcl-2 oncogenic protein expression. Am J Pathol 1992; 140:1327–1335.
3. Shia J, Teruya-Feldstein J, Pan D, et al. Primary follicular lymphoma of the gastrointestinal tract: a clinical and pathologic study of 26 patients. Am J Surg Pathol 2002; 26:216–224.
4. Fischbach W, Tacke W, Greiner A, Konrad H, Muller-Hermelink HK. Regression of immunoproliferative small intestinal disease after eradication of Helicobacter pylori. Lancet 1997; 349:31–32.
5. Lecuit M, Abachin E, Martin A, et al. Immunoproliferative small intestinal disease associated with Campylobacter jejuni. N Engl J Med 2004; 350:239–248.
6. Rosenberg SA. Validity of the Ann Arbor staging classification for the non-Hodgkin's lymphomas. Cancer Treat Rep 1977; 61:1023–1027.
7. Rohatiner A, d'Amore F, Coiffier B, et al. Report on a workshop convened to discuss the pathological and staging classifications of gastrointestinal tract lymphoma. Ann Oncol 1994; 5:397–400.
8. Pavlick AC, Gerdes H, Portlock CS. Endoscopic ultrasound in the evaluation of gastric small lymphocytic mucosa-associated lymphoid tumors. J Clin Oncol 1997; 15:1761–1766.
9. Nakamura S, Matsumoto T, Suekane H, et al. Predictive value of endoscopic ultrasonography for regression of gastric low grade and high grade MALT lymphomas after eradication of Helicobacter pylori. Gut 2001; 48:454–460.
10. Nathwani BN, Anderson JR, Armitage JO, et al. Marginal zone B-cell lymphoma: a clinical comparison of nodal and mucosa-associated lymphoid tissue types. Non-Hodgkin's Lymphoma Classification Project. J Clin Oncol 1999; 17:2486–2492.
11. Isaacson P, Wright DH. Malignant lymphoma of mucosa associated lymphoid tissue. A distinct type of B-cell lymphoma. Cancer 1983; 52:1410–1416.
12. Isaacson PG, Spencer J. Malignant lymphoma of mucosa-associated lymphoid tissue. Histopathology 1987; 11:445–462.
13. Dierlamm J, Pittaluga S, Wlodarska I, et al. Marginal zone B-cell lymphomas of different sites share similar cytogenetic and morphologic features. Blood 1996; 87:299–307.
14. Wotherspoon AC, Ortiz-Hidalgo C, Falzon MR, Isaacson PG. Helicobacter pylori-associated gastritis and primary B-cell gastric lymphoma. Lancet 1991; 338:1175–1176.
15. Doglioni C, Wotherspoon AC, Moschini A, DeBoni M, Isaacson PG. High incidence of primary gastric lymphoma in northeastern Italy. Lancet 1992; 339:834–835.
16. Parsonnet J, Hansen S, Rodriguez L, et al. Helicobacter pylori infection and gastric lymphoma. N Engl J Med 1994; 330:1267–1271.
17. Zucca E, Bertoni F, Roggero E, et al. Molecular analysis of the progression from Helicobacter pylori-associated chronic gastritis to mucosa-associated lymphoid-tissue lymphoma of the stomach. N Engl J Med 1998; 12:804–810.
18. Peng H, Ranaldi R, Diss TC, Isaacson PG, Bearzi I, Pan L. High frequency of CagA+ Helicobacter pylori infection in high-grade gastric MALT B-cell lymphomas. J Pathol 1998; 185:409–412.
19. Hussell T, Isaacson PG, Crabtree JE, Spencer J. Helicobacter pylori-specific tumor-infiltrating T cells provide contact dependent help for the growth of malignant B cells in low-grade gastric lymphoma of mucosa-associated lymphoid tissue. J Pathol 1996; 178:122–127.
20. Du M, Diss TC, Xu C, Peng H, Isaacson PG, Pan L. Ongoing mutation in MALT lymphoma immunoglobulin gene suggests that antigen stimulation plays a role in clonal expansion. Leukemia 1996; 10:1190–1197.
21. Qin Y, Greiner A, Trunk MJ, Schmausser B, Ott MM, Muller-Hermelink HK. Somatic hypermutation in low-grade mucosa-associated lymphoid tissue-type B-cell lymphoma. Blood 1995; 86:3528–3534.
22. Streubel B, Lamprecht A, Dierlamm J, et al. T(14;18)(q32;q21) involving IGH and MALT1 is a frequent chromosomal aberration in MALT lymphoma. Blood 2003; 101:2335–2339.
23. Wotherspoon AC, Finn TM, Isaacson PG. Trisomy 3 in low-grade B-cell lymphomas of mucosa-associated lymphoid tissue. Blood 1995; 85:2000–2004.

24. Dierlamm J, Baens M, Wlodarska I, et al. The apoptosis inhibitor gene API2 and a novel 18q gene, MLT, are recurrently rearranged in the t(11;18)(q21;q21) associated with mucosa-associated lymphoid tissue lymphomas. Blood 1999; 93:3601–3609.
25. Maes B, Baens M, Marynen P, De Wolf-Peeters C. The product of the t(11;18), an API-MLT fusion, is an almost exclusive finding in marginal zone cell lymphoma of extranodal MALT-type. Ann Oncol 2000; 11:521–526.
26. Ott G, Katzenberger T, Greiner A, et al. The t(11;18)(q21;q21) chromosome translocation is a frequent and specific aberration in low-grade but not high-grade malignant non-Hodgkin's lymphomas of the mucosa-associated lymphoid tissue (MALT-) type. Cancer Res 1997; 57:3944–3948.
27. Ye H, Liu H, Attygalle A, et al. Variable frequencies of t(11;18)(q21;q21) in MALT lymphomas of different sites: significant association with CagA strains of H Pylori in gastric MALT lymphoma. Blood 2003; 102:1012–1018.
28. Starostik P, Patzner J, Greiner A, et al. Gastric marginal zone B-cell lymphomas of MALT type develop along 2 distinct pathogenetic pathways. Blood 2002; 99:3–9.
29. Willis TG, Jadayel DM, Du MQ, et al. Bcl10 is involved in t(1;14)(p22;q32) of MALT B cell lymphoma and mutated in multiple tumor types. Cell 1999; 96:35–45.
30. Zhang Q, Siebert R, Yan M, et al. Inactivating mutations and overexpression of BCL10, a caspase recruitment domain-containing gene, in MALT lymphoma with t(1;14)(p22;q32). Nat Genet 1999; 22:63–68.
31. Du MQ, Peng H, Liu H, et al. BCL10 gene mutation in lymphoma. Blood 2000; 95:3885–3890.
32. Zhou H, Wertz I, O'Rourke K, et al. Bcl10 activates the NF-kappaB pathway through ubiquitination of NEMO. Nature 2004; 427:167–171.
33. Maes B, Demunter A, Peeters B, De Wolf-Peeters C. BCL10 mutation does not represent an important pathogenic mechanism in gastric MALT-type lymphoma, and the presence of the API2-MLT fusion is associated with aberrant nuclear BCL10 expression. Blood 2002; 99:1398–1404.
34. Liu H, Ye H, Dogan A, et al. T(11;18)(q21;q21) is associated with advanced mucosa-associated lymphoid tissue lymphoma that expresses nuclear BCL10. Blood 2001; 98:1182–1187.
35. Ruland J, Duncan GS, Elia A, et al. Bcl10 is a positive regulator of antigen receptor-induced activation of NF-kappaB and neural tube closure. Cell 2001; 104:33–42.
36. Wotherspoon AC, Doglioni C, Diss TC, et al. Regression of primary low-grade B-cell gastric lymphoma of mucosa-associated lymphoid tissue type after eradication of Helicobacter pylori. Lancet 1993; 342:575–577.
37. Bayerdorffer E, Neubauer A, Rudolph B, et al. Regression of primary gastric lymphoma of mucosa-associated lymphoid tissue type after cure of Helicobacter pylori infection. MALT Lymphoma Study Group. Lancet 1995; 345:1591–1594.
38. Roggero E, Zucca E, Pinotti G, et al. Eradication of Helicobacter pylori infection in primary low-grade gastric lymphoma of mucosa-associated lymphoid tissue. Ann Intern Med 1995; 122:767–769.
39. Steinbach G, Ford R, Glober G, et al. Antibiotic treatment of gastric lymphoma of mucosa-associated lymphoid tissue. An uncontrolled trial. Ann Intern Med 1999; 131:88–95.
40. Fischbach W, Goebeler-Kolve ME, Dragosics B, Greiner A, Stolte M. Long term outcome of patients with gastric marginal zone B cell lymphoma of mucosa associated lymphoid tissue (MALT) following exclusive Helicobacter pylori eradication therapy: experience from a large prospective series. Gut 2004; 53:34–37.
41. Liu H, Ruskon-Fourmestraux A, Lavergne-Slove A, et al. Resistance of t(11;18) positive gastric mucosa-associated lymphoid tissue lymphoma to Helicobacter pylori eradication therapy. Lancet 2001; 357:39–40.
42. Liu H, Ye H, Ruskone-Fourmestraux A, et al. T(11;18) is a marker for all stage gastric MALT lymphomas that will not respond to H. pylori eradication. Gastroenterology 2002; 122:1286–1294.
43. Ye H, Liu H, Raderer M, et al. High incidence of t(11 ;18)(q21 ;q21) in Helicobacter pylori-negative gastric MALT lymphoma. Blood 2003; 101:2547–2550.
44. Yeh KH, Kuo SH, Chen LT, et al. Nuclear expression of BCL10 or nuclear factor kappa B helps predict Helicobacter pylori-independent status of low-grade gastric mucosa-associated lymphoid tissue lymphomas with or without t(11;18)(q21;q21). Blood 2005; online publication.
45. Rudolph B, Bayerdorffer E, Ritter M, et al. Is the polymerase chain reaction or cure of Helicobacter pylori infection of help in the differential diagnosis of early gastric mucosa-associated lymphatic tissue lymphoma? J Clin Oncol 1997; 15:1104–1109.
46. Thiede C, Wundisch T, Alpen B, et al. Long-term persistence of monoclonal B cells after cure of Helicobacter pylori infection and complete histologic remission in gastric mucosa-associated lymphoid tissue B-cell lymphoma. J Clin Oncol 2001; 19:1600–1609.
47. Thiede C, Alpen B, Morgner A, et al. Ongoing somatic mutations and clonal expansions after cure of Helicobacter pylori infection in gastric mucosa-associated lymphoid tissue B-cell lymphoma. J Clin Oncol 1998; 16:3822–3831.
48. Fischbach W, Goebeler-Kolve M, Starostik P, Greiner A, Muller-Hermelink HK. Minimal residual low-grade MALT-type lymphoma after eradication of Helicobacter pylori. Lancet 2002; 360:547–548.
49. Raderer M, Streubel B, Woehrer S, et al. High relapse rate in patients with MALT lymphoma warrants lifelong follow-up. Clin Cancer Res 2005; 11:3349–3352.

50. Morgner A, Miehlke S, Stolte M, et al. Development of early gastric cancer 4 and 5 years after complete remission of Helicobacter pylori associated gastric low grade marginal zone B cell lymphoma of MALT type. World J Gastroenterol 2001; 7:248–253.
51. Pinotti G, Zucca E, Roggero E, et al. Clinical features, treatment and outcome in a series of 93 patients with low-grade gastric MALT lymphoma. Leuk Lymphoma 1997; 26:527–537.
52. Thieblemont C, Dumontet C, Bouafia F, et al. Outcome in relation to treatment modalities in 48 patients with localized gastric MALT lymphoma: a retrospective study of patients treated during 1976–2001. Leuk Lymphoma 2003; 44:257–262.
53. Schechter NR, Portlock CS, Yahalom J. Treatment of mucosa-associated lymphoid tissue lymphoma of the stomach with radiation alone. J Clin Oncol 1998; 16:1916–1921.
54. Noy A, Yahalom J, Zaretsky L, Brett I, Zelenetz AD. Gastric mucosa-associated lymphoid tissue lymphoma detected by clonotypic polymerase chain reaction despite continuous pathologic remission induced by involved-field radiotherapy. J Clin Oncol 2005; 23:3768–3772.
55. Tsang RW, Gospodarowicz MK, Pintilie M, et al. Localized mucosa-associated lymphoid tissue lymphoma treated with radiation therapy has excellent clinical outcome. J Clin Oncol 2003; 21:4157–4164.
56. Hammel P, Haioun C, Chaumette MT, et al. Efficacy of single-agent chemotherapy in low-grade B-cell mucosa-associated lymphoid tissue lymphoma with prominent gastric expression. J Clin Oncol 1995; 13:2524–2529.
57. Wohrer S, Drach J, Hejna M, et al. Treatment of extranodal marginal zone B-cell lymphoma of mucosa-associated lymphoid tissue (MALT lymphoma) with mitoxantrone, chlorambucil, and prednisone (MCP). Ann Oncol 2003; 14:1758–1761.
58. Bertoni F, Conconi A, Capella C, et al. for the International Extranodal Lymphoma Study Group and the United Kingdom Lymphoma Group. Molecular follow-up in gastric mucosa-associated lymphoid tissue lymphomas: early analysis of the LY03 cooperative trial. Blood 2002; 99:2541–2544.
59. Jager G, Neumeister P, Brezinschek R, et al. Treatment of extranodal marginal zone B-cell lymphoma of mucosa-associated lymphoid tissue type with cladribine: a phase II study. J Clin Oncol 2002; 20:3872–3877.
60. Streubel B, Ye H, Du MQ, Isaacson PG, Chott A, Raderer M. Translocation t(11;18)(q21;q21) is not predictive of response to chemotherapy with 2CdA in patients with gastric MALT lymphoma. Oncology 2004; 66:476–480.
61. Raderer M, Jager G, Brugger S, et al. Rituximab for treatment of advanced extranodal marginal zone B cell lymphoma of the mucosa-associated lymphoid tissue lymphoma. Oncology 2003; 65:306–310.
62. Conconi A, Martinelli G, Thieblemont C, et al. Clinical activity of rituximab in extranodal marginal zone B-cell lymphoma of MALT type. Blood 2003; 102:2741–2745.
63. Martinelli G, Laszlo D, Ferreri AJ, et al. Clinical activity of rituximab in gastric marginal zone non-Hodgkin's lymphoma resistant to or not eligible for anti-Helicobacter pylori therapy. J Clin Oncol 2005; 23:1979–1983.
64. Al-Saleem T, Al-Mondhiry H. Immunoproliferative small intestinal disease (IPSID): a model for mature B-cell neoplasms. Blood 2005; 105:2274–2280.
65. Malekzadeh R, Kaviani MJ, Tabei SZ, et al. Lack of association between Helicobacter pylori infection and immunoproliferative small intestinal disease. Arch Iran Med 1999; 2:1–4.
66. Baddoura FK, Unger ER, Muffarrij A, Nassar VH, Zaki SR. Latent Epstein-Barr virus infection is an unlikely event in the pathogenesis of immunoproliferative small intestinal disease. Cancer 1994; 74:1699–1705.
67. el Saghir NS. Combination chemotherapy with tetracycline and aggressive supportive care for immunoproliferative small-intestinal disease lymphoma. J Clin Oncol 1995; 13:794–795.
68. Celik AF, Pamuk GE, Pamuk ON, Uzunismail H, Oktay E, Dogusoy G. Should we suppress the antigenic stimulus in IPSID for lifelong? Am J Gastroenterol 2000; 95:3318–3320.
69. Salimi M, Spinelli JJ. Chemotherapy of Mediterranean abdominal lymphoma. Retrospective comparison of chemotherapy protocols in Iranian patients. Am J Clin Oncol 1996; 19:18–22.
70. Shih LY, Liaw SJ, Dunn P, Kuo TT. Primary small-intestinal lymphomas in Taiwan: immunoproliferative small-intestinal disease and nonimmunoproliferative small-intestinal disease. J Clin Oncol 1994; 12:1375–1382.
71. Armitage JO, Weisenburger DD for the Non-Hodgkin's Lymphoma Classification Project. New approach to classifying non-Hodgkin's Lymphomas: clinical features of the major histologic subtypes. J Clin Oncol 1998; 16:2780–2795.
72. Koch P, del Valle F, Berdel WE, et al. for the German Multicenter Study Group. Primary gastrointestinal non-Hodgkin's lymphoma: I. Anatomic and histologic distribution, clinical features, and survival data of 371 patients registered in the German multicenter study GIT NHL 01/92. J Clin Oncol 2001; 19:3861–3873.
73. Ibrahim EM, Ezzat AA, Raja MA, et al. Primary gastric non-Hodgkin's lymphoma: clinical features, management, and prognosis of 185 patients with diffuse large B-cell lymphoma. Ann Oncol 1999; 10:1441–1449.
74. Ibrahim EM, Ezzat AA, El-Weshi AN, et al. Primary intestinal diffuse large B-cell non-Hodgkin's lymphoma: clinical features, management, and prognosis of 66 patients. Ann Oncol 2001; 12:53–58.

75. Shipp et al. The International Non-Hodgkin's Lymphoma Prognostic Factors Project. A predictive model for aggressive non-Hodgkin's lymphoma. N Engl J Med 1993; 329:987–994.
76. Cortelazzo S, Rossi A, Roggero E, et al. for the International Extranodal Lymphoma Study Group (IELSG). Stage-modified international prognostic index effectively predicts clinical outcome of localized primary gastric diffuse large B-cell lymphoma. Ann Oncol 1999; 10:1433–1440.
77. Alizadeh AA, Eisen MB, Davis RE, et al. Distinct types of diffuse large B-cell lymphoma identified by gene expression profiling. Nature 2000; 403:503–511.
78. Fisher RI, Gaynor ER, Dahlberg S, et al. Comparison of a standard regimen (CHOP) with three intensive chemotherapy regimens for advanced non-Hodgkin's lymphoma. N Engl J Med 1993; 328:1002–1006.
79. Coiffier B, Lepage E, Briere J, et al. CHOP chemotherapy plus rituximab compared with CHOP alone in elderly patients with diffuse large B-cell lymphoma. N Engl J Med 2002; 346:235–242.
80. Feugier P, Van Hoof A, Sebban C, et al. Long-term results of the R-CHOP study in the treatment of elderly patients with diffuse large B-cell lymphoma: a study by the Groupe d'Etude des Lymphomes de l'Adulte. J Clin Oncol 2005; online publication.
81. Raderer M, Valencak J, Osterreicher C, et al. Chemotherapy for the treatment of patients with primary high grade gastric B-cell lymphoma of modified Ann Arbor stages IE and IIE. Cancer 2000; 88:1979–1985.
82. Wohrer S, Puspok A, Drach J, Hejna M, Chott A, Raderer M. Rituximab, cyclophosphamide, doxorubicin, vincristine and prednisone (R-CHOP) for treatment of early-stage gastric diffuse large B-cell lymphoma. Ann Oncol 2004; 15:1086–1090.
83. Fleming DM, Mitchell S, Dilawari RA. The role of surgery in the management of gastric lymphoma. Cancer 1982; 49:1135–1141.
84. Miller TP, Dahlberg S, Cassady JR, et al. Chemotherapy alone compared with chemotherapy plus radiotherapy for localized intermediate- and high-grade non-Hodgkin's lymphoma. N Engl J Med 1998; 339:21–26.
85. Horning SJ, Weller E, Kim K, et al. Chemotherapy with or without radiotherapy in limited-stage diffuse aggressive non-Hodgkin's lymphoma: Eastern Cooperative Oncology Group Study 1484. J Clin Oncol 2004; 22:3032–3038.
86. The Non-Hodgkin's Lymphoma Pathologic Classification Project. National Cancer Institute sponsored study of classifications of non-Hodgkin's lymphomas: summary and description of a working formulation for clinical usage. Cancer 1982; 49:2112–2135.
87. Miller TP, LeBlanc M, Spier C, et al. CHOP alone compared to CHOP plus radiotherapy for early stage aggressive non-Hodgkin's lymphoma: update of the Southwest Oncology Group (SWOG) randomized trial. Blood 2001; 98(suppl 1):3024a.
88. Miller TP, Unger JM, Spier C, et al. Effect of adding rituximab to three cycles of CHOP plus involved-field radiotherapy for limited-stage aggressive diffuse B-cell lymphoma (SWOG 0014). Blood 2004; 104(suppl 1):3263.
89. Maor MH, Velasquez WS, Fuller LM, Silvermintz KB. Stomach conservation in stages IE and IIE gastric non-Hodgkin's lymphoma. J Clin Oncol 1990; 8:266–271.
90. Alpen B, Kuse R, Parwaresch R, Muller-Hermelink HK, Stolte M, Neubauer A. Ongoing monoclonal B-cell proliferation is not common in gastric B-cell lymphoma after combined radiochemotherapy. J Clin Oncol 2004; 22:3039–3045.
91. Paulson S, Sheehan RG, Stone MJ, Frenkel EP. Large cell lymphomas of the stomach: improved prognosis with complete resection of all intrinsic gastrointestinal disease. J Clin Oncol 1983; 1:263–269.
92. Sheridan WP, Medley G, Brodie GN. Non-Hodgkin's lymphoma of the stomach: a prospective pilot study of surgery plus chemotherapy in early and advanced disease. J Clin Oncol 1985; 3:495–500.
93. Binn M, Ruskone-Fourmestraux A, Lepage E, et al. Surgical resection plus chemotherapy versus chemotherapy alone: comparison of two strategies to treat diffuse large B-cell gastric lymphoma. Ann Oncol 2003; 14:1751–1757.
94. Koch P, del Valle F, Berdel WE, et al. German Multicenter Study Group. Primary gastrointestinal non-Hodgkin's lymphoma: II. Combined surgical and conservative or conservative management only in localized gastric lymphoma – results of the prospective German multicenter study GIT NHL 01/92. J Clin Oncol 2001; 19:3874–3883.
95. Aviles A, Nambo MJ, Neri N, et al. The role of surgery in primary gastric lymphoma: results of a controlled clinical trial. Ann Surg 2004; 240:44–50.
96. Morgner A, Miehlke S, Fischbach W, et al. Complete remission of primary high-grade B-cell gastric lymphoma after cure of Helicobacter pylori infection. J Clin Oncol 2001; 19:2041–2048.
97. Chen LT, Lin JT, Shyu RY, et al. Prospective study of Helicobacter pylori eradication therapy in stage I(E) high-grade mucosa-associated lymphoid tissue lymphoma of the stomach. J Clin Oncol 2001; 19:4245–4251.
98. Kuo SH, Chen LT, Yeh KH, et al. Nuclear expression of BCL10 or nuclear factor kappa B predicts Helicobacter pylori-independent status of early-stage, high-grade gastric mucosa-associated lymphoid tissue lymphomas. J Clin Oncol 2004; 22:3491–3497.

99. Hashimoto Y, Nakamura N, Kuze T, Ono N, Abe M. Multiple lymphomatous polyposis of the gastrointestinal tract is a heterogeneous group that includes mantle cell lymphoma and follicular lymphoma: analysis of somatic mutation of immunoglobulin heavy chain gene variable region. Hum Pathol 1999; 30:581–587.
100. Lavergne A, Brouland JP, Launay E, Nemeth J, Ruskone-Fourmestraux A, Galian A. Multiple lymphomatous polyposis of the gastrointestinal tract. An extensive histopathologic and immunohistochemical study of 12 cases. Cancer 1994; 74:3042–3050.
101. Tamura S, Ohkawauchi K, Yokoyama Y, et al. Non-multiple lymphomatous polyposis form of mantle cell lymphoma in the gastrointestinal tract. J Gastroenterol 2004; 39:995–1000.
102. Raderer M, Puspok A, Birkner T, Streubel B, Chott A. Primary gastric mantle cell lymphoma in a patient with long standing history of Crohn's disease. Leuk Lymphoma 2004; 45:1459–1462.
103. Sucker C, Klima KM, Doelken G, Heidecke CD, Lorenz G, Stockschlaeder M. Unusual sites of involvement in non-Hodgkin's lymphoma: case 3. Intussusception as a rare complication of mantle cell lymphoma. J Clin Oncol 2002; 20:4397–4398.
104. Romaguera JE, Medeiros LJ, Hagemeister FB, et al. Frequency of gastrointestinal involvement and its clinical significance in mantle cell lymphoma. Cancer 2003; 97:586–591.
105. Sam JW, Levine MS, Farner MC, Schuster SJ, Alavi A. Detection of small bowel involvement by mantle cell lymphoma on F-18 FDG positron emission tomography. Clin Nucl Med 2002; 27:330–333.
106. Ruskone-Fourmestraux A, Delmer A, Lavergne A, et al. Multiple lymphomatous polyposis of the gastrointestinal tract: prospective clinicopathologic study of 31 cases. Groupe D'etude des Lymphomes Digestifs. Gastroenterology 1997; 112:7–16.
107. Mahe B, Moreau A, Moreau P, Le Tortorec S, Harousseau JL, Milpied N. High dose radiochemotherapy followed by autologous stem cell transplantation in four patients with multiple lymphomatous polyposis. Cancer 1995; 75:2742–2746.
108. Howard OM, Gribben JG, Neuberg DS, et al. Rituximab and CHOP induction therapy for newly diagnosed mantle-cell lymphoma: molecular complete responses are not predictive of progression-free survival. J Clin Oncol 2002; 20:1288–1294.
109. Lenz G, Dreyling M, Hoster E, et al. Immunochemotherapy with rituximab and cyclophosphamide, doxorubicin, vincristine, and prednisone significantly improves response and time to treatment failure, but not long-term outcome in patients with previously untreated mantle cell lymphoma: results of a prospective randomized trial of the German Low Grade Lymphoma Study Group (GLSG). J Clin Oncol 2005; 23:1984–1992.
110. Romaguera JE, Khouri IF, Kantarjian HM, et al. Untreated aggressive mantle cell lymphoma: results with intensive chemotherapy without stem cell transplant in elderly patients. Leuk Lymphoma 2000; 39:77–85.
111. Romaguera JE, Fayad L, Rodriguez MA, et al. Rituximab plus Hypercvad (R-HCVAD) alternating with rituximab plus high-dose methotrexate-cytarabine (R-M/A) in untreated mantle cell lymphoma (MCL): prolonged follow-up confirms high rates of failure-free survival and overall survival. Blood 2004; 104:[abstract #128].
112. Khouri IF, Romaguera J, Kantarjian H, et al. Hyper-CVAD and high-dose methotrexate/cytarabine followed by stem-cell transplantation: an active regimen for aggressive mantle-cell lymphoma. J Clin Oncol 1998; 16:3803–3809.
113. Mangel J, Leitch HA, Connors JM, et al. Intensive chemotherapy and autologous stem-cell transplantation plus rituximab is superior to conventional chemotherapy for newly diagnosed advanced stage mantle-cell lymphoma: a matched pair analysis. Ann Oncol 2004; 15:283–290.
114. Gianni AM, Magni M, Martelli M, et al. Long-term remission in mantle cell lymphoma following high-dose sequential chemotherapy and in vivo rituximab-purged stem cell autografting (R-HDS regimen). Blood 2003; 102:749–755.
115. Ganti AK, Bierman PJ, Lynch JC, Bociek RG, Vose JM, Armitage JO. Hematopoietic stem cell transplantation in mantle cell lymphoma. Ann Oncol 2005; 16:618–624.
116. Dreyling M, Lenz G, Hoster E, et al. Early consolidation by myeloablative radiochemotherapy followed by autologous stem cell transplantation in first remission significantly prolongs progression-free survival in mantle-cell lymphoma: results of a prospective randomized trial of the European MCL Network. Blood 2005; 105:2677–2684.
117. Gopal AK, Rajendran JG, Petersdorf SH, et al. High-dose chemo-radioimmunotherapy with autologous stem cell support for relapsed mantle cell lymphoma. Blood 2002; 99:3158–3162.
118. Khouri IF, Lee MS, Saliba RM, et al. Non-ablative allogeneic stem-cell transplantation for advanced/recurrent mantle cell lymphoma. J Clin Oncol 2003; 21:4407–4412.

30 Palliative Surgery in Advanced Gastrointestinal Malignancies

Colette R. J. Pameijer
Division of Surgical Oncology and Colon and Rectal Surgery, State University of New York at Stony Brook, Stony Brook, New York, U.S.A.

Lawrence D. Wagman
Liver Tumor Program, Division of Surgery, City of Hope National Medical Center, Duarte, California, U.S.A.

Palliation has been part of surgical practice since the dawn of medicine, yet the meaning of palliative surgery has evolved over time and varies from surgeon to surgeon. In the past, palliative surgery simply meant "not curative." Today, we define palliative surgery as any operation that removes symptom(s) or impending symptom(s). Thus, a palliative operation that completely eradicates disease can also be curative. The terms are not mutually exclusive, and refer to different oncologic goals. As people are living longer with advanced or metastatic disease due to newer chemotherapeutic agents, issues of quality-of-life (QOL), and effective palliation, become more and more important.

There are multiple case series and one prospective study (1) that demonstrate that surgery can effectively palliate the symptoms that accompany advanced cancer. The rates of morbidity associated with major procedures in these patients are typically high, on the order of 25% or more. Yet a majority of patients will obtain symptom-specific relief for the remainder of their life. Issues that have been difficult to standardize are the selection of patients for palliative surgery and outcome measurement. There are few well-designed studies that prove which prognostic criteria should be used to select patients. However, several important questions need to be addressed when contemplating surgery in patients with advanced gastrointestinal (GI) malignancies: the likelihood of effective palliation from the procedure, the morbidity of the procedure, the ratio of remaining life expectancy versus the recovery time from the procedure, and the patient's and family's wishes. It is important that the patient and surgeon have realistic expectations of the outcome of the proposed intervention.

The symptoms of advanced GI malignancies can be distilled down to a few broad categories: bowel obstruction, hemorrhage, pain, jaundice, and ascites. The evidence for management of each of these symptoms will be reviewed.

BOWEL OBSTRUCTION

Bowel obstruction is a common occurrence in patients with GI malignancy. The true incidence is unknown, but has been estimated to occur in 10% to 28% of patients (2). The management options for malignant bowel obstruction (MBO) include resection or bypass, ostomy formation, tube decompression (e.g., gastrostomy, jejunostomy, or cecostomy), stent placement, or medical management of the symptoms of obstruction.

The presence of a bowel obstruction in a patient with a history of cancer does not necessarily indicate recurrence. A small but significant percentage of patients will have a benign etiology of their obstruction. The rates described range from 3% to 35%, and represent adhesions, radiation enteritis, or benign diseases such as diverticulitis. Patients with true malignant bowel obstruction are well described in multiple case series in the literature, although different authors reach different conclusions from often similar data. Patients may have a short survival time and high morbidity rate after surgical intervention. This data leads some to believe that surgery is of little benefit in these patients, yet others cite up to 80% palliation of obstruction, often lasting until death. A recent Cochrane Review of surgery for the symptoms of bowel obstruction in advanced gynecological and GI cancer was performed, reviewing 25 different studies. The methodological quality of all the studies was low, and only a qualitative review was possible. There were several problems encountered when reviewing the literature on malignant bowel obstruction, including variability in patient population, a lack of consistency in outcome measures, and a lack of consistency in the definition of these measures. The conclusion from review of these reports was that the role of surgery remained controversial, and no definite conclusions could be drawn.

There is much surgical lore on the subject of patient selection and MBO, but little data. Factors such as advanced age, ascites, carcinomatosis, previous radiation, and multilevel obstruction are often cited as poor prognostic factors. However, there are no case series demonstrating this, let alone higher quality studies. Furthermore, the outcome being measured is usually survival, which is not a primary goal of palliative surgery. The parameter of a global performance status has been studied, specifically in patients with bowel obstruction and malignancy. In a retrospective review, there was a clear correlation between a patient's performance status and resolution of their obstruction, as well as their survival (3). Disease-free interval (DFI) can also indicate a patient's prognosis. If the interval between cancer diagnosis and bowel obstruction is less than one year, the patient has a particularly poor prognosis (4), and surgical intervention needs to be very carefully considered. Another retrospective review suggested that a small bowel obstruction (vs. large), a noncolorectal primary, and the presence of ascites were predictors of poor palliation with surgical intervention. The authors selected a functional indicator (the ability to tolerate solid food) as the definition of palliation in this series (5). This may be considered the "gold standard" for resolution of obstruction.

Once the decision has been made to operate on a patient with MBO, further intraoperative decisions need to be made. Often the anatomy of the obstruction will make the decision easy, that is, an unresectable pelvic lesion will mandate a colostomy. The situation can be more complicated with an asymptomatic but locally advanced pancreatic or gastric cancer, where the chance of a curative resection is unlikely. Several case series advocate resecting the primary rather than performing a bypass, as the patients will have a better outcome. The outcome measured is survival, rather than any QOL indicator. These studies are significantly flawed in that they represent the natural history of each patient's disease, and not the impact of our surgical intervention. Bearing these methodological inconsistencies in mind, the rates of palliation from surgical intervention range from 42% to 81%. The morbidity rate varies widely, but is as high as 42%.

A colostomy may be performed as the primary procedure of choice for a distal obstructing lesion, or when a patient is determined intraoperatively to be unresectable. There is no literature specifically concerning the effectiveness of colostomy for malignant bowel obstruction; however, colostomy is used as a historical control in several studies evaluating colonic stents. It is often assumed that a colostomy decreases a patient's QOL, but this is controversial. A recent review of 1400 patients in 11 different studies determined that no firm conclusions could be drawn on this question. Six studies concluded that the QOL was the same for abdominoperineal resection (APR) versus anterior resection, but four studies concluded that QOL was significantly worse after APR (6). All studies included in this review utilized validated QOL questionnaires, and 10 of 11 studies were rated as 2b data.

For proximal (esophagus to duodenum) or distal (rectal) GI obstruction, stenting is an alternative to surgical bypass. There is one prospective randomized trial comparing stents to bypass, and multiple case series that demonstrate low morbidity, good palliation, and lower cost for stenting gastric, duodenal, or rectal obstruction (7–17). The randomized trial involved 22 patients with unresectable malignant rectosigmoid obstruction, randomly assigned to either a colonic stent or a colostomy. The rates of morbidity and mortality were similar for the two groups, but the stented patients had a shorter length of stay and shorter time to oral intake (16). Unfortunately, this trial does not give any long-term outcomes, such as patency rates of the stent or duration of palliation of either group. Most of the case series do not evaluate the median duration of patency of the stents, and the median survival of the patients is typically three months. Up to 36% of patients will require further procedures, either additional endoscopic procedures or surgery to manage unresolved symptoms or stent complications. The most common complications from stent placement include migration, perforation, and tumor ingrowth causing reobstruction. Intestinal stenting is a good alternative to surgical intervention in patients who are not surgical candidates, or have a life expectancy of only a few months.

Gastrostomy tubes provide comfortable decompression for patients who have a proximal bowel obstruction and are not candidates for any other intervention. Multiple case series describe good relief of the symptoms of bowel obstruction with placement of a percutaneous (PEG) or operative gastrostomy tube (18–20). The median survival of the patients selected for this intervention is on the order of days to weeks, but they can often tolerate small amounts of liquids, and obtain relief from nausea and vomiting. The reported morbidity of this procedure is close to zero.

Some practitioners opt for a PEG tube only when patients have failed medical management and no other operative options exist. The concept of medical management of a bowel obstruction can be foreign to surgeons, yet is well described in nonsurgical literature. A combination of pain medication, antiemetics and antisecretory drugs can palliate the symptoms of bowel obstruction in patients who have no other options. Octreotide can be effective in reducing GI secretions, thereby reducing the symptoms of bowel obstruction. In small case series, most patients obtained relief from vomiting with the addition of octreotide, with no significant side effects (21,22). The drawback to this drug is its cost.

HEMORRHAGE

Hemorrhage is a less common consequence of advanced GI malignancy, occurring in 6% to 10% of these patients. Malignant hemorrhage can be catastrophic, or a persistent ooze. The approach to a patient with a malignant hemorrhage will depend on the location of the bleeding, the volume of bleeding, the patient's overall status, and the status of the malignant process. Management options include endoscopic intervention, embolization, radiation, medication, and resection or bypass of the bleeding segment. Often more than one technique is needed, as some interventions are appropriate for acute control of bleeding, and others for definitive long-term control. There are multiple case series describing the outcome of specific interventions in various malignancies, but there are few comparisons of one therapy with another in similar clinical scenarios.

Esophageal bleeding may be due to primary esophageal tumors, or from varices due to large liver tumors or cirrhotic changes. Much of the literature on management of esophageal varices concerns patients without cancer, but the data is applicable. Esophageal bleeding is amenable to several endoscopic techniques, including injection of epinephrine or sclerosing agents, band ligation, thermal coagulation, and yttrium aluminum garnet (YAG) laser coagulation. The initial success rate of hemorrhage control is 67% to 90%, but 33% to 80% of patients will rebleed. Endoscopy provides good initial control of bleeding, and provides a window of opportunity to fully evaluate the patient and make a definitive plan in the event that the patient rebleeds. Medical therapy with vasopressin, somatostatin, or a somatostatin analog can also control esophageal variceal bleeding. One meta-analysis comparing ligation, sclerotherapy, and medical therapy concluded that ligation is superior to other interventions, with sclerotherapy and medical therapy being equivalent (23). A review of this meta-analysis found several methodological problems, and the reviewer states that the study's conclusions are suspect and should be approached with caution. A second methodologically more reliable meta-analysis reviewed 15 randomized controlled trials (RCTs) involving cirrhotic patients with active variceal bleeding, comparing sclerotherapy with a variety of medical treatments (24). Their conclusion is that sclerotherapy is not significantly better than medical therapy in terms of controlling bleeding, and may have a higher incidence of adverse outcomes. The medical therapies included in this analysis were vasopressin, terlipressin, somatostatin, and octreotide. Arterial embolization can be considered, if other interventions have failed. There is no data for this other than single case reports. Embolization requires that the bleeding vessel be technically approachable, and not an end-artery such that organ ischemia will result from arterial occlusion.

The therapeutic options for gastric or duodenal bleeding are similar to those for esophageal bleeding. In addition to endoscopic and medical therapies, gastroduodenal bleeding is generally more amenable to surgical intervention than esophageal bleeding with easier access to the bleeding site and a better defined anatomy for ligation and direct suture placement. There are no studies comparing surgical to nonsurgical interventions and as would be expected the two approaches are implemented based on patient acuity and specific bleeding etiology. Radiation therapy can be considered for control of slower bleeding or as a follow-up to the acute control of a bleeding tumor.

Hepatocellular carcinoma (HCC) can precipitate hemorrhage through direct tumor invasion of surrounding organs, invasion of the biliary system leading to hemobilia, spontaneous rupture of tumor, or esophageal varices, as discussed earlier. Up to 26% of patients with HCC will develop bleeding of some sort, with tumor rupture being the most common cause. Several case series describe the outcome of this patient group, with retrospective comparisons of several treatment approaches. Arterial embolization is effective in achieving control of hemorrhage from either rupture or hemobilia, and may serve as the definitive intervention (25). Lesions as large as 32 cm can be embolized successfully. Resection can be the primary intervention or can follow embolization, and has been suggested for patients with single, small lesions. In a series of 18 patients, those managed initially with surgery alone had a 100% in-hospital mortality rate, compared to 0% for those managed initially with embolization (26). We would recommend arterial embolization first, with a careful consideration of surgical intervention if needed. Published selection criteria for surgery for HCC should be utilized in evaluating patients for resection. Criteria indicating a good prognosis include tumor size (usually <5 cm), number of tumors, lack of hepatic or portal vein involvement, Child-Pugh score, α-feto protein level, and a planned negative margin resection.

Bleeding from colorectal neoplasms is common, yet there is a paucity of data on the incidence and management of this problem. A review of 1333 patients with lower GI bleeding found that 19% had a cancer or polyp accounting for their bleed (27). Patients with bleeding colorectal malignancies are often candidates for resection, which will definitively control the problem. In patients who are technically unresectable, a colostomy may also be effective in controlling bleeding, although there is no data available to establish the rate of success of colostomy. A few case series describe Nd:YAG laser treatment of rectal malignancies. These series were usually for symptoms of obstruction although few patients with bleeding are included (28,29). The rate of palliation in this small number of patients is very high, with little or no treatment-related morbidity or mortality. Radiation therapy should also be considered for patients who have chronic bleeding and who are poor surgical candidates. Radiation can be used in conjunction with stenting to both improve the patency of the stent and control bleeding. Radiation can be effective in controlling hemorrhage in up to 85% of patients (30).

Rectal bleeding can also occur with radiation proctitis, a troublesome consequence of the treatment of pelvic malignancies. This may occur in the absence of recurrent disease. A colostomy can often be avoided in these patients with the application of topical agents. A prospective case series and a prospective randomized trial of sucralfate enemas versus steroid enemas both concluded that sucralfate enemas are highly effective in controlling the symptoms of radiation proctitis (i.e., pain, diarrhea), although the control of bleeding is not specifically addressed (31,32). Two case series evaluate the effectiveness of rectal formaldehyde in the control of bleeding from radiation proctitis (33,34). The application of 4% formaldehyde in one or two treatments will control bleeding in 81% to 100% of patients. To safely perform the procedure, patients are placed in the lithotomy position and do not require sedation. The perineum and anal canal should be protected with ointment, and an anoscope is used to visualize the area. Gauze should be placed proximal to the hemorrhage to protect normal mucosa. Cotton balls soaked with 4% formaldehyde are applied to the bleeding rectal mucosa until it turns white and stops bleeding. The rectum is then irrigated with saline. The treatment can be repeated in three weeks if necessary, and if applied precisely is not associated with any complications (34).

PAIN

The indications for surgical intervention for pain from advanced or recurrent GI cancer are limited. The etiology of this pain is usually related to direct invasion of surrounding soft tissue and neural structures, making a negative margin resection difficult. While any advanced GI malignancy may cause pain, there is some data to support surgical intervention for patients with advanced or recurrent rectal or pancreatic cancer.

Pelvic exenteration is a radical operation that has been utilized as a palliative procedure in patients with rectal cancer, for symptoms of bleeding, obstruction, or pain. Several case series describe pelvic exenteration for patients with advanced or recurrent rectal cancer, many of whom undergo surgery for palliation of pain. Two series quote high rates of palliation from exenteration, ranging from 50% to 83%, with pain being the major symptom palliated (35,36). The morbidity is quite high at 47% or more, with a significant percentage of these being major complications such as sepsis, renal failure, or pulmonary embolism. What is missing from these earlier reports is the duration of palliation. The exact etiology of this pain is not specified. A later (2003) case series looked at 105 exenterations, 20 of which were performed for pain. While seven of 20 patients were relieved of pain at 30 days, by the end of the follow-up period (minimum two years or death) 67% of the 24 palliative patients had persistent or recurrent pain (37). The large percentage of patients with pain as a component of recurrent pelvic malignancies highlights the importance of local control at the time of primary intervention. Furthermore, the failure of radical operations to palliate successfully emphasizes the need for a multimodality approach to this pain syndrome.

The impact of pain on a patient's QOL and the impact of various treatments on that pain are well described in a prospective study of 45 patients with locally recurrent rectal cancer, who were assessed regularly for pain and QOL using validated instruments (38). Patients underwent a variety of treatments, with 30 undergoing resection and many receiving chemotherapy or chemoradiotherapy. The authors conclude that there are several predictors of a poor QOL after treatment for recurrent rectal cancer, including pain at initial presentation, female sex, pelvic exenteration (vs. less surgery), and bony resection. Although a majority of surgical patients reported mild to moderate pain during the first three years postoperatively, there was a slow improvement in QOL scores. Patients treated nonsurgically reported moderate to severe pain after the first three months of treatment, with a worsening QOL. Post-treatment pain is pervasive in this group of patients, and they continue to require aggressive management. Thus, exenteration may offer short-term relief of pelvic pain, but the cost is high and there is a significant chance of new or other symptoms arising. Pelvic exenteration is rarely warranted for isolated symptoms of pain, but can be considered with the presence of other symptoms.

As radiation has been adopted as a standard component of primary rectal cancer treatment for stage II and III disease, the use of radiation in the setting of recurrent disease is limited. Re-irradiation strategies have been developed utilizing a careful review of previous port films, collimated techniques, computed tomography (CT) planning and conformal techniques. A case series of 52 patients who were re-irradiated includes 40 of whom had pain. Re-irradiation doses ranged from 20 to 40 Gy, with total cumulative doses ranging from 67 to 105 Gy. The acute toxicity was no worse than Grade 3 (severe diarrhea, perineal skin breakdown, or mucositis), occurring in 31% of patients. Palliation of pain was high, with 65% having a complete response and an additional 28% a partial response, for a median of nine months (39).

The patient with pelvic pain secondary to recurrent cancer should be considered for surgical resection when the pain is coupled with other symptoms such as obstruction, and for radiation when an adequate treatment dose is possible and pain is a unique symptom.

Pain in patients with pancreatic cancer is a particularly ominous sign. In a prospective study of patients with newly diagnosed pancreatic cancer, pain was an independent predictor of survival, regardless of whether the patient underwent resection or not (40). Often, systemic analgesics (including nonsteroidal anti-inflammatory drugs and opiates) are inadequate, or they lead to GI distress, constipation, nausea, or vomiting. Several prospective and randomized studies have evaluated the efficacy of celiac plexus block versus systemic analgesia alone (41–45). These studies largely come to the same conclusions. The utilization of neurolytic celiac plexus block (NCPB) significantly reduces the need for other analgesics, and is associated with significantly fewer side effects than from the standard narcotic analgesics. The duration of pain relief is fairly short, typically about four weeks. Celiac plexus block does not seem to impact long-term pain control, and the impact of celiac plexus block on QOL has been less consistently demonstrated. One randomized trial concluded that although the NCPB significantly lowered pain, there was no difference in QOL (41). Another study documented a fairly stable QOL after NCPB, versus a deterioration in QOL in patients receiving systemic therapy alone (43). NCPB can be performed at the time of laparoscopy or laparotomy, or can be done percutaneously in otherwise nonoperative candidates.

It might be possible to improve the efficacy of NCPB. A recent prospective series sought to improve the efficacy of NCPB. Twelve patients had a celiac catheter placed, and after the standard alcohol block they received either a second block or intermittent bupivicaine as needed. The authors describe a significant decrease in opioid consumption and improved QOL (46).

NCPB may be an effective adjunct to systemic management of pain in patients requiring high doses of opioids, although the true benefit is probably in reducing the side effects of opioids.

JAUNDICE

The treatment options for jaundice resulting from malignant obstruction of the bile duct include surgical bypass, percutaneous transhepatic stenting, or endoscopic biliary stenting. There are five prospective randomized trials comparing surgical bypass with stents (47–51). The earliest trial used percutaneous transhepatic stents, and the remaining trials used endoscopic stents. Although the numbers vary slightly, all the trials lead to the same conclusions. Both procedures are successful in alleviating biliary obstruction, with stents having slightly higher overall success rates than surgery. Recurrence rates are higher with stents, ranging from 0% to 38%. Recurrence rates after surgery range from 0% to 15%. While surgical bypass provides more long-lasting relief, it is at the cost of a higher morbidity rate. Stenting is associated with about a 10% morbidity rate, and surgery has close to a 20% morbidity rate.

The appropriate intervention for a patient with malignant obstructive jaundice should be determined within the scope of their disease, their performance status, and patient preference. For instance, if a patient is being explored and is found to be unresectable, it is reasonable to perform a biliary bypass. If a patient is deemed to be unresectable from the outset, the risks of an operation need to be weighed against the smaller risks of endoscopy and stent placement. If the anticipated life expectancy is on the order of months, endoscopic stent placement is a more appropriate intervention.

Several different types of biliary stents are available. The least desirable stent in our opinion is an external transhepatic drain. Patients can have significant fluid losses with subsequent electrolyte abnormalities from chronic drainage of bile. These stents may be placed temporarily, but should be internalized as soon as possible. Fixed diameter endoscopic stents are made of plastic. The plastic stents are relatively temporary, typically requiring replacement every few months due to being dislodged or becoming occluded. Expandable metal stents should be considered permanent, and can be placed in nonoperative candidates for biliary decompression. Metal stents can also become occluded with tumor in-growth, and stent placement may be accompanied by external beam radiation or brachytherapy.

In addition to biliary obstruction, the question of duodenal obstruction often needs to be addressed at the same time in these cases. Up to 23% of patients with malignant biliary obstruction will develop gastric obstruction as well. Several case series review the outcome of single versus double bypass for locally advanced pancreatic cancer (52,53), as well as the best choice of bypass procedure (54). Double bypass (gastric and biliary) is recommended over single bypass, as the patients are more effectively palliated. In addition, a choledochoduodenostomy seems to have the lowest rate of complications, with cholecystojejunostomy having a higher rate of sepsis and obstruction in the latter phases of the malignancy when the bile duct is engulfed or invaded by tumor. Loop versus Roux-Y gastrojejeunostomy have similar outcomes in this case series. Although no data exist, it is our experience that gastrojejeunostomies can be problematic in any scenario. They often do not work if the patient is not yet obstructed, and it may not work well even if the patient is obstructed due to gastroparesis from tumor invasion. Nevertheless, we advocate this palliative procedure.

ASCITES

Malignant ascites represents only 10% of all cases of ascites, but in a patient with a GI malignancy ascites likely indicates peritoneal spread of disease. The distinction between malignant and nonmalignant ascites is important for prognostic reasons as well as treatment planning. Ascitic fluid should be sent for cytology and chemistries, as up to one-third of patients with malignancy will have nonmalignant ascites. Cytology often yields the diagnosis. In addition, the presence of an elevated ascites:serum ratio of lactate dehydrogenase or tumor antigens indicates a malignant etiology.

Diuretics and sodium restriction are often used to control ascites in patients with cirrhosis; however, this regimen is not very effective for patients with malignant ascites. A comparison of plasma volume with ascites volume was undertaken in nine patients with peritoneal carcinomatosis, four with chylous malignant ascites, and three with portal hypertension and massive hepatic metastases. All patients were placed on diuretics and a sodium restricted diet. Both plasma and ascites volumes were calculated using an isotope dilution technique. The 13 patients with carcinomatosis or chylous ascites demonstrated approximately 0.4 to 0.5 kg/day weight loss with no significant change in the volume of ascites. The patients with portal hypertension and massive liver metastatses fared slightly better, with approximately 0.2 L/day improvement in ascites (55). Although diuretics and salt restriction will assist in total body water excretion, they typically result in dehydration without amelioration of ascites in this patient population, and we do not recommend this approach.

Tunneled drainage catheters can be placed to intermittently drain ascites. A permanent catheter is more appealing than repeated paracentesis, as patients can manage these catheters themselves. The drawback to external drainage of ascites is the protein loss and possible hypovolemia that can follow large volume drainage. Several case series describe low morbidity and 100% palliation of the symptoms of ascites with placement of either a Pleurex or Tenckhoff catheter (56,57). These catheters are typically patent until the death of the patient. If volume loss is a significant problem, it is possible to reinfuse the ascites. After draining a planned volume of ascites (usually one to three liters), we give a test dose of 100 cc of the ascites through a central venous catheter. If the patient tolerates this without difficulty, for example, no shortness of breath or chills, we reinfuse approximately the volume drained. There are a few studies of ascites reinfusion demonstrating that it is safe and effective in patients with nonmalignant ascites.

Several case series describe the outcome of peritoneovenous shunts (PVS) in malignant ascites. Most studies report similar results, with 64% to 75% of patients deriving relief from their ascites (58–61). One study reported that 18% of shunts required revision (60), and another study that the QOL after PVS was no different than after paracentesis (59). One case series with 116 patients reported mixed results for PVS in patients with malignant ascites. The mean patency was 83 days, 62% of patients obtained relief but 49% had one or more complications, and the shunt-related mortality rate was 13% (58). Nevertheless, a majority of patients obtain lasting relief from ascites with a PVS, provided patients are appropriately selected. Contraindications to PVS include bloody ascites or underlying coagulopathy. Blood in ascites tends to occlude the shunt quickly. As all patients become coagulopathic to some degree after placement of the shunt, with disseminated intravascular coagulation (DIC) being a potentially fatal complication of PVS, pre-existing coagulopathy, even if correctable, remains a contraindication. Furthermore, excellent cardiac and renal function is required to excrete the vascularized volume.

There are several well-designed prospective studies of debulking and intraperitoneal chemotherapy for carcinomatosis; however, the endpoint in all of these studies is survival. QOL or palliation of symptoms is not reported, and these studies will not be reviewed here.

REFERENCES

1. McCahill LE, Smith DD, Borneman T, et al. A prospective evaluation of palliative outcomes for surgery of advanced malignancies. Ann Surg Oncol 2003; 10:654–663.
2. Ripamonti C, De Conno F, Ventafridda V, Rossi B, Baines MJ. Management of bowel obstruction in advanced and terminal cancer patients. Ann Oncol 1993; 4:15–21.
3. Weiss SM, Skibber JM, Rosato FE. Bowel obstruction in cancer patients: performance status as a predictor of survival. J Surg Oncol 1984; 25:15–17.
4. Pameijer CR, Mahvi DM, Stewart JA, Weber SM. Bowel obstruction in patients with metastatic cancer: does intervention influence outcome? Int J Gastrointest Cancer 2005; 35:127–134.
5. Blair SL, Chu DZ, Schwarz RE. Outcome of palliative operations for malignant bowel obstruction in patients with peritoneal carcinomatosis from nongynecological cancer. Ann Surg Oncol 2001; 8:632–637.

6. Pachler J, Wille-Jorgensen P. Quality of life after rectal resection for cancer, with or without permanent colostomy. Cochrane Database Syst Rev 2005; CD004323.
7. Kaw M, Singh S, Gagneja H, Azad P. Role of self-expandable metal stents in the palliation of malignant duodenal obstruction. Surg Endosc 2003; 17:646–650.
8. Kim JH, Yoo BM, Lee KJ, et al. Self-expanding coil stent with a long delivery system for palliation of unresectable malignant gastric outlet obstruction: a prospective study. Endoscopy 2001; 33:838–842.
9. Born P, Rosch T, Bruhl K, et al. Long-term results of endoscopic treatment of biliary duct obstruction due to pancreatic disease. Hepatogastroenterology 1998; 45:833–839.
10. Lucas CE, Ledgerwood AM, Bender JS. Antrectomy with gastrojejunostomy for unresectable pancreatic cancer-causing duodenal obstruction. Surgery 1991; 110:583–589.
11. Yim HB, Jacobson BC, Saltzman JR, et al. Clinical outcome of the use of enteral stents for palliation of patients with malignant upper GI obstruction. Gastrointest Endosc 2001; 53:329–332.
12. Johnson R, Marsh R, Corson J, Seymour K. A comparison of two methods of palliation of large bowel obstruction due to irremovable colon cancer. Ann R Coll Surg Engl 2004; 86:99–103.
13. Mosler P, Mergener KD, Brandabur JJ, Schembre DB, Kozarek RA. Palliation of gastric outlet obstruction and proximal small bowel obstruction with self-expandable metal stents: a single center series. J Clin Gastroenterol 2005; 39:124–128.
14. Hunerbein M, Krause M, Moesta KT, Rau B, Schlag PM. Palliation of malignant rectal obstruction with self-expanding metal stents. Surgery 2005; 137:42–47.
15. Carne PW, Frye JN, Robertson GM, Frizelle FA. Stents or open operation for palliation of colorectal cancer: a retrospective, cohort study of perioperative outcome and long-term survival. Dis Colon Rectum 2004; 47:1455–1461.
16. Fiori E, Lamazza A, De Cesare A, et al. Palliative management of malignant rectosigmoidal obstruction. Colostomy vs. endoscopic stenting. A randomized prospective trial. Anticancer Res 2004; 24:265–268.
17. Maetani I, Tada T, Ukita T, Inoue H, Sakai Y, Nagao J. Comparison of duodenal stent placement with surgical gastrojejunostomy for palliation in patients with duodenal obstructions caused by pancreaticobiliary malignancies. Endoscopy 2004; 36:73–78.
18. Brooksbank MA, Game PA, Ashby MA. Palliative venting gastrostomy in malignant intestinal obstruction. Palliat Med 2002; 16:520–526.
19. Scheidbach H, Horbach T, Groitl H, Hohenberger W. Percutaneous endoscopic gastrostomy/jejunostomy (PEG/PEJ) for decompression in the upper gastrointestinal tract. Initial experience with palliative treatment of gastrointestinal obstruction in terminally ill patients with advanced carcinomas. Surg Endosc 1999; 13:1103–1105.
20. Cannizzaro R, Bortoluzzi F, Valentini M, et al. Percutaneous endoscopic gastrostomy as a decompressive technique in bowel obstruction due to abdominal carcinomatosis. Endoscopy 1995; 27:317–320.
21. Mercadante S, Spoldi E, Caraceni A, Maddaloni S, Simonetti MT. Octreotide in relieving gastrointestinal symptoms due to bowel obstruction. Palliat Med 1993; 7:295–299.
22. Muir JC, von Gunten CF. Antisecretory agents in gastrointestinal obstruction. Clin Geriatr Med 2000; 16:327–334.
23. Gross M, Schiemann U, Muhlhofer A, Zoller WG. Meta-analysis: efficacy of therapeutic regimens in ongoing variceal bleeding. Endoscopy 2001; 33:737–746.
24. D'Amico G, Pietrosi G, Tarantino I, Pagliaro L. Emergency sclerotherapy versus vasoactive drugs for variceal bleeding in cirrhosis: a Cochrane meta-analysis. Gastroenterology 2003; 124:1277–1291.
25. Ngan H, Tso WK, Lai CL, Fan ST. The role of hepatic arterial embolization in the treatment of spontaneous rupture of hepatocellular carcinoma. Clin Radiol 1998; 53:338–341.
26. Yoshida H, Onda M, Tajiri T, et al. Treatment of spontaneous ruptured hepatocellular carcinoma. Hepatogastroenterology 1999; 46:2451–2453.
27. Zuckerman GR, Prakash C. Acute lower intestinal bleeding. Part II: etiology, therapy, and outcomes. Gastrointest Endosc 1999; 49:228–238.
28. Tranberg KG, Moller PH. Palliation of colorectal carcinoma with the Nd-YAG laser. Eur J Surg 1991; 157:57–60.
29. von Ditfurth B, Buhl K, Friedl P. Palliative endoscopic therapy for rectal cancer with neodymium: YAG laser. Eur J Surg Oncol 1990; 16:376–379.
30. Pereira J, Phan T. Management of bleeding in patients with advanced cancer. Oncologist 2004; 9:561–570.
31. Gul YA, Prasannan S, Jabar FM, Shaker AR, Moissinac K. Pharmacotherapy for chronic hemorrhagic radiation proctitis. World J Surg 2002; 26:1499–1502.
32. Kochhar R, Patel F, Dhar A, et al. Radiation-induced proctosigmoiditis. Prospective, randomized, double-blind controlled trial of oral sulfasalazine plus rectal steroids versus rectal sucralfate. Dig Dis Sci 1991; 36:103–107.
33. Biswal BM, Lal P, Rath GK, Shukla NK, Mohanti BK, Deo S. Intrarectal formalin application, an effective treatment for grade III haemorrhagic radiation proctitis. Radiother Oncol 1995; 35:212–215.
34. Roche B, Chautems R, Marti MC. Application of formaldehyde for treatment of hemorrhagic radiation-induced proctitis. World J Surg 1996; 20:1092–1094.

35. Yeung RS, Moffat FL, Falk RE. Pelvic exenteration for recurrent and extensive primary colorectal adenocarcinoma. Cancer 1993; 72:1853–1858.
36. Brophy PF, Hoffman JP, Eisenberg BL. The role of palliative pelvic exenteration. Am J Surg 1994; 167:386–390.
37. Miner TJ, Jaques DP, Paty PB, Guillem JG, Wong WD. Symptom control in patients with locally recurrent rectal cancer. Ann Surg Oncol 2003; 10:72–79.
38. Esnaola NF, Cantor SB, Johnson ML, et al. Pain and quality of life after treatment in patients with locally recurrent rectal cancer. J Clin Oncol 2002; 20:4361–4367.
39. Lingareddy V, Ahmad NR, Mohiuddin M. Palliative reirradiation for recurrent rectal cancer. Int J Radiat Oncol Biol Phys 1997; 38:785–790.
40. Kelsen DP, Portenoy R, Thaler H, Tao Y, Brennan M. Pain as a predictor of outcome in patients with operable pancreatic carcinoma. Surgery 1997; 122:53–59.
41. Wong GY, Schroeder DR, Carns PE, et al. Effect of neurolytic celiac plexus block on pain relief, quality of life, and survival in patients with unresectable pancreatic cancer: a randomized controlled trial. JAMA 2004; 291:1092–1099.
42. Polati E, Finco G, Gottin L, Bassi C, Pederzoli P, Ischia S. Prospective randomized double-blind trial of neurolytic coeliac plexus block in patients with pancreatic cancer. Br J Surg 1998; 85:199–201.
43. Kawamata M, Ishitani K, Ishikawa K, et al. Comparison between celiac plexus block and morphine treatment on quality of life in patients with pancreatic cancer pain. Pain 1996; 64:597–602.
44. Mercadante S, Catala E, Arcuri E, Casuccio A. Celiac plexus block for pancreatic cancer pain: factors influencing pain, symptoms and quality of life. J Pain Symptom Manage 2003; 26:1140–1147.
45. Okuyama M, Shibata T, Morita T, et al. A comparison of intraoperative celiac plexus block with pharmacological therapy as a treatment for pain of unresectable pancreatic cancer. J Hepatobiliary Pancreat Surg 2002; 9:372–375.
46. Vranken JH, Zuurmond WW, de Lange JJ. Increasing the efficacy of a celiac plexus block in patients with severe pancreatic cancer pain. J Pain Symptom Manage 2001; 22:966–977.
47. Bornman PC, Harries-Jones EP, Tobias R, Van Stiegmann G, Terblanche J. Prospective controlled trial of transhepatic biliary endoprosthesis versus bypass surgery for incurable carcinoma of head of pancreas. Lancet 1986; 1:69–71.
48. Shepherd HA, Royle G, Ross AP, Diba A, Arthur M, Colin-Jones D. Endoscopic biliary endoprosthesis in the palliation of malignant obstruction of the distal common bile duct: a randomized trial. Br J Surg 1988; 75:1166–1168.
49. Andersen JR, Sorensen SM, Kruse A, Rokkjaer M, Matzen P. Randomised trial of endoscopic endoprosthesis versus operative bypass in malignant obstructive jaundice. Gut 1989; 30:1132–1135.
50. Dowsett J, Russell R, Hatfield A, et al. Malignant obstructive jaundice: a prospective randomized trial of by-pass surgery versus endoscopic stenting. Gastroenterology 1989; 96:128A.
51. Smith AC, Dowsett JF, Russell RC, Hatfield AR, Cotton PB. Randomised trial of endoscopic stenting versus surgical bypass in malignant low bileduct obstruction. Lancet 1994; 344:1655–1660.
52. Neuberger TJ, Wade TP, Swope TJ, Virgo KS, Johnson FE. Palliative operations for pancreatic cancer in the hospitals of the U.S. Department of Veterans Affairs from 1987 to 1991. Am J Surg 1993; 166:632–636.
53. Eastman MC, Kune GA. The objectives of palliative surgery in pancreas cancer: a retrospective study of 73 cases. Aust N Z J Surg 1980; 50:462–464.
54. Potts JR, III, Broughan TA, Hermann RE. Palliative operations for pancreatic carcinoma. Am J Surg 1990; 159:72–77.
55. Pockros PJ, Esrason KT, Nguyen C, Duque J, Woods S. Mobilization of malignant ascites with diuretics is dependent on ascitic fluid characteristics. Gastroenterology 1992; 103:1302–1306.
56. Barnett TD, Rubins J. Placement of a permanent tunneled peritoneal drainage catheter for palliation of malignant ascites: a simplified percutaneous approach. J Vasc Interv Radiol 2002; 13:379–383.
57. Rosenberg S, Courtney A, Nemcek AA, Jr, Omary RA. Comparison of percutaneous management techniques for recurrent malignant ascites. J Vasc Interv Radiol 2004; 15:1129–1131.
58. Schumacher DL, Saclarides TJ, Staren ED. Peritoneovenous shunts for palliation of the patient with malignant ascites. Ann Surg Oncol 1994; 1:378–381.
59. Gough IR, Balderson GA. Malignant ascites. A comparison of peritoneovenous shunting and nonoperative management. Cancer 1993; 71:2377–2382.
60. Edney JA, Hill A, Armstrong D. Peritoneovenous shunts palliate malignant ascites. Am J Surg 1989; 158:598–601.
61. Zanon C, Grosso M, Apra F, et al. Palliative treatment of malignant refractory ascites by positioning of Denver peritoneovenous shunt. Tumori 2002; 88:123–127.

Index